VETERINARY HISTOLOGY OF DOMESTIC MAMMALS AND BIRDS

5th Edition

Textbook and Colour Atlas

5m Publishing

VETERINARY HISTOLOGY OF DOMESTIC MAMMALS AND BIRDS

5th Edition

Textbook and Colour Atlas

Hans-Georg Liebich

Translated and revised by
Corinna Klupiec

5m Publishing

First published 2010

This edition published by 5m Publishing 2019

Authorised translation of the second German language edition of Hans-Georg Liebich, Funktionelle Histologie der Haussäugetiere und Vögel 5. Auflage © 2010 by Schattauer GmbH, Stuttgart/Germany

Corinna Klupiec asserts her right to be known as the translator of this work

Published by
5M Publishing Ltd,
Benchmark House,
8 Smithy Wood Drive,
Sheffield, S35 1QN, UK
Tel: +44 (0) 1234 81 81 80
www.5mpublishing.com

A Catalogue record for this book is available from the British Library

ISBN 9781789180091

Book layout by KPSM, Neville Lodge, Tettenhall, Wolverhampton

Printed and bound by CPI Group (UK) Ltd, Croydon, CR0 4YY

Photos and illustrations by Schattauer

Important note:
Medicine is an ever-changing science, so the contents of this publication, especially recommendations concerning diagnostic and therapeutic procedures, can only give an account of the knowledge at the time of publication. While utmost care has been taken to ensure that all specifications regarding drug selection and dosage and treatment options are accurate, readers are urged to review the product information sheet and any relevant material supplied by the manufacturer, and, in case of doubt, to consult a specialist. From both an editorial and public interest perspective, the publisher welcomes notification of possible inconsistencies. The ultimate responsibility for any diagnostic or therapeutic application lies with the reader.

Prof. Dr Klaus-Dieter Budras
Institut für Veterinär-Anatomie
Fachbereich Veterinärmedizin
Freie Universität Berlin
Koserstraße 20, D-14195 Berlin

Univ.-Prof. Dr Dr h.c. mult. Hans-Georg Liebich
Tierärztliches Fakultät
Ludwig-Maximilians-Universität München
Veterinärstraße 13, D-80539 München

Univ.-Prof. Dr Johann Maierl
Lehrstuhl für Anatomie, Histologie und Embryologie
Ludwig-Maximilians-Universität München
Veterinärstraße 13, D-80539 München

Priv.-Doz. Dr Sven Reese
Lehrstuhl für Anatomie, Histologie und Embryologie
Ludwig-Maximilians-Universität München
Veterinärstraße 13, D-80539 München

Dr Grammatia Zengerling
Lehrstuhl für Anatomie, Histologie und Embryologie
Ludwig-Maximilians-Universität München
Veterinärstraße 13, D-80539 München

Contents

Foreword

Veterinary Histology of Domestic Mammals and Birds is a translation of the 5th edition of the German volume *Funktionelle Histologie der Haussäugetiere und Vögel*, a combined textbook and colour atlas designed for students and practising veterinarians. For several decades, this format has been very well received. The publication of an English language version aims to extend its reach to an international audience.

Through previous German editions, this book has established a reputation as a high-quality text and striking pictorial work and has become recognised as a seminal resource for the study of fundamental microscopic anatomy.

The primary objective in developing this book was to help students, veterinary practitioners and researchers attain a better understanding of histology. A further goal was to take an interdisciplinary approach, creating links with macroscopic anatomy and physiology. This strategy made histology more accessible to students and clinicians and enabled the reader to develop a greater appreciation of the overarching relationships between the structure and function of organs and organ systems.

In the execution of this approach, descriptions of tissue and organ structure are integrated with references to the many functions of the building blocks of cells, tissues and organ systems to facilitate understanding of biological interactions and pathophysiological derangements.

The current edition highlights the considerable importance of histology as a foundation for comprehending related fields of science and medicine. With around 600 colour photos, a multitude of electron microscope images, comprehensive colour schematics and a generous supply of tabulated information, the book helps to create a 'picture' of the relationships between form and function, and draws attention to the aspects of histology that are most pertinent to students and practising veterinarians. This version, like its German language predecessors, is thus intended to be much more than just a 'histo book' that helps students to study and prepare for examinations.

An additional aim, in this inaugural English edition, is to augment the time-honoured combination of robust didactic text and quality atlas with the most recent developments in scientific research. In doing so, care has been taken to maintain a sense of proportion, to avoid losing focus on the information that is most applicable and accessible to veterinary students. More detailed explanations are left to the relevant specialised literature.

Translation of the 5th German edition has been carried out by Dr Corinna Klupiec BVSc PhD Grad Cert Ed Stud, a former lecturer in veterinary anatomy in the Faculty of Veterinary Science at the University of Sydney. It was most fortuitous to access the services of Dr Klupiec, a highly competent translator who approached the complexities of histology, including new developments in the field, with great meticulousness and vigour. I extend my sincere thanks to Dr Klupiec for her outstanding translation, and for the seamlessness of the collaboration between Munich and Sydney that enabled the completion of this project.

I would also like to express particular thanks to Dr Grammatia Zengerling and to Prof. Dr Budras, Prof. Dr Maierl and Dr Reese, whose suggestions regarding content have contributed to the success of this book.

Thanks are also due to Ms Christel Schura for digital colouring of the schematic representations and editing of the digital colour images. Through her fruitful efforts in improving colouring techniques, Ms Schura has developed a form of 'digital water colouring' that greatly facilitates the understanding of complex histological relationships.

Munich, Spring 2019

Hans-Georg Liebich

Translator's note

It is hard to conceive of a more detailed, intricate and evolving discipline than histology, particularly when one incorporates concepts of cellular and molecular biology. Adding to this complexity, in the veterinary field, is the histological variation observed among the domestic animal species. The production of a work such as *Funktionelle Histologie der Haussäugetiere und Vögel*, upon which this translation is based, thus represents a remarkable achievement. Also worthy of acknowledgement is the attention paid by the authors to both the educational and aesthetic aspects of the book, resulting in a work of substance and beauty.

In translating this text, I have attempted to do justice to the years of work devoted by the contributing authors to the five German language editions. I have also endeavoured to add salient updates from the contemporary literature. This undertaking can of course never be considered complete, as the body of knowledge grows on a daily basis and information frequently becomes superseded. Nevertheless, acknowledgment of new discoveries and perspectives is an important part of the scientific process.

The translation of several chapters was aided considerably by the expertise of colleagues experienced in teaching veterinary histology. Dr Susan Hemsley MVSc PhD Grad Cert Ed Stud, of the Centre for Veterinary Education at the University of Sydney, made invaluable contributions to the chapters on epithelial tissue, connective and supportive tissues, blood and haemopoiesis, the immune system and lymphatic organs, and the digestive system. I am indebted also to Dr Glenn Shea BVSc (Hons) PhD, senior lecturer in veterinary anatomy at the University of Sydney, for his pertinent and insightful comments on the chapters pertaining to the male reproductive and respiratory systems.

Completion of the translation would not have been possible without the contributions of Prof. Dr Hans-Georg Liebich, who addressed my many questions with patience and perseverance. It was a rewarding experience to work closely with the author of the original text.

It remains for me to express my heartfelt thanks to Ms Sarah Hulbert of 5M Publishing for her steadfast support throughout the completion of this project. I also thank the production team for bringing the translated text to publication.

Sydney, Autumn 2019
Corinna Klupiec

About the companion website

Please visit the companion website to this book at this link https://www.5mbooks.com/veterinary-histology

The website gives access to 900 supplementary colour images, including further information and exercises to test the reader's knowledge. The following subjects are covered:

01 The cell
02 Epithelial tissue
03 Connective and supportive tissue
04 Muscle tissue
05 Nervous tissue
06 Circulatory system
07 Blood cells
08 Lymphatic organs
09 Endocrine system
10 Digestive system
11 Respiratory apparatus
12 Urinary organs
13 Male reproductive organs
14 Female reproductive organs
15 Common integument
16 Sensory organs
17 Nervous system

The cell (cellula)

1

Eukaryotic cells contain a soluble matrix (cytosol) in which numerous organelles and inclusions are suspended. These cellular contents are referred to collectively as the cytoplasm. Cellular processes associated with metabolism, respiration, energy transformation, contractility and cell motility take place within the cytoplasm. These processes involve functional interactions between the cytosol and the organelles. The matrix is an aqueous gel incorporating variably sized molecules and structural elements in the form of a cytoskeleton.

Most organelles are bounded by a **biological membrane** that, by virtue of its specialised layered structure, separates the individual organelles from the surrounding matrix (**compartmentation**). This permits diverse metabolic processes to occur independently within the confines of the same cell. The cellular organelles can be subdivided as follows:

- membranous organelles:
  - nucleus,
  - endocytotic vesicles,
  - exocytotic vesicles,
  - endosomes,
  - lysosomes,
  - peroxisomes,
  - rough endoplasmic reticulum (rER),
  - smooth endoplasmic reticulum (sER),
  - Golgi apparatus,
  - mitochondria,
- non-membranous organelles:
  - ribosomes,
  - microtubules,
  - filaments (actin filaments, intermediate filaments) and
  - centrioles.

The **nucleus directs all of the functions of the cell** and **houses its genetic material**. Strands of deoxyribonucleic acid (DNA) within the nucleus store genetic information and serve as a regulatory and information-processing system for cellular metabolism. The intracellular organelles act synergistically, their combined actions giving rise to the specific functions of a particular cell. As these are clearly distinguishable under the light microscope, the **cytoplasm** and the **nucleus** are conventionally regarded as separate compartments. The nucleus is basophilic (= binds with basic stains, e.g. stains blue with haematoxylin), while the cytoplasm is predominantly acidophilic (binds with acidic stains, e.g. stains red with eosin). The cytoplasm is surrounded by a highly differentiated biological membrane, the **plasma membrane** (**plasmalemma**), that serves both to separate the cell from its surroundings and to establish a connection between the cell and its environment.

Cell membrane (cytolemma, membrana cellularis)

Cell membranes are biological membranes that constitute the structural foundation of most organelles and form the outer boundary of the cell. The outer (surface) membrane is highly specialised and is termed the plasmalemma.

All biological membranes have a similar basic structure (**unit membrane**) comprising layers of **phospholipid** and **protein molecules** held together by non-covalent bonds. Chains of lipid molecules form a **lipid bilayer** that encloses, or is traversed by, protein molecules and glycoproteins in a ratio of 2:1 (depending on cell type, this relationship varies from 4:1 to 1:4).

With a total thickness of 7.5 to 10 nm, the cell membrane can only be seen using electron microscopy. When prepared with osmic acid, the cell membrane appears as three layers: an electron-dense **outer layer** (**lamina externa**), an **inner layer** (**lamina interna**) and an electron-lucent **intermediate layer** (**lamina intermedia**).

On the outer surface of the plasmalemma, carbohydrates (oligosaccharide chains) attach to membrane proteins, forming glycoproteins, and to lipids of the bilayer, forming glycolipids. This gives rise to a layer known as the glycocalyx (cell coat).

Cell membrane structure

The cell membrane is a biological membrane (Figures 1.1 and 1.2) comprising lipid-protein layers covered on their external surface by oligosaccharide chains. The individual components of the cell membrane comprise:

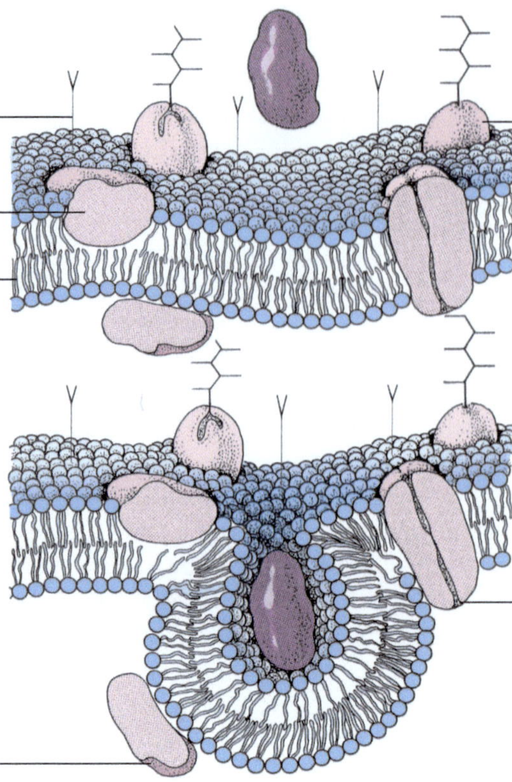

1.1 Structure of the cell membrane (schematic). The membrane consists of a lipid bilayer with associated membrane proteins. Carbohydrate side chains attach to the outer surface of the membrane, giving rise to the glycolipids and glycoproteins that make up the glycocalyx. During uptake of ligands (e.g. proteins), the membrane invaginates to form an endocytotic vesicle.

- a lipid bilayer,
- membrane proteins and
- surface polysaccharides.

Lipid bilayer

The lipid molecules of the cell membrane are arranged in a **double layer**. Phospholipids are the main component of the bilayer, with **cholesterol** and **glycolipids** present in smaller quantities. The lipids are amphipathic, with **one hydrophilic** (affinity for water, polar), electrically charged head group and **two hydrophobic** (water-repelling, non-polar) hydrocarbon tails. The hydrophobic tails consist alternately of saturated and unsaturated fatty acids. The hydrophilic head groups are oriented towards the outer surfaces of the membrane while the hydrophobic tails face towards each other. Due to their specific lipid molecule content, and the concentration of electric charge in the outer membrane components, most membranes are **asymmetrical** (Figure 1.1).

The structure of the cell membrane has important functional implications. The variable length of the saturated and unsaturated hydrocarbon chains, and their ability to move, influences the dynamics of the membrane, giving it a **fluid quality**.

At a molecular level, the fluidity of the membrane is determined by the ability of the phospholipids to **rotate** and **diffuse laterally** within the membrane. Less frequently, they also **flip-flop** between individual layers of the bilayer.

The fluidity of the cell membrane gives rise to the **plasticity** of the cell as a whole. Components of the membrane may be pinched off (e.g. by exocytosis or endocytosis) or replaced. Following interruption by external influences or cellular secretory activity, the lipid bilayer is re-established spontaneously within the aqueous microenvironment, thus restoring the continuity of the membrane.

Cholesterol is an important functional component of the membrane, serving to regulate the intramembranous movement of lipid chains and to increase the **mechanical strength of the bilayer**.

Glycolipids are present in the outer layer of the plasmalemma of all animal cells and contribute significantly to the asymmetry of the cell membrane. Their head groups, consisting of one or more polar sugar residues (oligosaccharides), project beyond the surface of the membrane. Glycolipids consist predominantly of neutral glycolipids (e.g. galactocerebroside within myelin sheaths) or gangliosides (e.g. sialic acids in cell receptors) (for further information refer to 'Membrane polysaccharides', below, and biochemistry texts).

Membrane proteins

The proteins of the cell membrane are incorporated into the lipid bilayer, where they perform membrane-specific functions (Figures 1–1 and 1–2). Membrane proteins include transport proteins, enzymes and specific receptor proteins. These are globular and, like the membrane lipids, amphipathic. Membrane proteins similarly exhibit hydrophobic inwardly oriented regions and hydrophilic moieties that project from one side or, more commonly, both sides of the membrane.

Several types of membrane proteins are recognised. These are named according to their functions:

- pumps: e.g. for amino acids, sugars, Na^+, Ca^{2+},
- channel proteins: passive diffusion of ions or molecules through the membrane,
- receptor proteins: cell recognition and binding of ligands (e.g. hormones, antibody reactions),
- linking proteins: binding with the intracellular cytoskeleton (e.g. actin filaments) or the extracellular matrix (e.g. fibronectins),
- enzymes: e.g. ATPase associated with the inner membrane of mitochondria, disaccharidases and dipeptidases involved in digestion and
- structural proteins: establish connections to the plasmalemma of neighbouring cells (e.g. between epithelial cells).

According to their location with respect to the lipid bilayer, a distinction is made between:

- integral membrane proteins and
- peripheral membrane proteins.

INTEGRAL MEMBRANE PROTEINS

Integral proteins span the **entire membrane**. They are difficult to extract, and project beyond the cell membrane on both sides (transmembrane proteins, intramembranous proteins and channel proteins). Their hydrophobic segments are bound to one or more fatty acid chains, thus anchoring them within the lipid bilayer.

Integral membrane proteins can move laterally within the membrane (**membrane fluidity**). Lateral movement of membrane proteins can be inhibited by certain structures including cytoskeletal components (actin filaments, intermediate filaments, microtubules), physical connections between cells (gap junctions, tight junctions) and lipid rafts.

PERIPHERAL MEMBRANE PROTEINS

Peripheral proteins penetrate the inner or outer lamina of the cell membrane to a variable extent and are easier to extract from the aqueous fraction during protein purification. These proteins are bound to fatty acids or integral membrane proteins.

Membrane polysaccharides

The outer surface of the plasmalemma is associated with a sugar residue coat of varying thickness (**glycocalyx; cell coat, surface coat**). The **glycocalyx** consists of **oligosaccharide chains** that are joined by covalent bonds with membrane proteins (forming glycoproteins) or, to a lesser extent, with lipids (forming glycolipids) (Figure 1.1). All membrane proteins, and about 10% of lipids, are associated with sugar residues. The accumulation of carbohydrates on the outer surface contributes to the asymmetry of the plasmalemma.

The structure of the oligosaccharide side chains is extremely complex. It comprises relatively few sugars (including glucose, fucose, mannose, glucosamine, galactose, sialic acids) that are interconnected in various ways. Sialic acid (N-acetyl neuraminic acid) imparts a negative charge to the cell surface. The glycocalyx, together with the plasmalemma, is constantly renewed by the cell. This process involves the delivery of sugars to the cell membrane by transport vesicles produced in the Golgi apparatus. In this way, the cell membrane contributes to the specificity of the cell surface.

The **glycocalyx** performs **various functions**. It forms a large number of receptors that receive information directly from other cells, or indirectly through messenger molecules (chemical signals such as hormones) and transmit the information to the cell. The glycocalyx contributes to recognition of endogenous or foreign cells and to the initiation of immune responses. Blood groups are determined by glycolipids in the glycocalyx of erythrocytes. The majority of processes occurring during cellular differentiation are also mediated by the glycocalyx.

Plasmalemma

The **plasmalemma** carries receptors for chemical signals from the extracellular compartment (e.g. hormones, neurotransmitters) and serves as a selective filter for regulation of intra- and extracellular electrolyte concentrations. In addition, the plasmalemma contributes to the uptake of nutrients and release of cellular products.

Through the expression of specific molecules, the plasmalemma mediates a large number of temporary associations among cells, contributes to adhesion between similar and unlike cells and participates in cell recognition. Direct connections between cells play an important role in growth and differentiation events, both during embryogenesis and in the adult animal. Cell adhesion molecules (CAM), which first appear on the plasmalemma during embryonic development, are fundamental in the formation of specialised intercellular junctions. Cell recognition is the critical first step in all immune responses; the surface molecules that develop for this purpose are components of the **major histocompatibility complex** (**MHC**).

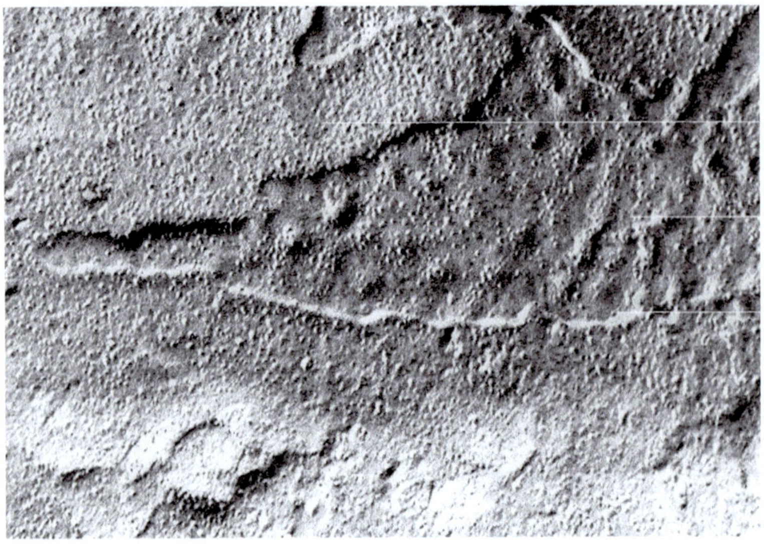

1.2 Freeze-fracture electron microscope image of the cell membrane (plasmalemma) of a lymphocyte showing the lipid bilayer and membrane proteins (x40,000).

At the **outer surface of the plasmalemma**, membrane proteins serve as **receptors** for **signalling molecules**. These include receptors involved in endocytosis and in recognition of other cells or cellular parasites (protozoa, viruses). Also present are receptors for substances that act as **primary messengers** in **signal transduction pathways**, including hormones, growth factors, cytokines and neurotransmitters.

These receptors are particularly significant in determining the function and structure of each cell, and in establishing its specificity. The structure of numerous receptors has been characterised, enabling detailed examination of cell structure and function by means of cloning, mutagenesis and transfection. **Protein tyrosine kinases** and **G-protein coupled receptors** represent two prominent groups of cell surface receptors that convey signals to regulatory systems within the cytoplasm.

Protein tyrosine kinases include receptors (receptor tyrosine kinases, RTKs) for growth factors such as epidermal growth factor (EGF) and insulin-like growth factor I (IGF-I). This receptor type is activated by binding of a ligand with endogenous kinase on the external surface of the plasmalemma. Subsequent autophosphorylation or phosphorylation of other proteins results in the stimulation of cell-specific metabolic reactions.

G-protein coupled receptors are activated by a range of ligands including hormones and neurotransmitters. This receptor type acts as a **membrane modulator** by regulating the activity of the membrane-associated enzyme adenylyl cyclase. G-protein coupled receptors thus influence production of the **second messenger cyclic AMP (cAMP)** within the cytoplasm (stimulation through G_s-proteins, inhibition through G_i-proteins). This diverse family of receptors includes adrenergic, cholinergic, dopaminergic and peptidergic receptors. The three components of the system – receptor, G-protein and enzyme – are able to **move freely** within the plane of the membrane. Binding of this group of receptors with ligands occurs as a result of random interactions (**mobile receptors**).

While the plasmalemma, with its lipid bilayer, serves as a barrier to the simple diffusion of most water-soluble molecules, passage of small molecules across the membrane is enabled by **membrane transport proteins** including **channel proteins** and **carrier proteins** (Fig. 1.3) (see below).

Channel proteins are components of **ionotropic neurotransmitter receptors**, in which receptor subunits form a centrally located ion conduit (**ion channel**). **Nicotinic acetylcholine receptors** are included in this group. Activation of the receptor results in opening of the ion channel and influx of Na^+, leading to membrane depolarisation. This mechanism is integral to the transmission of signals between **presynaptic cells** and **postsynaptic cell membranes**.

Transport facilitated by **carrier proteins** may be passive or active (see below). Other membrane proteins have enzymatic or catalytic functions.

Cellular metabolism

Cells are characterised by the capacity to engage in continuous synthesis, transformation, breakdown and, under certain circumstances, release of materials. To sustain such metabolic activity, the cell takes up organic and inorganic substances (**substrates**) from its surroundings and modifies these through a series of chemical reactions. These reactions take place within the cellular matrix or in association with cellular organelles.

Through this process, a diverse range of dietary nutrients enters the cell and undergoes enzymatic cleavage (**cellular digestion**). Substances such as monosaccharides, fatty acids and amino acids, as well as ions and vitamins, are incorporated into cellular metabolic processes. Oxygen also passes into the cell.

These mechanisms are subject to hormonal and neural control. The breakdown of substrates within the cell is associated with generation of mechanical, thermal, electrical or chemical energy. Eventually, the breakdown products are used to synthesise new structural elements and fuels. Cell-specific substances destined for **secretion** by the cell are also produced. Metabolic waste products are eliminated by **excretion**.

Mechanisms of substrate uptake

Substances that enter or leave the cell must pass through the boundary created by the plasmalemma. This occurs through membrane transport or vesicular transport.

Membrane transport

The structure of the cell membrane permits the uptake of low molecular weight and polar substances. This can occur via (Figure 1.3):

- simple diffusion or
- membrane protein transport, through binding with:
  - carrier proteins or
  - channel proteins.

Carrier proteins permit the transport of small, water-soluble molecules. These are usually **specific to certain types of molecules**. Upon coupling with a molecule, the protein undergoes conformational changes that result in carriage of the molecule across the membrane. This may involve active transport against a concentration gradient (e.g. Na^+/K^+ pumps) or passive transport (e.g. glucose).

Channel proteins also transport small water-soluble molecules. They are regulated by membrane potentials (e.g. in neurons), neurotransmitters (e.g. acetylcholine receptors on muscle cells) or mechanical forces (e.g. in the inner ear).

Vesicular transport

Numerous macromolecules pass into or out of the cell without compromising the integrity of the cell membrane. This occurs through the formation of membrane-bound **vesicles** that are pinched off from the plasmalemma (**vesicular transport**). Within the cell, the vesicles are able to transfer their contents to other cellular compartments. The formation of vesicles can be demonstrated using electron microscopy. Two types of vesicular transport are recognised:

- endocytosis (uptake of macromolecules) and
- exocytosis (release of macromolecules).

ENDOCYTOSIS

In the process of endocytosis, the plasmalemma surrounds the molecule before invaginating and budding off as a vesicle (Figures 1.4 and 1.5). The uptake of vesicular contents is often induced by an increase in the density of the plasmalemma in the vicinity of certain actin filament proteins (particularly clathrin, molecular weight 180,000 Da) (see below). These proteins subsequently coat the exterior surface of the vesicle (**coated vesicles**).

There are three mechanisms of endocytosis:

- pinocytosis,
- receptor-mediated endocytosis and
- phagocytosis.

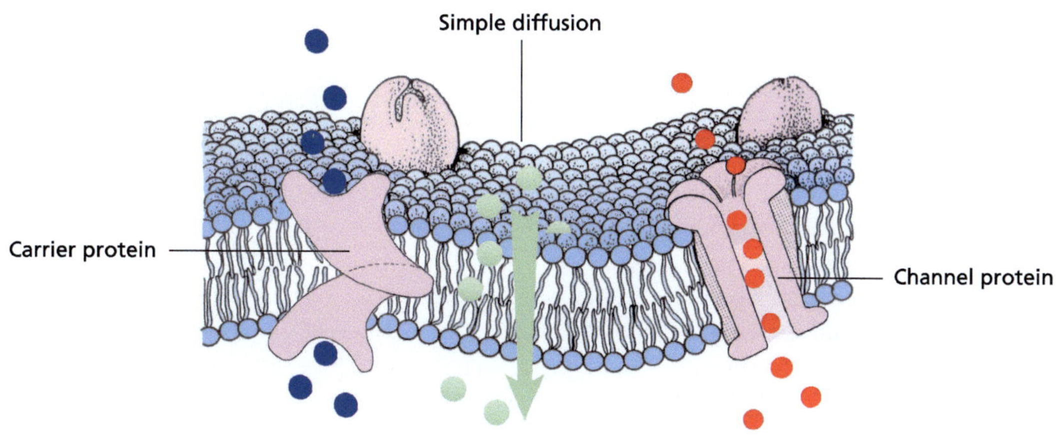

1.3 Transmembrane molecular transport (schematic).

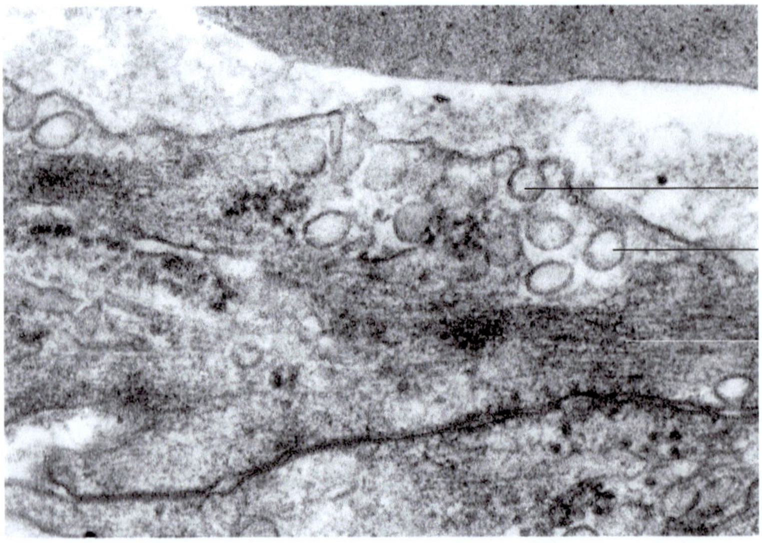

1.4 Endocytotic and exocytotic vesicles in a vessel wall (x20,000).

Pinocytosis

The term pinocytosis refers to the formation of small vesicles containing fluid or soluble macromolecules. Most cells are capable of this type of endocytosis. It is a continuous, dynamic process, supported by mechanoenzymes. Pinocytotic vesicles are particularly numerous in the endothelia of blood vessels and in smooth muscle cells. Pinocytosis is **clathrin-independent**.

Receptor-mediated endocytosis

Receptor-mediated endocytosis is observed in many types of cells. It involves **surface receptors for specific ligands** (e.g. Fc receptors for antigen–antibody complexes, LDL receptors for regulation of cellular cholesterol homeostasis, transferrin receptors for iron metabolism). The surface of erythrocytes contains embedded glycoprotein receptors. If these are lost, the affected cell is recognised as senile and is taken up by macrophages (part of the innate immune system).

In this form of endocytosis, uptake of molecules occurs in well-defined regions of the cell in which clathrin molecules are aggregated (**coated pits**). Interaction of clathrin with the receptor is mediated by adaptin, a vesicular transport adaptor protein. These membrane segments then become liberated from the plasmalemma forming '**coated vesicles**' (transport vesicles of clathrin-dependent receptor-mediated endocytosis) (Figure 1.5).

Phagocytosis

Phagocytosis involves the uptake of **solid particles**. Cellular ingestion of large particles (e.g. bacteria) or cell fragments results in the formation of vesicular inclusions

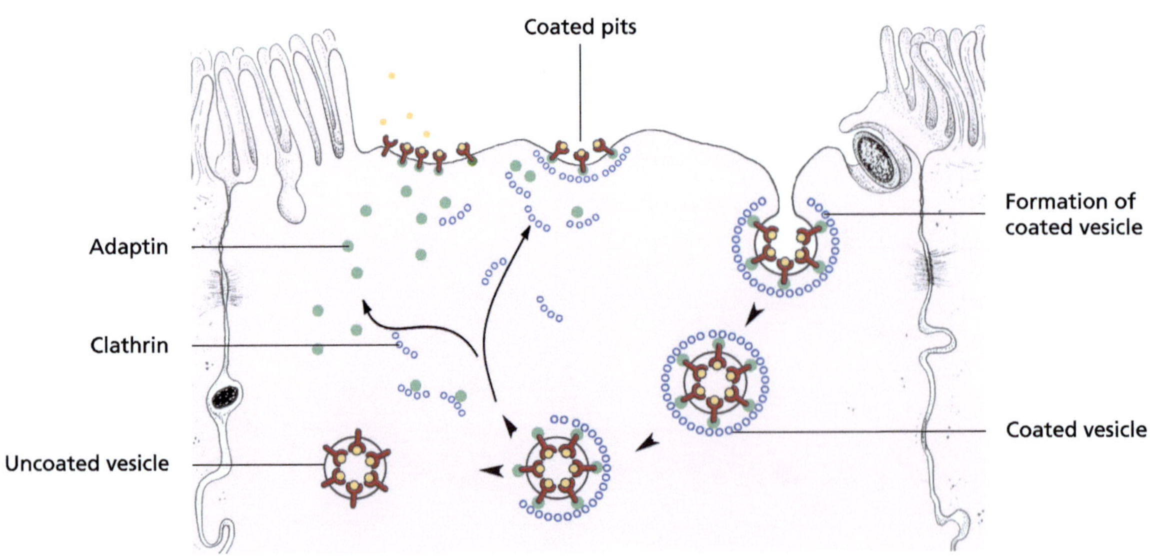

1.5 Receptor-mediated endocytosis (schematic).

(**vacuoles**). The internalised vesicles, which can reach 250 nm in diameter, are referred to as **phagosomes** (Figure 1.6). Phagocytosis is predominantly performed by specialised cells (phagocytes), particularly cells of the **mononuclear phagocytic system** (**MPS**).

Phagocytosis is typically a **receptor-mediated process** in which cell surface receptors recognise antibody fragments associated with invading microorganisms or cells. In the cell-mediated immune response, for example (see Chapter 8, 'Immune system and lymphatic organs'), bacteria become coated with antibody molecules that are recognised by receptors on macrophages. Binding of the antibody with the receptor stimulates the cell to engulf and phagocytose the microorganism.

In addition, phagocytes have the capacity to take up **non-biological materials** (e.g. inhaled pollutants) and cell fragments (e.g. from wounds, sites of inflammation and cell degeneration) **without the involvement of receptors**. Phagocytosis is usually associated with a reorganisation of intracellular actin filaments. Ingestion of substances by phagocytosis is thus a clathrin-independent actin-dependent form of endocytosis.

Vesicle formation occurs at varying rates in different cells. **Macrophages** are capable of internalising 100% of their cell surface in the form of vesicles within a period of half an hour. Since this does not alter the surface of the volume of the cell, it follows that the vesicles are extensively **recycled**, and reincorporated into the cell membrane. Membrane-associated release of materials by the cell is also part of this recycling process.

In most cases, vesicles formed by endocytosis enter the endosomal system (see below). In some cases, endocytotic vesicles are transported through the cell and released at another surface, without undergoing alteration. This process is referred to as **transcytosis** (**cytopempsis**).

EXOCYTOSIS

The mechanism of exocytosis is similar to that of endocytosis but **occurs in the opposite direction**. Cellular products are packaged into vesicles within the cell and transported to the surface. The vesicles fuse with the plasmalemma and deposit their contents into the surrounding medium. After fusion of the exocytotic vesicle with the plasmalemma, the membrane associated with the vesicle is reintroduced into the cytoplasm in a subsequent endocytotic event. Two exocytotic pathways are recognised:

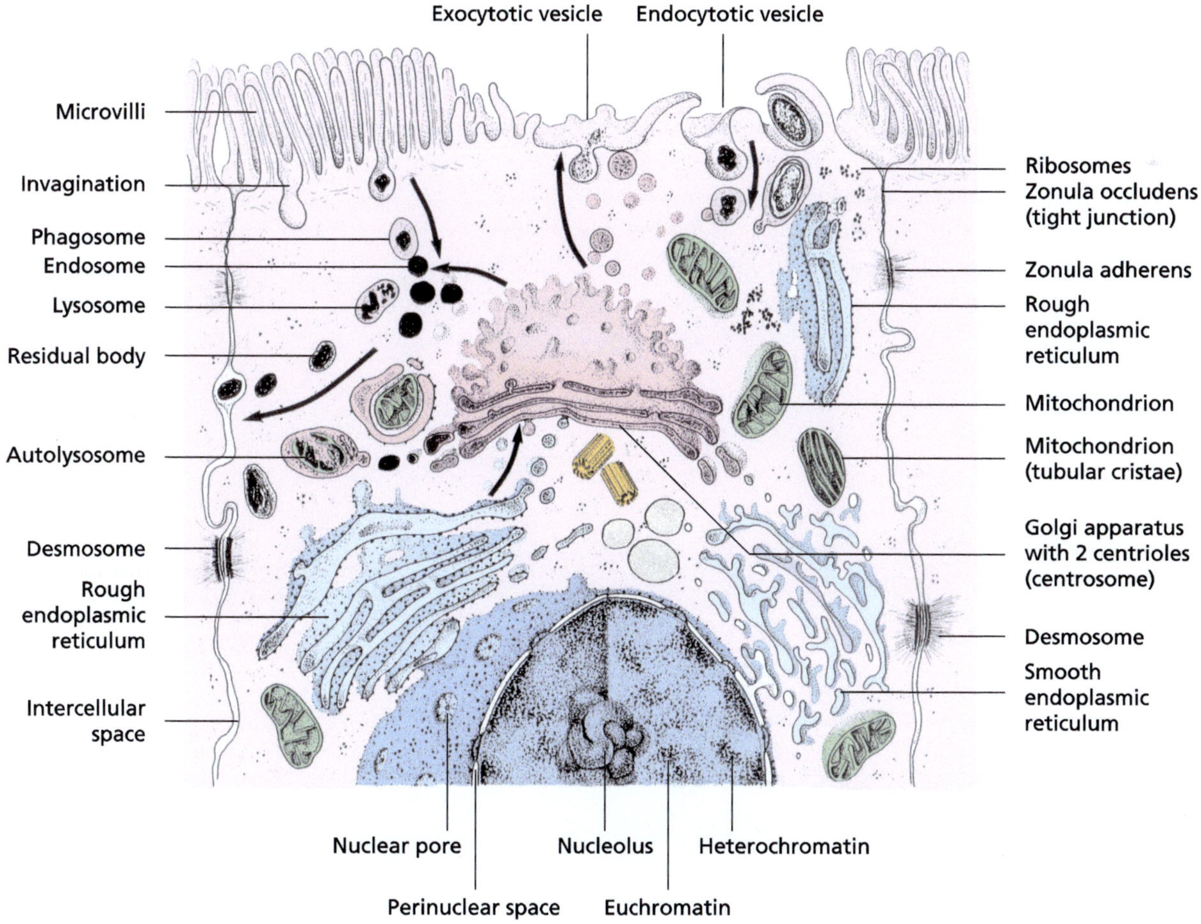

1.6 Overview of the principal cellular organelles and various types of cell surface specialisations.

- constitutive and
- regulated secretory.

In the constitutive pathway, substances intended for export from the cell are delivered continuously to the plasma membrane. This is exemplified by the secretion of certain proteins immediately after their synthesis in the Golgi apparatus (e.g. antibodies in plasma cells or collagen precursors in fibroblasts).

Regulated secretory exocytosis is performed by specialised cells (e.g. endocrine or exocrine gland cells, or nerve cells), in which hormones and other secretory products are stored in the form of secretory granules. The release of these granules is **Ca^{2+}-dependent** and is controlled by **hormonal** and **neural** mechanisms (e.g. the liberation of zymogen granules by chief cells of the gastric mucosa or acinar cells of the pancreas).

ENDOSOMAL SYSTEM

Within the cell, endocytosed vesicles become associated with a system of membrane-bound compartments known as **endosomes**. Early endosomes are usually located peripherally. Those located deeper in the cytoplasm (late endosomes) generally mature into **lysosomes**.

Two models exist to explain the endosomal system. According to one, endosomes are a stable component of the cytoplasm, while in the other they are formed from endocytotic vesicles. **Early endosomes** manifest as a **tubulovesicular structure**, subdivided into cisternae by invagination of their membranes. Proteins are transported from early endosomes to **late endosomes** by endosomal vesicles referred to as **multivesicular bodies**. These contain acid hydrolases, and are found in abundance in liver cells, epithelial cells of the epididymis and in Type II alveolar epithelial cells in the lung. After undergoing additional biochemical transformation, late endosomes (also referred to as **prelysosomes**) mature into **lysosomes**.

The primary function of endosomes is the sorting and recovery of proteins within the endocytotic vesicular transport system. Ligands are separated from receptors and the resulting components are directed into processing pathways for recycling or degradation.

Intracellular metabolism

Intracellular metabolic processes take place either in the cell matrix or in association with the cellular organelles, particularly ribosomes and the membrane-bound compartments of the endoplasmic reticulum. The nucleus plays a central role in coordinating the activity of these (and other) organelles.

Mitochondria and the Golgi apparatus also participate in intracellular metabolism, as do lysosomes and peroxisomes (see below).

Cell matrix (cytosol)

The cytosol is the site of most of the reactions that, in biochemical terms, constitute **intermediate** (**intermediary**) **metabolism**. This involves the liberation of energy (ATP) through the breakdown of small molecules and the synthesis of new macromolecules that contribute to the structure of the cell or maintenance of cellular metabolic processes.

The cytosol comprises over **half of the volume of the cell**. It contains enzymes involved in glycolysis and gluconeogenesis, and serves as the site of assembly of sugars, fatty acids, nucleotides and amino acids into complex organic molecules. In particular, a large portion of the **protein biosynthetic pathway** takes place within the cytosol. Structural proteins that contribute to the **stability**, **plasticity** and **motility** of the cell are formed here. The cell matrix has a high binding affinity for water and electrolytes.

In addition to enzymes, the cytosol contains dissolved proteins that confer upon the matrix the quality of a gel. The gel constantly changes its physical state by temporarily entering a liquid phase (**solgel state**).

While molecular components of cellular metabolism are typically not morphologically observable, individual **structures associated with the storage of products of intermediate metabolism** can be visualised with microscopy. In the synthesis of fat (triglycerides), fatty acids are stored in lipid droplets. Glycogen, a storage form of polymerised glucose, can be appreciated morphologically as glycogen granules. Structural proteins and lysosomes can also be identified.

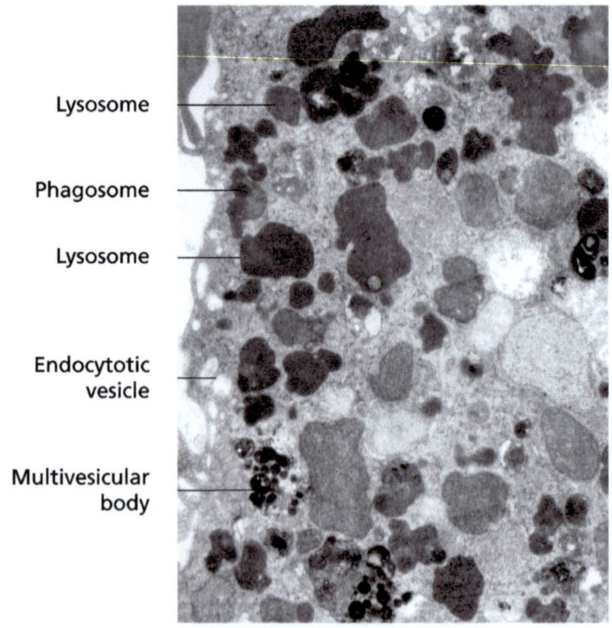

1.7 Components of lysosome biogenesis in a macrophage (x10,000).

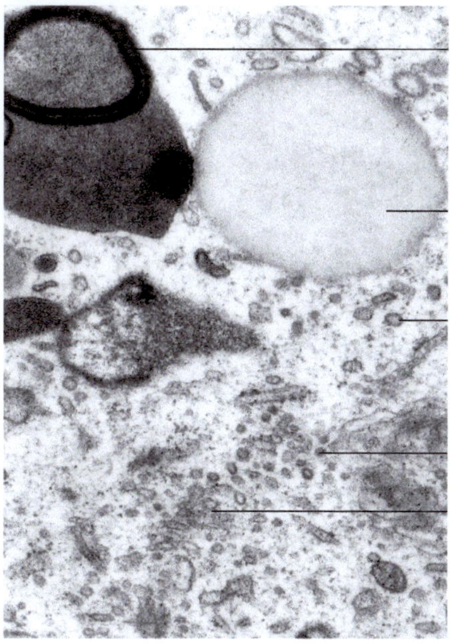

1.8 Lysosome with adjacent lipid droplet in a liver cell (x10,000).

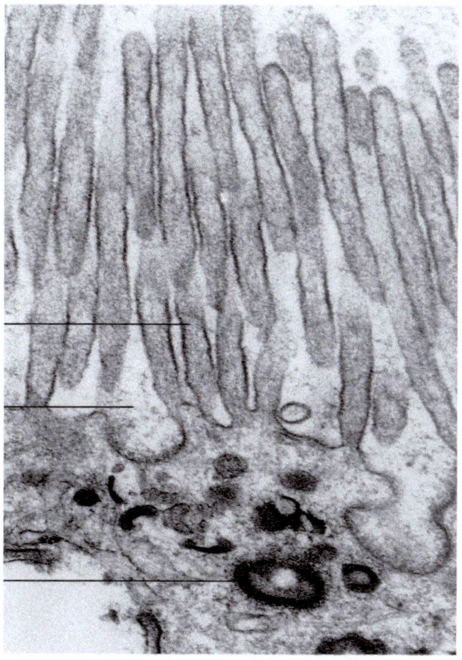

1.9 Lysosomes in the tubular epithelium of the kidney of a dog (x22,000).

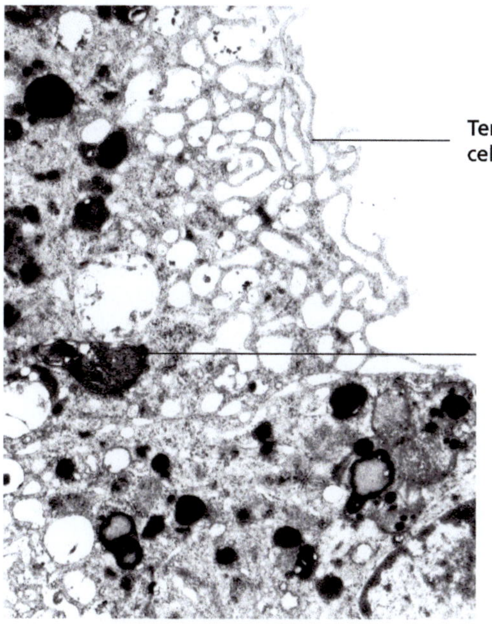

1.10 Lysosomes in a peritoneal macrophage (x4500).

Lysosomes (lysosoma)

Lysosomes are membrane-bound organelles responsible for intracellular digestion and enzymatic degradation of soluble and solid substances.

Lysosomes contain a large range of structurally diverse enzymes (acid hydrolases). These are synthesised in the rER and sorted in the Golgi apparatus. Depending on the function of the cell, lysosomal enzymes consist primarily of acid phosphatases, glycosidases, peptidases (proteases), esterases, sulfatases, deoxyribonucleases and ribonucleases (active at pH 5.0). The enzymes are separated from the surrounding cytosol by a phosphatide-glycolipid-protein membrane with a built-in proton-ATPase (proton pump).

Lysosomal enzymes are responsible for the **digestion of substances originating from inside and outside the cell**. The end products (nucleotides, amino acids or sugars) pass into the cell matrix where they are incorporated into cellular metabolic processes.

Material that cannot be digested enzymatically is retained within the lysosome as **residual bodies**. These may be ejected from the cell through the plasmalemma. Those that remain within the cell can lead to formation of **endogenous pigments** (e.g. lipofuscin).

Lysosomes are also involved in physiological processes associated with **embryogenesis** and play a role in **programmed cell death** (**apoptosis**).

Disruption of the integrity of the lysosomal membrane, by endogenous or exogenous factors, results in the release of lysosomal enzymes into the surrounding cytosol, leading to **degradation** of cellular components within the cytoplasm. Causative factors include oxygen deficiency, X- and UV radiation and various cytotoxins. This process, referred to as **autolysis**, usually results in **death of the cell**.

Abnormalities of lysosomal enzyme function can give rise to **lysosomal storage diseases**. These are characterised by the genetically determined absence of functional enzymes, resulting in accumulation of undigested substrates.

LYSOSOME STRUCTURE

Lysosomes are ovoid to spherical organelles (Figures 1.6 to 1.10). Their limiting membrane is reinforced by an abundance of glycolipids. The membrane permits egress of metabolic end products into the cytosol and facilitates

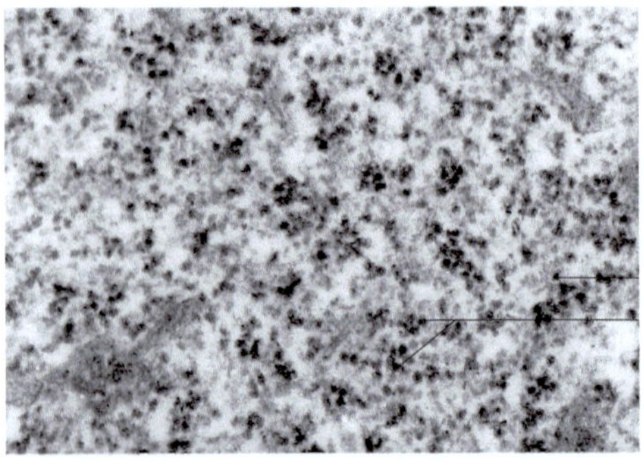

1.11 Ribosomes and polyribosomes in a canine liver cell (x45,000).

the entry of H^+ ions for activation of lysosomal enzymes. Lysosomes vary in size and in the density of their matrix. Most are 0.2–0.6 μm in diameter but may reach 5 μm in cells with high endocytotic activity.

For many years, lysosomes were considered to arise from the Golgi apparatus as primary lysosomes, which then merged with late endosomes to become secondary lysosomes. Recent findings suggest that lysosome biogenesis is a more complex process, involving merging of post-Golgi vesicles with the endocytic pathway. In this model, early endosomes or phagosomes containing internalised materials are converted into late endosomes, which mature into lysosomes. Lysosomes also feature in **autophagy**, the process by which intracellular components (organelles, membranes, excess cellular products) are degraded. These components are isolated and engulfed in a membrane to form an **autophagosome**. Fusion of an autophagosome with a lysosome gives rise to an **autolysosome** (autophagolysosome). Autophagy plays an important part in cell regeneration and in the recycling of organelles and cell membranes.

Under certain physiological conditions, lysosomes can be transferred out of the cell, becoming active in the extracellular compartment, e.g. breakdown of connective tissue and digestion of ground substance in bone (osteoclasts). Lysosomes also play an important role in lysis of tissue fragments in inflammatory reactions.

In polymorphonuclear neutrophilic granulocytes, aggregated lysosomes can be observed with the light microscope as azurophilic granules. They are frequently also identifiable in macrophages as phagocytosed fragments of bacteria or cell debris.

Peroxisomes (peroxisoma)

Peroxisomes (microbodies) are membrane-bound organelles that contain **oxidative enzymes** (e.g. D-amino acid oxidase, urate oxidase and catalase). They are present in almost all cells. Peroxisomes catalyse the breakdown (β-oxidation) of fatty acids producing acetyl-CoA. They also perform an important role in **detoxification reactions**, and thus are abundant in liver and kidney cells.

The oxidation of substrates by peroxisomes results in reduction of oxygen to hydrogen peroxide (H_2O_2). Produced by many intracellular oxidative reactions, hydrogen peroxide is harmful to the cell. This is broken down, and thus detoxified, by peroxisomal catalase.

Peroxisomes also contribute to lipid biosynthesis. They produce the lipid layer of the myelin membrane of neurons and synthesise the fatty components of sebaceous glands. Free acetyl groups are used by peroxisomes in the biosynthesis of cholesterol.

Peroxisomes measure 0.15–0.25 μm in diameter. Their generally homogeneous internal structure may be interrupted by crystalline or tubular inclusions. Peroxisomal membranes are formed by budding from the tubules of the smooth endoplasmic reticulum; the contents of the peroxisome are synthesised in the cytosol.

Organelles of anabolism

A major proportion of cellular metabolism involves organelles that function primarily to synthesise protein (**ribosomes** and **rough endoplasmic reticulum**) and lipid (smooth endoplasmic reticulum).

RIBOSOMES (RIBOSOMA)

Ribosomes are cytosolic ribonucleoprotein particles. Numerous enzymes involved in intermediate metabolism (multi-enzyme complexes) are synthesised in these organelles. Ribosomes translate the information encoded in messenger ribonucleic acid (mRNA) into amino acid sequences and link the individual amino acids to form polypeptide chains (for further information, refer to biochemistry texts).

RIBOSOME STRUCTURE

Ribosomes are spheroid to ovoid structures (diameter 15–30 nm). They consist of one larger and one smaller subunit. According to their sedimentation coefficients, the subunits are designated **60S** and **40S**. The larger subunit comprises two ribonucleic acids (RNA) and 45 different proteins. One ribonucleic acid and 33 proteins make up the smaller subunit. The overall structure and function of the ribosome is determined by interactions between ribosomal RNA (rRNA) and mRNA produced in the nucleus. The composition of ribosomes is around 40% rRNA and 60% associated protein.

Within the cytoplasm, ribosomes are either present as individual structures or are assembled into spiral chains referred to as **polyribosomes** (**polysomes, polyribosoma**). Polyribosomes consist of several individual ribosomes attached at intervals to a single mRNA molecule. Free ribosomes and polyribosomes primarily synthesise proteins that are required by the cell itself (e.g. structural proteins, enzymes) (Figures 1.6 and 1.11).

The number of ribosomes is related to the function of the cell. Rapidly growing cells or cells actively synthesising protein contain considerably more ribosomes than degen-

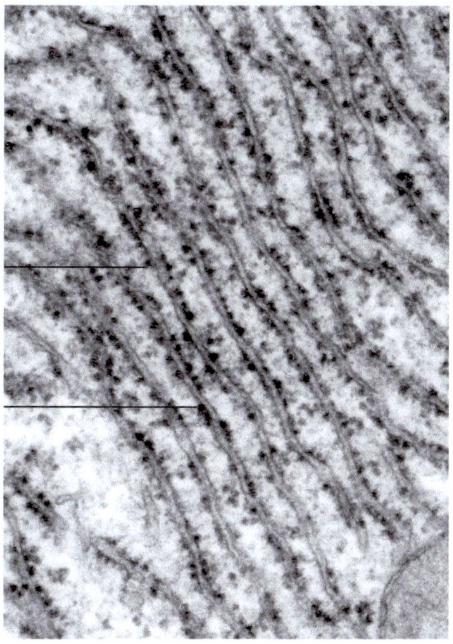

1.12 Rough endoplasmic reticulum (rER) in a liver cell (x14,000).

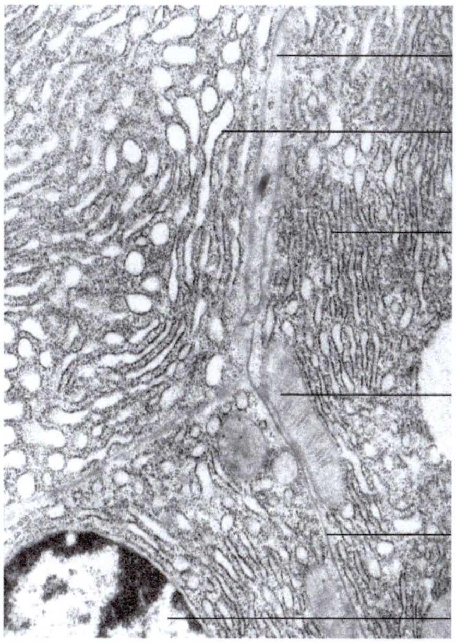

1.13 Rough endoplasmic reticulum (rER) in a cell of the exocrine pancreas (x8000).

erating cells. The density of the ribosome population influences the staining properties of the cell. Cytoplasm rich in ribosomal RNA is strongly basophilic as basic stains (e.g. methylene blue, toluidine blue) bind with the phosphate groups of free RNA. Ribosomes may also be attached to the cytoplasmic surface of the membranes of the endoplasmic reticulum (Figures 1.6, 1.12 to 1.14, 1.16).

ENDOPLASMIC RETICULUM (RETICULUM ENDOPLASMATICUM)

The endoplasmic reticulum (ER) is a system of membranes manifesting as stacks of flattened, interconnected cisternae and tubules (Figures 1.6, 1.12 to 1.16). These structures form an enclosed cavity that extends, typically in a parallel arrangement, throughout the cell.

The portion of the endoplasmic reticulum in which the outer surface of the membrane is studded with ribosomes is termed the rough (granular) endoplasmic reticulum (rER). Endoplasmic reticulum lacking ribosomes is referred to as smooth endoplasmic reticulum (sER).

Both of the key structural components of all cellular membranes – lipids (phospholipids and cholesterol) and proteins – are synthesised in large part at the membranes of the ER.

ROUGH ENDOPLASMIC RETICULUM (RETICULUM ENDOPLASMATICUM GRANULOSUM)

Rough endoplasmic reticulum is found in almost all nucleated cells and is particularly abundant in cells actively engaged in **protein synthesis** (Figures 1.6, 1.12 to 1.14, 1.16). These include secretory cells of the salivary glands and exocrine pancreas, nerve cells (as Nissl bodies) and lipid-producing cells of the mammary glands. Proteins produced by rER-associated ribosomes enter the lumen of the endoplasmic reticulum where they undergo post-translational modification. When proteins are produced in quantities exceeding the capacity of the rER to export them, **the cisternae become expanded**.

The rough endoplasmic reticulum may merge with the outer membrane of the nucleus, such that the lumen of the ER is continuous with that of the **perinuclear cistern** of the nuclear envelope. Transport vesicles arising from the free ends of the rER membrane carry specific molecules to other organelles or to the cell surface.

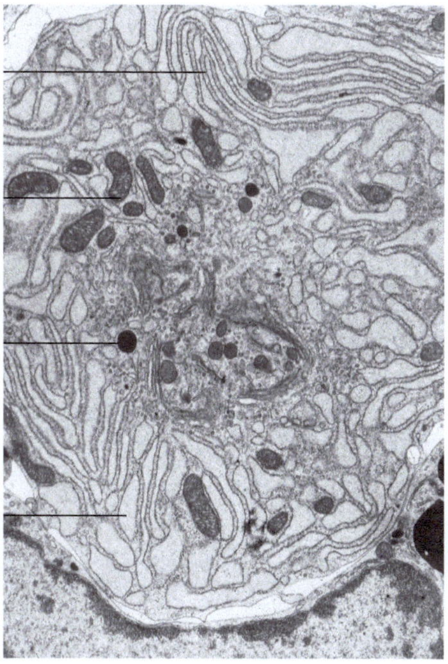

1.14 Rough endoplasmic reticulum (rER) (x5000).

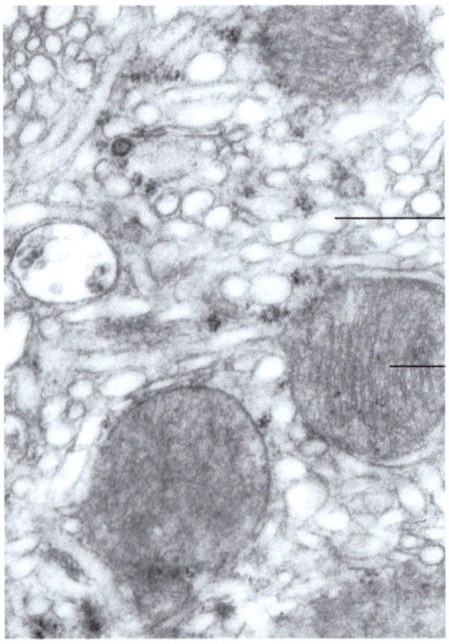

1.15 Smooth endoplasmic reticulum (sER) (x16,000).

Function: The rough endoplasmic reticulum plays a central role in intracellular metabolism. It synthesises cell-specific molecules from substances that have been endocytosed and broken down by the lysosomal enzyme system. Products of cytoplasmic metabolism make a significant contribution to this synthetic process, providing a range of 'building blocks' for new cellular products. At the ER membrane, these substrates are assembled into **macromolecules** that are required by other cellular organelles to perform their specific functions.

Ribosomes are integral in the synthesis of proteins by the rER. Newly synthesised ribosomal proteins pass through complex protein channels into the lumen of the ER, where they undergo modification including:

- folding,
- formation of disulfide bonds and
- initial glycosylation.

A degree of quality control also occurs in the rER, with incorrectly folded proteins being exported to the cytosol where they are degraded by proteases.

Glycosylation primarily takes place on the inner, luminal surface of the ER membrane, and is subsequently completed by the Golgi apparatus. Transport vesicles budding from the ER membrane pass to the Golgi apparatus, endosomes, lysosomes, peroxisomes, the plasmalemma and the nuclear membrane. Most of the proteins contained in these vesicles are glycosylated with oligosaccharide chains.

The proteins carried by the transport vesicles contribute to metabolism within the aforementioned organelles or are released from the cell as secretory product. They are also incorporated into cellular membranes. The rER thus assumes an important role in **intracellular transport** and **communication.**

Rough endoplasmic reticulum is particularly prominent in protein-secreting gland cells. Dense accumulations of ER-cisternae are present in the basal cytoplasm. Under the light microscope this portion of the cytoplasm appears as a basophilic region referred to as **ergastoplasm**.

SMOOTH ENDOPLASMIC RETICULUM (RETICULUM ENDOPLASMATICUM NONGRANULOSUM)

The smooth endoplasmic reticulum consists of predominantly short, interconnected **tubules** that do not have **ribosomes** on their surface (Figures 1.6 and 1.15).

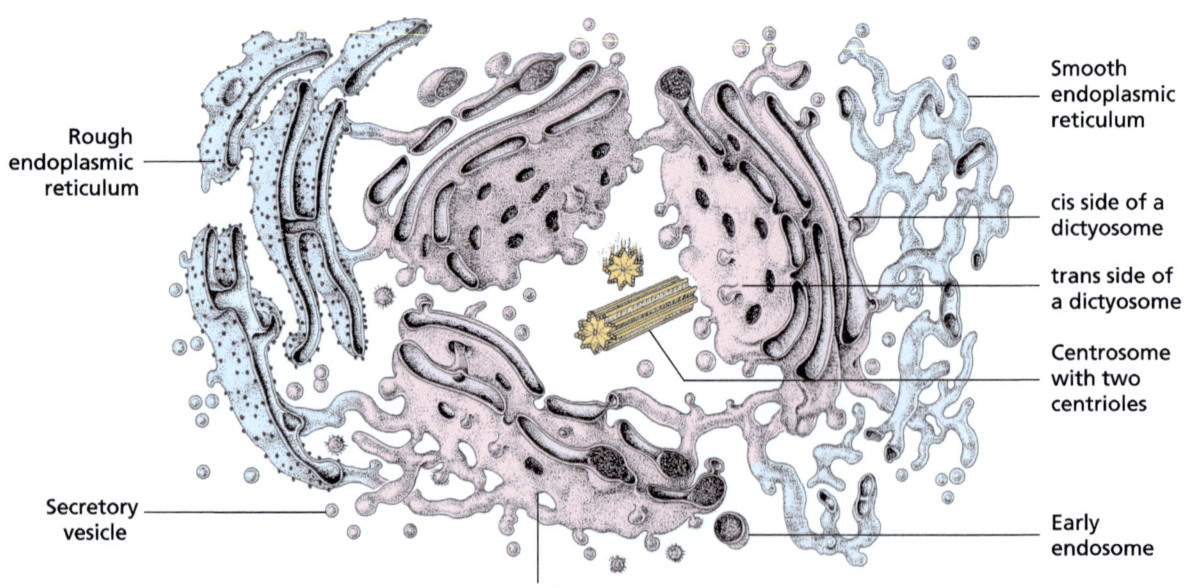

1.16 Golgi apparatus with central centriole pair and adjacent smooth and rough endoplasmic reticulum (schematic).

Function: Smooth ER is abundant in cells that are active in **lipid metabolism** (e.g. liver cells). The membrane of the sER contains enzymes involved in synthesis of lipoproteins and serves as an anchor for components of **gluconeogenesis**. In the liver, the sER contains enzymes involved in **detoxification** (e.g. of harmful hydrocarbons). **Steroid hormone synthesis** takes place in the smooth ER of cells of the adrenal cortex and corpus luteum. Muscle cells contain a modified form of sER (**sarcoplasmic reticulum**), in which Ca^{2+} ions are stored.

Smooth endoplasmic reticulum also participates in the **formation** and **recycling** of cellular membranes.

Organelles of protein modification and vesicular trafficking

All cells contain a vesicular trafficking system through which its various organelles are connected. This includes vesicles that enter the cytosol after budding from the membrane of the endoplasmic reticulum and the outer membrane of the nuclear envelope.

Cytoplasmic vesicles that arise through endocytosis, as well as endosomes and lysosomes, also contribute to transport of substances within the cell.

Most of these transport vesicles interact with a key organelle, the Golgi apparatus, which is responsible for sorting, packaging and directing of metabolic products within the cell. Vesicular transport is carefully controlled and takes place along the system of microfilaments within the cell (cytoskeleton).

GOLGI APPARATUS (COMPLEXUS GOLGIENSIS)

The Golgi apparatus is named after the Italian neurohistologist and Nobel prize winner, Camillo Golgi (1843–1926). With the aid of a similarly eponymous silver stain, Golgi observed what he described as an *apparato reticulare interno* within nerve cells derived from the cerebellum.

Structure: The Golgi apparatus is a compound structure composed of slightly curved clusters of stacked, flattened (plate-like) **membrane-bound cisternae** or **sacs**.

The membrane stacks have a smooth surface and are not in direct contact with one another. As in the endoplasmic reticulum, the membranes enclose a **lumen** that may be dilated, depending on the activity of the cell. Dilatations at the ends of the cisternae become pinched off to form **vesicles**. Individual membrane stacks are also referred to as **dictyosomes** (Figures 1.6, 1.16 to 1.18). Dictyosomes are **concentrated around the nucleus**. Most cells contain at least one Golgi apparatus. Depending on the type and function of the cell, multiple Golgi apparatuses may be present. This applies in particular to secretory cells (e.g. in salivary glands, intestinal glands, nerve cells and hepatocytes). Dictyosomes have a **forming**, or **cis**, **side** and a **maturing**, or **trans**, **side**.

Cis side: The cis side takes up membrane-bound, thin-walled transport vesicles originating from the endoplasmic reticulum. The vesicle membrane fuses with that of the Golgi apparatus and the vesicular contents enter the cisternal lumen. This process is repeated, with transport vesicles conveying materials from one cisterna to the next. Vesicles arising from the nuclear envelope pass into the Golgi

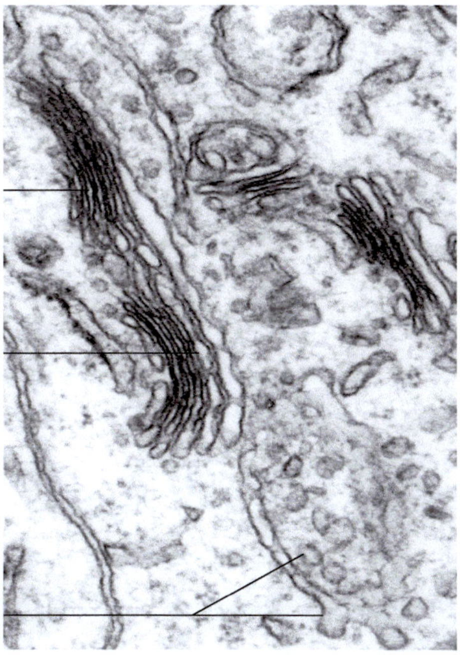

1.17 Dictyosomes in an actively secreting gland cell (x14,000).

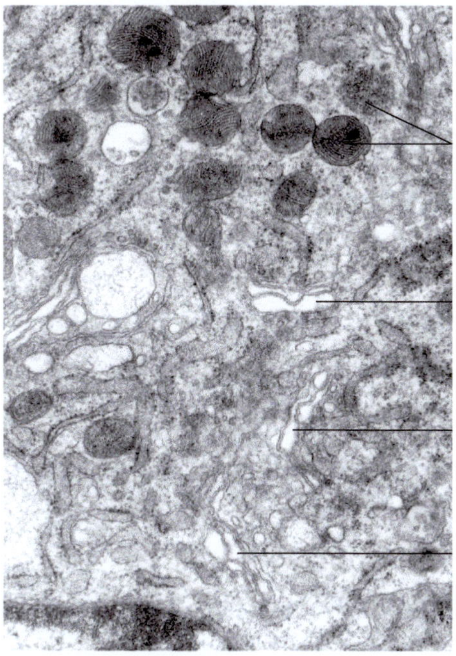

1.18 Dictyosomes of a Golgi apparatus in an actively secreting gland cell containing secretory granules (x9000).

apparatus in a similar manner. The cis side thus represents the side of substance uptake and growth of the dictyosome.

Trans side: The trans side features an accumulation of vesicles that are still in contact with, or have become detached from, the membrane. The proteins in these vesicles are destined for various locations including the apical cytoplasm (secretory proteins within **secretory vesicles**) and lysosomes (membrane proteins and enzymes). This side of the Golgi apparatus is thus responsible for sorting and vesicle distribution.

Function: The primary function of the Golgi apparatus is **terminal processing** of macromolecules and **targeted dispersal** of the resulting end products to their final destination. Proteins synthesised in the ER are glycosylated (with complex oligosaccharides and mannose-rich oligosaccharides) to form glycoproteins, proteoglycans and lysosomal proteins. Modification of lipoproteins also occurs in the Golgi apparatus.

In actively secreting cells, the Golgi apparatus serves to create a stockpile of **cellular secretions**. The concentration of secretory product allows for rapid release from the cell in response to increased demand. The Golgi apparatus therefore assumes cell-specific roles in **storage**, **transport** and **release of secretions**.

Secretory vesicles leave the **trans side** of the Golgi apparatus and travel, generally via a system of microtubules or microfilaments, to the cell surface. There, the outer membrane of the transport vesicle fuses with the plasmalemma and its contents are transferred into the extracellular environment (**exocytosis**). Secretion may be regulated by **neurotransmitters** (e.g. acetylcholine) or by **hormones** (e.g. cholecystokinin in the pancreas).

Other vesicles are delivered to the apical and basolateral regions of the cell, for incorporation into the plasma membrane, and to endosomes and lysosomes.

Membrane recycling: Fusion of the transport vesicle membrane with the plasmalemma results in an increase in the surface area of the cell. This phenomenon is limited by the simultaneous **invagination** and incorporation of segments of the plasmalemma into the cytoplasm where they are utilised in forming membranes of new transport vesicles.

Organelles of cellular respiration and energy production

The viability of a cell is sustained by metabolically active cellular organelles and by intracellular transport of solid and dissolved substances. To support these processes, the cell requires endogenous sources of energy. This is the role of the **mitochondria**.

MITOCHONDRIA

Mitochondria **supply energy** to the cell through two main mechanisms:

- energy release through cellular respiration (oxidative phosphorylation) and
- synthesis of specialised metabolic enzymes.

In a multi-stage process, culminating in **oxidative phosphorylation**, mitochondria break down sugars and fatty acids to form CO_2 and H_2O. This process is accompanied by the liberation of **adenosine triphosphate** (**ATP**), a molecule containing stored energy. Mitochondria also participate in other processes associated with metabolism e.g. components of lipogenesis, the urea cycle and gluconeogenesis. Structurally, mitochondria are differentiated into a number of compartments (see below).

Structure: Mitochondria are generally elongated, sometimes elliptical to spheroid organelles (Figures 1.6,

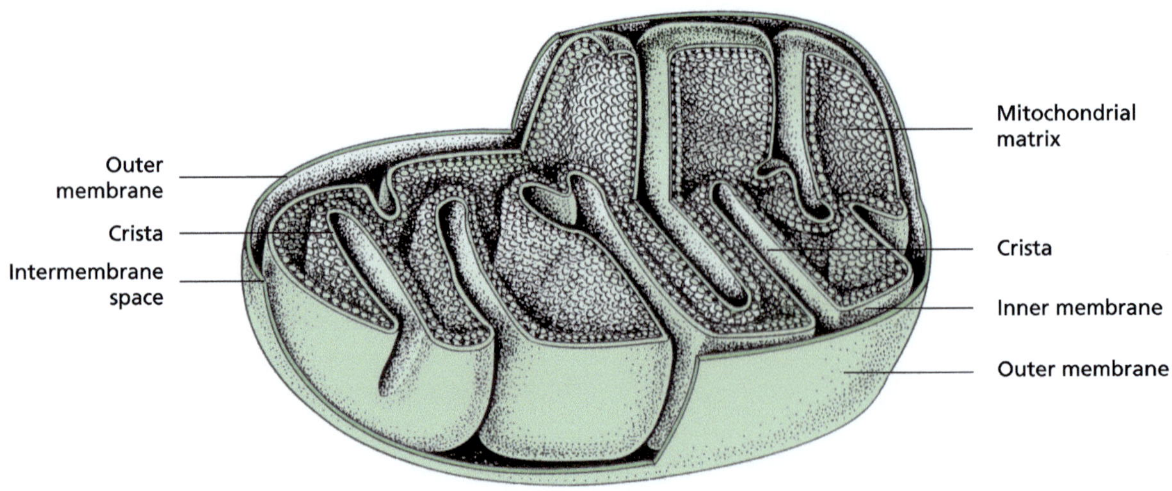

1.19 Mitochondrion (schematic).

1.19 to 1.22). They are typically 2–7 µm long and 0.2–2.0 µm wide. Mitochondria are capable of replicating by fission, a process that occurs particularly during increased metabolic activity and prior to mitosis. They have a lifespan of approximately 20 days and are broken down within the cell by autophagy. Mitochondria are composed of several compartments:

- mitochondrial matrix,
- inner membrane,
- outer membrane and the
- intermembrane space (spatium intermembranosum).

The functions of the mitochondria take place in the **matrix** and at the **inner membrane**. The **outer membrane** encases the inner, functional components. Between these two membranes is the narrow **intermembrane space** (Figures 1.19 and 1.20).

Mitochondrial matrix: The mitochondrial matrix appears finely granular and variable in density. Small **matrix granules** (30–50 nm) containing Ca^{2+} and Mg^{2+} ions increase in number when intramitochondrial concentrations of these cations are increased.

The mitochondrial matrix contains an abundance of the enzymes involved in the oxidation of **pyruvate** and **fatty acids**. Breakdown of these substrates results in formation of **acetyl-CoA** which enters the **citric acid cycle**, an enzyme-catalysed metabolic pathway that gives rise to CO_2, NADH, $FADH_2$ and CoA.

The matrix also contains **mitochondrial DNA (mtDNA)**, a specialised form of DNA that is synthesised **outside the nucleus**. The presence of extranuclear DNA supports the conclusion that mitochondria originated from **prokaryotes (bacteria)** and accounts for the observation that mitochondria synthesise some of their own structural proteins. The mitochondrial matrix also contains **ribonucleic acids (ribosomal, messenger** and **transfer RNA**).

Inner membrane: The inner mitochondrial membrane is typically arranged in folds referred to as cristae (Figures 1–19, 1.21 and 1.22). In some cells, these take the form of tubular projections (Figure 1.20). The number of cristae is determined by the type and function of the cell, and by the metabolic activity of the mitochondrion. Cells of the liver, muscles and kidney exhibit a particularly high density of cristae. During fasting, the number of cristae is reduced.

The tubular form (Figure 1.20) is the much less common type of mitochondrion. It is found principally in cells that produce steroid hormones (e.g. adrenal cortex, Leydig cells in the testes). A longitudinally prismatic arrangement of the cristal membrane is also recognised (e.g. glial cells).

The inner mitochondrial membrane contains a large number of **enzymes that are essential for sustaining life**, a feature that distinguishes it from other cell membranes. On the surface facing the matrix, the membrane carries enzymes associated with the **respiratory chain (electron transport chain)** and **oxidative phosphorylation**. The vast majority of energy for the cell is generated at the inner mitochondrial membrane, through the formation of ATP from adenosine diphosphate (ADP) and inorganic phosphate. The morphological entities associated with energy generation, referred to as **elementary particles**, consist of a globular enzyme-containing head and a stalk connected to the inner membrane by a foot-plate (Figure 1.23) (refer to biochemistry texts for further detail).

The inner mitochondrial membrane is impermeable to many molecules. Abundant embedded phospholipids limit the passage of ions through the membrane.

Outer membrane: The structure of the outer mitochondrial membrane is similar to that of other biological membranes. Specialised transmembrane proteins facilitate the uptake of lipids and small proteins. These substances, comprising mainly enzymes, enter the **intermembrane space**. As the inner membrane is impermeable to these molecules (without the aid of specific carriers), the

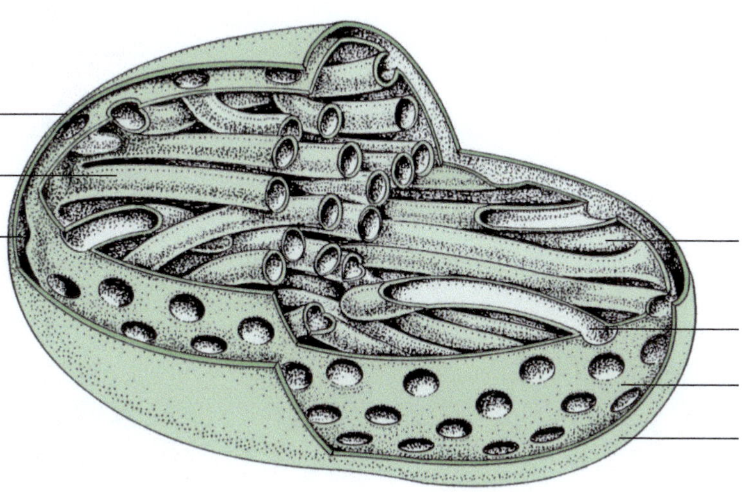

1.20 Mitochondrion with tubular projections (schematic).

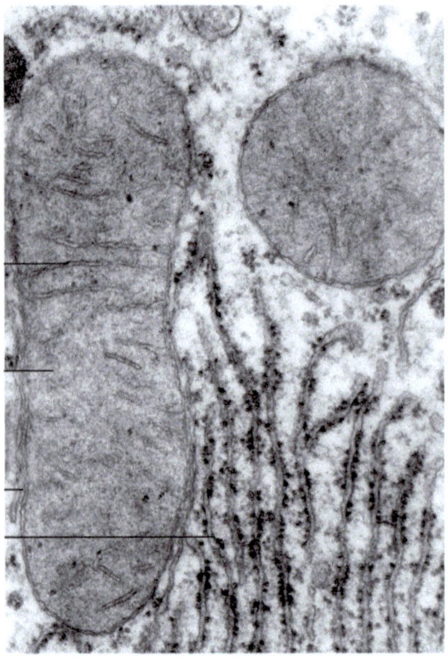

1.21 Mitochondrion (longitudinal and transverse sections, x12,000).

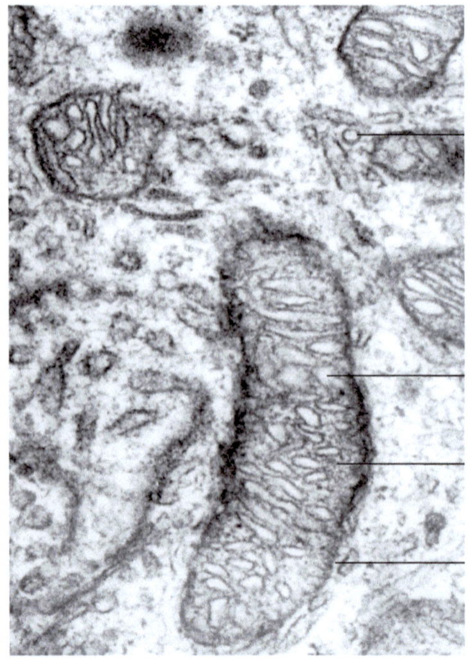

1.22 Mitochondrion (longitudinal and transverse sections, x8000).

molecular composition of the intermembrane space is similar to that of the cytosol.

NUMBER AND DISTRIBUTION OF MITOCHONDRIA

The number and density of mitochondria vary between cell types. Liver cells contain up to 3000 mitochondria, depending on of their level of metabolic activity. A sustained increase in energy metabolism results in an increase in the number and size of these organelles. Intoxication or oxygen deprivation leads to a rapid reduction in the number of mitochondria, which swell or undergo vacuolar degeneration.

Within the cytoplasm, mitochondria accumulate in regions where the energy demand is greatest. Their intracellular migration usually occurs along adjacent microtubules. In some instances, they become stacked at the base of the cell resulting in basal banding that can be seen with the light microscope (cells of the striated [secretory] duct of salivary glands and the proximal tubule of the nephron). In spermatozoa, they form spirals around the axonemal complex in the middle piece. Within skeletal muscle cells, mitochondria lie between, and oriented parallel to, bundles of myofilaments. In both spermatozoa and muscle, energy generated by the mitochondria is used for cellular contractility.

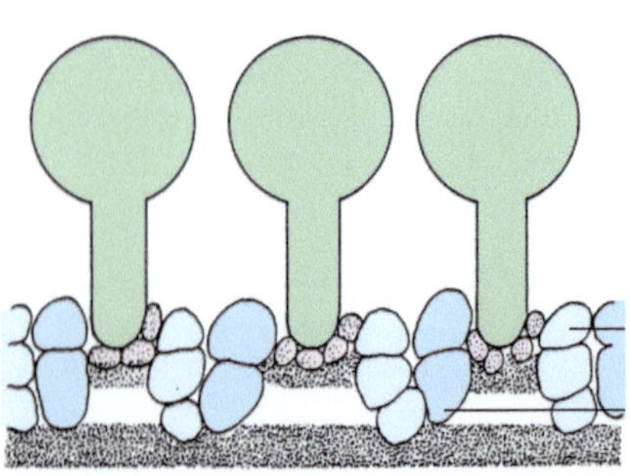

1.23 Inner mitochondrial membrane with elementary particles (schematic).

Cell contractility and motility

Living cells are characterised by the ability to alter their shape and to reposition their organelles through constant movement of the cytoplasm (intracellular transport). These functions are performed by a complex network of proteins embedded in the cytoplasm, collectively referred to as the cellular **cytoskeleton.** The cytoskeleton is composed of **three main structural proteins**:

- actin filaments (microfilaments),
- microtubules and
- intermediate filaments.

The cell also contains numerous proteins that are associated with the structural proteins of the cytoskeleton. These create interconnections among the structural proteins, establish connections with the plasmalemma and participate in interactions with other proteins (see below).

Actin filaments (microfilaments)

Actin is an abundant protein in all cells, particularly muscle cells. Actin filaments (diameter 6–8 nm) are thinner, more flexible and shorter than microtubules. They consist of two forms of actin: **free G-actin** (**globular actin**) and **polymerised F-actin** (**filamentous actin**).

Polymerisation occurs at the rapidly growing plus end of the filament. This process requires K^+, Mg^{2+} and ATP and is regulated by various actin-binding proteins (ABP) (see below).

Actin filaments form a dense network that interconnects individual organelles. The filaments extend into peripheral cell processes and provide **structural support** for the cytoplasm. In addition, they act together with **myosin** (**tropomyosin**) **filaments** to bring about cell contraction and associated motility. The specialised **actin–myosin complex of muscle cells** is described in more detail in Chapter 4, 'Muscle tissue'. Based on their diameter (5–7 nm), actin filaments are also referred to as microfilaments.

Actin filaments undergo constant reorganisation according to the functional demands of the cell. A number of actin-binding proteins participate in this process (see also text box below). Cross-linking of actin filaments into parallel bundles by the actin-bundling protein **fimbrin** gives rise to the structural core of specialised cell surface projections known as **microvilli** and **stereocilia** (Figures 1.24 and 1.25). Aggregates of actin filaments contribute to the contractile ring that divides the cell during the final phase of mitosis. Actin filaments mediate processes associated with endo- and exocytosis, facilitate intramembranous movement of transport proteins and expedite cellular movement. By combining with filamin and α-actinin to form a flexible mesh, actin also contributes to the **gel-like nature of the cytoplasm**.

Examples of non-muscle actin-binding proteins can be summarised as follows:

- **fimbrin**, **villin** and **fascin**: actin-bundling proteins as seen in microvilli,
- **filamin**: cross-links with actin giving rise to gel-state of cytoplasm,
- **gelsolin**: usually initiates polymerisation of actin, but in the presence of high Ca^{2+} concentrations causes severing of actin filaments, thus converting the gel-like cytoplasm into a fluid state,
- **vinculin**: binds actin filaments to the plasmalemma, and
- **spectrin**, **ankyrin**, **adductin**, **protein 4.1** and **protein 4.9**: actin cross-linking proteins, studied particularly in the cytoskeleton of erythrocytes, in which they contribute to the stability of the cell membrane.

Actin filaments are **not inherently contractile**. It is the interaction with numerous actin-binding proteins that alters the spatial conformation of the filaments. The proteins give the actin filaments specific characteristics, enabling them to participate in a **number of functions within the cell**, including:

- anchoring (and regulation of mobility) of membrane proteins – actin filaments form a three-dimensional network throughout the cell and contribute to specialised lateral intercellular adhesions and other types of anchoring junctions (e.g. focal adhesions),
- formation of the structural framework of microvilli,
- formation of the 'terminal web' beneath the cell surface,
- cellular locomotion (e.g. migrating cells and tumour cells) and
- formation of cell processes (e.g. filopodia) and contribution to cytoplasmic streaming.

Microtubules

Microtubules (Figures 1.26 and 1.30) are **impermanent structures** that can be rapidly assembled and dismantled. Arising from the **microtubule-organising centre** (**MTOC**) (containing the centrioles), microtubules are formed by end-to-end attachment of **free tubulin molecules**. These molecules originate from the disassembly of microtubules elsewhere in the cell. Microtubules also grow outward from **basal bodies**, the organising centre for cilia and flagella (see below).

Microtubules are **not contractile**, rather they serve as attachment sites for contractile proteins.

Structurally, microtubules manifest as elongated, narrow **protein cylinders** with a consistent diameter of 25 nm. Measuring up to several micrometres in length, they extend throughout the cell in an organised, cell-specific manner, thus contributing substantially to the morphology of the cell. When a cell undergoes a change in shape,

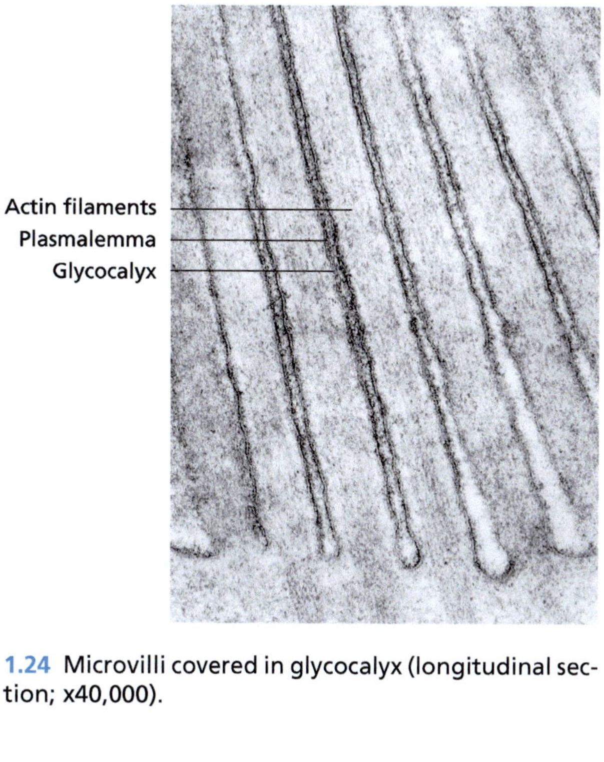

1.24 Microvilli covered in glycocalyx (longitudinal section; x40,000).

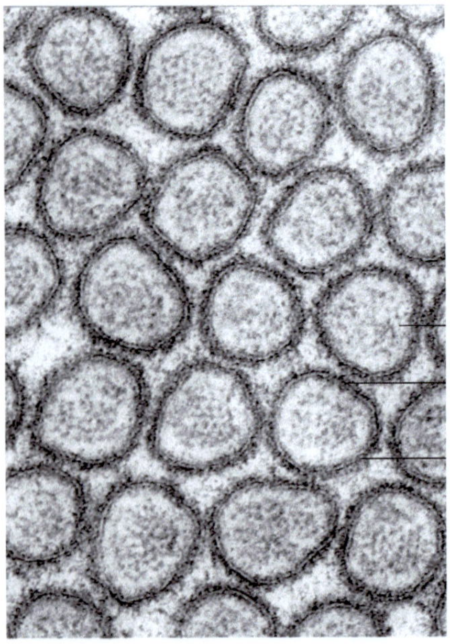

1.25 Microvilli covered in glycocalyx (transverse section, x40,000).

new microtubules are formed in one location; elsewhere, others are broken down.

Microtubules are inherently flexible. Binding with other microtubules or with other cellular components increases their rigidity, contributing to the structural integrity of the cell. Microtubules also participate in a range of other functions including:

- intracellular vesicular transport (e.g. secretory vesicles, endosomes, lysosomes),
- attachment of chromosomes to the mitotic spindle and movement of chromosomes during mitosis and meiosis,
- movement of cilia and flagella,
- elongation and motility of cells and
- maintenance of cell shape.

Microtubules play an important role in the movement of individual organelles within the cytoplasm, and in movement of the cell as a whole. They **guide** the movement of intracellular organelles and serve as '**tracks**' for transport vesicles and vacuoles passing between metabolically active organelles and the cell surface.

Microtubule-associated transport proteins direct **intracellular movement** of organelles and cytoplasmic inclusions towards their intended destination. Entities destined for the cell surface (e.g. secretory vesicles) are bound to microtubules by **kinesin**. **Dynein** carries intracellular structures towards the centre of the cell and to the nucleus. **Axonemal dyneins** are responsible for the movement of cilia and flagella.

Microtubules are composed of the **globular polypeptide tubulin**, which in turn consists of two polypeptide subunits: α- and β-tubulin (each molecular weight 50,000 Da).

The tubulin dimers (formed from free cytoplasmic α- and β-tubulin molecules) polymerise end-to-end, the α-subunit of one molecule binding to the β-component of another. The resulting chains are termed **protofilaments** (Figure 1.30). Thirteen protofilaments combine to form the wall of the microtubule.

Formation of microtubules is promoted by Mg^{2+} and by calmodulin binding of Ca^{2+}. Microtubules are highly labile (dynamically unstable) structures that can quickly be disassembled (Table 1.1). At low temperatures, or in high Ca^{2+} environments, they spontaneously depolymerise and can then be reassembled into new microtubules in another location, under different conditions. Agents such as **colchicine**, **colcemid** and **vinblastine** prevent the ordered polymerisation of tubulin into microtubules. They are used in research and therapeutics as antimitotic agents (**formation of the mitotic spindle** during cell division is inhibited, blocking mitosis in metaphase).

Microtubules can be identified with light microscopy using special stains (labelled anti-tubulin antibodies), polarisation microscopy and phase contrast microscopy. Due to their limited resolution under light microscopy, they may erroneously be described as fibres or fibrils (e.g. the mitotic spindle).

Microtubules can become arranged into ordered, complex structures, forming the structural basis of:

- the centriole and
- cilia.

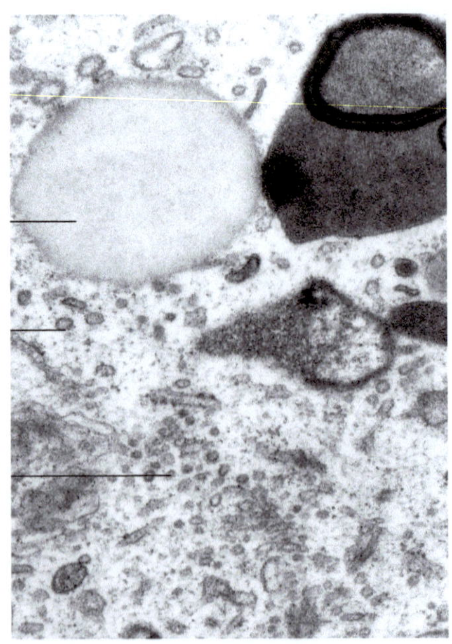

1.26 Fine structure of microtubules (x10,000).

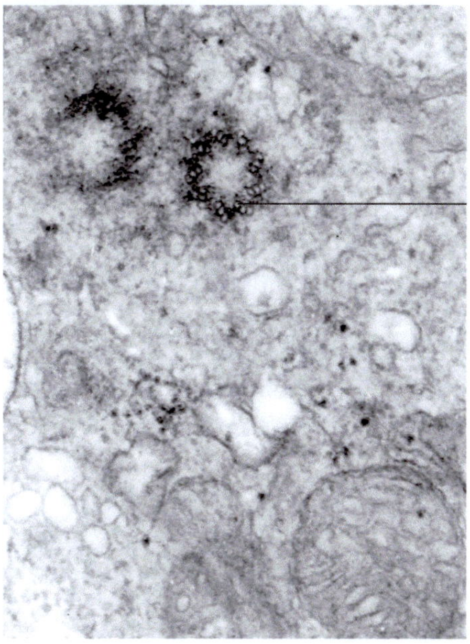

1.27 Fine structure of a centriole (x34,000).

Centriole (centriolum)

The functions of the centriole include:

- formation of basal bodies from which cilia develop and
- formation of the mitotic spindle.

Centrioles, along with the nearby Golgi apparatus, are present in almost all cells (Figures 1.6 and 1.27). They are **cylindrical** in shape (length 0.3 μm, diameter 0.1 μm). The cylinder wall is composed of **nine microtubule triplets (9×3 pattern)** (Figure 1.27). Each triplet contains a complete, cylindrical microtubule (**A-subfibre**) fused with two incomplete hemi-cylindrical microtubules (**B-** and **C-subfibre**). The nine triplets are connected by protein bridges, giving rise to the cylindrical form of the centriole. These cross-linkages confer a high degree of stability.

Centrioles usually occur in perpendicularly oriented pairs (Figure 1.6). Located in the vicinity of the nucleus and closely associated with the Golgi apparatus, they form part of the **MTOC**. Prior to mitotic cell division, these organelles undergo duplication. In this process, nine single microtubules are formed initially; these subsequently expand into triplets.

The known functions of centrioles include organisation of **intracellular microtubules**. This is particularly important in coordinating the formation of the mitotic spindle during cell division. Microtubules do not arise directly from the wall of the centriole. Instead, they extend from the so-called pericentriolar material surrounding the central portion of the centrioles. The location of the centriole in the cytocentre directs the polarity of the cell. Duplication of centrioles is one of the pathways for the formation of **basal bodies**, from which cilia and flagella develop (Figures 1.28 and 1.29).

Microtubule-organising centre (MTOC)

The microtubule-organising centre (cytocentre, centrosome) incorporates both the centrioles and the pericentriolar material. Most microtubules are associated with the MTOC. The MTOC controls the number, polarity, direction and organisation of microtubules formed during cell division. If centrioles are absent, the MTOC

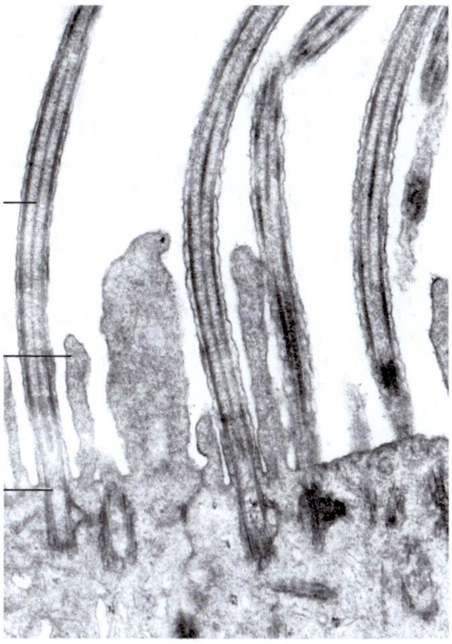

1.28 Apical surface of an epithelial cell with longitudinally sectioned cilia (x8000).

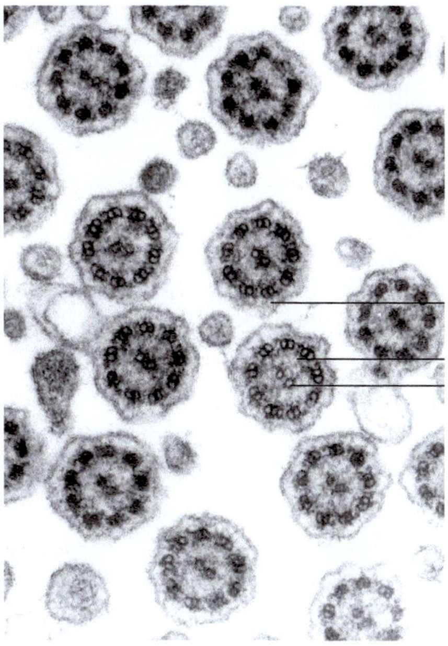

1.29 Cilia in cross-section (x20,000).

disappears. The MTOC also coordinates the formation of new microtubules. The many proteins found in the pericentriolar material of the MTOC include γ-tubulin, which serves as the starting point for formation of new microtubules. The α- and β-tubulin dimers attach in a specific orientation to the γ-tubulin molecules.

Cilia

Cilia and flagella are polar processes that extend as **cellular evaginations** from the free surface of the cell. The structural feature responsible for motility of cilia is a central axoneme composed of a **pair of microtubules surrounded by nine peripheral microtubule doublets** (**9×2+2**).

Cilia and flagella are bounded by the plasmalemma. Both have the same structure and are distinguished by their length (cilia 2–10 μm, flagella up to 200 μm) (Figures 1.28 to 1.30).

Intermediate filaments

Intermediate filaments are polypeptide chains that provide structural support for the cell. They are considered to be the least soluble components of the cytosol. Intermediate fibres are typically arranged in parallel, passing along lines of pressure and tension within the cytoplasm. Their diameter (8–10 nm) lies between that of actin filaments and microtubules (hence 'intermediate' filament). Intermediate filaments are particularly well developed in

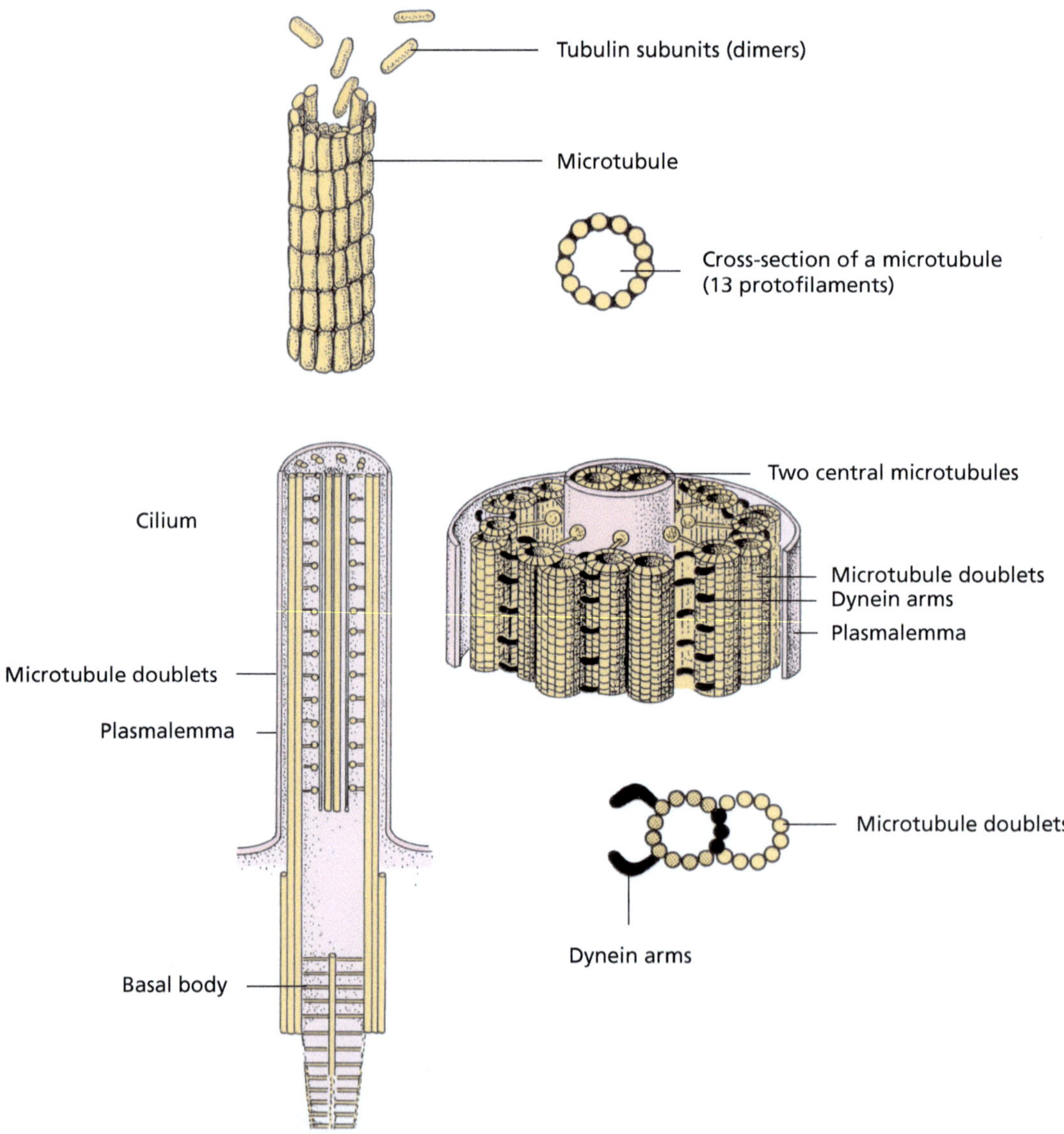

1.30 Representations of a microtubule and cilium (schematic). Microtubules are composed of tubulin subunits (tubulin dimers) that join together to form a hollow cylinder. Within cilia, microtubules form the axoneme, consisting of two central microtubules surrounded by nine microtubule doublets. Radial spokes connect the doublets to a central sheath, while dynein arms interconnect the microtubule pairs.

superficial cells subjected to large mechanical forces (surface epithelia), in axons and at junctions between adjacent myofibril bundles (at the Z line) (Table 1.1).

Intermediate filament-associated proteins play an important role in the cytoskeleton. Some (e.g. plectins) bind to actin filaments and microtubules while others (e.g. desmoplakins or plakoglobulins) form attachment plaques for the cytoskeleton, which are constituents of desmosomes and hemidesmosomes.

In contrast to actin filaments and microtubules, intermediate filaments do not disassemble and reform. Instead, they constitute substantial, **permanent structural elements** of the cell. They contribute to the integrity of cell-to-cell junctions and to connections between the cell and the extracellular matrix. The composition of the polypeptide chain of intermediate filaments exhibits **considerable cell specificity**. Several classes are recognised (Table 1.2), including:

- Class I and II: keratins,
- Class III: vimentin and vimentin-like filaments,
- Class IV: neurofilaments and
- Class V: lamins.

Keratins (cytokeratins, tonofilaments)

This group includes more than 50 different **cell-** and **tissue-specific** isoforms and subtypes. Keratins are found particularly in cells of epithelial origin. Their **component keratin proteins** form an **intracellular network**, organised along mechanical lines, that inserts on desmosomes at the plasmalemma. Through these cellular junctions, the filaments extend functionally into neighbouring cells and serve to increase the strength of the epithelium as a whole. Based on their mechanical properties, keratin filaments are also referred to as **tonofilaments**. Those found in hair, horn, claws and hooves are termed hard, or structural, keratins.

Vimentin and vimentin-like proteins

This class includes various subtypes, the most common being vimentin filaments found in **connective tissue cells** (**fibroblasts**). Vimentin-like proteins are found in glial cells (glial fibrillary acidic protein), muscle cells (desmin) and in association with the nuclear envelope.

Neurofilaments

Neurofilaments are permanent constituents of the cell processes of **neurons** (dendrites and axons). They are composed of neurofilament-triplet-proteins and provide structural support.

Lamin A and lamin B

Lamin A and lamin B are found in the cell nucleus.

Exogenous and endogenous cellular inclusions

Exogenous inclusions are taken up from the exterior of the cell (e.g. by phagocytosis). Endogenous inclusions are those formed within the cell as by-products of cellular metabolism. Together, these inclusions are sometimes termed **paraplasm**. They are **highly heterogeneous** (Figures 1.31 and 1.32) and are subdivided into:

- **storage and reserve materials** (e.g. glycogen, fats, proteins) and
- **pigments**:
  - endogenous (e.g. ferritin, haemosiderin, melanin) and
  - exogenous (e.g. dust, heavy metals).

Characteristic inclusions include intracellular fat droplets, glycogen (Figure 1.31), protein crystals and pigments. Pigments (see below) represent a special form of inclusion.

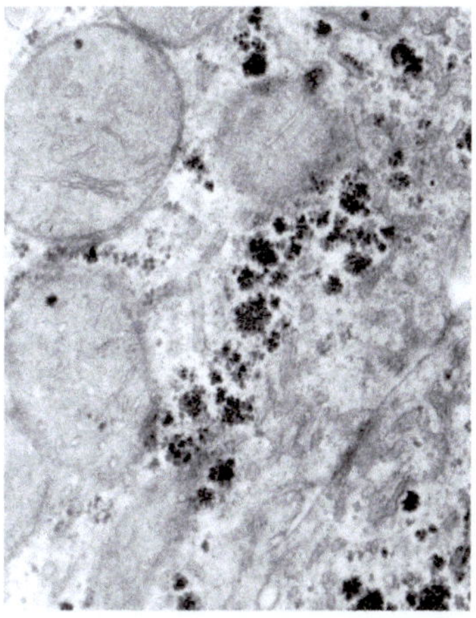

1.31 Electron microscope image showing glycogen in a liver cell (x27,000).

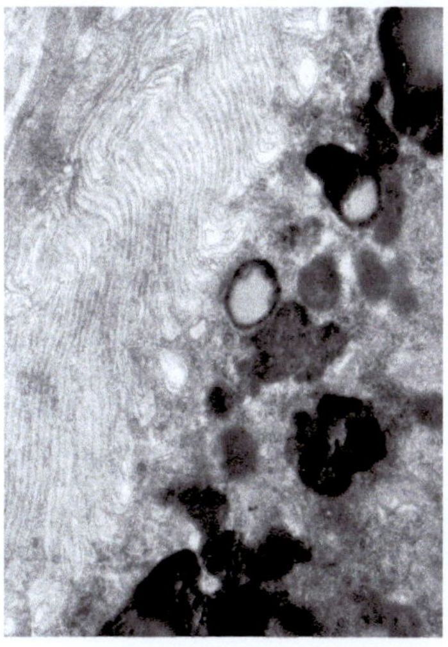

1.32 Melanin in the retinal pigment epithelium in the fundus of the eye (x18,000).

Endogenous pigments

Endogenous pigments are **coloured products of cellular metabolism**. In animal cells, these include haemoglobin, myoglobin and iron reservoirs such as ferritin and haemosiderin. Haemosiderin, a product of haemoglobin degradation, is stored in splenic macrophages or Kupffer cells in the liver.

Melanin is an endogenous pigment present in skin, the retinal pigment epithelium and in the meninges. In epidermal melanocytes, melanin is contained within membrane-bound organelles termed melanosomes. Differentiated melanosomes contain tyrosinase for synthesis of melanin. As a dark pigment, melanin is photoprotective. The role of melanin in the function of the retinal pigment epithelium (Figure 1.32) is described in Chapter 16, 'Receptors and sense organs'.

Residual bodies arising from fat metabolism are also considered a form of endogenous pigment (lipofuscin). Lipofuscin is often observed as a sign of ageing in cardiac myocytes and in kidney and liver cells.

Exogenous pigments

Exogenous pigments are primarily taken up **from the air** via the lungs. They subsequently become concentrated within tissue cells (e.g. soot particles or heavy metals in the lungs or lymph nodes).

Nucleus

The nucleus (Figure 1.6) is an essential component of animal cells, occurring in all cells other than mature mammalian erythrocytes. It is the repository of **genetic information**, which is stored in coded form in chromosomes containing **deoxyribonucleic acid** (**DNA**).

Table 1.2 Composition and occurrence of protein classes (I–V) associated with intermediate filaments.

Type of protein	Molecular weight	Occurrence
Class I & II		
Keratins:		
– acid cytokeratins	40–64	All epithelial cells
– basic cytokeratins	52–68	All epithelial cells
Class III		Cells of mesodermal origin (including endothelial cells, myofibroblasts)
Vimentin and vimentin-like proteins:		
– vimentin	55	
– desmin	53	Muscle cells
– glial fibrillary acidic protein	50–52	Neuroglia (oligodendroglia, astrocytes, microglia, ependymal cells), Schwann cells, pituicytes
– peripherin	54	Neurons
Class IV		
Neurofilament (L)	68	Neurons
Neurofilament (M)	110	Neurons
Neurofilament (H)	130	Neurons
Synemin	182	Muscle cells
Paranemin	178	Muscle cells
Nestin	240	Muscle cells
Class V		Nucleus of most differentiated cells
Lamin A	62–72	
Lamin B	65–68	Nucleus of all nucleated cells

Table 1.1 Characteristics of the cytoskeleton.

	Actin filaments	Microtubules	Intermediate filaments
Appearance	Helical double strand	Hollow cylinder	Cord-like bundles
Diameter	6–8 nm	20–25 nm	8–10 nm
Main protein(s)	Actin	Tubulin	Various
Structural features of filaments	Thin, flexible	Dynamic, transient (labile)	Permanent (stable)
Location	Microvilli, terminal web, contractile units of muscle cells	Cilia, centriole, spindle apparatus, contractile ring during cell division	Desmosomes, hemidesmosomes, in association with nuclear envelope
Main function	Key element of the cytoskeleton	Intracellular transport, movement of cilia, cell shape and movement, attachment of chromosomes to spindle	Structural

Information held within the nucleus is carried by **messenger ribonucleic acid** (**mRNA**).

The nucleus is the functional centre of the cell, directing information exchange and metabolism and regulating the processes of cell differentiation and maturation.

The nucleus is delimited by a double membrane termed the **nuclear envelope** (Figures 1.33 and 1.34). This segregation of genetic material from the cytoplasm distinguishes **animal eukaryotic cells** from **prokaryotic cells** (**bacteria**), in which the nuclear envelope is absent. The nuclear envelope separates the processes of DNA replication and RNA synthesis (**transcription**) within the nucleus from ribosomal protein synthesis (**translation**) in the cytoplasm.

Chemical signals that bind with specific receptors at the surface of the cell are transported by intracellular carrier substances to the nuclear envelope, through which they pass into the nucleoplasm. In this way, extracellular stimuli such as nerve impulses and hormonal signals are able to influence nuclear coordination and regulation of cellular processes. The nucleus exists only as a discrete organelle in cells that are not undergoing division (see 'Mitotic (M) phase'). During this period, it is also referred to as the **intermitotic** or **interphase nucleus**. From a functional perspective, this is termed the **metabolic nucleus** or **nucleus of synthesis**. During mitosis, the nuclear matrix incorporating the chromosomes (**nucleoplasm**) mixes with the cytosol.

The structure of the nucleus varies between cell populations. Differences include chromatin distribution, protein, nucleic acid and water content, enzyme types and metabolic activity. This structural diversity is determined by genetic, chemical, physical and functional factors.

Number, size, shape and position

While each cell (except mature mammalian erythrocytes) typically contains **one nucleus**, cells containing **two nuclei** are regularly found in liver cells, cells lining the glandular gastric mucosa, sweat glands and in the epithelium of the urinary passages. Some cell types, including striated muscle cells and osteoclasts, are **multinucleated**. Cells containing multiple nuclei are also distinguished by a large amount of cytoplasm (giant cells).

The **volume of the nucleus** is directly proportional to the **volume of the cell** (**nuclear/cell volume**). Each cell population has a characteristic nuclear/cell volume that lies within a certain range. The size of the nucleus is determined by the number and size of the chromosomes. An increase in the number of chromosomes (e.g. in endomitosis) is associated with a corresponding rise in the volume of the nucleus. Enlargement of the nucleus can also result from increased uptake of fluids or metabolites (**functional nuclear growth**). The size of the nucleus can further be influenced by daily rhythms (e.g. nutrient intake), age and sex. The nucleus of spermatozoa is notably small and dense, its metabolic activity being very low.

The **shape** of the nucleus also varies between cells, generally conforming to the shape of the cytoplasm. In spherical, cuboidal and polygonal cells, the nucleus is usually spheroid. The nucleus of columnar cells assumes an

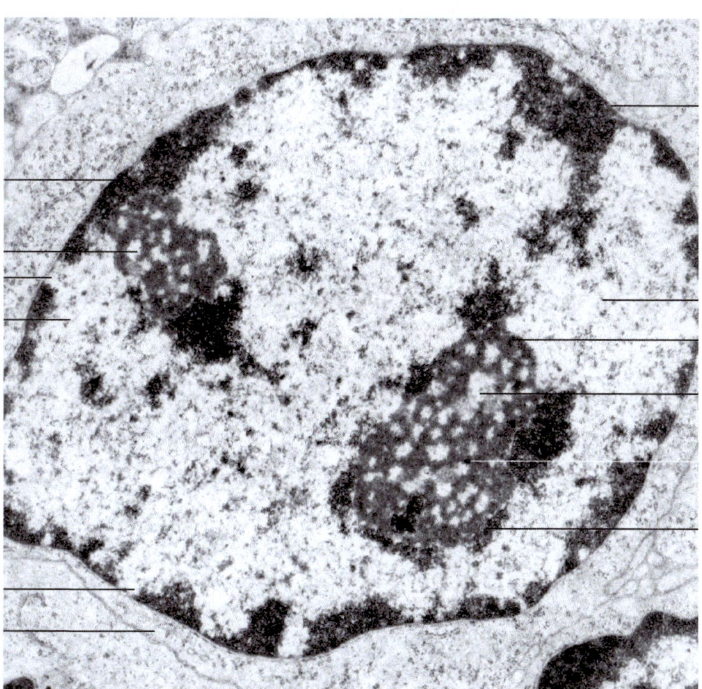

1.33 Electron microscope image of a reticular cell with two nucleoli, euchromatin and peripherally located, dense heterochromatin (x4000).

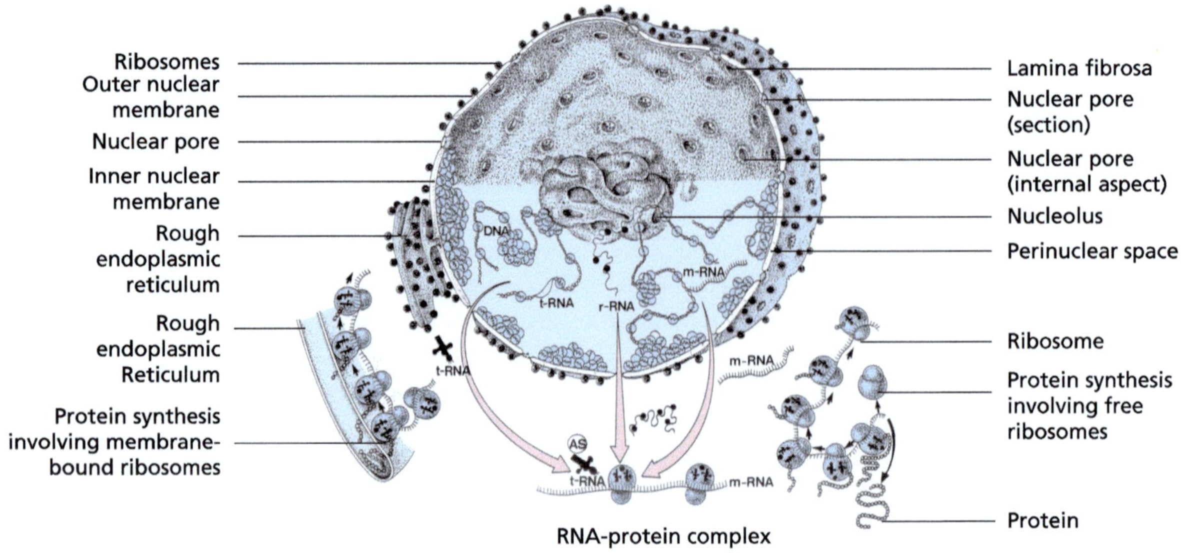

1.34 Nucleus with adjacent rough endoplasmic reticulum, and ribosomal protein synthesis (schematic).

ovoid, elliptical form, aligned with the longitudinal axis of the cell. Flattened endothelial cells have a similarly compressed nucleus. Depending on the age of the cell the nucleus may appear rod-shaped or segmented (e.g. in granulocytes); in mature spermatozoa it is flat and bilaterally compressed. Within particular cell populations, the shape of the nucleus is generally consistent and can be used for identifying cell types.

The **location** of the nucleus within the cytoplasm exhibits considerable variation. In free or cuboidal cells, it is usually located centrally. Within fat cells, the paraplasmic inclusions (lipid droplets) displace the nucleus to the periphery. In glandular epithelial cells, the position of the nucleus is influenced by the type of secretory product (peripheral in cells producing mucous secretions, more central in serous cells). The nucleus of skeletal striated muscle cells is exclusively located adjacent to the plasmalemma (subplasmalemmal), while that of smooth muscle cells and cardiac myocytes lies in the centre of the cytoplasm. The functional state of the cell may also influence the location of the nucleus.

Nuclear envelope (nucleolemma)

The nucleus is surrounded by a nuclear envelope consisting of **two concentric unit membranes** (Figures 1.33 and 1.34). The **inner membrane** (**membrana nuclearis interna**) encloses the nucleoplasm. A **nuclear lamina** (**lamina fibrosa**) composed of fine filaments is usually present on the internal aspect of the inner membrane. The **outer membrane** (**membrana nuclearis externa**) is lined with ribosomes and is continuous with the rough endoplasmic reticulum. Between the two membranes is a perinuclear space (**perinuclear cistern, cisterna nucleolemmae**) of variable width (20–60 nm) that opens into the interior of the rER.

The direct connection between the compartments of the nucleus and rER facilitates the regulatory functions of the nucleus. Components of the ER can be used for synthesis of the nuclear envelope – a regular occurrence during mitosis.

The electron-dense **fibrous lamina** on the internal surface of the inner membrane has a dual function. In addition to its structural role in shaping the nucleus and stabilising the nuclear pores (see below), specific regions of the lamina regulate the interaction between chromosomes (chromatin) and the inner nuclear membrane. The fibrous lamina may also control the breakdown of the nuclear membranes during mitosis.

The nuclear envelope is interrupted at regular intervals by **nuclear pores** (**pori nucleares**) (diameter 50–80 nm; Figures 1.33 and 1.34). The pores are formed by fusion of the inner and outer membranes and are surrounded on both sides of the nuclear envelope by a ring of granular material. Together, the pore and its associated ring are termed the **nuclear pore complex**. The nuclear pore complex contains a central opening through which large proteins are actively transported. Additional water-filled channels allow for the transport of small water-soluble molecules.

The number and size of the nuclear pores reflected the activity of the nucleus. The permeability of the pores allows the exchange of substances, particularly RNA molecules, between the nucleus and the cytosol.

Nucleoplasm (nucleoplasma)

The nucleoplasm (Figures 1.33 and 1.34) is variably defined as the entirety of the contents of the nuclear envelope, including matrix, genetic material (chromatin, chromosomes) and nucleoli, or as just the matrix itself. The nuclear matrix is the fluid component of the interior of the nucleus (consisting of soluble RNA, ions, glycoproteins and metabolites) in which the chromatin and nucleoli are embedded.

Chromatin (chromatinum)

The term **chromatin** encompasses all of the components of the chromosomal DNA within the nucleus. Also referred to as DNA–protein (nucleoprotein) complexes, these components consist of approximately one-third DNA and two-thirds basic and acidic proteins (histones and non-histones), phospholipids, ions (Ca^{2+}), glycoproteins and small quantities of RNA.

Histones are **structural proteins** that bind with the DNA double helix due to their positive charge. They stabilise the DNA strand and regulate various reactions involving the DNA chain. Histones are responsible for packaging 5 cm-long DNA molecules that make up a chromosome into smaller units (nucleosomes).

In this process, the DNA double helix is repeatedly wound around a histone complex. The structure of the resulting nucleosome chain resembles a string of pearls ('beads-on-a-string chromatin', Figure 1.35).

Short non-nucleosomal segments of DNA are interposed between nucleosomes at regular intervals. The **nucleosome** chains form strand-like complexes by aggregating with other proteins in continually varying arrangements. These complexes are termed chromatin fibrils (diameter 30 nm). Relatively large segments of the chromatin fibrils become arranged in folds composed of irregular coils. During mitosis these undergo additional condensation to form a discrete chromosome (Figure 1.35).

The term **chromosome** refers to the DNA molecule and its associated protein scaffold. Depending on the stage of the cell cycle, the structural organisation of the chromosome varies, ranging from chromatin fibres to the condensed form that manifests during mitosis. The genetic information contained within the chromosome is carried by the DNA molecule.

During **interphase**, chromatin can be subdivided based on morphological criteria (independently of association with a particular chromosome) into euchromatin and heterochromatin.

EUCHROMATIN (EUCHROMATINUM)

Segments of chromatin fibres can undergo extensive **unfolding**, forming a loose, filamentous ball known as **euchromatin** (Figures 1.6 and 1.33). Functionally, euchromatin represents the genetically active DNA of the chromosome which is largely devoid of nucleosome complexes. Euchromatic nuclei stain weakly; their individual chromatin fibres are discernible only by using electron microscopy.

The presence of a large amount of euchromatin in the nucleus indicates a high degree of cellular metabolic activity, underpinned by an increase in transcription of nucleic acids. Euchromatic chromatin is subject to hormonal activation, resistant to breakage and sensitive to radiation (e.g. X- and UV radiation).

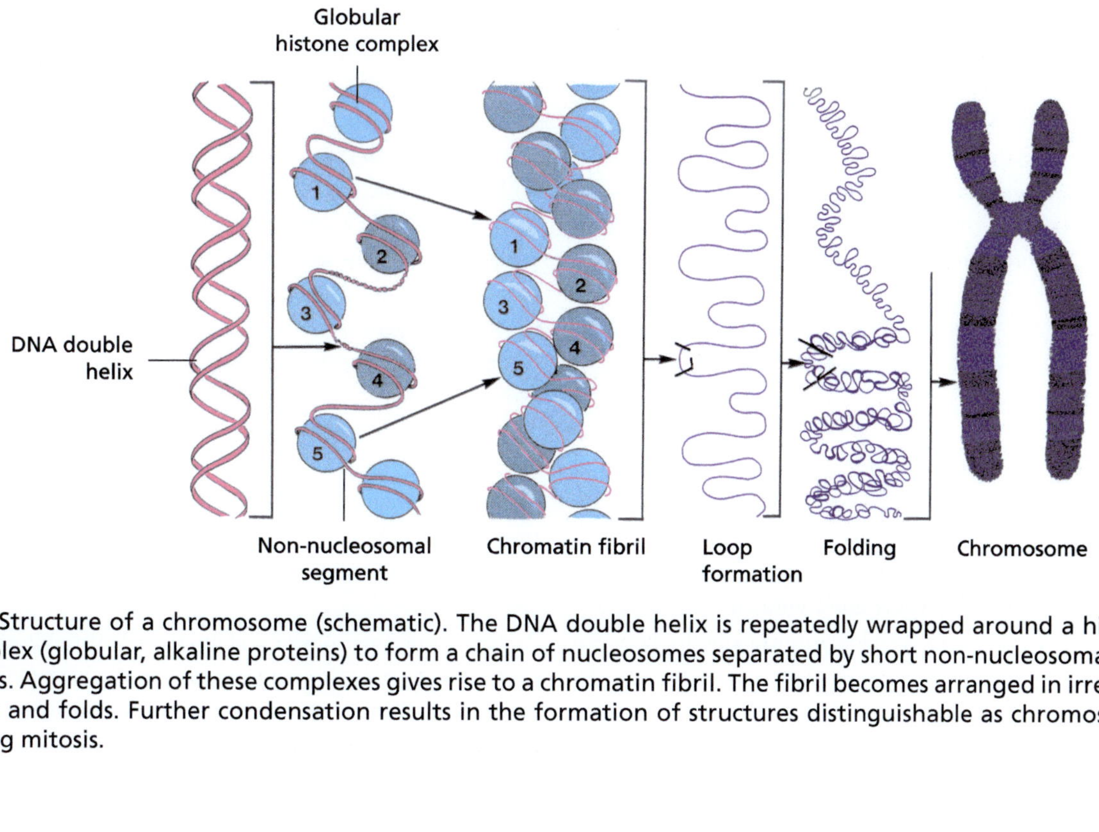

1.35 Structure of a chromosome (schematic). The DNA double helix is repeatedly wrapped around a histone complex (globular, alkaline proteins) to form a chain of nucleosomes separated by short non-nucleosomal segments. Aggregation of these complexes gives rise to a chromatin fibril. The fibril becomes arranged in irregular loops and folds. Further condensation results in the formation of structures distinguishable as chromosomes during mitosis.

HETEROCHROMATIN (HETEROCHROMATINUM)

In **heterochromatin**, large portions of chromatin are strongly coiled and folded (Figures 1.6 and 1.33). Histologically, heterochromatic regions of the nucleus appear irregularly granular, are frequently darkly staining (basophilic) and can be selectively identified using various histological techniques. A high proportion of heterochromatin signifies a relatively **low level of cellular metabolic activity**. Heterochromatin is predominantly located peripherally but can also be widely distributed throughout the nucleus.

Heterochromatin is not under hormonal control, is sensitive to breakage and exhibits a high rate of mutation. In contrast to euchromatin, it is highly resistant to the effects of radiation (e.g. X- and UV radiation).

Sex chromatin represents a specialised form of chromatin found in female cells. This component of the X-chromosome remains condensed during interphase and can be identified histologically as a typically peripherally located region of dense chromatin or, in neutrophils, as a drumstick-shaped nuclear appendage.

While the amount of euchromatin and heterochromatin varies from cell to cell, the relative proportion of each type of chromatin is consistent within particular cell populations and can thus be used as a diagnostic aid. Cells with a **'light'** (**euchromatic**) **nucleus** are usually metabolically active, while those with a **'dark'** (**heterochromatic**) **nucleus** are relatively quiescent.

Nucleolus

The nucleolus is a spherical to ovoid, strongly basophilic nuclear inclusion that is present exclusively during **interphase**. It arises after mitosis from the nucleolar organising centre of various different chromosomes and disintegrates shortly before cell division begins.

Nucleoli (diameter 3 μm) are found as free structures within the nucleoplasm or in contact with the inner nuclear membrane (Figures 1.6 and 1.36). They are not enclosed by a membrane. With the light microscope, nucleoli appear particularly dense and homogeneous, and are strongly refractive. They can be subdivided into three regions:

- granular component (pars granulosa): consists primarily of pre-ribosomal RNA particles (10–15 nm); peripherally located,
- dense fibrillar component (pars fibrosa): contains RNA transcripts, usually forms central clumps and
- fibrillar centres: regions containing DNA components (intra- and perinucleolar chromatin) involved in RNA synthesis.

The fibrillar and granular components form a sponge-like network (**nucleolonema**). Intra- and perinucleolar chromatin is present in the spaces between the anastomosing strands of the nucleolonema. Some cells (e.g. oocytes) have a ring-shaped nucleolus in which there is a distinct separation of the two RNA components.

The nucleolus is a centre of RNA synthesis. Ribosomes are produced here and, once assembled, are released into the cytoplasm. The size of the nucleolus reflects the amount of stored RNA and is a morphological indicator of cellular protein biosynthesis. As synthetic activity increases, the granular components of the nucleolus expand. The presence of several nucleoli in one nucleus reflects a high level of protein metabolism (e.g. in nerve cells, pancreatic cells, embryonic cells and tumour cells).

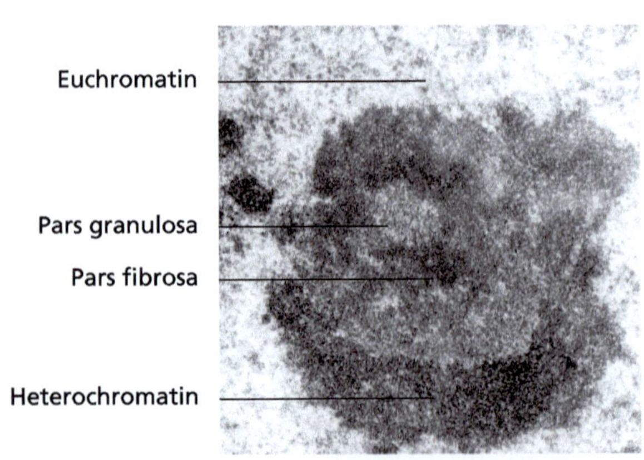

1.36 Electron microscope image of a nucleolus (x28,000).

Cell growth and division

Cellular growth and division are defining features of living organisms. As the lifespan of each cell is finite, it must be equipped with the genetic machinery to replicate itself. In order to maintain vital physiological processes, an equilibrium exists within the body between cell death and the production of new cells. Only during physical growth, phases of cell or organ renewal, or during physiological derangements does this balance shift towards a net increase in cell production.

The bulk of the lifespan of a cell is taken up by the **growth phase** (**interphase**). The period during which division occurs accounts for only a few hours of the existence of the cell. During the growth phase, the cell increases (often doubles) in size, and its organelles are replicated, in preparation for the production of a viable daughter cell. During this phase, the cell also performs the various functions that are characteristic for that cell type. The growth phase thus incorporates the synthesis of endogenous and extracellular substances, as well as cell differentiation. At the end of the growth phase, most cells enter the **mitotic phase**.

There are several different types of cell division. By far the most common is the division of a mother cell into two genetically identical daughter cells that exhibit the same morphological and functional characteristics. In this

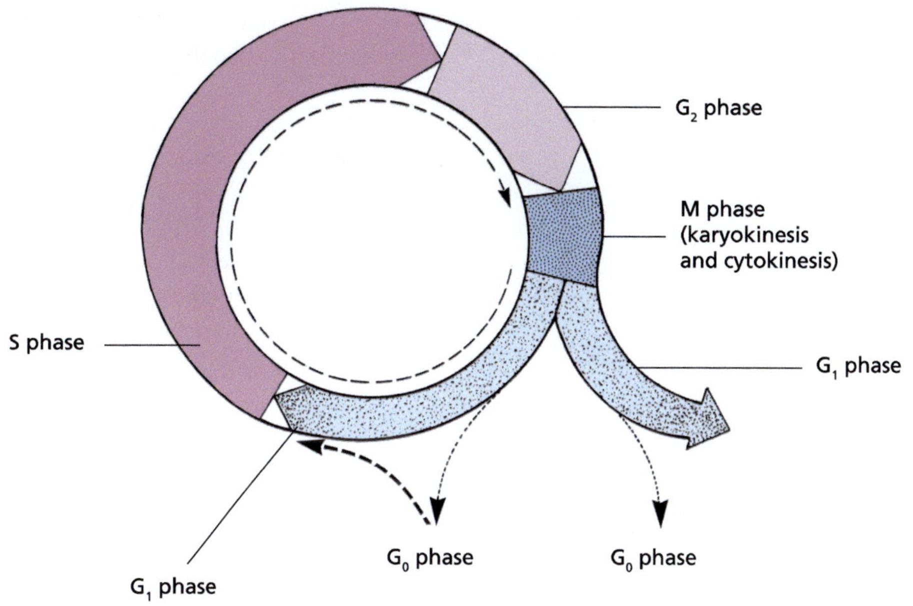

1.37 Cell cycle (schematic).

process, known as mitosis, both daughter cells receive an identical copy of the genes contained in the nucleus of the parent cell. The term mitosis is derived from the threadlike appearance of the chromosomes during nuclear division (Gk *mitos* = thread). Division of the nucleus (karyokinesis) is followed by division of the cytoplasm (cytokinesis), leading to complete division of the cell.

Replication of the chromosome set without subsequent nuclear or cellular division is referred to as **endomitosis.** The term **amitosis** describes the doubling of genetic material and subsequent division of the nucleus and cytoplasm without the formation of recognisable chromosomes. Male and female germ cells undergo a specialised form of cell division, referred to as **meiosis**, in which the chromosome set is halved (haploidy). The full set of chromosomes (diploidy) is re-established only when an ovum is fertilised.

Cell cycle

For most cells of the body, growth and division are regularly recurring processes. The cell cycle begins with division (mitosis), then enters a metabolically active growth phase (**interphase**) before ending with another cell division. Each of these phases can be further subdivided into phases that differ in their chronological progression (Figure 1.37). The features of these phases may also vary considerably in different cell populations.

Interphase

Interphase encompasses three phases:

- **G_1 phase** (precedes DNA duplication, G = gap),
- **S phase** (DNA duplication, S = synthesis) and
- **G_2 phase** (between DNA duplication and mitosis).

These three consecutive phases typically account for over 90% of the duration of the cell cycle. In rapidly growing cells, the cell cycle can be completed within 16–24 hours, of which 1–2 hours are taken up by mitosis.

The duration of the cell cycle is cell-specific. Epithelial cells (e.g. those lining deep intestinal crypts) constantly undergo rapid cycles of division, each being completed within 8–11 hours. Other cell populations are characterised by cell cycles lasting days, weeks or years (e.g. cartilage cells, bone cells and muscle cells).

The **G_1 phase** is the period in which the cell performs the functions that are specific to that cell type. It is dominated by RNA production and protein biosynthesis. The duration of this phase is particularly variable, ranging from hours to years, depending on cell type. In preparation for the subsequent S phase, the G_1 phase involves the production of enzymes and proteins required for chromosome assembly. The supply of these molecules results in transition to the synthesis phase and the end of the G_1 phase.

An exception to this sequence of events is observed in postmitotic cells that have lost the capacity for division. These include mature nerve cells, which, despite being highly metabolically active, do not progress to the S phase. Such cells are described as being in the **G_0 phase**.

The **S phase** (duration 6–8 hours) is characterised by the duplication of genetic material (replication of the DNA double helix). The double helix divides asymmetrically into single strands (Y-shaped replication fork) and, through complementary base pairing, is copied to form two new DNA strands. Each chromosome now consists of two identical chromatin strands (sister chromatids). The S phase concludes when all of the cellular DNA is replicated. From the end of the S phase until the beginning of mitosis, the DNA content of the cell is doubled (4d).

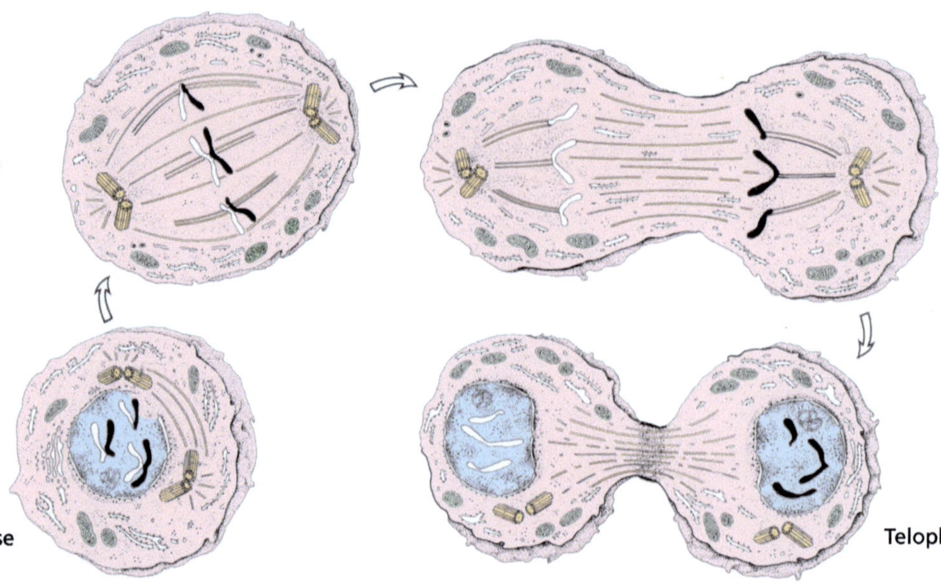

1.38 Processes occurring during mitosis (schematic).

The G_2 **phase** (duration 1–2 hours) is the interval between the end of DNA duplication (during S phase) and the initiation of nuclear division. During this phase, there is increased synthesis of materials required for mitosis. This includes division of the paired centrioles and production of microtubules that will form the mitotic spindle.

Towards the end of the G_2 phase, elaboration of kinase results in dissolution of the lamina fibrosa of the nuclear envelope. Increased phosphorylation of nucleosomes brings about gradual condensation of the chromosomes; if present, cell surface features such as microvilli begin to regress.

Mitotic (M) phase: nuclear division (karyokinesis) and cytoplasmic division (cytokinesis)

The processes occurring during mitosis ensure the equal distribution of genetic information contained within the DNA strands (that were duplicated during S phase) among the two daughter cells. Morphologically, this replication of genetic material at the molecular level manifests as the assembly of chromatin into chromosomes. During cell division, the chromosomes (containing duplicated DNA) become organised and their identical thread-like chromatin strands (chromatids) are separated and displaced to opposite poles of the cell. This is followed by division of the cytoplasm, in which the cytosol and organelles are evenly divided among the two resulting daughter cells (Figure 1.38). While these processes are confluent, cell division is conventionally subdivided into four phases:

- prophase,
- metaphase,
- anaphase and
- telophase.

PROPHASE

In prophase, chromatin threads **condense** and move towards the centre of the nucleus (Figures 1.38 and 1.39). This intense condensation of genetically identical chromatids eventually gives rise to visible chromosomes. The chromatids are held together by the **centromere**.

As the chromosomes continue to condense, the **nucleolus** begins to break down. The membrane stacks of the Golgi apparatus and the endoplasmic reticulum similarly undergo regression. By the end of this phase, **lysis of the nuclear envelope** is complete and **longitudinal separation of the chromosomes into two separate chromatids** commences.

Initiation of mitotic spindle formation is a further key feature of prophase. The mitotic spindle becomes organised around the two centriole pairs (centrosomes) formed by duplication of centrioles during the S phase (see 'Centriole', 'Microtubule-organising centre'). Each centriole pair forms the centre of a **star-shaped arrangement of microtubules.** As prophase progresses, the centriole pairs and associated microtubules migrate over the outer surface of the nuclear membrane to form the bipolar mitotic spindle. As the centriole pairs separate, polar microtubules (microtubules that pass between the two sets of centrioles) become visible with the light microscope.

METAPHASE

Complete lysis of the nuclear envelope and disappearance of the nucleoli mark the beginning of **metaphase** (Figures 1.38 and 1.39). Remnants arising from the breakdown of various membranes remain in the vicinity of the mitotic spindle. Concurrently, the **matrix of the nucleus and the cell begin to mix**. Chromosomes become attached to **kinetochore microtubules**, so named because they

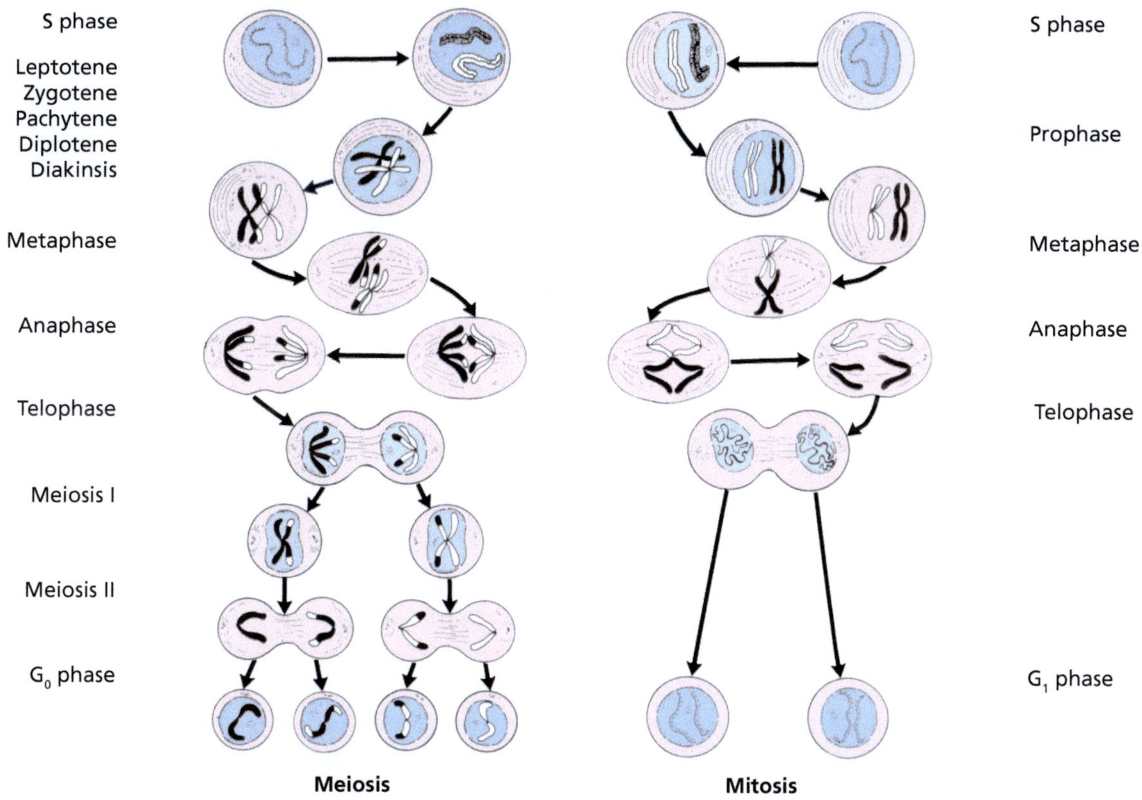

1.39 Meiosis, mitosis and cytokinesis (schematic).

bind to protein complexes (kinetochores) located on each chromatid near the centromere. The kinetochore microtubules are responsible for producing **ordered movement of the chromosomes**. During metaphase, **longitudinal separation of the chromosomes** continues. Guided by the kinetochore microtubules, the chromosomes become aligned along a plane in the equatorial region of the cell, forming the **metaphase plate**.

ANAPHASE

During anaphase, the **chromatids of each chromosome are separated from one another** (Figures 1.38 and 1.39). The two kinetochores of each chromosome break apart and the chromatids are drawn towards the poles. This involves shortening of the kinetochore microtubules, with concurrent lengthening of the fibres making up the spindle. The poles move further apart, and the cell takes on an ovoid shape. As the chromatids move towards the poles, their free ends are oriented towards the equator, while the centromere faces the poles.

TELOPHASE

Telophase begins when the chromatids have reached the poles of the spindle (Figures 1.38 and 1.39). The kinetochore microtubules break down and the spindle fibres further increase in length. Concurrently, a new nuclear envelope is formed from the **membranes of the endoplasmic reticulum**. An ion-rich, strongly hypertonic nuclear environment is thus re-established. The previously condensed and now separated **chromatids begin to uncoil** and eventually can no longer be detected with histological stains. During the formation of the nuclear envelopes, the **nucleoli** develop from specific segments of the chromatids. With the resumption of RNA synthesis, nuclear division is concluded.

CYTOKINESIS

Commencing in late anaphase, furrowing of the plasma membrane continues in telophase (Figures 1.38 and 1.39) resulting in random distribution of organelles between the two daughter cells. The **cleavage furrow** is produced by a ring of **actin filaments**, which forms at the level of the equator. The furrow deepens until the remains of the spindle fibres in the middle of the cell become compressed. This compacted central area is only maintained for a short period. Its separation gives rise to two daughter cells.

The two new cells are genetically identical to the mother cell and contain a similar complement of organelles. However, these are smaller than the mother cell and may not be of equal size. During the subsequent growth phase (interphase), the cell increases in volume and commences its specific processes of differentiation and metabolism. A full cell cycle of growth and division is thus complete.

Endomitosis

Endomitosis is an incomplete internal form of division that bears only partial similarity with mitosis. After replicating during the S phase, the chromatids appear and separate, but **subsequent nuclear and cell division does not occur**. In contrast to mitosis the **nuclear envelope does not disintegrate**, and a **mitotic spindle is not formed**.

As the chromatids are not divided among two nuclei, the nucleus retains double the usual number of chromosomes. Repeated endomitoses may occur, resulting in a high degree of **polyploidy**. This is usually accompanied by the formation of multiple nucleoli, an increase in nuclear volume, elevated metabolic activity and growth in cell volume. The nuclei of highly differentiated cells, such as megakaryocytes of the bone marrow or particular liver cells, often undergo maturation through endomitosis.

Amitosis

In contrast to all of the previously described processes of cell division, **amitosis** is characterised by direct division of the nucleus and cytoplasm **without the formation of visible chromosomes** or breakdown of the nuclear envelope. Division of the nucleus is brought about by microtubules that form a 'drawstring' around the nucleus, separating it into two portions of equivalent volume. The original organelle population is retained.

Amitosis frequently results only in nuclear division, giving rise to multinucleate cells.

Meiosis

Mammalian **fertilisation** (**syngamy**, **karyogamy**) occurs through union of the nuclei of male and female gametes (oocytes and spermatozoa). In order to prevent doubling of the number of chromosomes with each generation, the diploid set of chromosomes in the germ cells must be reduced by half to become **haploid**. This is achieved by **meiosis**.

Meiosis involves two nuclear divisions. In the diploid germ cell (2n), homologous chromosomes (equivalent chromosomes of maternal and paternal origin) each form genetically identical **chromatid pairs** (**4d**). These exchange genetic material ('crossing over') before becoming separated in an initial division (**meiosis I**, **reductional division**). This gives rise to a haploid gamete in which the number of chromosomes and the amount of DNA is halved (**1n**, **2d**). In a subsequent division, **meiosis II** (**equatorial division**), the amount of DNA (but not the number of chromosomes) is halved again. This is achieved, as in mitosis, by the separation of sister chromatids. In contrast to mitosis, however, this division is not preceded by (further) duplication of DNA (Figure 1.39).

Meiosis I (reductional division)

Meiosis I begins with a prolonged **prophase** (**prophase I**) that is subdivided into five stages (Figure 1.39). While variation exists in the events that are ascribed to each stage, the stages are consistently referred to as:

- leptotene (= thin strand),
- zygotene (= yoke-like strand),
- pachytene (= thick strand),
- diplotene (= double strand) and
- diakinesis.

In the **leptotene stage**, chromatin fibrils undergo condensation to form elongated, **thin chromatin strands** (containing DNA that was duplicated in the previous S phase). Homologous pairs of **sister chromatids** draw near to one another (homologous pairing) and become connected by point-like **synaptonemal complexes** (**zygotene**). The chromatin strands become shorter and thicker. In the **pachytene stage** the homologous chromatid pairs are very closely associated. There is exchange of genetic material between maternal and paternal chromosomes (**crossing over**). In the final stage of prophase I (**diplotene**), **homologous chromosomes** begin to separate. Junctions between the chromosomes (**chiasmata**) represent sites at which crossing over has occurred.

Towards the end of prophase, the nuclear envelope disintegrates and chromosomes become recognisable as separate entities. During this stage (**diakinesis**), kinetochore and spindle microtubules are formed.

The subsequent phases (metaphase, anaphase and telophase) proceed in a similar manner to their counterparts in mitosis. In contrast to mitosis, however, the centromeres that connect sister chromatids do not split. Consequently, it is homologous chromatid pairs (rather than sister chromatids) that become separated. This results in halving of the number of chromosomes (Figure 1.39).

Meiosis II (equatorial division)

The sequence of events during meiosis II is similar to that occurring during **mitosis**, with the exception that only a haploid set of chromosomes undergoes separation (Figure 1.39). In contrast to meiosis I, the **centromeres of each chromatid pair become separated**, allowing sister chromatids to be detached from one another. Division of the two nuclei thus results in **four haploid gametes** (**1n**, **1d**). When the male and female gametes fuse at **fertilisation**, the two haploid nuclei combine to form a diploid somatic cell with a full complement of DNA (2n, 2d).

Cell death

A physiological equilibrium exists in multicellular organs and tissues between the number of proliferating and degenerating cells. Abnormalities can result in an increase in cell number (e.g. hyperplasia, neoplasia, autoimmune disease) or a reduction in the cell population (e.g. atrophy, degenerative disease). There are two mechanisms of cell death:

- necrosis (accidental cell death [pathological]) and
- apoptosis (programmed cell death).

Necrosis (Figure 1.40) results from **irreversible exogenous** or **endogenous injury** caused by noxious physical or chemical factors (e.g. radiation, trauma, toxins, hypothermia, ischaemia) that cause **disruption of the plasmalemma** and **swelling of the cytoplasm**. Following rupture of the cell membrane, organelles are **broken down** by lysosomal enzymes (**autolysis**).

The cell fragments enter the extracellular space, and the nuclear material condenses (**pyknosis**) and eventually undergoes complete dissolution (**karyolysis**). Cellular necrosis is often accompanied by damage to adjoining tissue and initiation of inflammation.

In contrast, **apoptosis** is a form of **programmed cell death**. The processes involved in apoptosis are regulated by the cell itself. The stages in apoptosis are shown in Figure 1.41:

- a reduction in cell volume due to shrinking of the cytoplasm and arrangement of the cytoskeleton into concentric bundles; loss of mitochondrial function with release of cytochrome c (resulting in activation of a cascade of proteolytic enzymes [caspases]),
- fragmentation of nuclear DNA into oligonucleosomal pieces (due to endonuclease activity within the intact nuclear envelope),
- modification of the plasmalemma through translocation of intramembrane molecules to the external surface ('membrane blebbing') and
- cell breakdown with formation of membrane-bound apoptotic bodies containing organelles and nuclear material – apoptosis is not associated with the induction of inflammation.

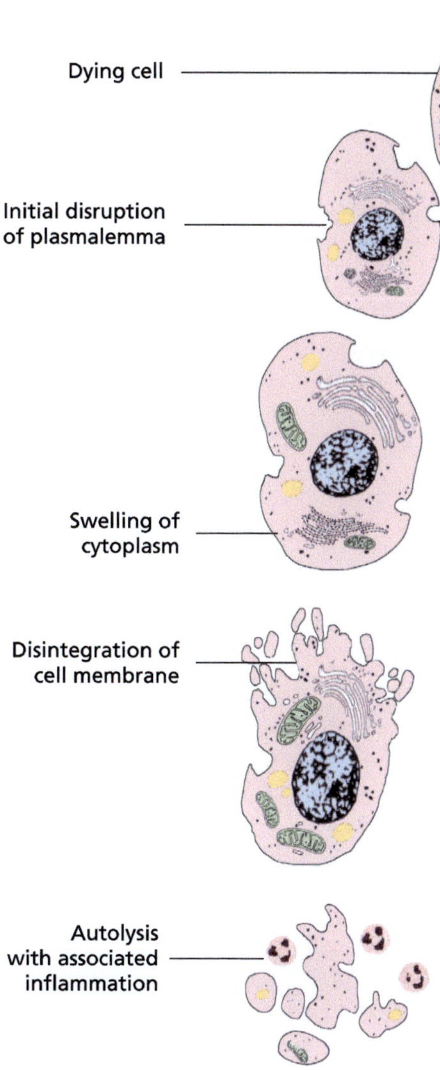

1.40 Necrosis (schematic).

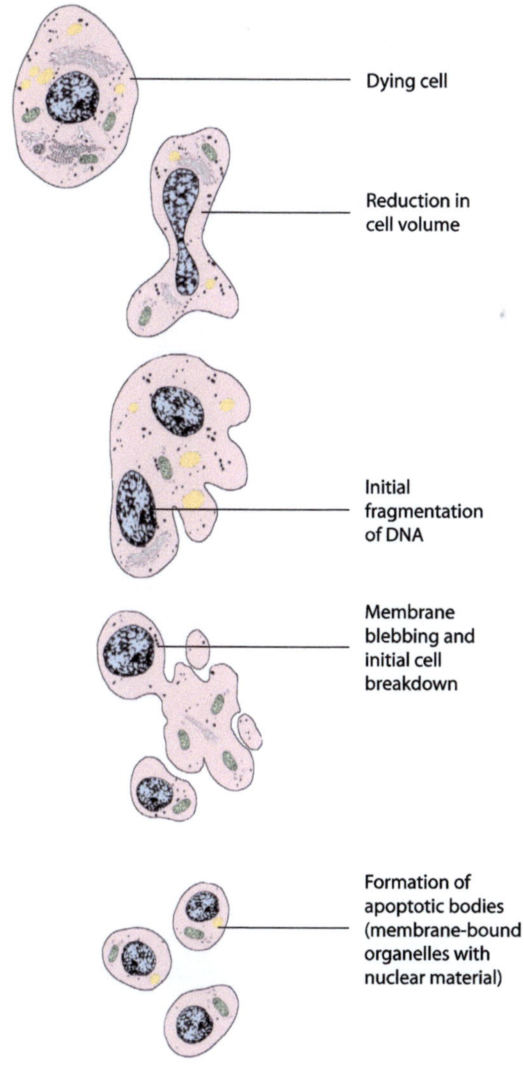

1.41 Apoptosis (schematic).

Apoptosis can be triggered by specific **factors** (tumour necrosis-factor, TNF) and by certain neurotransmitters, free radicals, oxidants and UV radiation. In addition to these external factors, cells contain genes and proteins (e.g. Bcl-2 family) that have a regulatory role in apoptosis (e.g. Bax [Bcl-associated X] protein is pro-apoptotic).

Apoptosis is a **physiological process**. During embryonic development of tissues and organs, it serves to eliminate cells that are no longer required. Mammary gland involution also occurs through apoptosis.

Cell surface specialisations

With the exception of free cells (e.g. blood cells), the cells of the body are interconnected to form organs and tissues. As a result of cell-to-cell connections, most cells of the body have a structural and functional relationship with neighbouring cells. The existence of several different types of cellular connections reflects the diversity of cellular functions.

In the case of epithelial cells, specialised structures are also present on the apical cell surface. Cell surface specialisations are subdivided into:

- free (apical) surface structures,
- lateral surface structures and
- basal surface structures.

Apical surface specialisations

The free surface of epithelial cells is lined by an electron microscopically amorphous layer of proteins, glycoproteins and sugar residues referred to as the **glycocalyx**. These proteins contribute to epithelial cell function by acting as sites of cell recognition and adhesion.

Several epithelia exhibit specialised cell surface modifications. These include enzymes such as hydrolases, ion channels and carrier proteins (e.g. for glucose transport). Surface modifications may be temporary or permanent, depending on the function of the cell.

Sac-like **invaginations** of the plasmalemma occur as impermanent, variable structures. These are associated with the uptake of material by the cell (**phagocytosis** or **pinocytosis**). Cellular **evaginations**, including **microvilli** (see below) and **microplicae**, extend in the opposite direction. These serve to enhance absorption by the cell. Permanent cell surface modifications (Figures 1.42 to 1.46) include:

- microvilli: generally uniform, mostly non-motile cytoplasmic processes,
- cilia (kinocilia): long, motile cytoplasmic processes and
- stereocilia: particularly long, often secretory cytoplasmic process (also described as very long microvilli).

Microvilli

Microvilli are long, finger-like surface projections. They are generally consistent in length (see below) and are covered by a well-developed **glycocalyx** (Figures 1.42 and 1.43). Intestinal microvilli are richly endowed with sugar-cleaving enzymes. Microvilli are involved in absorption;

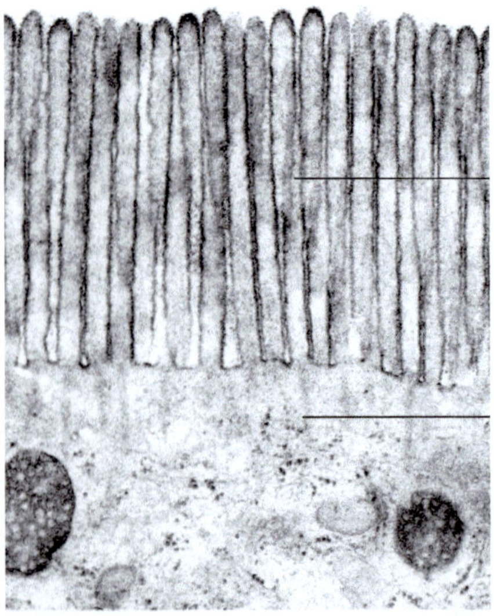

1.42 Microvilli forming a brush border on the apical surface of a cell (x40,000).

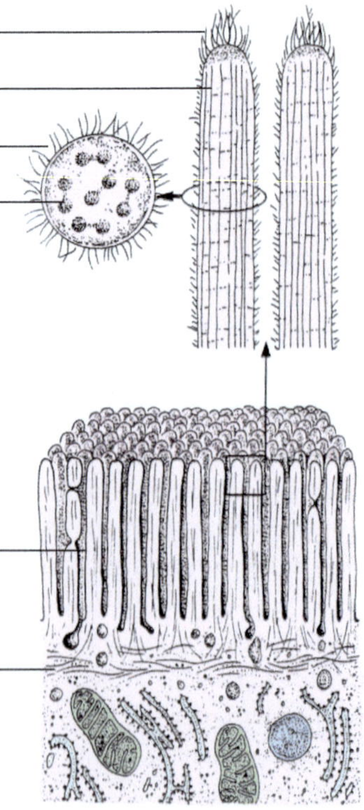

1.43 Apical cell surface with brush border of microvilli (schematic).

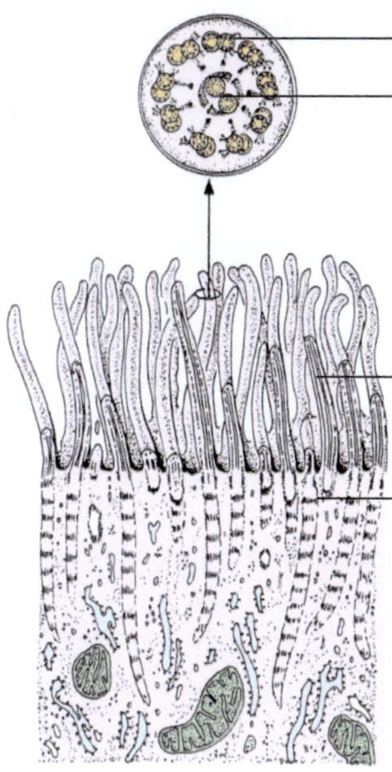

1.44 Apical cell surface with cilia (schematic).

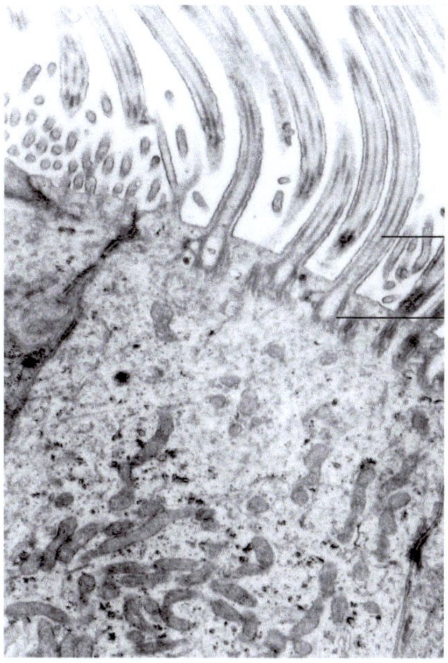

1.45 Apical cell surface with cilia and basal bodies. Epithelial cell of oviduct, sheep (x24,000).

their number and appearance are usually correlated with the absorptive capacity of the cell. In cell types exhibiting little transcellular transport they may be short and irregular. In others, they are more uniform. On the surface of cells that function primarily in trans-epithelial fluid transport (e.g. in the intestine and renal tubules), microvilli form a tightly packed **brush border** that is visible with the light microscope.

Microvilli contain actin filaments that are stabilised and interconnected by fimbrin, fascin, espin and myosin I. At the tip of the microvillus, the filaments are secured to the actin-bundling protein villin. The base of the actin filament bundle is linked to a horizontal network of filaments (terminal web) that is connected by spectrin to the plasmalemma. Contraction of the terminal web (enabled by the presence of myosin II and tropomyosin) causes the microvilli to diverge.

Cilia (kinocilia)

The term cilium is generally used to refer to a motile cell process, though non-motile forms also exist. Cilia measure up to 10 μm in length. In the tracheobronchial tree, they mobilise mucus and transport individual foreign particles towards the pharynx. The cilia of the oviduct transport fluids and ova in the direction of the uterus (Figures 1.28 to 1.30, 1.44 and 1.45) (see also 'Cell contractility and motility').

Cilia contain an axoneme composed of two central microtubules and nine peripheral microtubule doublets (9×2+2) connected by radial protein spokes (Figures 1.30 and 1.44). At the base of the cilium, the nine microtubule doublets are connected to a modified centriole, or **basal body** (**kinetosome**). Similar in structure to a centriole, the basal body coordinates the uniform, rhythmic movement of the cilia.

The basal body consists of a ring of nine microtubule triplets. Two microtubules of each triplet are continuous with the nine peripheral microtubule pairs of the axoneme. The two central microtubules of the axoneme arise from the top of the basal body. Protein complexes interconnect the microtubules of the axoneme, contributing to the stability and motility of the cilium.

The microtubule doublets of the axoneme consist of two components, A and B microtubules. The **A microtubule** is composed of 13 tubulin subunits, arranged side-by-side and a **B microtubule** containing ten tubulin subunits. The A and B microtubules are connected, at intervals of approximately 90 nm, by a passive elastic component referred to as **nexin**.

At intervals of 24 nm, each doublet is associated with a pair of '**arms**' composed of **ciliary dynein.** The **radial spokes** connecting the nine doublets with the two central microtubules are located at 29 nm intervals.

Cilia exhibit a synchronously undulating motion, during which the dynein arms of the microtubule doublet form temporary cross-links with the B microtubule of an adjacent doublet. Using energy derived from the hydrolysis of ATP, these dynein bridges move smoothly along the B microtubule. During this process, the passive elastic connections involving nexin and the radial spokes accumulate energy that is used for the subsequent reverse movement.

Cilia are found on many cells of the body. Their principal function is to transport fluids and solid materials, including mucus, dust and dead cells, along the cell surface. Accordingly, cilia are abundant in the epithelium of the respiratory tract and the oviduct. A modified cilium (flagellum) found on spermatozoa is responsible for the forward movement of the cell.

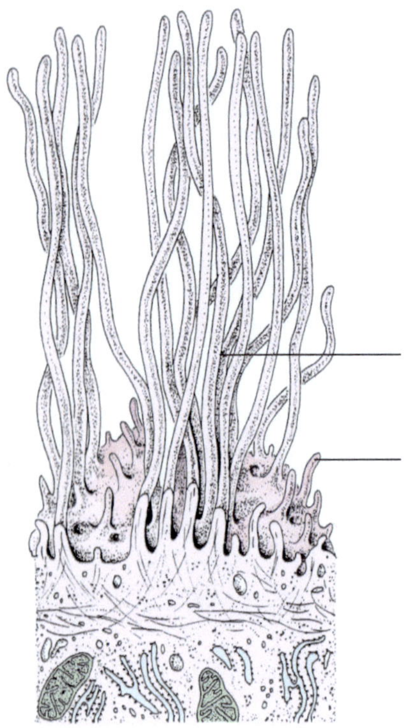

1.46 Apical cell surface with stereocilia (schematic).

Stereocilia

Stereocilia are elongated cell processes (5–7 μm). They resemble microvilli and are often described as particularly long versions of these structures (Figure 1.46). Stereocilia lack a microtubular substructure. They occur in bundles and serve to increase surface area and participate in absorption and secretion by epithelial cells.

Stereocilia are found in the epididymis, in proximal portions of the ductus deferens and on the sensory hair cells of the inner ear. The stereocilia of the epididymis are particularly long cellular extensions that arise from apical cell protrusions. Similar to microvilli, they incorporate actin filament bundles interconnected by proteins (e.g. fimbrin). The stereocilia of the hair cells of the ear act as sensory mechanoreceptors.

Lateral surface specialisations

Firm connections between the lateral surface of adjacent cells are essential for maintaining the functional integrity of surface epithelia. As well as reinforcing the mechanical strength of the cell layer, these connections have an important role in intercellular transport.

In the plasmalemma of laterally adjacent cell walls, cell adhesion molecules (CAMs; see below) form an important component of specialised cell junctions. The content and composition of the proteins and lipids of the lateral cell membrane differ substantially from those of the apical membrane. The connections between cells fall into two categories, direct and indirect:

- direct contacts:
  - interdigitations and
- indirect contacts:
  - occluding junctions (zonula occludens, tight junction),
  - anchoring junctions (zonula adherens, macula adherens [desmosome]) and
  - communication junctions (gap junction, nexus).

Direct contacts

The lateral and basal cell surfaces of many epithelial cells exhibit irregularly developed **folds and invaginations** that form interdigitations or interleaving zipper-like connections between neighbouring cells.

These are particularly pronounced in surface epithelia associated with intensive ion exchange (e.g. cells of proximal renal tubules or the cells of the striated [secretory] duct of salivary glands). The plasmalemma projects into the cell in the form of irregular, often elongated infoldings. The lateral and particularly basal surface area available for molecular transport is thus considerably increased.

The **width of the intercellular space** has important functional implications. Usually manifesting as a narrow cleft (20–25 nm), the intercellular space contains substances required for cellular metabolism (including carbohydrates, glycoproteins, amino acids, ions). In the actively absorbing epithelia of the small intestine and gall bladder, these intercellular spaces may be greatly expanded due to active transport of sodium and water.

Indirect contacts

ZONULA OCCLUDENS (TIGHT JUNCTION)

In zonulae occludentes (tight junctions), the outer layers of adjacent cell membranes become fused, eliminating the intercellular space. Tight junctions are usually located apically, where they serve as a vital physiological barrier (Figure 1.47). By forming a tight **seal** between neighbouring epithelial cells, they restrict the movement of water or molecules into the intercellular space.

The zonula occludens forms a '**belt**' around the apical region of epithelial cells, thus preserving the integrity of the apical and lateral domains of the cell. The junctions themselves are formed by a variably dense **anastomosing intramembranous network** of ridges comprised of linear arrays of transmembrane proteins (e.g. occludin). Transmembrane protein-associated zona occludens proteins ZO-1, ZO-2 and ZO-3 have a **regulatory** role in zonula occludens formation. Moreover, ZO-1 and ZO-3 facilitate interaction between occludin and the actin cytoskeleton, thus stabilising the intercellular junction.

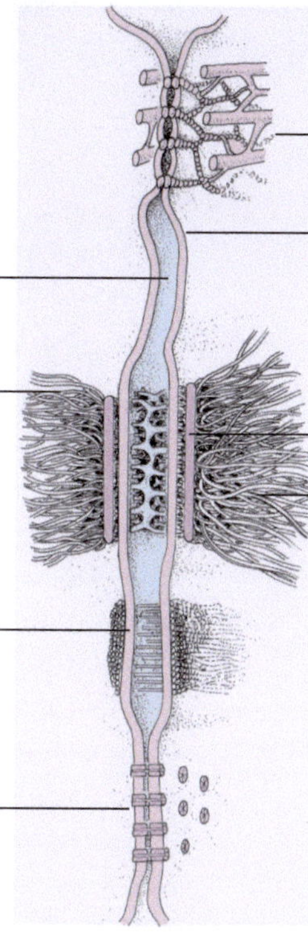

1.47 Intercellular junctions associated with the lateral cell surface (schematic).

It appears that the density of the zonula occludens can be regulated and is related to the metabolic requirements of the cell. A relatively large number of ridges (up to ten) results in a high degree of impermeability (e.g. epithelium of the bladder and intestine). If the ridges are sparsely elaborated, as in the renal tubules, greater transport of water, electrolyte and soluble materials is possible. Many noxious agents (e.g. toxins) target the zonula occludens membrane proteins, causing an abnormal increase in permeability.

The zonula occludens separates the **intercellular compartment into apical and basal regions**, thus contributing to cell polarity. Passage of substances into the intercellular space across the zonula occludens is referred to as the **paracellular pathway**. Substances may also reach the intercellular space by being transported across first the apical and then lateral cell membranes, below the zonula occludens. This is known as the **transcellular pathway**.

ZONULA ADHERENS AND DESMOSOME (MACULA ADHERENS)

Cell-to-cell contacts in which proteins connect the cytoskeletons of adjacent epithelial cells are referred to as **anchoring junctions**. Their function is to **impart mechanical strength** to the epithelium. Specific transmembrane proteins (cell adhesion molecules, CAMs) located at predetermined sites are connected by intracellular proteins to cytoskeletal filaments. Two types of anchoring junctions are recognised:

- zonula adherens – interacts with actin filaments and
- desmosome (macula adherens) – interacts with intermediate filaments (keratin filaments).

Additional forms of anchoring junctions (focal adhesions, hemidesmosome), incorporating the cell adhesion molecule integrin, are described under 'Basal surface specialisations'.

The zonula adherens surrounds the epithelial cell below the zonula occludens. Its belt-like configuration (width 0.1–0.5 µm), resembles that of the zonula occludens. Within the zonula adherens, the intercellular space is reduced to 15–20 nm.

The **zonula adherens** incorporates the cell adhesion molecule **E-cadherin**. The cytoplasmic segment of E-cadherin is attached to **catenin**, forming a complex that binds to **vinculin** and **α-actinin** and is responsible for interaction with the actin filaments of the cytoskeleton. The E-cadherin–catenin–actin–vinculin complex is continuous with the actin filaments of the **terminal web**.

Contraction of the actin filament bundles increases the mechanical strength of adjoining cells and may lead to widening of the intercellular space. These interactions are largely Ca^{2+}-dependent: withdrawal of Ca^{2+} results in breakdown of the junction.

While the zonula occludens allows the epithelium to act as a physiological barrier, facilitating compartmentali-

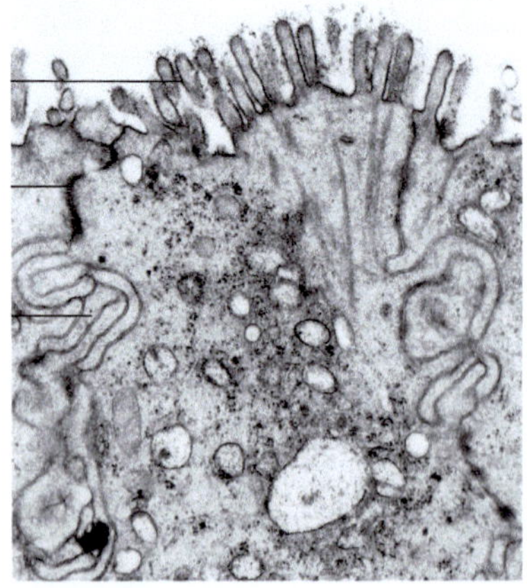

1.48 Electron micrograph of a zonula occludens adjoined by interdigitating cell processes (x21,000).

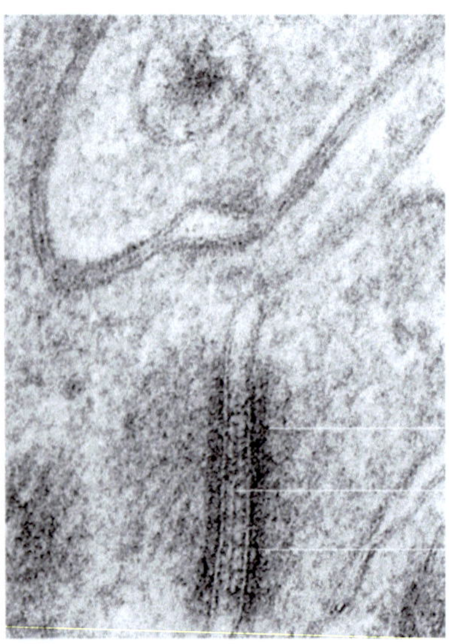

1.49 Electron micrograph of a desmosome (x45,000).

sation and selective restriction of the passage of substances through the epithelium, the zonulae adherentes (and desmosomes) perform a purely mechanical function. The presence of zonula occludens and zonula adherens in close proximity gives rise to **junctional complexes**. When viewed with light microscopy, these appear as a network referred to as the **terminal bar**.

Intercellular junctions in which membrane proteins interact with intermediate filaments (keratin filaments) include desmosomes (lateral cell membrane) and hemidesmosomes (basal cell membrane).

Desmosomes (Gk *desmo* = connection, *soma* = body) (diameter 0.3–0.5 μm) are disc-like plates that serve primarily to strengthen intercellular connections. At these sites, the apposing surface membranes condense. **Intracytoplasmic bundles of intermediate (keratin) filaments** attach at these locations, enhancing the strength of the cell-to-cell contact (Figures 1.47 and 1.49). The mechanical function of desmosomes is supported by the **ring-like** zonula adherens.

Desmosomes are the sole form of anchoring junction found in the stratified epithelia of the skin. In cuboidal and columnar epithelia, desmosomes and zonula adherens usually occur together. Desmosomes (diameter 0.4 × 0.25 μm) do not surround the cell as a continuous structure, rather they form **spot-** or **plaque-like** connections between neighbouring cells.

While they are found primarily in epithelia, they also occur between cardiac muscle cells. The width of the space between segments of plasma membrane joined by a desmosome is 20–40 nm.

On the cytoplasmic side of desmosomes, various **plaque proteins** (e.g. **desmoplakin**, **plakoglobins**, **desmocalmin**) aggregate to form a dense structure (desmosomal attachment plaque) in which the intermediate filaments are anchored. Between the two desmosomal plaques is an integrated band (**intermediate line**) containing the extracellular portions of Ca^{2+}-dependent transmembrane glycoproteins of the cadherin family (desmogleins, desmocollins).

The **intermediate** (**keratin**) **filaments** connected to the desmosome also serve as part of the supportive cytoskeleton, extending throughout the cytoplasm along lines of mechanical force.

GAP JUNCTION (NEXUS)

Gap junctions are **communicating junctions** that permit direct exchange of **chemical** or **electrical signals** between adjacent cells (e.g. in surface epithelia, smooth muscle).

Gap junctions are widely distributed through tissues and organs, particularly in epithelia, smooth muscle tissue, cardiac muscle and nervous tissue. Their diverse functions include **coordination of the activity** of adjacent cells (e.g. epithelia involved in fluid transport and electrolyte exchange, vascular and intestinal smooth muscle) and facilitation of the passage of regulatory molecules and smaller metabolites between cells. The intercellular space in gap junctions is very narrow (2–5 nm), appearing electron microscopically as a mere 'gap'.

Gap junctions are composed of **channel proteins** arranged in a circle to form the wall of a pore. Referred to as **connexons**, these protein complexes consist of six integral membrane subunits (connexins) configured to form a tunnel in the plasmalemma of each adjoining cell. The connexons in apposing membranes line up to form a channel that connects the two cells. The number of pores (up to 2 nm wide, 20 nm long) within a gap junction varies widely, up to several hundred. Their ability to open and close reversibly is integral to their function.

Basal surface specialisations

The basal cell domain exhibits several modifications:

- infolding of the basal cell membrane to increase surface area,
- junctions that anchor epithelial cells to the underlying extracellular matrix and
- the basement membrane.

The basal surface of most fluid-transporting epithelial cells is characterised by deep, irregular infoldings. These are particularly pronounced in the metabolically active cells of the proximal and distal renal tubules and in the striated (secretory) ducts of the salivary glands. Mitochondria are usually associated with the folds, providing a source of energy.

Connections between the base of the cell and the extracellular matrix strengthen the association between the epithelium and the underlying connective tissue. These include:

- focal adhesions – anchor long cytoskeletal actin filament bundles to the basement membrane and
- hemidesmosomes – anchor intermediate filaments of the cytoskeleton to the basement membrane; include transmembrane adhesion proteins of the integrin class.

Focal adhesions

By virtue of their actin filament component, focal adhesions play an important role in the dynamic processes associated with epithelial cells (e.g. **cell migration during wound healing**). Within transmembrane connecting zones, an attachment forms on the cytoplasmic side between **transmembrane proteins** (**mainly integrins**) and actin-binding proteins (α-actinin, vinculin, talin, paxillin), and with regulatory proteins (e.g. tyrosine kinase). Extracellularly, integrins are anchored to the basement membrane via glycoproteins (laminin and fibronectin), thus binding the epithelial cell to the underlying connective tissue.

Hemidesmosomes

Hemidesmosomes are similar in structure to desmosomes. They are found at the base of epithelia that are subjected to mechanical forces, serving to anchor the epithelial cells to the basement membrane. These include the epithelium of the skin, cornea, oral cavity, oesophagus, forestomachs and vagina.

The plaque found on the cytoplasmic side of hemidesmosomes incorporates desmoplakin-like proteins connected to cytoplasmic intermediate filaments. On the extracellular face, anchoring fibrils connect integrins with type III collagen of the basement membrane. This connection is supported by transmembranous collagen type XVII, via laminin and collagen type IV in the basal lamina.

Basement membrane (membrana basalis)

All epithelial cells rest upon a layer that can be demonstrated with the light microscope using periodic-acid Schiff staining or silver salt impregnation. In the context of light microscopy, this layer is referred to as the basement membrane.

Electron microscopic examination of the region occupied by the basement membrane of epithelia reveals three layers:

- lamina lucida (lamina rara interna),
- lamina basalis (basal lamina, lamina densa) and
- lamina fibroreticularis.

In some sources, the terms basement membrane and basal lamina are used interchangeably. Throughout this text, the material present between epithelial cells and underlying connective tissue is referred to as the basal lamina, except in specific circumstances.

LAMINA LUCIDA

The **lamina lucida** appears as a relatively light zone, up to 40 nm in width, between the base of the epithelium and the lamina basalis. This zone contains the extracellular portions of cell adhesion proteins of the integrin class (fibronectin receptors). These transmembrane proteins are connected to the cytoskeleton of the epithelial cell and, via collagens and laminins, to the lamina fibroreticularis. Some evidence suggests that the lamina lucida may not be a true layer, instead representing an artifact of fixation in which epithelial cells have shrunk away from underlying macromolecules.

LAMINA BASALIS

The **lamina basalis**, or basal lamina, is a thin (50–150 nm) filamentous layer of extracellular matrix between the base of the epithelium and the underlying connective tissue stroma (Figure 1.50). The filaments are woven into a network, forming an electron dense layer (hence its alternative term **lamina densa**). At least four groups of **structural proteins** are found in the lamina basalis including collagens, proteoglycans, laminins and glycoproteins (entactin/nidogen, fibronectin).

Type IV collagen is the predominant fibre type in the basal lamina. In contrast to other forms of collagen, which are synthesised by fibrocytes, type IV collagen of the basal lamina is **produced by epithelial cells**. An additional type of collagen (VII) serves to anchor the basal lamina to the lamina fibroreticularis, with reinforcement from fibronectin and other glycoproteins.

Proteoglycans (heparin sulfate and chondroitin sulfate) form the bulk of the matrix, which, due to its anionic nature, is heavily hydrated. The high proteoglycan content plays an important role in regulation of the passage of ions through the basal lamina. Both proteoglycans and laminin are considered products of the epithelial cells.

Laminin contributes substantially to the integration of the basal lamina with the base of the epithelium. Entactin (nidogen) and fibronectin stabilise the basal lamina and form part of the connection with the lamina fibroreticularis.

The basal lamina has **several functions**. As well as attaching the epithelium to the underlying connective tissue, it serves to compartmentalise superficial tissue layers, acting as a structural barrier between the epithelium (also muscle and nerve tissue, see below) and the connective tissue. In addition, the basal lamina functions as a selective filter, regulating the transport of substances via integral spaces and charge-dependent mechanisms. In the glomerulus of the kidney, the plasma filtrate traverses the capillary wall before passing through a well-developed basal lamina to enter the urinary space (blood–urine barrier, filtration barrier). In tissue repair, the basal lamina serves as a guide for regeneration.

Many individual, non-epithelial cells also have a basal lamina. These include muscle cells and peripheral nerve-supporting cells. In these cases, the basal lamina is sometimes referred to as the external lamina.

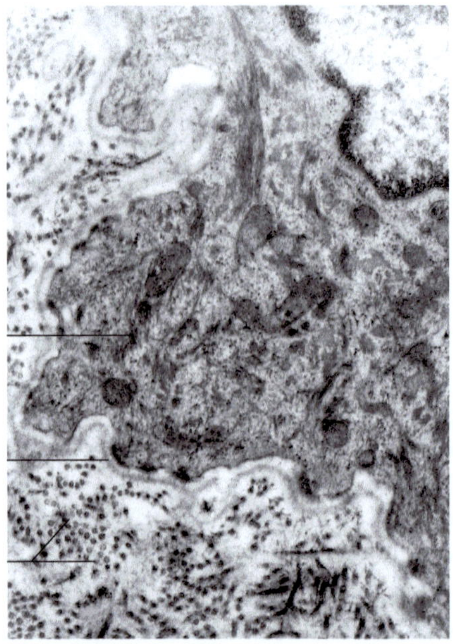

1.50 Basal lamina of an epithelial cell with underlying connective tissue (x5000).

LAMINA FIBRORETICULARIS

In certain instances, the basal lamina is associated with an additional dense layer comprising reticular (type III collagen) fibres and amorphous glycoproteins (**lamina fibroreticularis**). The lamina fibroreticularis, or reticular lamina, is in direct contact with the collagen fibres of the loose connective tissue layer.

While it is sometimes described as a secondary layer of the basement membrane, the reticular lamina is a component of the connective tissue. It comprises a three-dimensional network composed primarily of small subunits of collagen **type III** (reticular fibres) and **type VII**. The lamina fibroreticularis acts to link the basal lamina to underlying connective tissue layers.

Epithelial tissue (textus epithelialis)

2

Epithelial tissue consists of sheets of closely apposed cells. With few exceptions, it forms a boundary between the internal or external surfaces of the body and the underlying connective tissue. As such, epithelium coats the external body surfaces and lines internal cavities (including the luminal surface of vessels). It also lines the tracts that connect the internal organs with the exterior (gastrointestinal, respiratory and urogenital tracts) and constitutes the secretory component of glands.

In addition, epithelial tissues serve as receptors in organ systems associated with sensation (taste, touch, hearing, balance and vision).

The epithelium thus represents a **boundary** between biologically distinct compartments. Its **specific functions** are correspondingly numerous and varied, and can be used as the basis for dividing epithelia into tissue that:

- facilitates transport of substances along cellular surfaces by means of cilia (transport epithelia), e.g. in the respiratory mucosa,
- secretes various chemical substances into ducts that lead to the exterior (exocrine) or into the blood (endocrine) (secretory epithelium), e.g. (respectively) the pancreas and the thyroid gland,
- serves to eliminate harmful substances (excretory epithelia), e.g. in the kidney (Figure 2.1),
- lines the internal surface of vessels and body cavities, enabling transport of substances and fluids, e.g. endothelium and mesothelium (transport epithelium),
- fulfils a sensory role (sensory epithelium), e.g. taste buds in the oral cavity and
- performs a specialised role in the differentiation and maturation of male and female gametes (germinal epithelium).

As well as forming a selective barrier between the connective tissue compartment and other environments (the exterior, internal body cavities, the lumen of blood and lymph vessels), epithelia covering internal and external surfaces are vital for limiting the loss of fluid from the body.

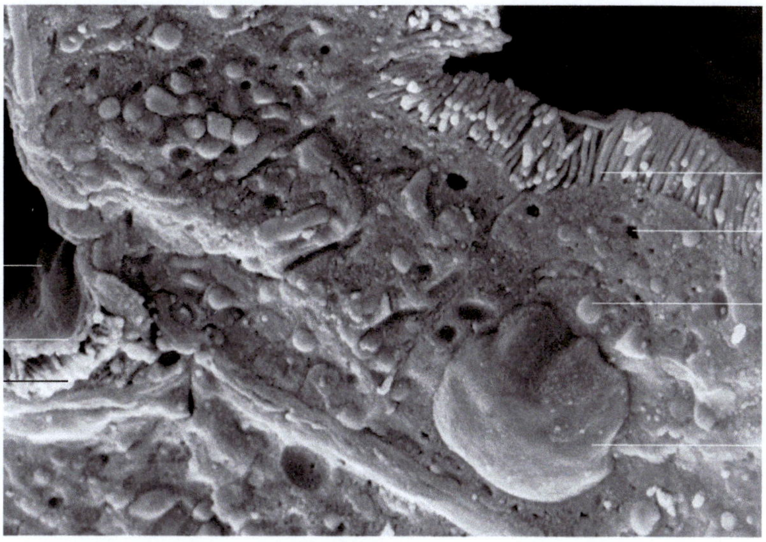

2.1 Scanning electron micrograph of the low columnar epithelium of a renal tubule in a dog (x5500).

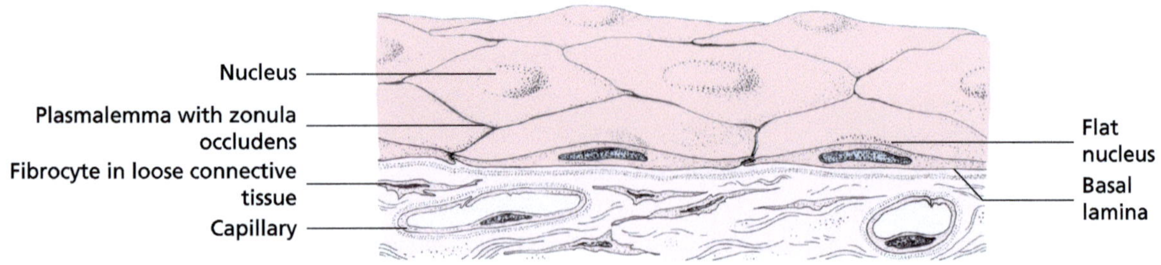

2.2 Simple squamous epithelium underlaid with basal lamina and lamina propria (schematic).

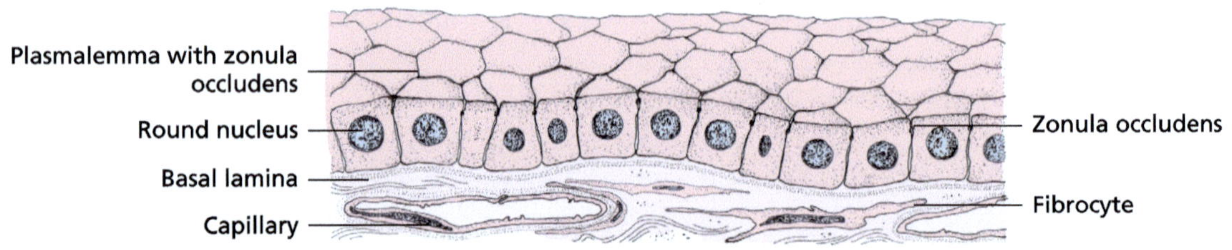

2.3 Simple cuboidal epithelium underlaid with basal lamina and lamina propria (schematic).

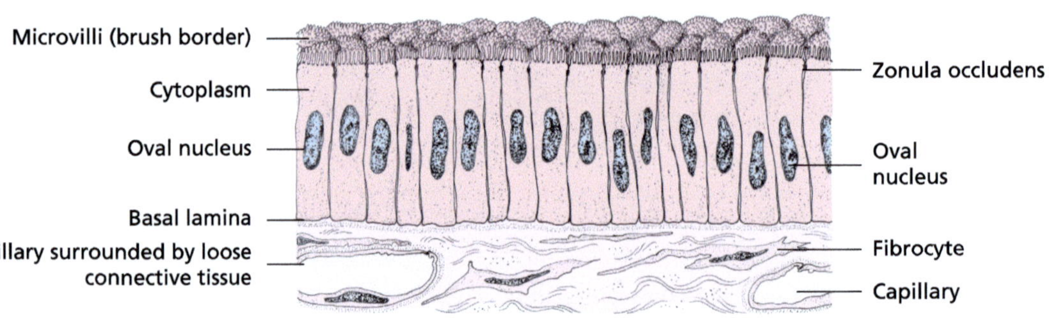

2.4 Simple columnar epithelium underlaid with basal lamina and lamina propria (schematic).

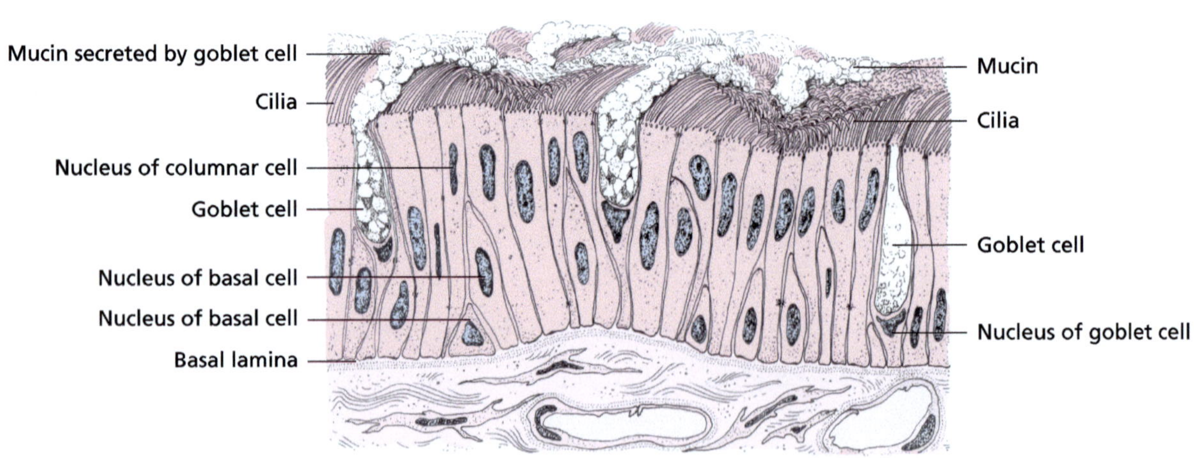

2.5 Ciliated pseudostratified epithelium with goblet cells (unicellular mucous glands), underlaid with basal lamina and lamina propria (schematic).

Epithelial tissue is further characterised by the following.

- It rests upon a basal lamina.
- It consists of cells that are closely apposed, held together by specialised intercellular junctions.
- Features of particular sections of the cell membrane give rise to morphological and functional cellular polarity.

In descriptions derived from electron microscopy, the layer upon which the basal surface of epithelial cells rests is referred to as the **basal lamina**. Using special stains (e.g. PAS), this acellular layer, composed of proteins and polysaccharides, can be visualised with the light microscope. In this context it is termed the **basement membrane** (see Chapter 1, 'The cell').

In a small number of locations, the epithelia have lost their association with a free surface and with the basal lamina. At these sites they are referred to as **epithelioid tissue** and are generally associated with **endocrine glands** (e.g. interstitial Leydig cells in the testes, luteal cells in the ovary, islets of Langerhans in the pancreas, the parenchyma of the adrenal gland and the hypophysis). Epithelioid cells are also present in the thymus.

Histogenesis

Epithelia can be distinguished based on their embryonic origin. They arise from all three primary germ layers.

Tissues arising from the **ectoderm** include the skin (epidermis) and its derivatives (e.g. sebaceous glands and sweat glands), epithelial components of the oral and nasal cavities, and parts of the visual, olfactory, gustatory and auditory systems.

The **mesoderm** gives rise to simple (single-layered) epithelia that line body cavities (thoracic, abdominal and pelvic cavities) and cover the external surface of internal organs as serosae. Epithelium of mesodermal origin also forms the internal lining of the circulatory and lymphatic systems (endothelium).

The **endoderm** differentiates into a multitude of epithelia that primarily line the interior of hollow organs or become part of parenchymatous organs. These endodermal cells subsequently determine organ function. Epithelia of endodermal origin are found, for example, throughout much of the gastrointestinal and respiratory tracts, in the bladder and accessory sex glands and in the middle ear (internal lining). The epithelium of exocrine glands (e.g. pancreas) and endocrine glands (e.g. thyroid gland and parathyroid gland) is also derived from endoderm.

Classification

Based on the structure and function of individual cells, epithelium can be classified as:

- surface epithelium,
- glandular epithelium or
- sensory or neuroepithelium.

Surface epithelium (epithelium superficiale)

Surface epithelium is located on the surface of tissues and organs and forms the sheet-like covering of the outer and inner surfaces of the body. The structure of these epithelia is largely determined by the demands of their environment (Table 2.1). The outer layers of the skin (epidermis) are subjected not only to mechanical forces, but also to radiation and changes in temperature and humidity. The internal lining of the respiratory tract is exposed to humidified air, while the organs responsible for conveying urine, including the bladder and urethra, are frequently in contact with strongly hypertonic fluid. In the gut, the intestinal epithelium encounters a wide range of nutrients. Reflecting these varied conditions, surface epithelia exhibit a range of specialisations.

Surface epithelia are classified according to the **number of cell layers** present and the **shape of the epithelial cells** (Figures 2.2 to 2.21). They may consist of one or more cell layers and are thus divided into:

- single-layered (simple and pseudostratified) epithelium and
- multi-layered (stratified) epithelium.

Single-layered epithelium (epithelium simplex)

Single-layered epithelium is found primarily on surfaces involved in absorption or secretion. It offers little resistance to mechanical forces yet can undergo distension. The shape of the epithelial cell varies with function and may be:

- squamous,
- cuboidal or
- columnar.

SIMPLE SQUAMOUS EPITHELIUM (EPITHELIUM SIMPLEX SQUAMOSUM)

In simple squamous epithelia, the cytoplasm of the epithelial cells is spread out (i.e. the cell is flat) (Figure 2.2). The typically flattened nuclei may bulge above the free surface of the cell. This type of epithelium facilitates passive diffusion across internal bodily surfaces. It forms the internal lining of vessels, where it is referred to as **endothelium**. Due to its conformability, it can accommodate changes in intraluminal volume. The presence of pores also allows for increased permeability and associated acceleration of metabolic processes.

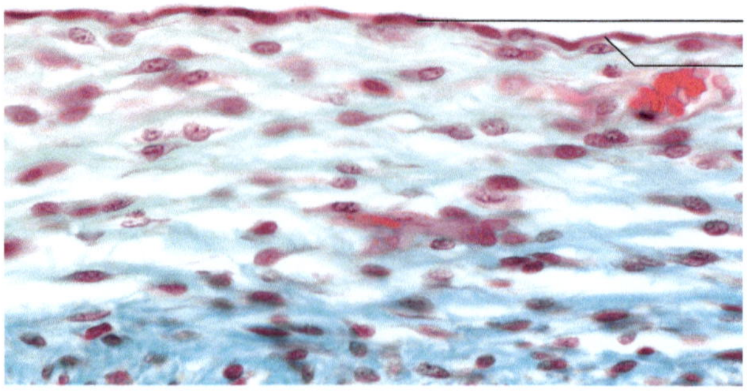

2.6 Simple squamous epithelium, parietal peritoneum (dog). The nuclei are largely flattened and the cytoplasm is spread out. Simple squamous epithelium forms the endothelial lining of vessels and the mesothelial lining of body cavities (e.g. pleural, peritoneal and pericardial cavities). Goldner's Masson trichrome stain (x480).

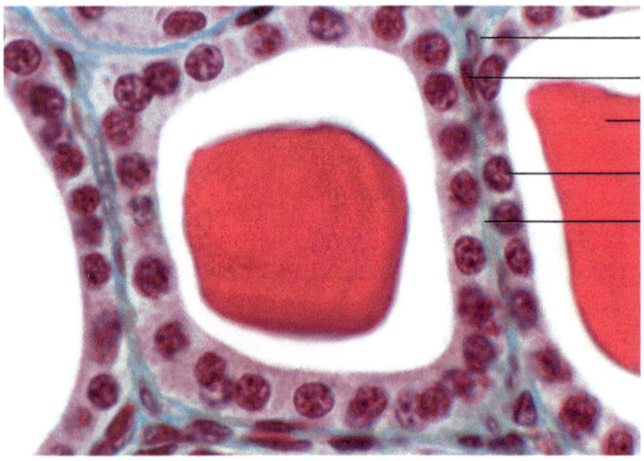

2.7 Simple cuboidal epithelium, thyroid follicle (pig). The height and width of the cell are similar, and the nucleus is round in cross-section. The cell boundaries are typically poorly distinguishable. The epithelium rests upon connective tissue containing numerous fibrocytes. Goldner's Masson trichrome stain (x100).

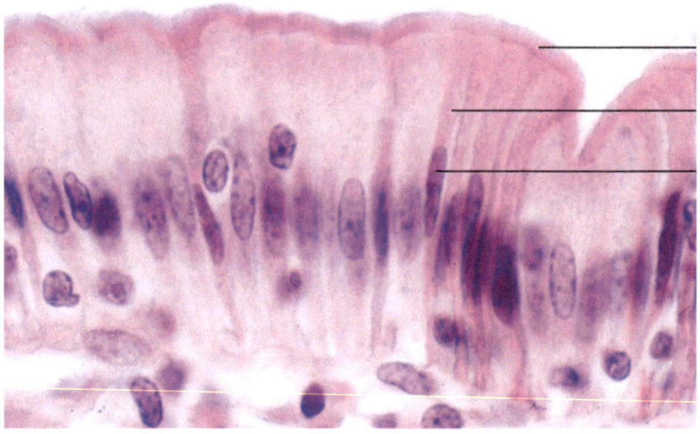

2.8 Simple columnar epithelium, small intestine (horse). Variation in the cytoplasmic staining in the tall narrow cells reflects differences in their functional state. The presence of a brush border on the free surface increases the absorptive capacity of the epithelium. The nuclei are oval (the long axis aligned with the apical–basal axis of the cell) with loose chromatin (euchromatin). Haematoxylin and eosin stain (x1000).

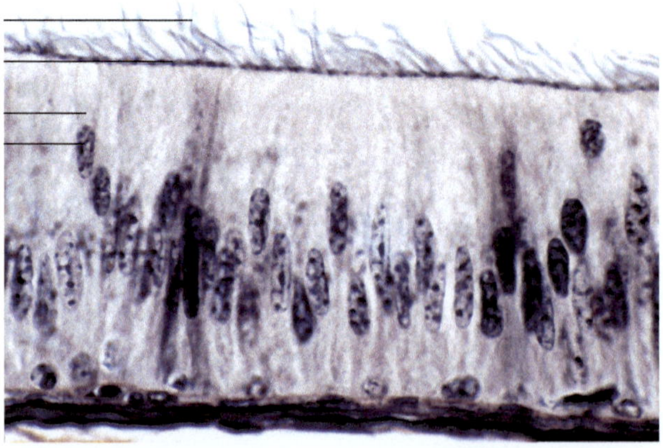

2.9 Epididymal duct, ox. In the pseudostratified type of surface epithelium, all the cells are in contact with the basal lamina though not all reach the free surface. Basal cells are visible at the base of the epithelium, while the nuclei of the other cells are located at various levels. In the epididymis, stereocilia are present at the surface. Iron haematoxylin stain (x480).

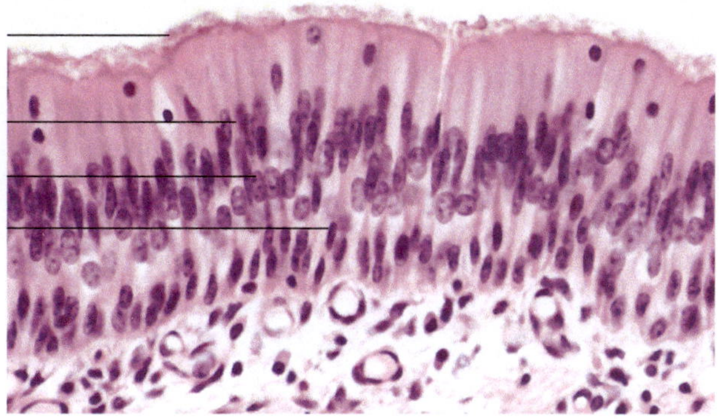

2.10 Pseudostratified columnar epithelium, nasal septum (calf). All cells are in contact with the basement membrane. However, based on the position of the nucleus, the cells appear to be arranged in at least three 'rows'. Haematoxylin and eosin stain (x480).

Simple squamous epithelium lines all the body cavities, where it is referred to as **mesothelium** (e.g. abdominal cavity, thoracic cavity, pericardial cavity, posterior corneal epithelium within the anterior chamber). In these locations, simple squamous epithelium, together with the underlying vascular connective tissue, serves to regulate gas and fluid exchange, and contributes to local non-specific immunity via phagocytosis (Figures 2.2 and 2.6).

SIMPLE CUBOIDAL EPITHELIUM (EPITHELIUM SIMPLEX CUBOIDEUM)

In simple cuboidal epithelium, the width of the epithelial cells is similar to their height; the usually spherical nucleus is located centrally (Figures 2.3 and 2.7). This form of epithelium is found in the ducts of glands, in several types of renal tubule and in the retinal pigment epithelium. It also appears on the surface of the ovary as germinal epithelium, on the surface of the lens and in small bile ducts. On the luminal surface of many glands, simple cuboidal epithelium undergoes constant functionally dependent development and regression. Accordingly, the epithelium in these locations can range in height from little more than squamous to low columnar.

SIMPLE COLUMNAR EPITHELIUM (EPITHELIUM SIMPLEX COLUMNARE)

Simple columnar epithelium (Figures 2.4 and 2.8) consists of cells that are distinctly taller than they are wide. The nuclei are predominantly oval (their long axis being aligned with the apical–basal cell axis) and may occupy a basal, central or apical position. As with cuboidal cells, the shape of columnar cells nevertheless varies according to their location and functional state. Simple columnar epithelium is typically associated with **absorption** or **secretion**. Absorptive simple columnar epithelium occurs throughout the gastrointestinal tract (from the gastric opening to the anal canal), where the free surface of the epithelial cells is densely populated with **microvilli** (0.5–1.0 μm in length; 3000 per cell in the small intestine). This type of epithelium also contains cells that support the function of the surrounding tissue, either through exocrine secretory activity (e.g. goblet cells) or endocrine secretion of substances such

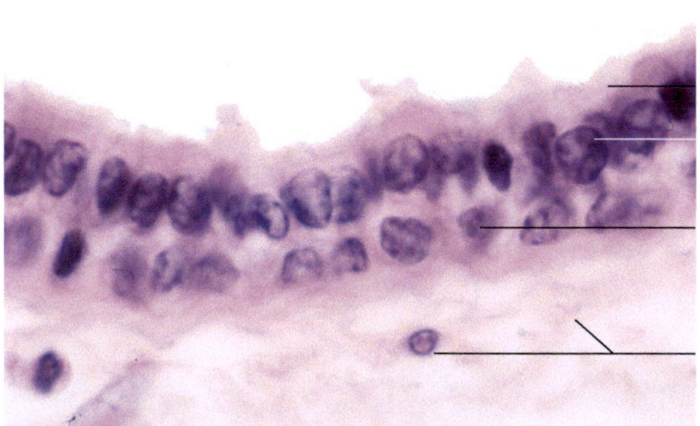

2.11 In this bi-stratified cuboidal epithelium, the nuclei are predominantly round and the cell borders are indistinct. Salivary gland duct (ox). Haematoxylin and eosin stain (x100).

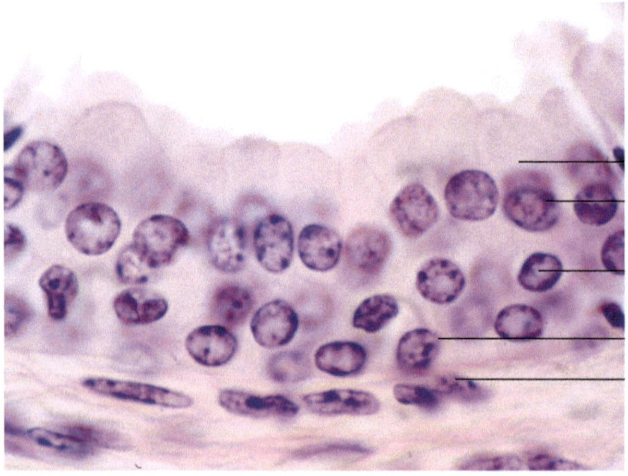

2.12 Stratified cuboidal to columnar epithelium. The round nuclei appear stacked on top of one another, clearly illustrating the layering of cells within this surface epithelium. Loose connective tissue containing fibrocytes underlies the epithelium. Salivary gland duct (ox). Haematoxylin and eosin stain (x100).

as biogenic amines and hormones. Simple columnar epithelium is also found on the luminal surface of the gall bladder, the uterine tube and the uterus.

PSEUDOSTRATIFIED EPITHELIUM (EPITHELIUM PSEUDOSTRATIFICATUM)

Pseudostratified epithelium is a special form of single-layered surface epithelium in which all cells are in contact with the basal lamina, yet not all reach the free surface. The cell nuclei lie at different levels, such that the cells appear to be arranged in two or more 'rows'. This creates the false impression that the epithelium is multi-layered (stratified). Those cells that do not reach the surface comprise undifferentiated basal reserve (or replacement) cells. The remaining cells, located between the basal cells, are columnar. Pseudostratified epithelium is widespread in the respiratory tract (respiratory epithelium) where the apical cell surface features numerous cilia. The epididymal duct is lined by pseudostratified epithelium bearing stereocilia (Figures 2.5, 2.9 and 2.10).

Multi-layered (stratified) epithelium (epithelium stratificatum)

Stratified epithelium consists of two or more cell layers, of which only the deepest layer rests on the basement membrane (Figures 2.11 to 2.17). The primary role of stratified epithelium is **protection**. The amount of mechanical stress to which it is subjected determines the morphology of the epithelium.

Based on the **shape of the cell in the surface layer**, irrespective of the shape of underlying cells, stratified epithelium is classified as:

- stratified cuboidal or columnar epithelium,
- stratified squamous epithelium:
  - non-keratinised stratified squamous epithelium and
  - keratinised stratified squamous epithelium.

The term **transitional epithelium** is used to describe an additional, specialised form of stratified epithelium.

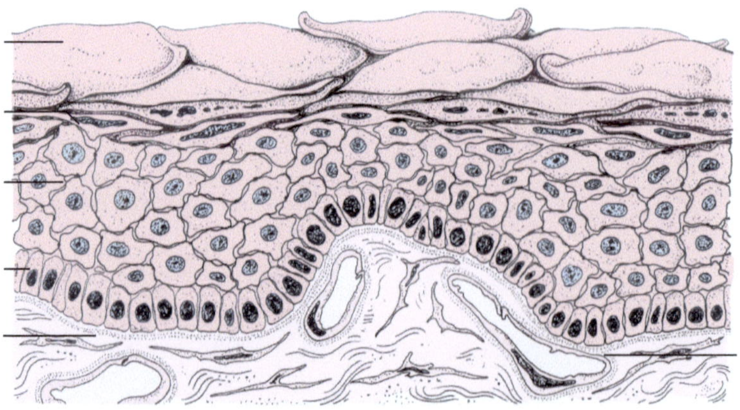

2.13 Non-keratinised stratified squamous epithelium, resting upon the basal lamina and lamina propria (schematic).

STRATIFIED CUBOIDAL OR COLUMNAR EPITHELIUM (EPITHELIUM STRATIFICATUM CUBOIDEUM/ COLUMNARE)

Stratified cuboidal or columnar epithelium is found in relatively few locations in the body. These include the lining of the larger excretory ducts of glands (e.g. parotid salivary gland) (Figures 2.11 and 2.12).

STRATIFIED SQUAMOUS EPITHELIUM (EPITHELIUM STRATIFICATUM SQUAMOSUM)

In stratified squamous epithelium, the cells of the basal layer (**stratum basale**) are primarily cuboidal to columnar. They undergo constant mitosis, forming new polygonal cells. As they mature, these cells are pushed towards the surface into the **stratum spinosum**.

Near the surface, the cells become flattened and the nucleus increases in density (pyknosis). These cells are constantly replaced by cells rising from the basal layer. The superficial cells may undergo partial or complete keratinisation before desquamating. The period that elapses between the formation of a new cell in the stratum basale through mitosis to its desquamation at the surface of the epithelium is generally 30 days.

In some regions, the protective function of stratified squamous epithelium is reinforced by the presence of basal epithelial pegs that interdigitate with **papillae** projecting from the underlying connective tissue of the dermis to form a particularly strong connection between these two tissue layers (Figures 2.14 and 2.15). As well as mechanical strength, this arrangement facilitates nourishment of the epidermis by increasing the surface area across which diffusion can take place.

NON-KERATINISED STRATIFIED SQUAMOUS EPITHELIUM (EPITHELIUM STRATIFICATUM SQUAMOSUM NONCORNIFICATUM)

Non-keratinised stratified epithelium consists of a single-layered stratum basale overlaid by multiple cell layers in the stratum spinosum. The surface of the epithelium is lined by a flat layer, the stratum superficiale. Despite the

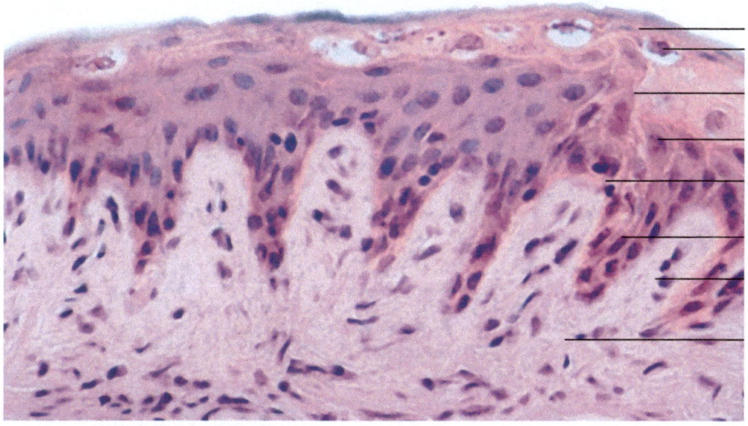

2.14 Stratified squamous epithelium with prominent connective tissue papillae, ruminal papilla (ox). Haematoxylin and eosin stain (x100).

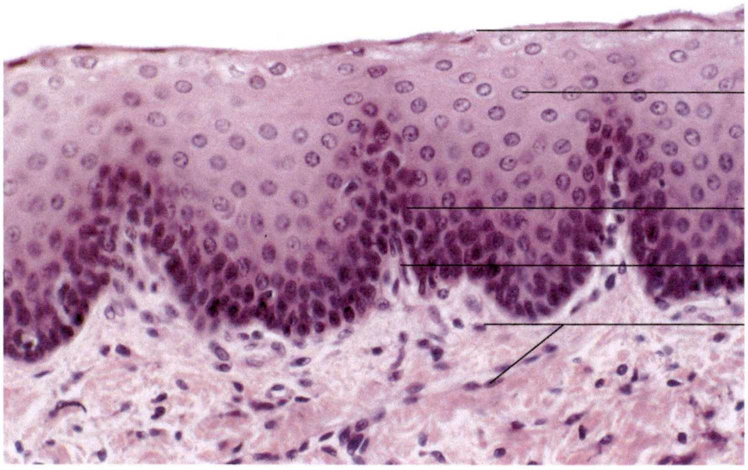

2.15 Stratified squamous epithelium, oesophagus (sheep). Connective tissue papillae protrude into epithelium from the lamina propria. Haematoxylin and eosin stain (x480).

classification of this epithelium as non-keratinised, the superficial cells may contain some keratin. However, unlike the outermost cells of keratinised epithelium, they retain their nucleus. As this type of epithelium is prone to dehydration, it is found in locations that experience relatively weak mechanical forces and are kept moist by glandular secretions. Depending on species, diet and other factors, these may include the oral cavity, pharynx, oesophagus, anal canal and vagina (Figures 2.13 to 2.15).

Keratinised stratified squamous epithelium (epithelium stratificatum squamosum cornificatum)

Keratinised stratified squamous epithelium forms the outer layer of the skin, the epidermis (see also Chapter 15, 'Common integument'). It consists of up to five distinct strata that become keratinised towards the surface and vary in their thickness depending upon the location of the epithelium within the body (Figures 2.16 and 2.17).

The basal stratum (stratum basale) is composed of basophilic, cuboidal to columnar cells that are firmly connected to the basal lamina by hemidesmosomes. The epithelium is thus securely anchored to the underlying connective tissue. Varying numbers of melanin granules may be present within the cytoplasm of basal cells. These cells (melanocytes) are responsible for pigmentation of the epithelium. The stratum basale also contains specialised cells that have immunological and/or phagocytic activity (Langerhans cells) as well as tactile cells (Merkel cells).

The **stratum spinosum** (**prickle cell** or **spinous layer**) is composed primarily of cuboidal polygonal cells that are tightly interconnected by numerous desmosomes (maculae adherentes), located at the end of cytoplasmic extensions. Under light microscopy this gives the cells a spiny appearance, from which this layer derives its name. This effect is often enhanced by the presence of large intercellular spaces and a high concentration of intracytoplasmic tonofilaments. The latter are arranged in a lattice

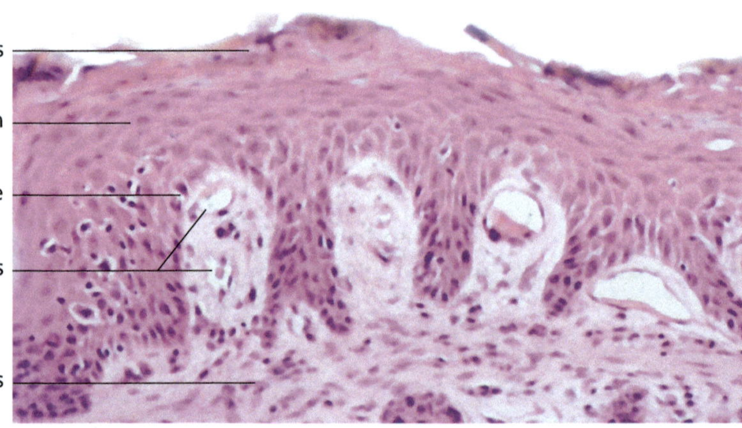

2.16 Stratified squamous epithelium; ruminal papilla (ox). Prominent connective tissue papillae are evident. Haematoxylin and eosin stain (x100).

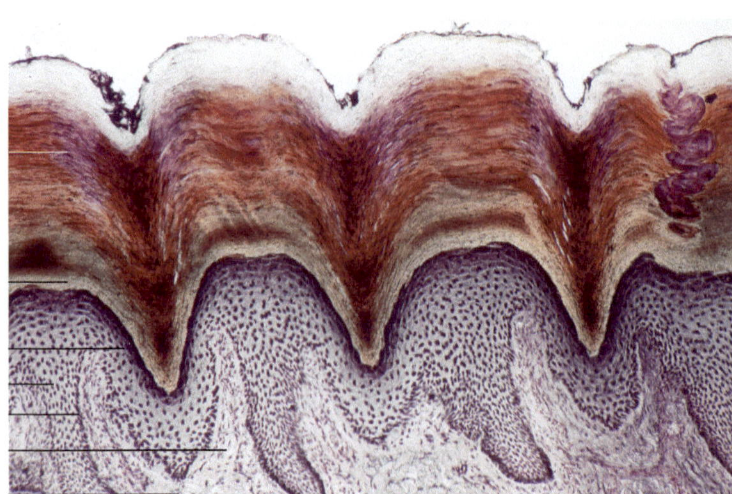

2.17 Keratinised stratified squamous epithelium with prominent dermal papillae; digital pad. Section prepared according to Schefthaler and Mayet (x80).

in which the orientation of filaments reflects the prevailing forces of pressure and tension. This contributes to the structural integrity of the epithelium.

By the time cells reach the **stratum granulosum** they are considerably flattened. Three to five layers of cells are present in this layer, depending on the degree of keratinisation. The cells are characterised by the accumulation of strongly basophilic granules containing keratohyalin (a histidine-rich protein), the appearance of lamellar bodies, a high density of tonofilaments and early degradation of the nucleus and other organelles. These morphological features represent the commencement of the keratinisation process (see Chapter 15, 'Common integument').

The **stratum lucidum** is a highly refractive layer in which the organelles barely take up any stain. The cytoplasm is comprised of compacted bundles of filaments in a homogeneous eosinophilic matrix. A stratum lucidum is found primarily in areas where the epidermis is thickened. It serves to shield the deeper epithelial layers from external influences (e.g. noxious agents) and to protect against dehydration of the epidermis and loss of body fluid.

The process of keratinisation is completed in the **stratum corneum**. Features associated with this layer include a thickening of the cell membrane, the dissolution of the nucleus and other organelles and the formation of keratin (a type of scleroprotein) from keratohyalin and tonofilaments.

The deeper layers of the epidermis (stratum basale, spinosum and granulosum) are nourished by diffusion and are pervaded by free nerve endings.

TRANSITIONAL EPITHELIUM (EPITHELIUM TRANSITIONALE)

Transitional epithelium is a specialised form of stratified epithelium. Its deepest (basal) layer consists of cuboidal to columnar cells that are connected to the basal lamina. These cells are overlaid by irregular 'mushroom-shaped' cells that become rounder towards the surface, forming caps over the deeper cell layers. The cytoplasmic processes of these more superficial cells are not necessarily in contact with the basal lamina. Transitional epithelium is found in the excretory passages of the urinary system (renal pelvis, ureter, bladder, urethra). As these structures are subjected to constant changes in pressure and distension, the epithelium can undergo rapid changes in height (Figures 2–18 to 2.21).

Glandular epithelium (epithelium glandulare)

Epithelial tissue involved in the **synthesis** and **secretion** of specific substances (**secreta**) is termed **glandular epithelium**. It is composed of a group of individual secretory cells. The secretory product is usually created in the form of **granules** that are released from the cell by various mechanisms. When a number of secretory cells combine to form an organ, the resulting tissue is referred to as a gland (e.g. salivary gland, lacrimal gland).

Glands can be classified according to various criteria, including their location, the way in which their secretory product is distributed, the number of cells, their morphology, the mechanism by which their secretory product is released and the composition of the secretion (Figures 2.22 and 2.23). Based on the distribution of secretory product, there are two main types of glands (Figure 2.24):

- endocrine glands and
- exocrine glands.

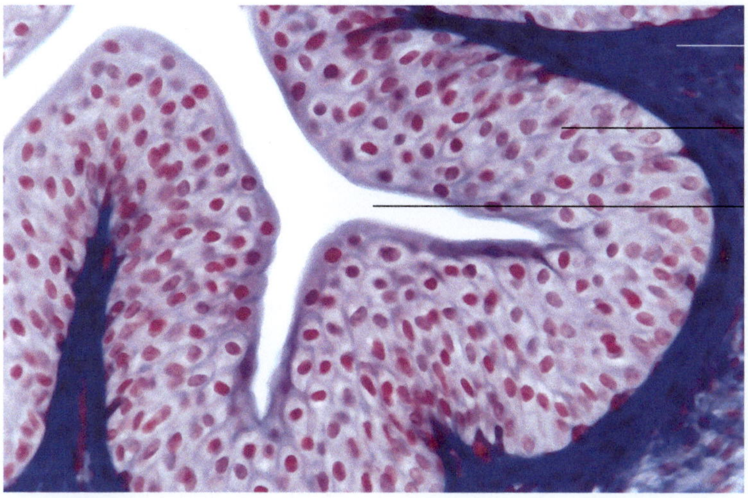

2.18 Bladder (dog). Transitional epithelium lines the excretory passages of the urinary system, including the renal pelvis (peripheral portion), the ureters, the bladder and the urethra. Azan stain (x100).

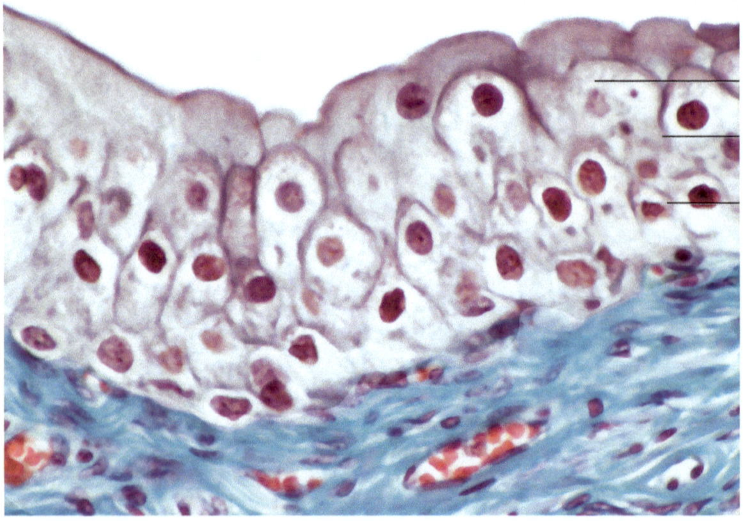

2.19 Bladder, non-distended (dog). Transitional epithelium can be considered a specialised form of stratified epithelium. While the deeper cells are in constant contact with the basal lamina, the superficial cells lose this connection (they may be in contact with the base of the epithelium via fine cytoplasmic processes). This epithelium is limited to the urinary passages. Goldner's Masson trichrome stain (x440).

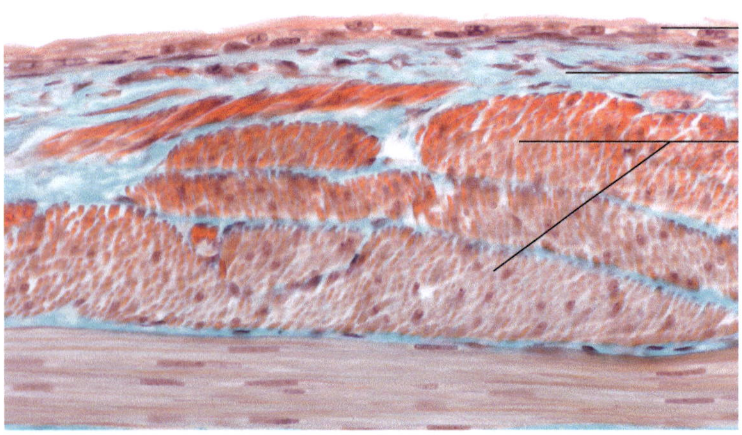

2.20 Bladder, distended (dog). When a urinary passage undergoes distension, the transitional epithelium may become considerably reduced in height. The basal epithelial cells become broader, remaining in contact with the basal lamina. Goldner's Masson trichrome stain (x440).

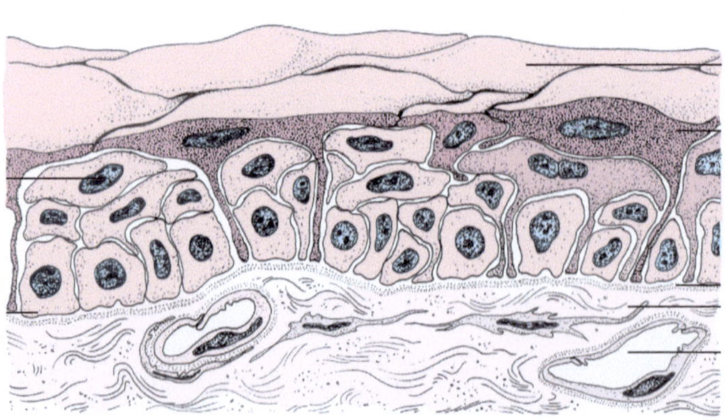

2.21 Transitional epithelium (schematic).

Table 2.1 Classification of surface epithelium based on morphology.

Epithelium	Layering	Occurrence
Squamous	Simple	Lining of body cavities (= serosa, mesothelium), lining of internal surface of vessel walls (= endothelium), posterior corneal epithelium
	Stratified	a) keratinised, e.g. body surface (epidermis) b) non-keratinised, e.g. oral cavity
Cuboidal	Simple	Many small ducts of glands, renal tubules, follicular epithelium of the thyroid gland, germinal epithelium of the ovary.
	Stratified	Ducts of salivary glands.
Columnar	Simple	Non-ciliated, e.g. gastrointestinal tract, gall bladder; ciliated, e.g. oviduct; non-ciliated pseudostratified, e.g. parts of ducts of glands; ciliated pseudostratified, e.g. respiratory mucosa; stereociliated, e.g. epididymal duct.
	Stratified	Large salivary gland ducts
Transitional		Variable in height, e.g. renal pelvis, ureter, bladder and urethra

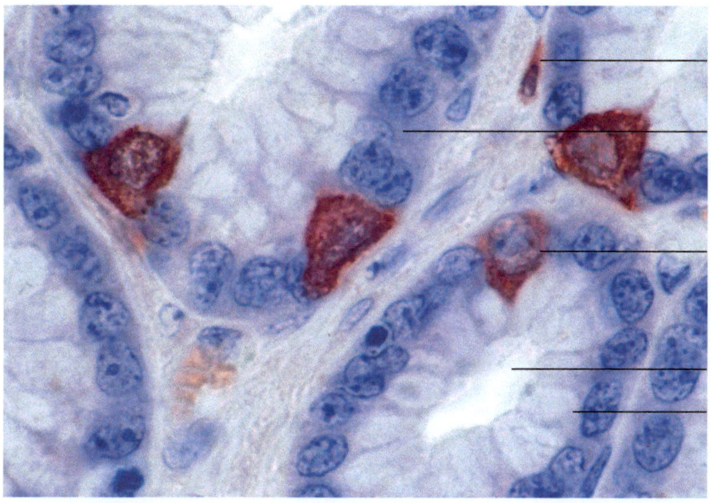

2.22 Proper gastric (fundic) gland region of the stomach (horse). Endocrine glands in the form of single intra-epithelial cells (enteroendocrine cells) are found in the wall of the gastric mucosa. Methylene blue stain (x100).

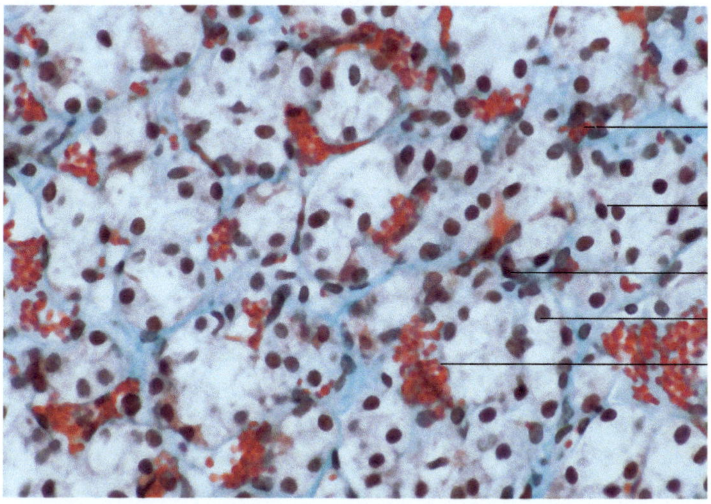

2.23 Parathyroid gland (goat). Endocrine glands release their specific secretory products (hormones) into the intercellular fluid, from which they are taken up primarily by capillaries. Simplest in structure is the parathyroid gland, in which clumps of secretory cells are surrounded by a dense capillary network. Goldner's Masson trichrome stain (x480).

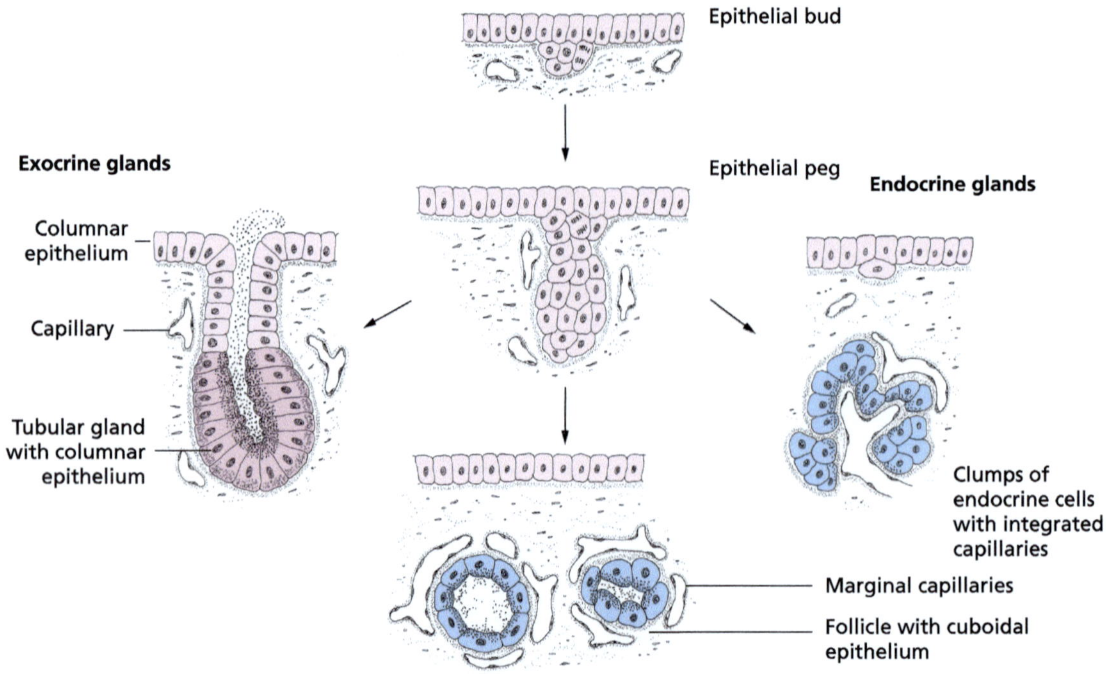

2.24 Differentiation of an exocrine extra-epithelial tubular gland and various types of endocrine glands from an ectodermal anlage (schematic).

Endocrine glands (glandulae endocrinae)

The cells of endocrine glands are typically surrounded by a **dense capillary network**. The glandular secretions, known as **hormones**, are released into the surrounding connective tissue from which they are typically taken up through the wall of a capillary and transported by the bloodstream to their target organ. There, they either bind to specific receptors on the target cell membrane or diffuse through the plasmalemma to reach receptors located within the cytoplasm. Thereupon, the hormones are able to influence cellular metabolism. Examples of endocrine glands include the pituitary, thyroid and adrenal glands.

In certain epithelia, hormonal secretions do not pass into the circulatory system. Instead, after diffusing into the extracellular compartment, they exert their effect directly on surrounding cells (tissue hormones e.g. neurotensin,

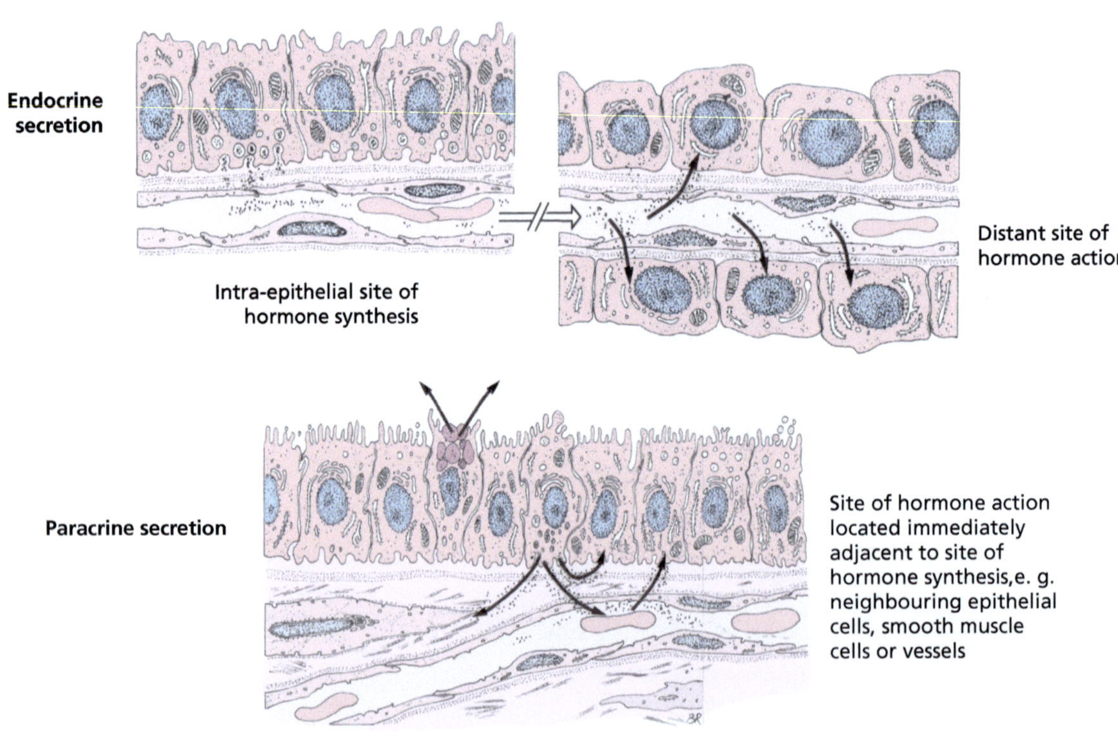

2.25 Endocrine and paracrine modes of cellular communication (schematic).

prostaglandins) (Figure 2.25). This form of secretion is referred to as **paracrine**. It is employed, for example, by enteroendocrine cells of the gastro-intestinal tract.

In the **autocrine** mode of secretion, the hormone acts upon the cell by which it was secreted (e.g. Leydig cells in the testes) (see also Chapter 9, 'Endocrine system').

Exocrine glands (glandulae exocrinae)

Exocrine glands are glands in which the secretory product is transported to the surface of the epithelium (Figures 2.31 to 2.44). Consisting of mucin, enzymes or other materials, the secretion reaches its destination in one of two ways: by passing directly to the internal or external body surface, or by travelling through a single duct or complex system of ducts. The composition and concentration of the secretory product may undergo modification during its passage to the surface. Exocrine glands include the mammary, salivary and bronchial glands. A summary of the structural elements of exocrine glands is provided in Table 2.3. Based on their relationship to the surface epithelium, exocrine glands are classified as:

- intra-epithelial glands (glandulae intraepitheliales) or
- extra-epithelial glands (glandulae exoepitheliales).

INTRA-EPITHELIAL GLANDS (GLANDULAE INTRAEPITHELIALES)

Intra-epithelial glands may consist of a single cell or a group of cells.

Goblet cells are typical **single-cell intra-epithelial exocrine glands** (Figures 2.26 to 2.30). They are club-shaped cells with a narrow base. The secretory product, **mucinogen**, is synthesised by the endoplasmic reticulum and Golgi apparatus, and accumulates in the apical region of the cell in the form of membrane-bound secretory granules.

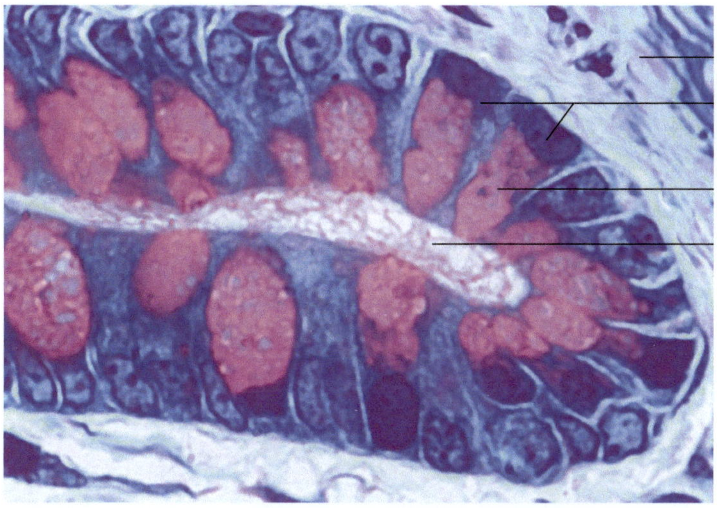

2.26 Small intestine (dog). The simplest form of exocrine gland is an intra-epithelial monocellular gland (goblet cell). Using methylene blue and safranin, the mucinogen/mucin stains red. Mucin creates a protective coat over the epithelial surface. Mucinogen fills much of the interior of the goblet cells, displacing the nucleus towards the base. Methylene blue and safranin stain (x600).

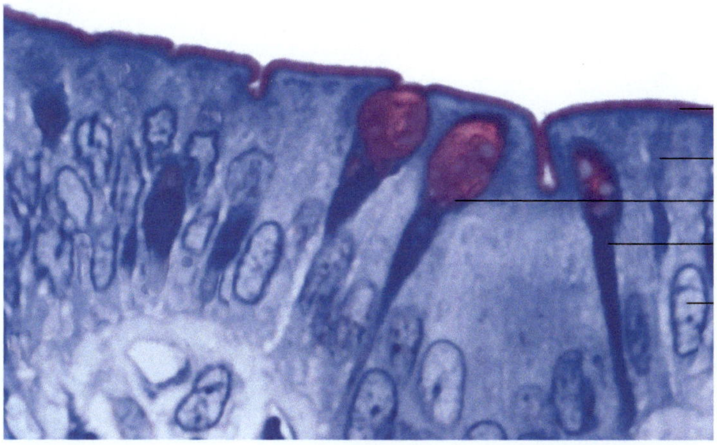

2.27 Small intestine (dog). Goblet cells collapse after releasing their secretory product; the cytoplasm stains more deeply and the nucleus appears elongated. Methylene blue and safranin stain (x600).

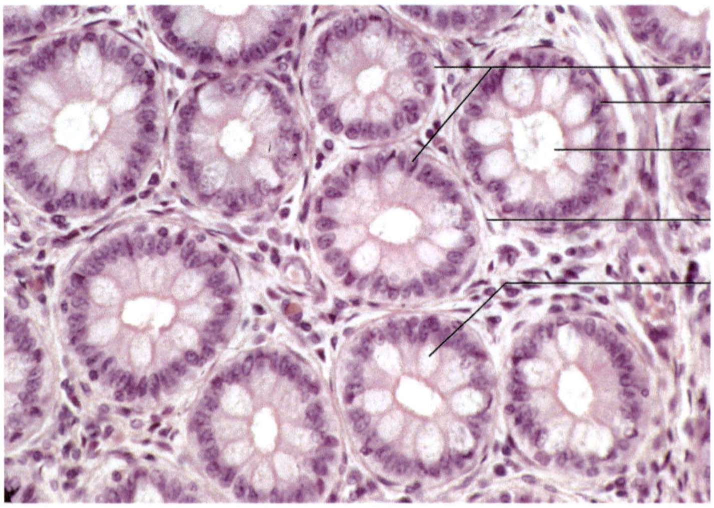

2.28 Large intestine (dog). In cross-section, the cells of exocrine tubular glands form a ring around a central lumen into which the secretory product is deposited. Goblet cells within the epithelium stain lightly with haematoxylin and eosin. Haematoxylin and eosin stain (x100).

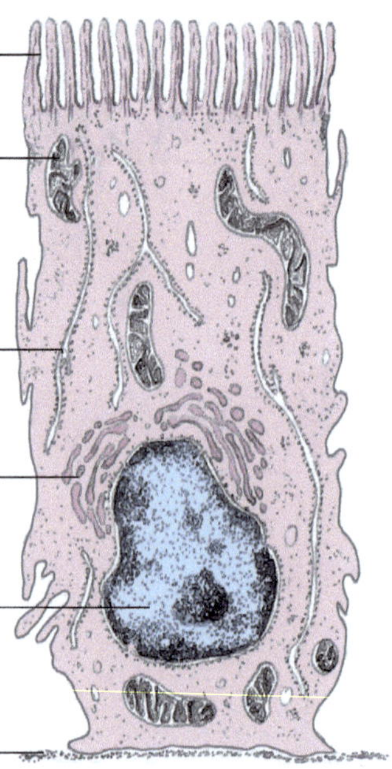

2.29 Columnar epithelial cell in the small intestine of a dog (schematic).

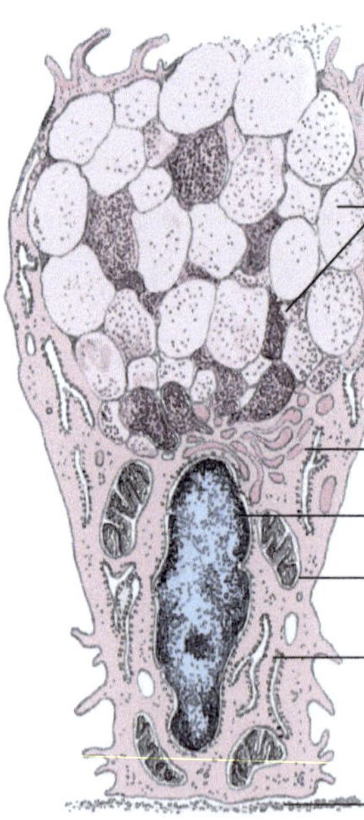

2.30 Goblet cell (schematic).

With the use of mucin special stains (PAS, mucicarmine), these granules selectively stain bright red–magenta. The secretory product is released by exocytosis.

Multicellular intra-epithelial exocrine glands are found in the pseudostratified epithelium of the airways of birds.

EXTRA-EPITHELIAL GLANDS (GLANDULAE EXOEPITHELIALES)

Extra-epithelial glands are located in the connective tissue underlying the epithelium. They are always multicellular. Their secretions are produced in **secretory units** (**secretory end pieces**) and are conveyed to the surface of the epithelium by ducts. Exocrine glands consisting of a (usually) single secretory unit and a single unbranched or minimally branched duct are termed **simple glands** (e.g. sweat glands).

Those in which multiple secretory units are connected to the surface by a highly branched system of ducts are referred to as **compound glands**.

The following criteria for categorising types of glands are discussed in more detail below:

- shape of the secretory unit,
- structure of the duct system,
- mode of secretion and
- chemical composition of the secretory product.

Shape of the secretory unit

Based on the shape of the lumen, secretory units (Figures 2.31 to 2.33) may be described as:

- tubular (resembling a hose or pipe),
- acinar (spherical, berry-shaped) or
- alveolar (vesicular) or
- mixed types, such as tubulo-alveolar or tubulo-acinar (often associated with compound glands).

The walls of the secretory units are comprised of secretory cells. Generally, the secretory end pieces consist of a single layer of glandular epithelium. Sebaceous glands, in which multiple cell layers are present, are an exception (Figure 2.39).

In some glands, the base of the secretory units is surrounded by **myoepithelial cells** that function as contractile elements. Embryologically, these are modified epithelial cells containing bundles of myofilaments. These cells may be arranged in parallel, or as a branching network, adjacent to the basal surface of the cells. Contraction of myoepithelial cells assists in expelling the secretory product into the duct. These cells are found particularly in sweat glands, the alveolae of the mammary glands and the salivary glands (Figure 2.33).

Structure of the ducts

In **simple exocrine glands** consisting of a single multicellular secretory unit and an unbranched duct, the secretory unit is typically tubular. Examples include the sweat glands of the skin. In **branched simple glands**, several secretory units empty into a single duct (e.g. gastric glands).

Compound glands are usually divided into lobules containing groups of secretory units that exhibit an organ-specific structure. The secretory product enters a complex system of strongly branching ducts, before emptying into a single excretory duct. This type of gland is exemplified by the large salivary glands (Figure 2.33).

Mode of secretion

The various modes in which the secretory product is released from the epithelial cells include:

- merocrine secretion (also referred to as eccrine),
- apocrine secretion and
- holocrine secretion.

Merocrine secretion (Figure 2.37) involves the release of substances that have been stored in the apical cytoplasm in the form of membrane-bound secretory granules. The

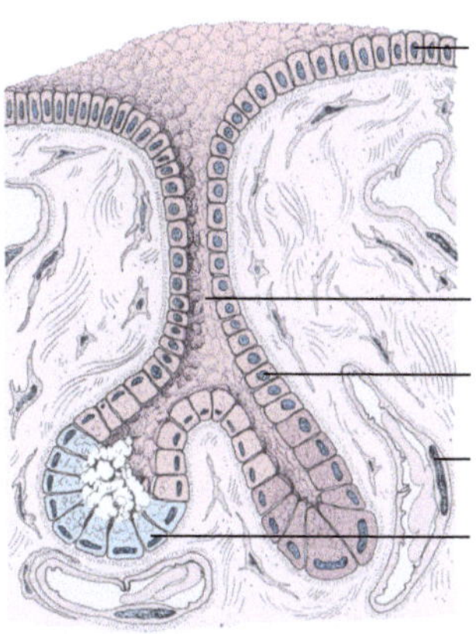

2.32 Acinar and tubular secretory units with associated duct (schematic).

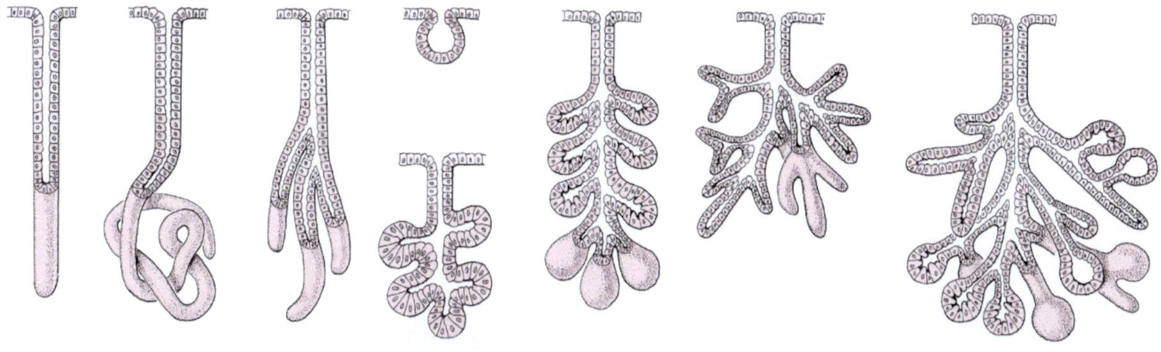

2.31 Types of exocrine tubular and alveolar glands (schematic), illustrating varying degrees of differentiation (simple, simple branched, compound).

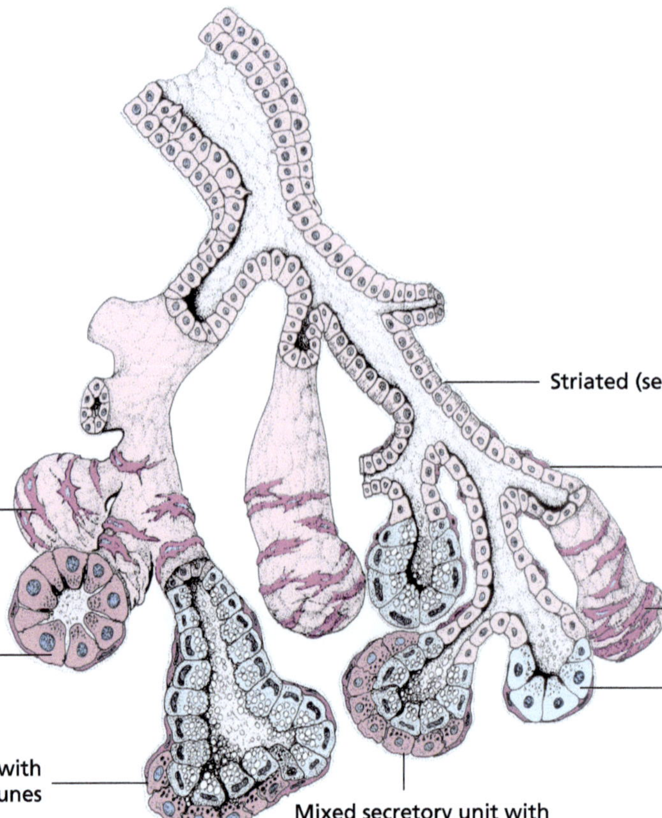

2.33 Serous, mucous and mixed secretory units of a compound tubulo-acinar gland with myoepithelial cells (schematic). See also Chapter 10, 'Digestive system'.

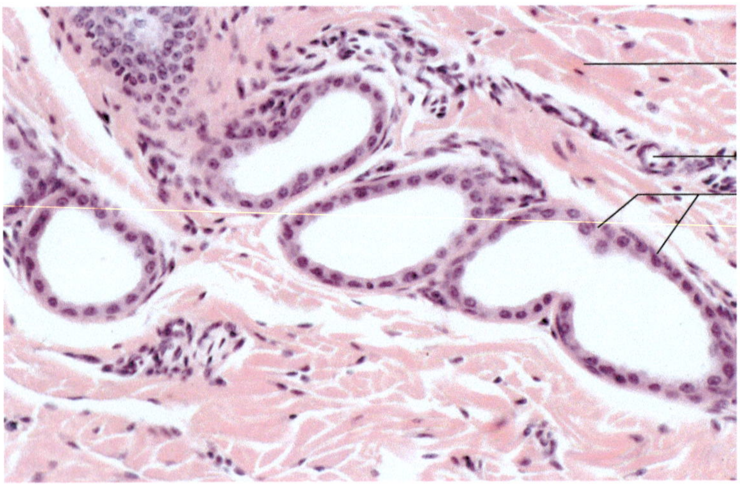

2.34 Sweat gland, skin (calf). Sweat glands are typically simple coiled tubular glands. In this histological section, several cross-sections of the same gland are evident. The gland is lined by a single layer of cuboidal epithelium that produces a watery secretion (sweat). Sweat glands are classified as extra-epithelial, exocrine, tubular merocrine or apocrine glands. Haematoxylin and eosin stain (x250).

content of the granules is released at the cell surface by exocytosis. In this process, the membrane of the secretory vesicle fuses with the apical plasmalemma and the secretory product is discharged into the extracellular space. The cell structure thus remains intact. This type of secretion is usually continuous. It is the most common secretory mechanism and occurs in the exocrine pancreas and in the endocrine glands.

In **apocrine secretion** (Figures 2.35, 2.36 to 2.38), the secretory granule is pinched off from the free cell surface together with a small amount of cytoplasm. Secretory granules are formed in the supranuclear region of the

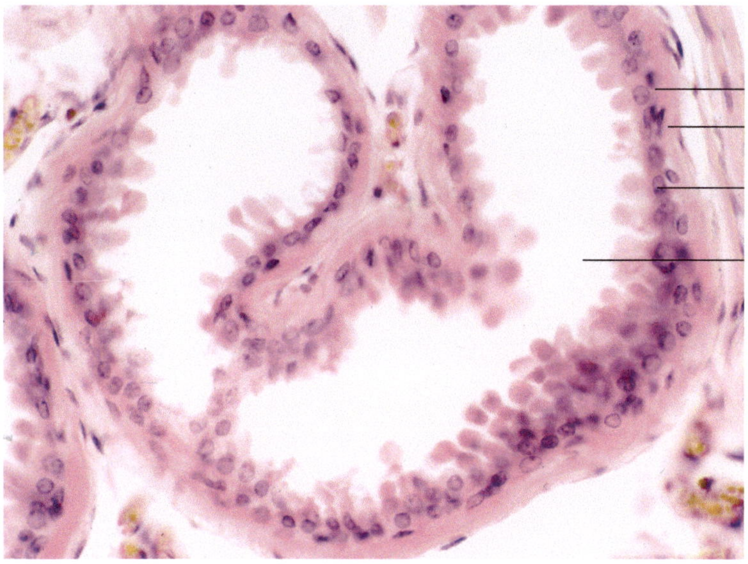

2.35 Apocrine secretion in a sweat gland, skin (pig). The cell surface bulges into the lumen of the tubular gland and the plasmalemma constricts around the secretory granule and adjacent cytoplasm, eventually separating both from the cell surface. Apocrine sweat glands produce scents used in communication. Haematoxylin and eosin stain (x480).

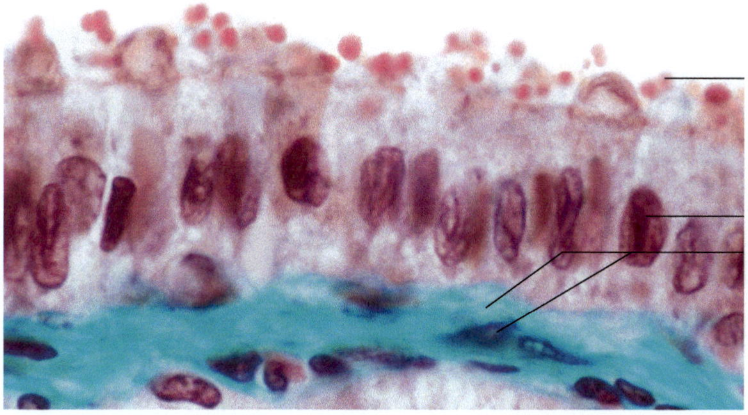

2.36 Apocrine secretion by columnar epithelial cells, epididymal duct (bull). Secretion occurs by vesicular constriction of the plasmalemma around the secretory product and adjacent cytoplasm. Goldner's Masson trichrome stain (x720).

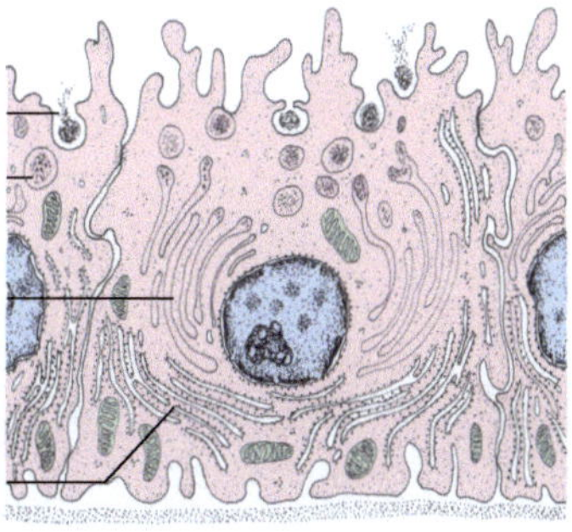

2.37 Merocrine mode of secretion (schematic). The secretion is discharged at the cell surface.

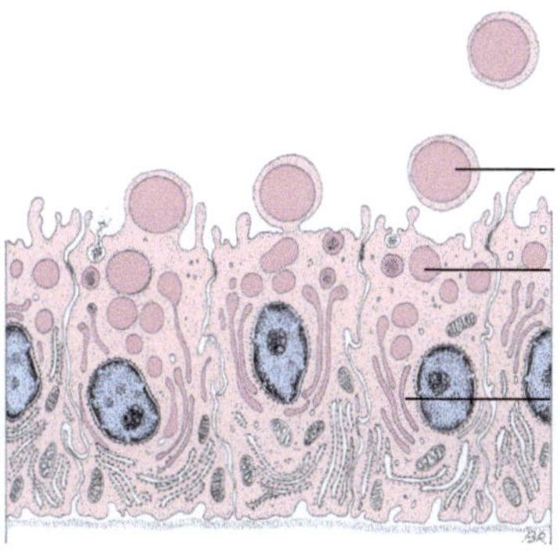

2.38 Apocrine mode of secretion (schematic). The secretion is surrounded by plasmalemma.

cytoplasm before migrating towards the apical cell surface. During the subsequent secretory process the cell changes in shape, its apical surface bulging into the lumen, but retains its functional integrity. Most sweat glands are of the apocrine type (Figure 2.35). Apocrine glands also occur in the eyelids and form the lining of the alveolae of the mammary gland and prostate gland.

In the **holocrine** mode of secretion, the secretory product is produced via fatty degeneration of the cell with the cell remnants forming part of the secretion (e.g. sebaceous gland). Characteristic features of this cellular transformation include the continuous accumulation of fat droplets and the shrinking and subsequent disintegration of the nucleus (pyknosis and karyorrhexis) in the apical portion of the cell (Figures 2.39 to 2.42).

CHEMICAL COMPOSITION OF THE SECRETION

Based on the **chemical composition of the secretion** and the **structure of the cells in the secretory unit**, exocrine glands may be classified as (Tables 2.2 and 2.3):

- serous,
- mucous or
- seromucous (mixed) glands.

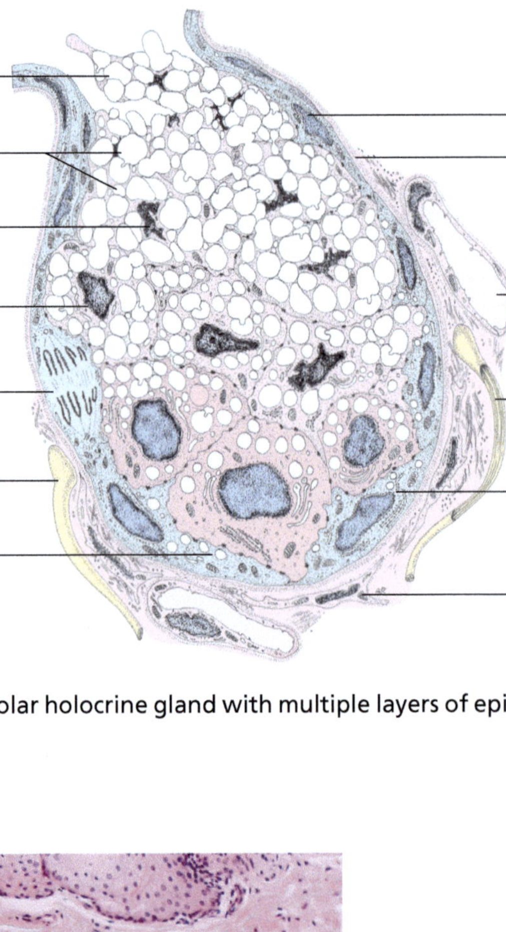

2.39 Exocrine, extra-epithelial, alveolar holocrine gland with multiple layers of epithelial cells (sebaceous gland; schematic).

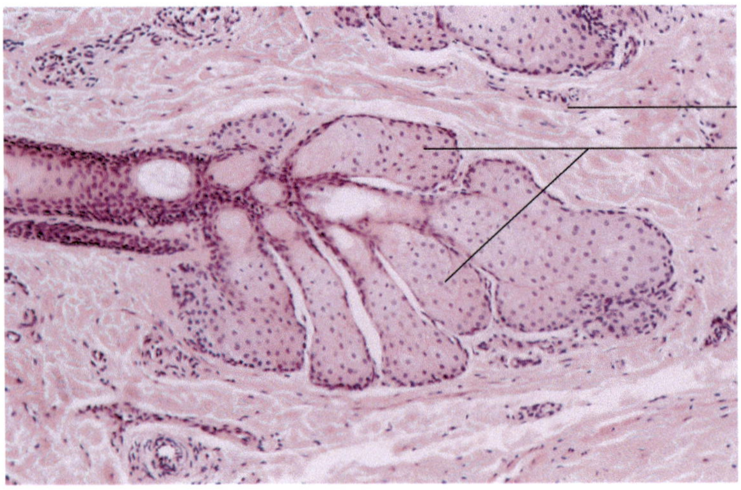

2.40 Skin (dog). In sebaceous glands, lipid produced by the Golgi apparatus is secreted together with the components of the disintegrating cell, as sebum. The secretion passes via a short duct to be deposited onto the surface of an associated hair. Sebaceous glands are classified as extra-epithelial exocrine, alveolar, holocrine glands. Haematoxylin and eosin stain (x200).

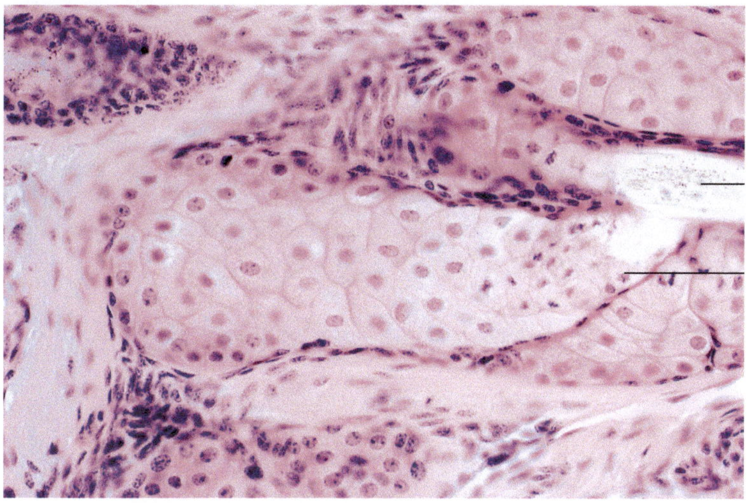

2.41 Skin (dog). Sebaceous gland with adjacent hair shaft. Haematoxylin and eosin stain (x480).

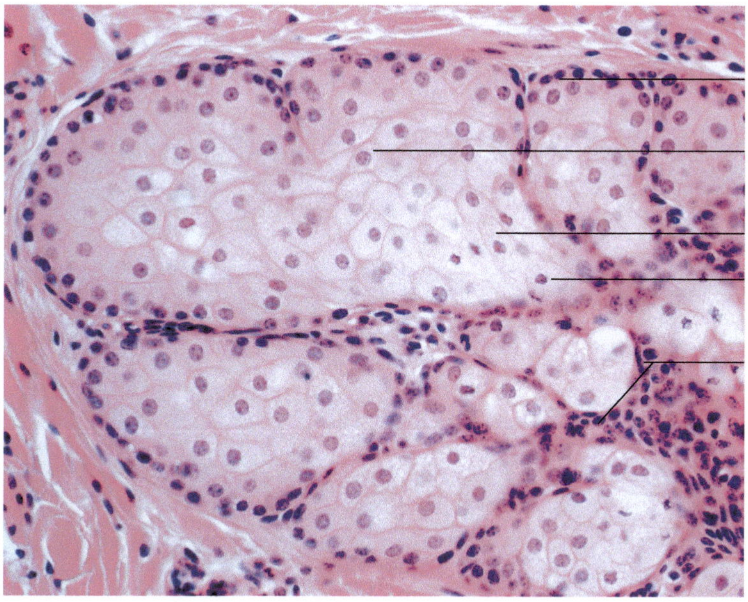

2.42 Skin (dog). Partial sections of numerous sebaceous glands illustrating basal epithelial cells, mature epithelial cells and fragmentation of the nucleus and cytoplasm in the formation of sebum. Haematoxylin and eosin stain (x480).

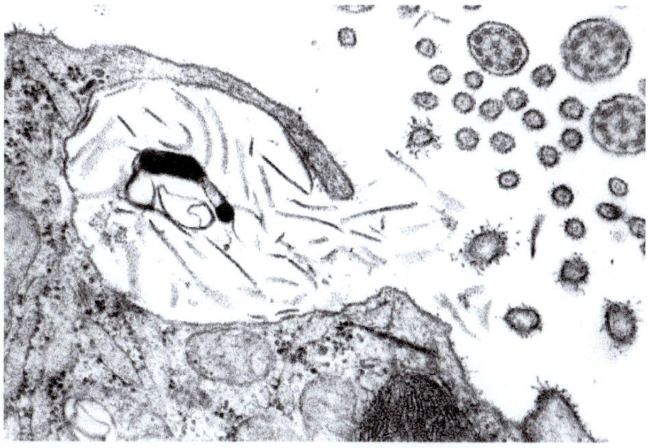

2.43 Merocrine secretion of predominantly lamellar material at the free surface of the epithelium. Oviduct, sheep (x16,000).

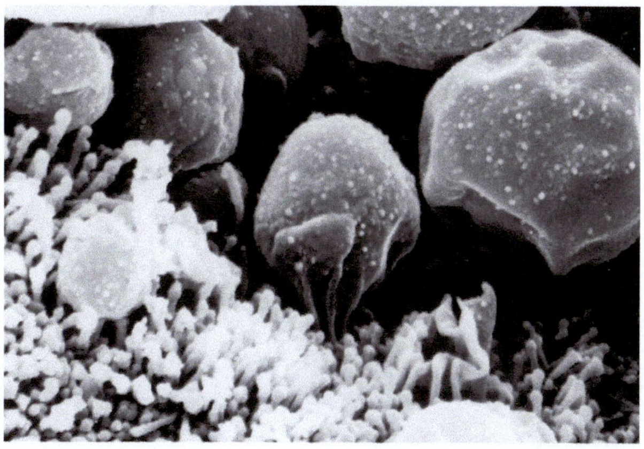

2.44 Scanning electron micrograph showing apocrine secretory granules with underlying microvilli of glandular cells. Gastric mucosa, dog (x15,000).

Serous glands (glandulae serosae) produce a watery secretion rich in protein and enzymes. The nuclei of the cells of the secretory units are usually spherical and are located centrally or slightly towards the base of the cell. Secretory granules of serous glands have a dense centre and a paler rim. The cytoplasm of the secretory cells is acidophilic and the lumen of the secretory unit is narrow. Other morphological cellular features include pronounced infolding of the basement membrane and finger-like interdigitations between neighbouring cells. Intercellular channels (**secretory capillaries**) bounded by zonulae occludentes may be present apically, permitting a transient increase in the secretory surface of the cell. Microvilli are present on the luminal surface (Figures 2.33, 2.45 and 2.46).

Mucous glands (glandulae mucosae) produce **mucin**, a glycoprotein with side chains containing oligosaccharides (incorporating glucose, galactose, mannose, N-acetylhexosamine and sialic acid). The secretory cells of mucous glands are usually arranged in a single layer and are pyramidal in shape, with a blunted point at their apical surface. The cell borders are well demarcated, and the lumen of the secretory unit is relatively wide. Typically, basophilic, densely staining flattened nuclei lie at the base of the cell. The cytoplasm has a foamy, vacuolated appearance, as the mucinogen (mucin precursor) within the cell is largely lost during histological processing (Figures 2.33, 2.47 and 2.48). Mucin stains pale blue with haematoxylin and eosin, and bright magenta with the PAS technique. Mucin also stains strongly with alcian blue, due to the high sialic acid and polysaccharide content of the mucin molecule. Mucin is found in many glandular secretions, particularly those of the salivary glands. It serves as both a protectant and a lubricant. The protein component of the mucinogen molecule is produced by the rER, while the carbohydrate portion is synthesised by the Golgi apparatus. Mucinogen is stored within the cell in pro-secretory granules. On secretion into the lumen of the secretory unit, mucinogen is hydrated to form mucin.

Seromucous (**mixed**) **glands** (glandulae seromucosae) contain both serous cells and mucous cells. The former produce a secretion high in protein; the latter secrete proteoglycans and mucin. The serous secretory units appear to form half-moon-shaped caps (**serous demilunes, crescents of Gianuzzi**) around the mucous units. However,

Table 2.2 Structural differences between serous and mucous gland cells.

Characteristic	Serous gland cell	Mucous gland cell
Shape of cell	Wedge-shaped to pyramidal, broader at base than apex	Columnar or pyramidal
Shape and position of nucleus	Spherical (round in cross-section), lightly staining, central to basal half of cell	Flattened, densely staining, at margin of cell base
Staining of cytoplasm	Haematoxylin and eosin: basophilic (blue) in basal region, eosinophilic (red) apically	Basophilic in basal region, pale in supranuclear region
Function	Protein synthesis	Mucin synthesis

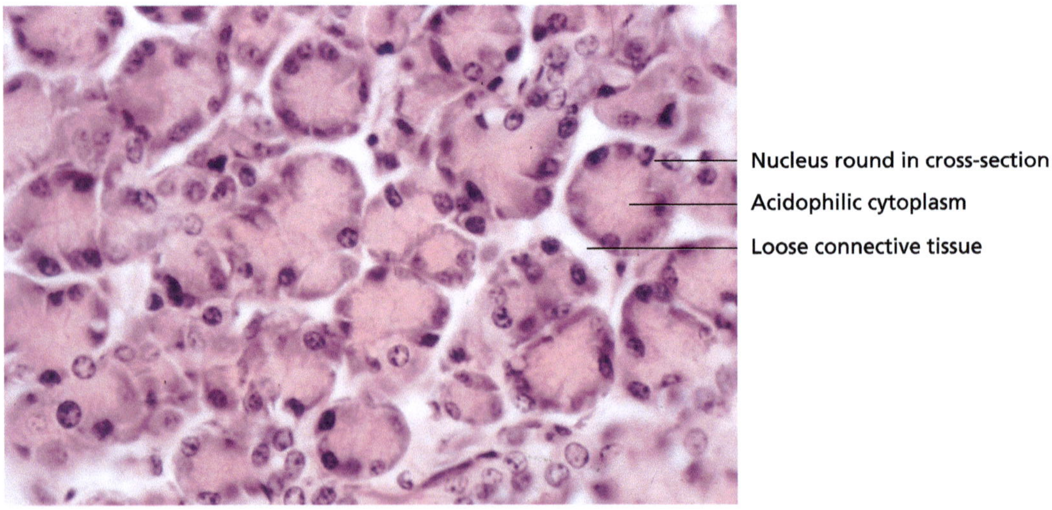

2.45 Parotid gland, horse. The serous secretory units are acinar. The cytoplasm of the secretory cells is acidophilic and the nuclei are spherical. The lumen into which the thin, watery secretion is discharged is often collapsed and is difficult to identify on histological sections. Haematoxylin and eosin stain (x480).

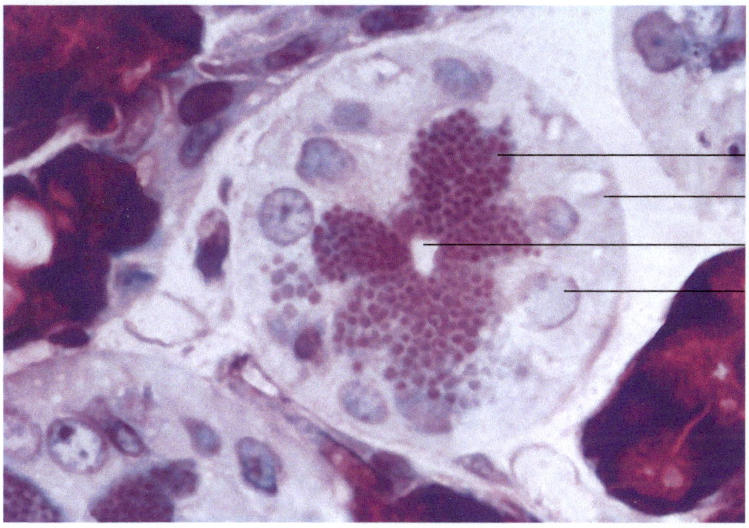

2.46 Parotid gland (dog). Serous secretory units are characterised by a narrow lumen and spherical nuclei. As seen in this image, the secretory granules can be clearly demonstrated with methylene blue and safranin staining (x720).

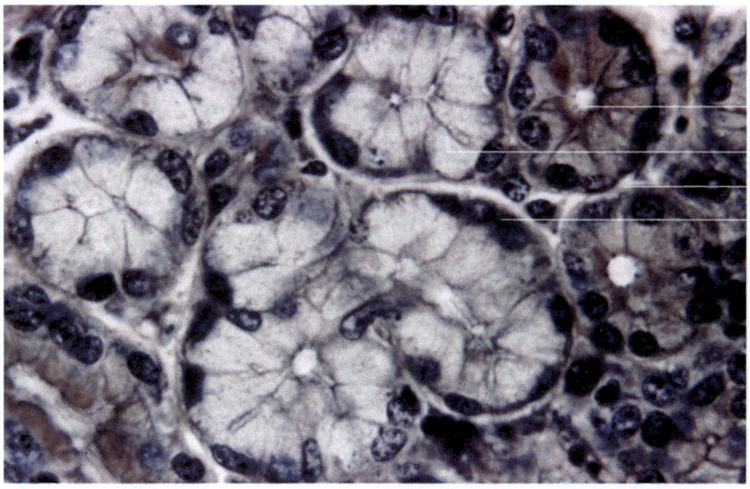

2.47 Labial gland, dog. Mucous secretory units are distinguished by a relatively large lumen (for the collection and transport of the thick secretory product), pale cytoplasm filled with mucinogen and marginally positioned, flattened nuclei. Iron haematoxylin stain (x600).

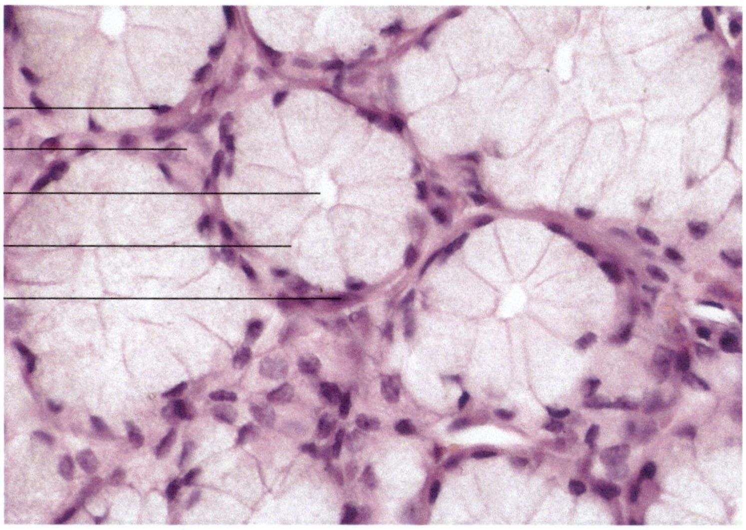

2.48 Mandibular gland (dog). The lumen of mucous secretory units is typically relatively wide, facilitating the transport of the mucous secretion. This is further supported by the contractile function of the peripherally located myoepithelial cells. Haematoxylin and eosin stain (x720).

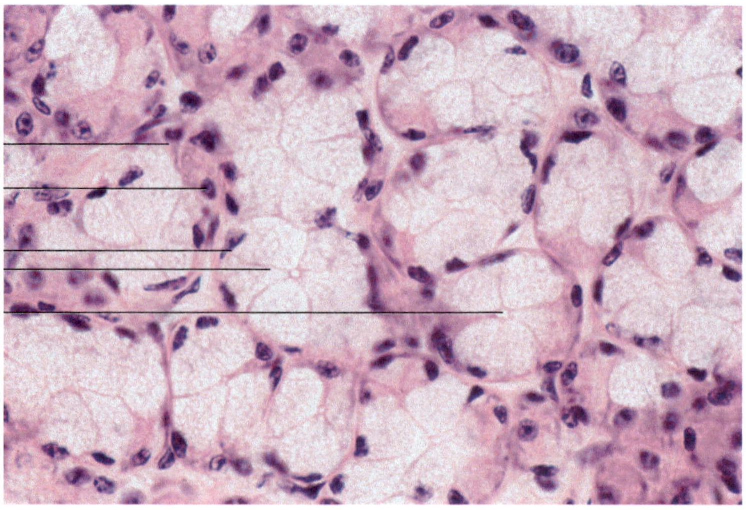

2.49 Sublingual gland (ox). Mixed secretory units of seromucous glands are characterised by a predominantly lightly staining mucous portion and an acidophilic serous component (serous demilune). Haematoxylin and eosin stain (x480).

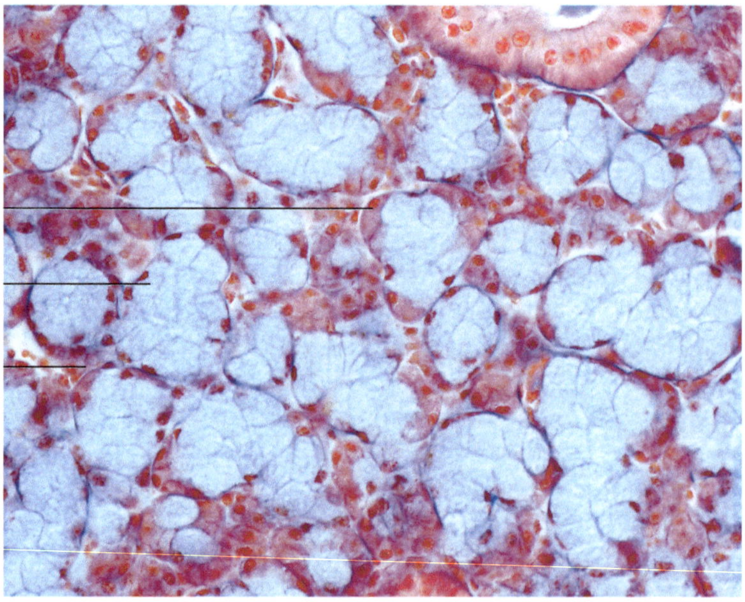

2.50 Sublingual gland (ox). The cap-like arrangement of the serous component of mixed (seromucous) glands can be demonstrated clearly using the Azan staining method, in which the mucous portions stain blue. Azan stain (x400).

recent findings based on electron microscopy techniques suggest that these cells occupy the same row as the mucous cells.

In some cases, mixed glands contain cells that produce both serous and mucous secretory product.

Based on the **chemical composition of the secretion**, exocrine glands may also be classified as **homocrine** or **heterocrine**. Homocrine glands produce only one type of secretion (e.g. the serous secretory product of the parotid gland of the horse). Heterocrine glands contain different types of secretory units and produce a mixed secretion (e.g. mixed secretion of the sublingual gland of the ox).

Germinal epithelia and epithelial tissue featuring specialisations for sensation, excretion and transport are described in subsequent relevant chapters.

Table 2.3 Structural elements of exocrine glands.

Morphological feature	Gland type	Examples
Number of secretory cells	Unicellular	Goblet cells
	Multicellular	Salivary gland
Location of the secretory cells with respect to the surface epithelium	Intra-epithelial glands	Goblet cells
	Extra-epithelial glands	All large exocrine glands
Shape of the secretory unit	Tubular	Glands of large intestine
	Acinar	Parotid gland, exocrine pancreas
	Alveolar	Sebaceous glands
	Tubulo-alveolar/tubulo-acinar	Sublingual gland
Structure of duct system	Single secretory units with a duct opening onto an epithelial surface	Sweat glands
	Branched glands with multiple secretory units that open into an unbranched duct	Gastric glands
	Compound glands in which multiple secretory units open into a strongly branched duct system	All large salivary glands
Mode of secretion	Merocrine (eccrine)	Most exocrine glands
	Apocrine	Scent (apocrine sweat) glands, mammary gland
	Holocrine	Sebaceous glands
Chemical composition of secretion	Serous	Parotid gland, exocrine pancreas
	Mucous	Pyloric glands
	Seromucous	Sublingual gland, mandibular gland, glands of the airways

3

Connective and supportive tissues (textus connectivus)

Connective and supportive tissues include a structurally and functionally diverse range of tissues that, except for the ectodermally derived connective tissue of the rostral head, originate from mesoderm. Thus, they are never located on the surface of the body. Connective and supportive tissues are integral in forming the framework of the body and the structure of organs. They perform mechanical and supportive roles, and participate actively in the exchange of substances between the vascular system and specific tissues. Connective tissue is also involved in cellular and humoral defence mechanisms, and contributes to thermoregulation and hydroregulation. Several connective tissues permanently retain their mesodermally derived capacity for regeneration and transformation.

Structure of connective and supportive tissues

Morphologically, connective and supportive tissues consist of:

- cells and
- intercellular matrix.

Cells

The cells of the connective and supportive tissues are derived from **embryonic mesenchymal cells**. Through their multiple processes, these cells form a loose, predominantly three-dimensional network. Their oval nucleus contains little heterochromatin.

Embryonic mesenchymal cells are **pluripotent,** capable of differentiating into either **resident cells** (cells that remain fixed within connective and supportive tissue) or **transient** or **wandering cells** (cells that enter the tissue in response to particular stimuli).

Resident cells

Resident cells of connective tissue include fibroblasts and adipocytes. Connective tissue macrophages (histiocytes) and mast cells are also fixed residents of connective tissue. However, as these are derived from the blood, they are considered in some classification systems to be wandering ('free') cells. Chondroblasts and osteoblasts are permanent residents of the supportive tissues, cartilage and bone.

Fibroblasts, chondroblasts and osteoblasts produce fibres, cartilage and bone, respectively, before differentiat-

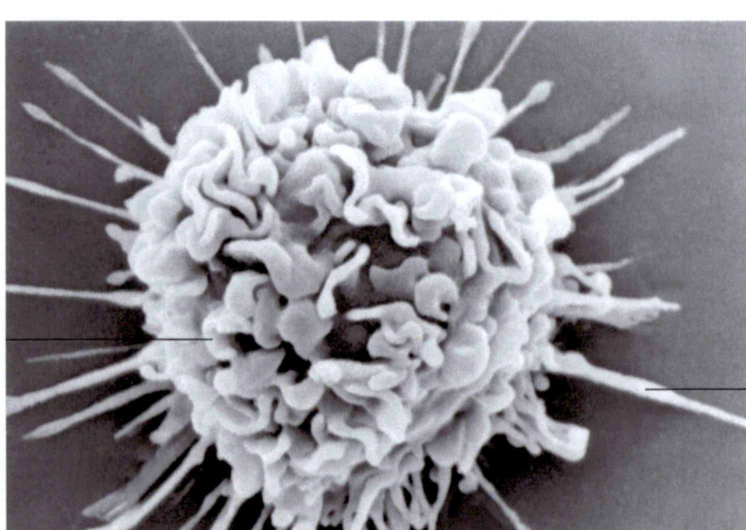

3.1 Scanning electron micrograph of a macrophage isolated from peritoneal fluid (x1000).

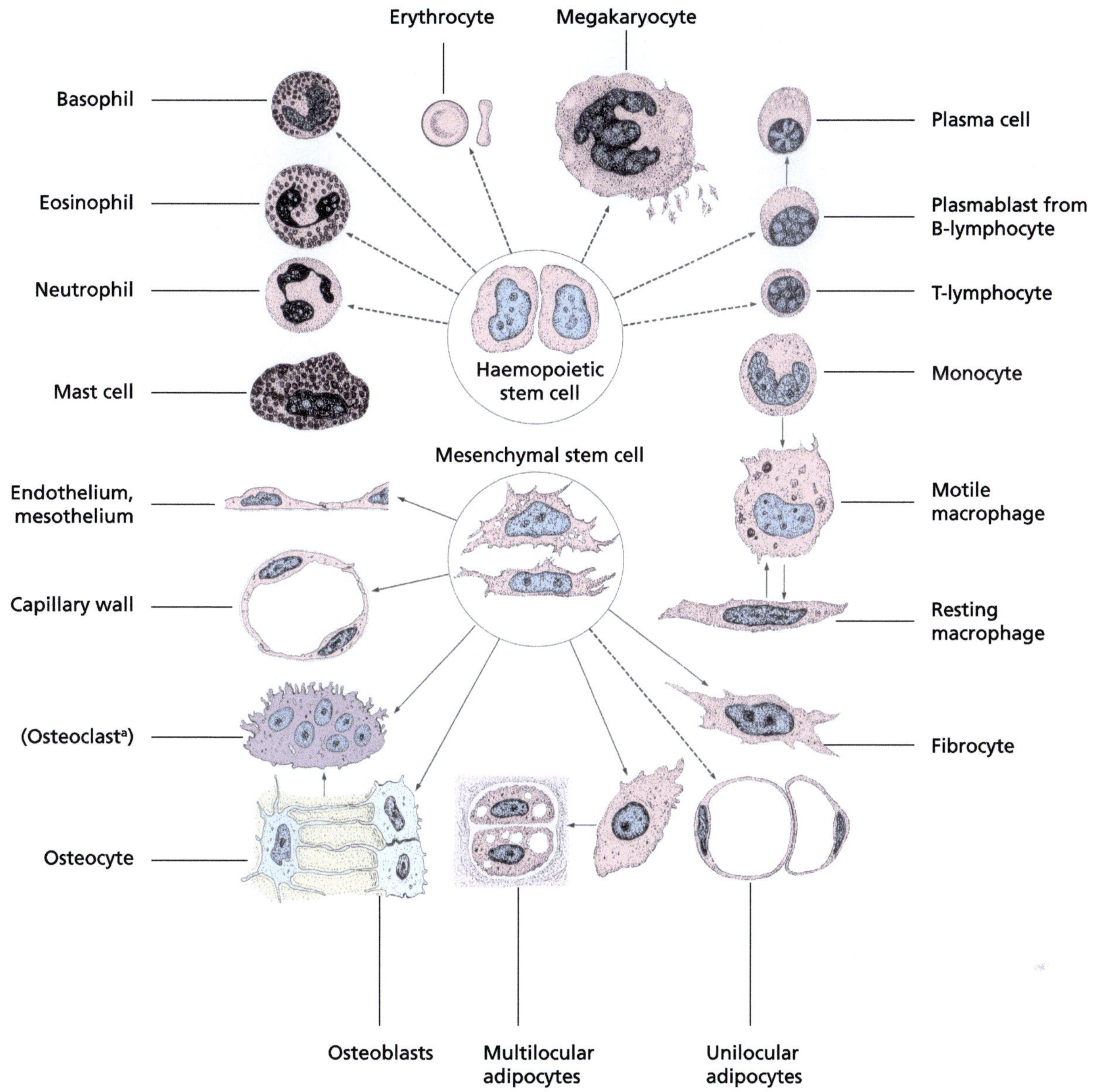

3.2 Differentiation of cells from the mesoderm (schematic). [a] Via fusion of mononuclear precursor cells of granulocyte-monocyte line.

ing further into mature, less active fibrocytes, chondrocytes and osteocytes.

Fibroblasts have irregularly developed cell processes and nuclei rich in euchromatin. Their cytoplasm contains numerous organelles that are dedicated primarily to protein biosynthesis (rough endoplasmic reticulum, ribosomes, Golgi apparatus). Fibroblasts synthesise the fibres and ground substance of the extracellular matrix.

Fibrocytes are small, spindle-shaped cells that usually lie between bundles of fibres. Under the light microscope their nuclei appear dense and elongated. The cytoplasm is weakly acidophilic with few metabolically active organelles.

Histiocytes, or **connective tissue macrophages**, are derived from circulating monocytes that enter the tissue and differentiate into macrophages (Figure 3.1). They are relatively numerous in loose connective tissue where, in their resting form, they may be difficult to distinguish from fibroblasts. The primary function of histiocytes is localised phagocytosis. Histiocytes can move freely in an amoeboid fashion through the tissue. Their nucleus is round to oval and the cell surface appears irregular due to the presence of numerous processes (pseudopodia). The cytoplasm contains granules (lysosomes). In addition to their endo- and phagocytic function, histiocytes (macrophages) have a role in antigen presentation and the immune response. They synthesise proteins (e.g. interferon, complement, cytokines) that act as immune mediators (see Chapter 8, 'Immune system and lymphatic organs'). The lifespan of active macrophages is approximately 2–3 months.

Mast cells are large cells (20–30 μm) found in loose connective tissue, particularly around blood vessels (Figure 3.3). They are typically ovoid with dense, ellipsoid nuclei. The cytoplasm encloses numerous basophilic metachromatic granules containing substances including **histamine**, **heparin** and **chemotactic factors**. In addition, mast cells synthesise **prostaglandins**, **leukotrienes** and **platelet-stimulating factors** through which they influence the diameter and permeability of vessels. The surface of mast cells expresses specific receptors for immunoglobulin E. Under certain circumstances, antigenic substances bind with these receptors, triggering the sudden release of chemical mediators from the cell (allergic reaction). A distinction is made between mucosal and connective tissue mast cells. Mast cells have a long lifespan, surviving weeks to months.

Chondroblasts, osteoblasts and adipocytes are described below. Other cell types sometimes included in the resident cell population of connective tissue are reticular cells (see below) and pericytes (see Chapter 6, 'Circulatory system').

Transient cells

Transient (wandering) cells are found primarily in loose connective tissue, in which the fibre content is relatively low. These cells continuously undergo active migration from the blood and lymphatic vascular systems into the extravascular space, where they pass through spaces in the interstitium. They are capable of amoeboid motility, which some use to re-enter the circulatory system. Transient cells include:

- lymphocytes,
- plasma cells,
- monocytes and
- granulocytes.

Lymphocytes are small spherical cells (8 μm). Their strongly basophilic nucleus is surrounded by a thin band of cytoplasm that appears pale under light microscopy.

Medium (10–18 μm) to large (15–25 μm) lymphocytes are also present in connective tissue. Lymphocytes are found in epithelia, the blood and lymphatic vascular systems, in subepithelial tissue and in lymphatic organs. They are involved primarily in acquired **cell-mediated** and **humoral immunity**. Pluripotent haemopoietic cells originating from the bone marrow differentiate into lymphocytic progenitor cells that pass to the thymus, where they differentiate further and reach a state of immunocompetence (**T lymphocytes**). These are the agents of **cell-mediated immunity**. Other lymphocytic stem cells differentiate in the bone marrow, Peyer's patches and tonsils (in mammals) or the bursa of Fabricius (birds) into immunocompetent **B lymphocytes**, which are responsible for the **humoral immune response** (see Chapter 7, 'Blood and haemopoiesis' and Chapter 8, 'Immune system and lymphatic organs').

Plasma cells are ovoid basophilic cells (20 μm) derived from B lymphocytes. The heterochromatin is concentrated in peripheral clumps, giving the nucleus a 'cartwheel' appearance. Plasma cells synthesise antibodies (**immunoglobulins**). This is reflected in the abundant endoplasmic reticulum and numerous free ribosomes within the cytoplasm. In the presence of chronic infection, the endoplasmic reticulum may contain acidophilic inclusions (Russell bodies).

Plasma cells are routinely found in subepithelial connective tissue of the gastric and intestinal mucosa, in germinal centres within lymphatic organs and in excretory glands. They possess limited amoeboid motility and most have a lifespan of 10–30 days.

Monocytes are predominantly ovoid cells (20 μm) with an indented, kidney-shaped heterochromatin-rich nucleus (Figure 3.4). The abundant cytoplasm contains large

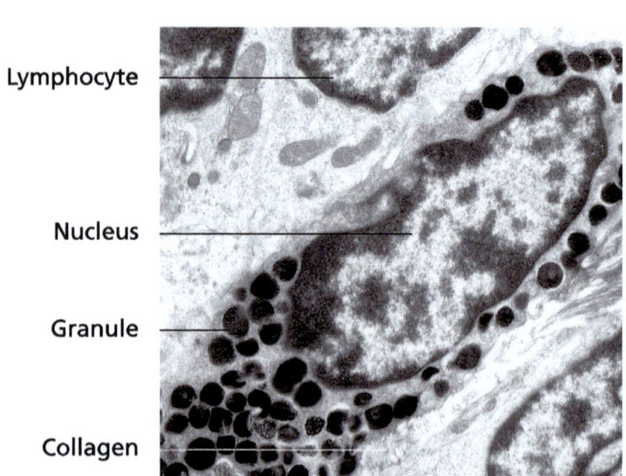

3.3 Tissue mast cell with numerous granules and adjacent lymphocytes (x3000).

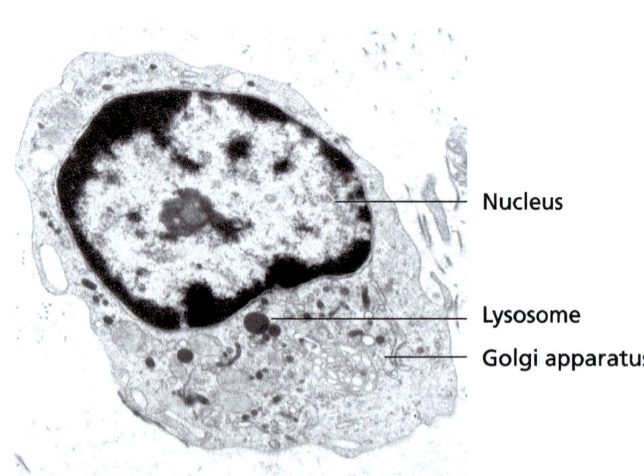

3.4 Monocyte in loose connective tissue (x6000).

numbers of metabolically active organelles (mitochondria, Golgi apparatus, ER) as well as azurophilic granules (lysosomes). Monocytes migrate from the blood vessels into the tissue, where they differentiate into macrophages.

Granulocytes are described in Chapter 8, 'Immune system and lymphatic organs'.

Intercellular matrix (substantia intercellularis)

The intercellular matrix is composed of **fibres** and **amorphous ground substance**. Both are produced by **connective tissue cells**, particularly **fibroblasts.** Other, closely related, cells, such as chondroblasts and osteoblasts, are also capable of synthesising intercellular matrix. The function of the extracellular matrix is determined by its biochemical composition: the proportion of fibres has a significant impact on the pliability, elasticity and flexibility of the tissue, while the amount of glycosaminoglycans in the amorphous ground substance influences the capacity for binding of extracellular water molecules. The metabolic activity of the connective tissue is regulated by hormones, particularly growth hormone, corticosteroids and oestrogens.

Fibroblasts (Figures 3.5 and 3.6) synthesise:

- **fibres**:
  - collagen fibres,
  - reticular fibres,
  - elastic fibres,
- **amorphous ground substance**:
  - proteoglycans and
  - structural glycoproteins.

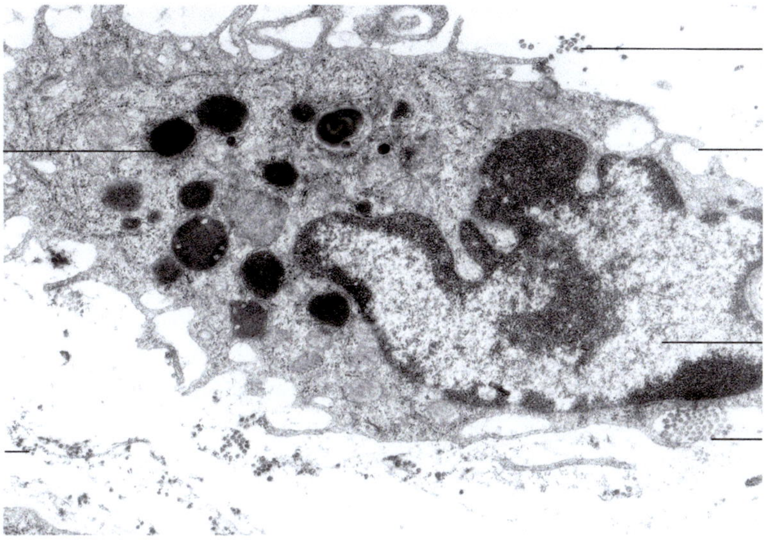

3.5 Fibroblast with dense granules, multiple cell processes and bundles of collagen fibrils (x5000).

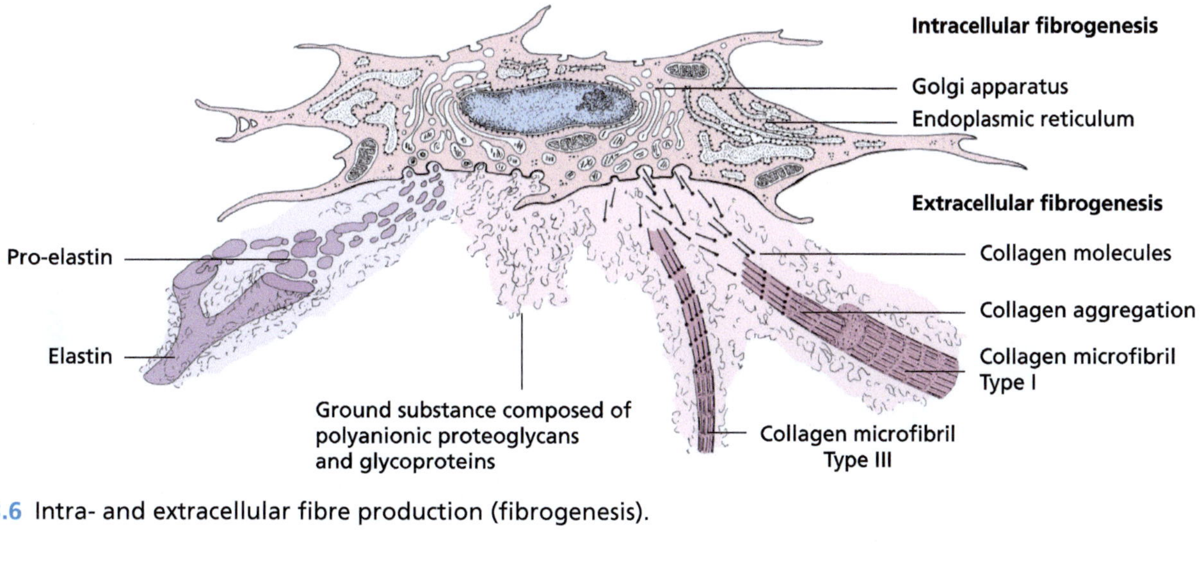

3.6 Intra- and extracellular fibre production (fibrogenesis).

Connective tissue fibres

COLLAGEN FIBRES (FIBRA COLLAGENOSA)

The scleroprotein collagen is the most commonly occurring type of connective tissue fibre. It performs specific **protective** and **supportive functions** in several tissues (e.g. skin, neuronal sheaths, tendons and ligaments, cartilage and bone). Collagen fibres also make up the **interstitial connective tissue** surrounding nerves and vessels, and form the **stroma** that binds together the functional tissue (parenchyma) of various organs.

Collagen fibres (Figures 3.7 and 3.10) have characteristic chemical and physical properties: they swell in acid environments, undergo partial digestion in gastric secretions (pepsin) and dissolve completely in alkali. Under polarised light, collagen fibres are uniaxially birefringent (anisotropic). This is attributable to their transverse banding (Figure 3.10; see also below). Due to their molecular structure, collagen fibres have a high tensile strength with a maximum stretching capacity of only 5% (Table 3.1).

The **arrangement** of collagen fibres varies with the type of connective tissue. Particularly in loose connective tissue, the fibres exhibit an undulating course. In dense irregular connective tissue such as fascia and aponeuroses, they are generally interwoven in a criss-crossing pattern. The collagen fibres of tendons are predominantly arranged in parallel (Figures 3.20 and 3.21).

Collagen fibres are synthesised by specific cells, including fibroblasts, chondroblasts and osteoblasts. The process of collagen production includes an intra- and an extracellular phase (Figures 3.5 and 3.6).

In the intracellular phase, the polypeptide collagen precursor **pro-collagen** is formed. Initially, structurally similar chains of over 1000 amino acids (α_1- and α_2-chains) are produced by the **ribosomes** of the **rough endoplasmic reticulum**. The resulting pro-α-chains are primarily composed of glycine, proline and alanine, with non-helical extensions (pro-peptides) at each end.

Within the endoplasmic reticulum, the proline and lysine residues are hydroxylated and the pro-α-chains are joined to form **triple** (**super**) **helices**. Galactosyl and glucosyl residues are added in the **Golgi apparatus**. The completed pro-collagen molecule is released from the Golgi apparatus within secretory vesicles that pass along microtubules to the cell surface before being released by exocytosis into the **extracellular space**.

This is followed by cleavage of the pro-peptides by the enzyme pro-collagen peptidase. The shortened triple helices, termed **collagen molecules** (formerly **tropocollagen**), are approximately 280 nm in length. Collagen molecules aggregate by polymerisation to form **collagen fibrils**. In this process, individual collagen molecules join end to end (with a gap between consecutive molecules) to form a microfibril. Covalent cross-linkages are also formed between adjacent microfibrils. It is thought that the formation of microfibrils is initiated by **electrostatic attraction** between neighbouring collagen molecules, which results in a staggered arrangement of the microfibrils (thus, also, staggering of the gaps between collagen molecules). As a result, collagen fibrils exhibit a distinctive **transverse banding pattern** when viewed using electron microscopy. The cross-linking of adjacent microfibrils contributes significantly to the mechanical strength of collagen fibres (Figure 3.10).

Microfibrils (diameter 20–300 nm) combine to form collagen fibrils (diameter 0.2–0.5 μm). Aggregation and cross-linking of fibrils give rise to **collagen fibres** (diameter 1–20 μm). These fibres are unbranched and typically form bundles of varying size.

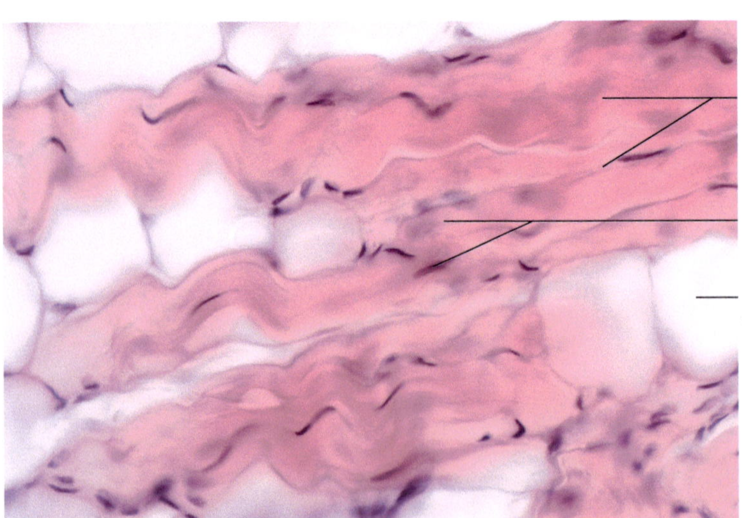

3.7 Skin (dog). Type I collagen fibres in the loose connective tissue are predominantly arranged in parallel; they follow a wave-like course and are unbranched. The nuclei of fibrocytes are flattened and conform to the arrangement of the fibres. Haematoxylin and eosin stain (x480).

Collagen fibres stain with eosin (red), aniline blue (blue) and with the dye light green (from Masson's trichrome; green). They can also be identified using polarised light microscopy based on their banding pattern. Biochemically, collagen fibres are divided into many different types, of which at least five are currently considered of morphological significance. Their distinguishing features include the amino acid sequence of the pro-α-chain and the number of saccharide residues.

Type I collagen is the most abundant form of body collagen (90%), occurring in tendons, fascia, bones, vessels, internal organs and dentin. It consists of two identical chains (α_1) and an additional, different, chain (α_2).

Types II and III consist of three α_1-chains that vary in their amino acid composition (e.g. in hydroxyproline, hydroxylysyl or cysteine residues). **Type II collagen** forms the structural collagen of hyaline cartilage. **Type III collagen** occurs in the walls of vessels, in internal organs (e.g. liver, kidney, spleen), in skin and in embryonic connective tissue. **Type IV** is found in basal laminae. **Type V collagen** is also associated with the basal lamina, and is distributed throughout connective tissue stroma. Types IV and V collagen are rich in hydroxyproline.

RETICULAR FIBRES (FIBRA RETICULARIS)

Reticular fibres derive their name from their finely branched, mesh-like arrangement (Figure 3–8). They form flexible three-dimensional networks within various organs and tissues (liver, kidney, glands, vessels), are associated with basal laminae and form a meshwork around tendons, ligaments and muscle fibres. Reticular fibres play an important supportive role in lympho- and haemoreticular tissues (spleen, lymph nodes, bone marrow) by providing a flexible scaffold.

Immunohistochemical techniques reveal that reticular fibres are composed of type III collagen. Precursor forms are produced within fibroblasts, with polymerisation and formation of microfibrils occurring in the extracellular

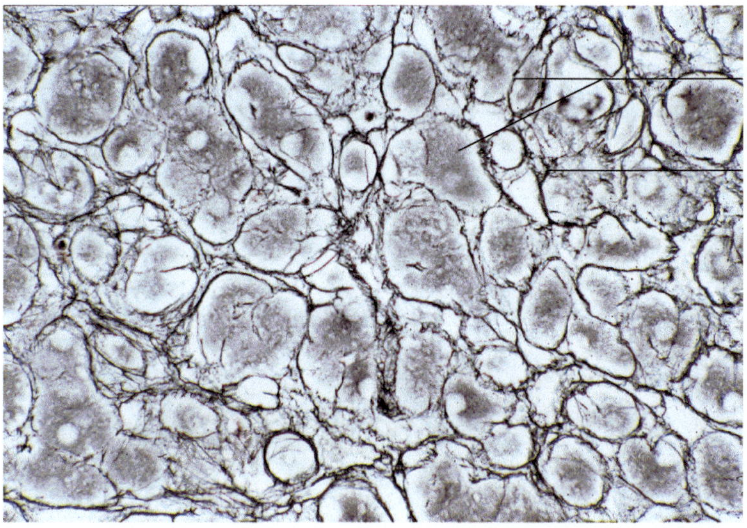

3.8 Ovary (cat). Reticular fibres are branched and can be impregnated with silver salts (argyrophilic fibres). They are composed of type III collagen. Reticular fibres form three-dimensional networks in various organs and in haemo- and lymphoreticular tissues. Achucarro method (x480).

Table 3.1 Comparative characteristics and morphological features of collagen, reticular and elastic fibres.

Characteristic	Collagen fibre	Reticular fibre	Elastic fibre
Soluble in water	Yes	No	No
Soluble in acids	Yes	No	No
Soluble in alkali	Yes	No	No
Digestible by pepsin	Yes	No	No
Digestible by trypsin	Yes	Yes	No
Branching of fibres	No	No	Yes
Branching of fibrils	Yes	Yes	No
Cross-striation	Yes	Yes	No
Refractivity	Weak	Strong	Strong
Resistant to tension	Yes	Yes (?)	No
Elastic under tension	No	Yes (?)	Yes
Elastic	No	No	Yes

space (Figure 3.6). In lymphoreticular tissues, reticular fibres are produced by specialised reticular cells with which they are in close contact.

Reticular fibrils (diameter 20–40 nm) exhibit cross-striations with a periodicity of 64–68 nm (as do collagen type I fibrils). Reticular fibres are delicate, measuring just 0.2–1 µm in diameter. Their surface is coated with proteoglycans and glycoprotein-rich substances (Table 3.1).

Under light microscopy, reticular fibres can be identified using the PAS reaction, or by superficial impregnation with silver salts (**argyrophilic staining**).

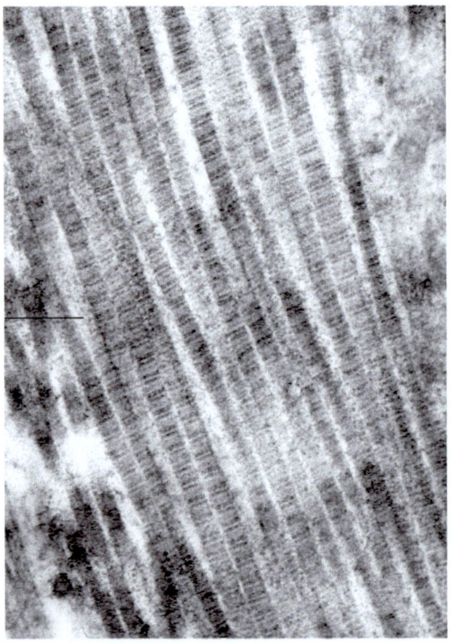

3.10 Collagen fibre bundle with distinct cross-striation of individual fibrils (x20,000).

ELASTIC FIBRES (FIBRA ELASTICA)

Elastic fibres are primarily distinguished from collagen fibres by their pronounced **elasticity** (can be stretched to 150% of their original length) and their marked **refractivity** (Figure 3.9). Elastic fibres exhibit branching and combine to form irregularly expanded networks or fenestrated membranes. They vary in diameter from 0.5 to 5 µm. This fibre type is resistant to acid and alkaline environments.

Elastic fibres are composed of a **central amorphous mass** (pars amorpha) surrounded by a network of **microfibrils** (pars filamentosa). The amorphous substance consists of **elastin**, a substance rich in glycine, alanine and proline.

Elastic fibres are synthesised by fibroblasts and, in some instances, smooth muscle. The cells produce pro-elastin which, as with collagen synthesis (cf. Figure 3.6), is polymerised in the extracellular matrix and deposited on a scaffold of microfibrils. Elastic fibres consist of a three-dimensional network of randomly distributed chains, and therefore lack the cross-striations seen in collagen and reticular fibres (Table 3.1 and Figure 3.9).

Elastic fibres occur in connective tissue as individual fibres or in bundles. They form the foundation for elastic tissues (e.g. elastic cartilage, wall of the aorta, internal and external elastic membranes of arteries) and elastic ligaments (e.g. nuchal ligament, ligamentum flavum). Elastic fibres can be specially stained using resorcin (red), aldehyde fuchsin (dark blue), van Gieson stain (red) and orcein (black).

An overview of the characteristics of the different connective tissue fibres is provided in Table 3.1, which illustrates that collagen and elastic fibres are consistently different while reticular fibres exhibit certain similarities with both of the other fibre types.

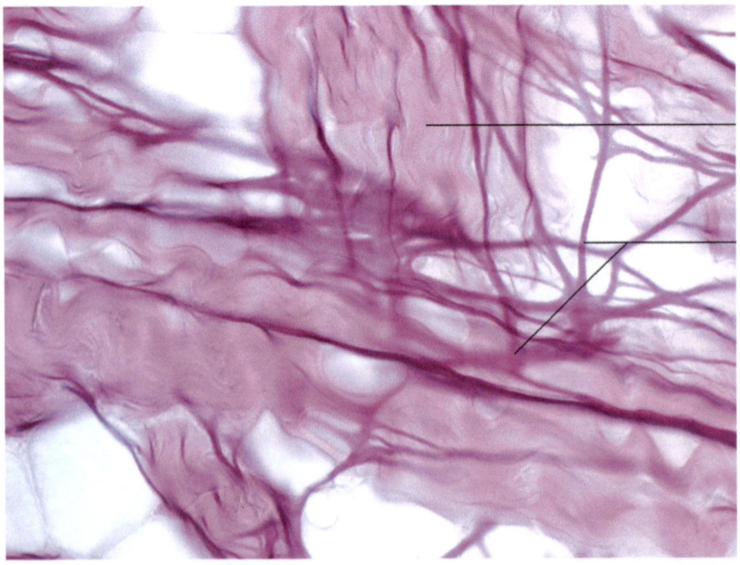

3.9 Skin (dog). Elastic fibres form web-like membranes. Even without staining, elastic fibres are strongly refractive. They do not exhibit cross-striations. Resorcin fuchsin stain (x480).

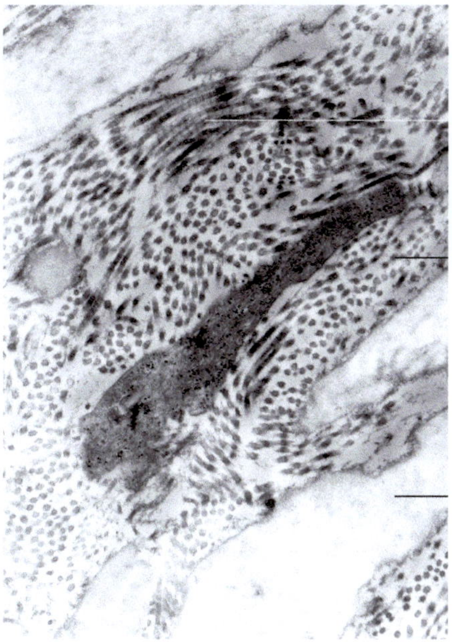

3.11 Collagen fibre bundles (longitudinal and transverse section) with enclosed elastic fibre (x6000).

Ground substance

The cells and fibres of connective and supportive tissues are embedded in a viscous, amorphous ground substance. The nature of the ground substance contributes to the characteristics of the tissue (e.g. the suppleness of connective tissue proper, the pliant yet pressure-resistant nature of cartilage or the mechanical strength of bone). All substances passing between the lumen of capillaries and the target organs of the body, be they solids, liquids or gases, must traverse the ground substance of the connective tissue.

Biochemically, ground substance is composed of polyanionic proteoglycans and structural glycoproteins. Proteoglycans contain a considerably greater proportion of carbohydrate than protein. They contain linear (unbranched) chains of disaccharide units comprising one of two acetylated sugars (glucosamine and galactosamine) and a uronic acid. Based on their high content of uronate and sulfate esters, these molecules are referred to as acid mucopolysaccharides, or glycosaminoglycans.

Glycosaminoglycans vary considerably in both their sulfate content and degree of acetylation. Consequently, there are various types (e.g. chondroitin sulfate, dermatan sulfate, keratin sulfate and [non-sulfated] hyaluronate) that bestow different characteristics on particular connective tissues. The synthesis of ground substance is hormonally regulated.

The chemical structure of the glycosaminoglycans permits binding of large quantities of cations and water molecules. In addition, the proteoglycan molecules are extensively interconnected. The combination of ground substance and collagen fibres thus forms a metabolically active permeable barrier that regulates extracellular transport of water-soluble molecules. The hydrophilic properties of glycosaminoglycans also allow the fluid content of the connective tissue to be increased or decreased. Connective tissue therefore also serves as a water reservoir (turgor).

Structural glycoproteins are composed of conjugated proteins bound covalently with carbohydrates (monosaccharides). These occur in tendons, cartilage, bone, vessel walls and basal laminae. They are involved in the regulation of connective tissue regeneration and calcification.

Types of connective tissue

Common to most types of connective tissue is their derivation from the **mesoderm**. Definitive classification of the different types of connective tissue is difficult, as they vary greatly and often manifest in transitional forms. Nevertheless, connective tissue is conventionally categorised as:

- embryonic connective tissue:
  - mesenchymal connective tissue,
  - mucous (or gelatinous) connective tissue,
- specialised connective tissue:
  - lymphoreticular connective tissue (lymphatic tissue),
  - haemoreticular connective tissue (haemopoietic tissue),
  - adipose tissue,
- connective tissue proper:
  - loose connective tissue (low fibre content) and
  - dense connective tissue (high fibre content) (Figure 3.12).

Embryonic connective tissue (textus connectivus embryonalis)

In the embryo, the mesoderm gives rise to mesenchymal and mucous connective tissue. Embryonic connective tissue consists of relatively poorly differentiated, widely spaced cells and gel-like ground substance.

The cells of **mesenchymal connective tissue** (**mesenchymal cells**) are predominantly stellate to polymorphous (7–10 μm) with long processes that form a three-dimensional network (Figures 3.13 and 3.14). The nucleus is relatively large and heterochromatic. Cell division is common. The cells, which are capable of phagocytic activity, can detach from the surrounding tissue and migrate through the typically amorphous ground substance in an amoeboid fashion. Mesenchymal cells give rise to the various connective and supportive tissues and their derivatives, most of the muscle cells, the vessels and the endo- and mesothelia.

Mucous connective tissue is derived from mesenchymal tissue. It is found around the umbilical vessels

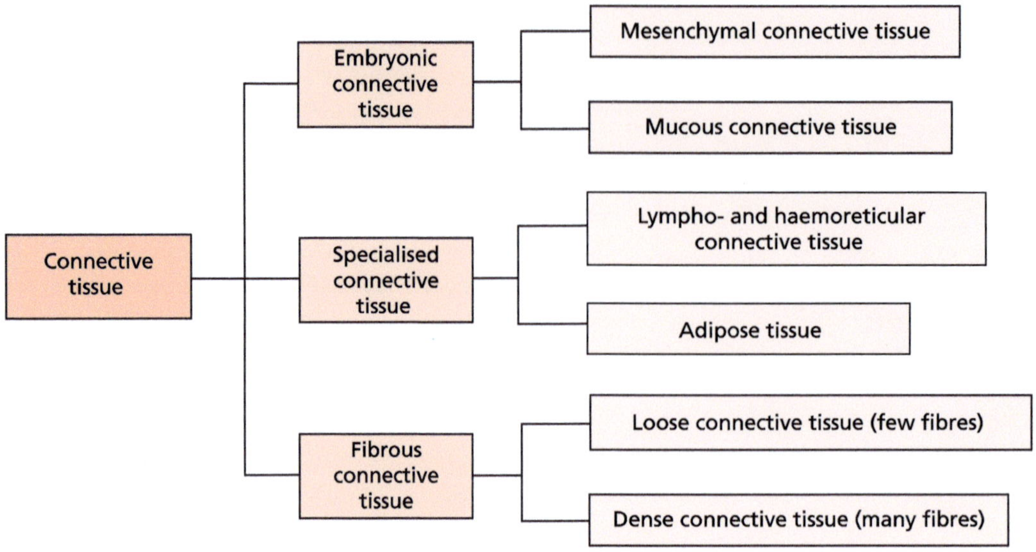

3.12 Classification of connective tissue (schematic).

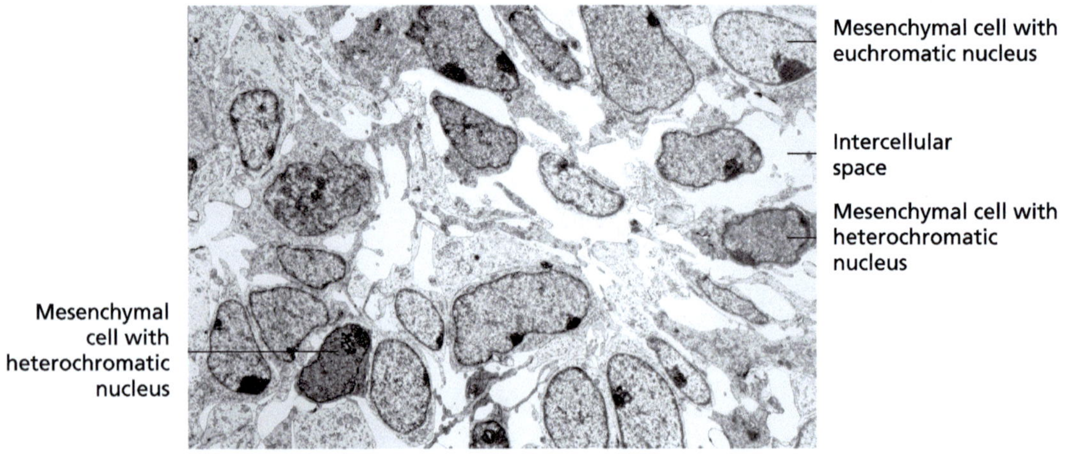

3.13 Fine structure of loosely arranged mesenchymal cells in mesenchymal connective tissue (x3000).

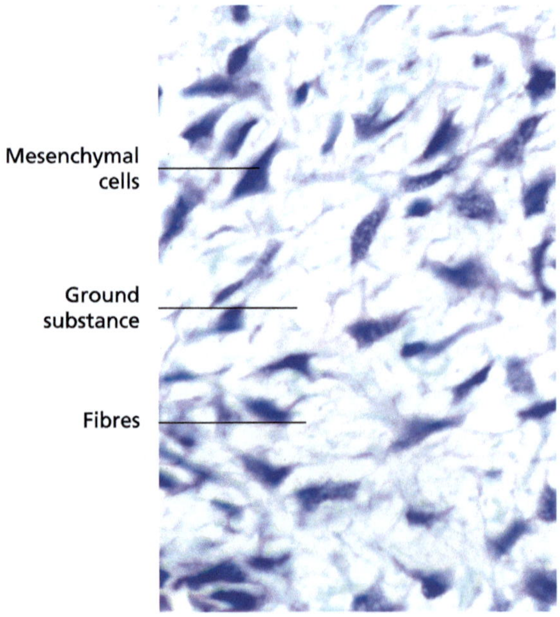

3.14 Mesenchyme (dog). Present mainly during embryonic development, mesenchymal connective tissue forms the foundation of most of the connective and supportive tissues of the body. The cells are connected by delicate cell processes and produce the relatively abundant ground substance. Methylene blue stain (x100).

(Wharton's jelly) and in dental pulp. It consists of a network of fibroblasts and mesenchymal cells that fill the large intercellular spaces with scant quantities of collagen fibrils and larger amounts of amorphous, hyaluronan-rich ground substance. This increases the mechanical strength and water-binding capacity of the tissue. Recent evidence indicates that some of the cells in Wharton's jelly have the potential to differentiate further (Wharton's jelly mesenchymal stem cells). A role for Wharton's jelly (umbilical cord) in cell-mediated immunity has been postulated.

Reticular connective tissue (textus connectivus reticularis)

Reticular connective tissue largely retains the characteristics of undifferentiated mesenchyme. It is composed of an open meshwork of reticular cells and delicate reticular fibres, as well as undifferentiated ground substance.

Reticular cells usually have a large euchromatic nucleus that can increase in density based on the functional status of the cell (**nuclear pleomorphism**). These cells synthesise reticular fibres and phagocytose dead cells and foreign particles. In addition, reticular cells are capable of recognising antigens on the cell surface and signalling this information to immunocompetent cells. With its networks of closely interlinked reticular cells and fibres, reticular connective tissue forms the structural framework of numerous organs (e.g. lymphatic organs, liver, genital organs, subepithelial layers of the gastrointestinal tract).

Lymphoreticular connective tissue (textus connectivus lymphoreticularis)

Lymphoreticular connective tissue (also referred to as lymphatic tissue) is reticular tissue in which the wide intercellular spaces have become populated with **free cells** (macrophages, lymphocytes, plasma cells, monocytes) (Figure 3.15). This tissue forms the stroma of lymphatic organs (lymph nodes, spleen, tonsils, thymus). Lymphoreticular tissue is a significant component of the adaptive and innate immune system (see Chapter 8, 'Immune system and lymphatic organs').

Haemoreticular connective tissue (textus connectivus haemopoeticus)

Reticular connective tissue containing **free blood cells**, or their **stem** or **progenitor cells**, is referred to as **haemoreticular connective tissue** (or haemopoietic tissue, e.g. in bone marrow). Although it is a specialised tissue, it retains its relationship with reticular tissue and may revert to this tissue type or undergo conversion to adipose tissue (see Chapter 7, 'Blood and haemopoiesis').

Adipose tissue (textus adiposus)

Adipose tissue consists of a homogeneous population of fat cells (**adipocytes**) that develop from undifferentiated mesenchymal cells through the intracellular accumulation of lipid droplets (Figures 3.16 to 3.19). Adipocytes occur either individually or in groups (lobules), thus forming a component of other tissues or organs. Adipose tissue has an abundant blood supply.

The functions of adipose tissue are manifold. In the context of **energy metabolism**, it is capable of relatively rapid storage and, as required, release of energy-rich substrates. Preferential sites of fat storage include subcutaneous tissue, the abdominal skin, the axilla and the inguinal region.

Adipose tissue undergoes constant proliferation (triglyceride synthesis, **lipogenesis**) and regression (triglyceride hydrolysis, **lipolysis**). Some of the fatty acids released during lipolysis are re-esterified with glycerol 3 phosphate (intracellular cycling).

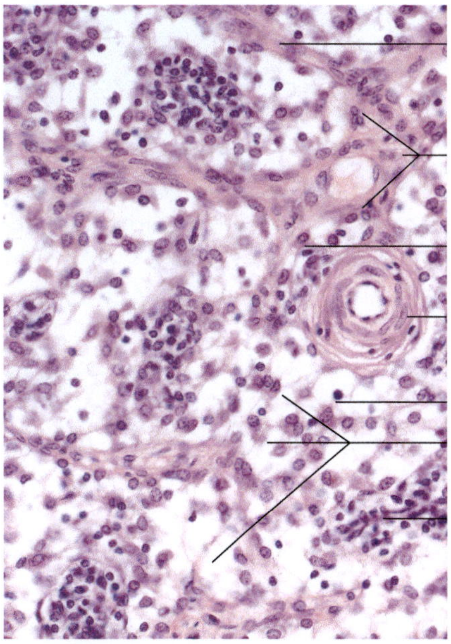

3.15 Lymph node (dog). Lymphoreticular tissue develops between connective tissue septa, giving rise to a three-dimensional meshwork of reticular cells and free lymphoid cells. The connective tissue septa are composed of fibroblasts, fibrocytes and collagen fibres. Haematoxylin and eosin stain (x480).

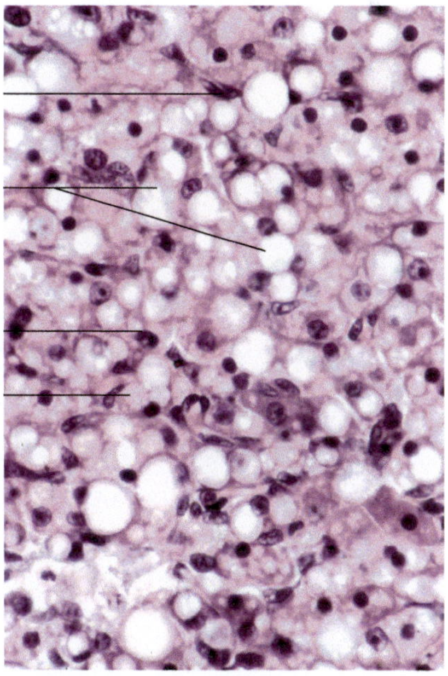

3.16 Renal fat (juvenile dog). Embryonic (brown) adipose tissue is characterised by the development of multiple lipid droplets within individual cells (multilocular adipose tissue). Haematoxylin and eosin stain (x300).

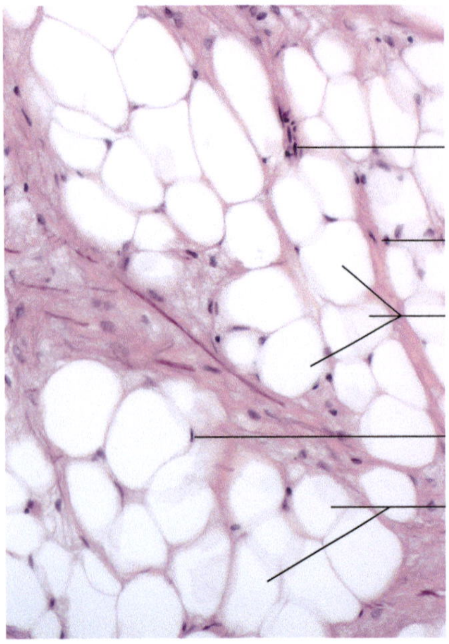

3.17 Foot pad (cat). In white adipose tissue, adipocytes contain only a single lipid droplet (unilocular adipose tissue). The organelles are displaced to the periphery of the cell; thus, the cell boundaries appear as distinct lines. The nucleus occupies a marginal position. Haematoxylin and eosin stain (x300).

Fat metabolism is regulated by neurotransmitters produced by **sympathetic nerve fibres**, and by **hormones**. Insulin and prostaglandin E_1 inhibit the release of fatty acids from fat cells by blocking adenylate cyclase cAMP-receptors on the plasmalemma (lipogenesis). In contrast, noradrenaline, adrenaline, ACTH, TSH, GH and glucagon promote lipolysis by activating the adenylate cyclase cAMP system. This results in cleavage of glycerol from triglyceride molecules, with the release of free fatty acids into the capillaries.

A notable functional feature of adipose tissue is its tendency to revert to less differentiated tissue (following depletion of stored fat). In ageing adipose tissue, the deposition of mucopolysaccharides can give rise to large vesicular, honeycomb-like fat cells (**serous fat**).

As a poor conductor of heat, adipose tissue acts as a thermal insulator thus contributing to **thermoregulation**. It also plays an important role in withstanding mechanical forces. Adipose tissue surrounds the kidney and has a cushioning effect in the foot pads and the orbit (retrobulbar fat). In addition, fat contributes to the structural integrity of organs and, in association with various joints, participates in shock absorption. Moreover, adipose tissue plays a role in **hydration**.

During embryonic development, adipose tissue serves as a **placeholder** for subsequently developing tissues. Fat also fills lympho- and haemoreticular tissues (e.g. thymus, bone marrow) after these have undergone physiological regression or pathological degeneration.

Based on differences in structure and function, as well as colour, location and vascularisation, adipose tissue can be divided into:

- pluri- or multilocular adipose tissue (brown fat) and
- unilocular adipose tissue (white fat).

Pluri- or multilocular adipose tissue (textus adiposus fuscus)

In pluri- or multilocular (brown) fat, the cytoplasm of adipocytes contains numerous fat droplets of varying size (Figures 3.16 and 3.18). This type of adipose tissue develops from strands of cells containing large numbers of mitochondria with abundant cytochrome (hence 'brown' fat). The individual **adipocytes** are smaller (15–25 μm) than in white adipose tissue (see below), with a predominantly centrally located nucleus and numerous glycogen and fat vacuoles. Adrenergic nerve fibres extend to the cell surface, accompanied by a dense network of capillaries. Brown fat is found in birds, hibernating animals and rodents (e.g. in the pectoral girdle). It also constitutes 5% of the body mass of newborn mammals (e.g. near the thyroid gland and at the renal hilus). The primary functions of brown fat are to **generate heat** and **provide a source of energy**.

Unilocular adipose tissue (textus adiposus albus)

In unilocular fat cells, lipid droplets deposited in the cytoplasm of **lipoblasts** (developing fat cells) coalesce to form a **single, large lipid droplet** from which the tissue derives its name (Figures 3.17 and 3.19).

Unilocular fat occurs as single cells or as clusters of cells joined into lobules by loose connective tissue. The cells may appear round or polyhedral (25–100 μm). **Individual adipocytes** are almost completely filled by the lipid droplet (which is stabilised by a coating of microfilaments), with only a rim of cytoplasm remaining. The organelles are thus displaced to, and concentrated at, the periphery of the cell. Consequently, the nucleus is marginally located and flattened.

The adipocytes are surrounded by a delicate network of reticular fibres and a dense capillary network. Fine periarteriolar plexuses of adrenergic nerve fibres regulate metabolic processes within the tissue.

Adipose cells do not divide. However, new cells can form from other mesenchymal cells. The colour of unilocular fat, which ranges from white (hence '**white fat**') to yellow, is determined by the quantity of exogenous fat-soluble pigments (e.g. carotenoids) in the tissue.

Connective tissue proper (textus connectivus collagenosus)

Throughout the body, connective tissue undergoes structural and functional adaptations, based on the mechanical

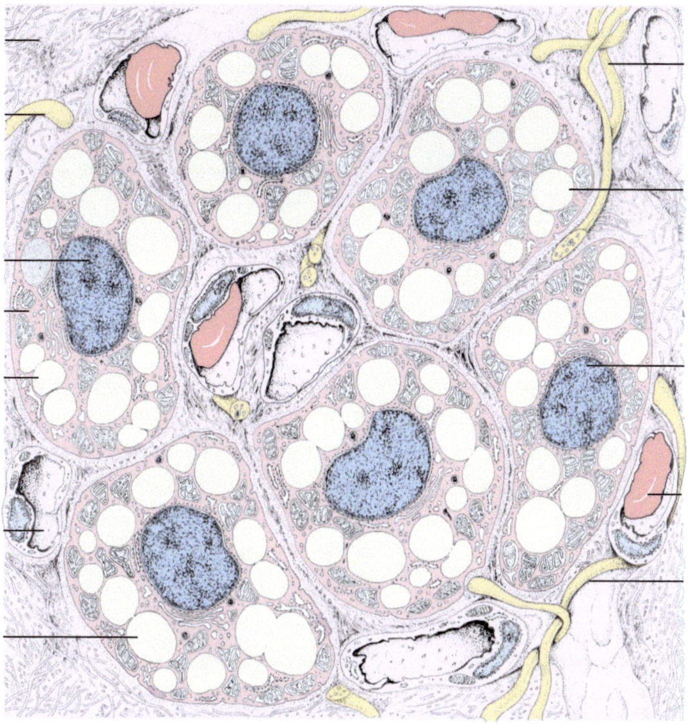

3.18 Multilocular (embryonic or brown) adipose tissue with capillary network and free nerve endings in loose connective tissue (schematic).

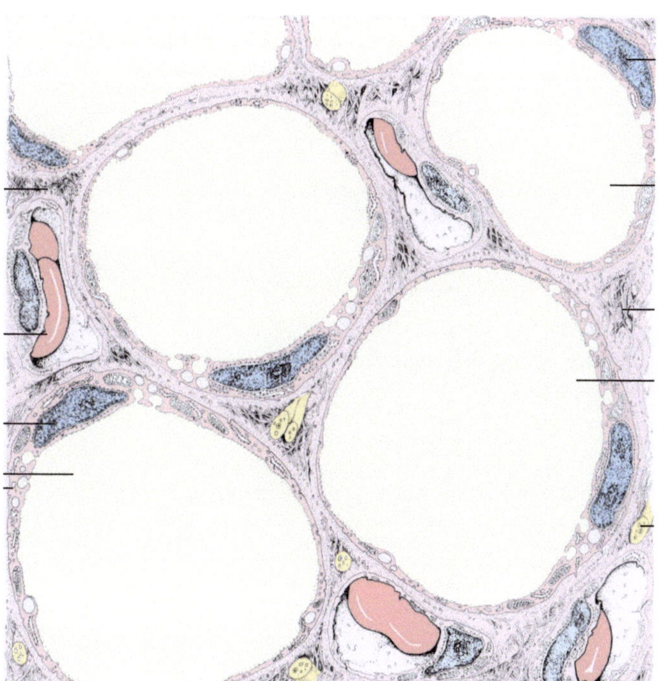

3.19 Unilocular (white) adipose tissue with capillary network and free nerve endings in loose connective tissue (schematic).

forces to which it is subjected. On this basis, connective tissue is categorised as:

- loose connective tissue (low fibre content) or
- dense connective tissue (high fibre content).

Loose connective tissue (textus connectivus collagenosus laxus)

Loose connective tissue is widely distributed throughout the body in the form of **interstitial connective tissue**. The collagen fibres are generally arranged in a grid-like fashion, allowing the tissue to adapt to functionally determined changes in tension. As well as forming a **flexible framework** (**stroma**) for the organs, it connects and separates individual organ segments and provides channels for nerves and vessels.

Loose connective tissue underlies epithelial tissue, from which it is separated only by the basal lamina. It is of functional significance in the exchange of metabolic substances between the capillaries and the parenchyma of organs.

The wide spaces between the collagen, reticular and elastic fibres facilitate intercellular transport, aided by the high water content of the hydrophilic glycosaminoglycans within the abundant **ground substance**. In this way, loose connective tissue plays an important part in **regulating the water content of the body**.

The cells of loose connective tissue consist primarily of flattened fibroblasts and fibrocytes. Their shape conforms to the course of the surrounding collagen fibres. Loose connective tissue frequently contains histiocytes, mast cells and transient cells (e.g. lymphocytes, plasma cells). These are responsible for **local immune responses**.

Dense connective tissue (textus connectivus collagenosus compactus)

Dense connective tissue is composed predominantly of collagen and elastic fibres, with relatively little ground substance and smaller cell populations (fibrocytes).

According to the functional requirements of the tissue, the fibre bundles are closely apposed, their alignment corresponding with the prevailing forces of tension and pressure. Dense connective tissue is more common in parts of the body subjected to relatively large mechanical forces. According to the arrangement of the collagen fibres, it is divided into:

- dense irregular connective tissue and
- dense regular connective tissue.

DENSE IRREGULAR CONNECTIVE TISSUE

Dense irregular connective tissue primarily forms the framework of organ capsules, fascia and aponeuroses, and the pericardium. The **perichondrium**, parts of the **periosteum** (**stratum fibrosum**) and joint capsules are composed of sheets in which collagen fibre bundles are configured in a lattice (crossing each other at various angles). This arrangement allows the tissue to adapt rapidly to changes in the shape of associated tissue (e.g. distension or constriction of a hollow organ, or contraction of a muscle). Dense irregular connective tissue contains little ground

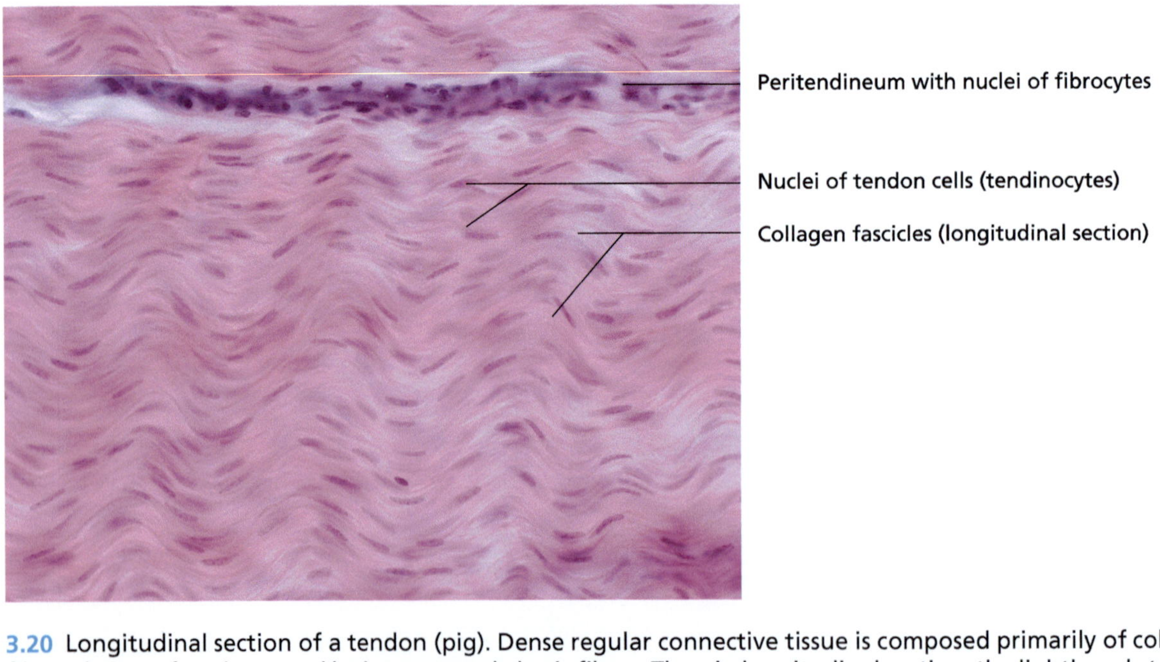

3.20 Longitudinal section of a tendon (pig). Dense regular connective tissue is composed primarily of collagen fibres that are foreshortened by interspersed elastic fibres. Thus, in longitudinal section, the lightly red-staining collagen fibres are arranged in waves. The shape of the tendinocytes (fibrocytes associated with tendons) conforms to the course of the surrounding fibres. Haematoxylin and eosin stain (x480).

substance. The shape of the fibrocytes conforms to the arrangement of the surrounding fibres.

DENSE REGULAR CONNECTIVE TISSUE

Regular dense connective tissue is characterised by the arrangement of fibre bundles in one predominant direction. **Tendons** and **ligaments** are the principal examples of this tissue type. They consist mainly of collagen or elastic fibres (Figures 3.20 to 3.23).

Tendons and most **ligaments** are composed primarily of parallel arrays of collagen fibres enmeshed in a sparse network of reticular fibres (Figure 3.20). The spaces between fibre bundles contain elongated **fibroblasts** (**tendinocytes**) recognisable with the light microscope by their basophilic nuclei (Figure 3.20). The shape of these cells is determined by the surrounding fibre arrangement; thus, they are narrow and irregularly flattened. The parallel bundling of collagen fibres serves to withstand forces of tension.

In tendons, the collagen fibrils and fibre bundles are separated by layers of loose connective tissue. The innermost sheath, termed the **endotendineum**, is formed by tendinocytes. Groups of collagen fascicles are surrounded by the **peritendineum**. The outer layer, or **epitendineum**, encloses the entire tendon (Figure 3.23).

Compared with other types of connective tissue, dense regular connective tissue exhibits little metabolic activity, with limited vascularisation of fibrous subunits. In addition, the dense arrangement of fibres inhibits the diffusion of nutrients.

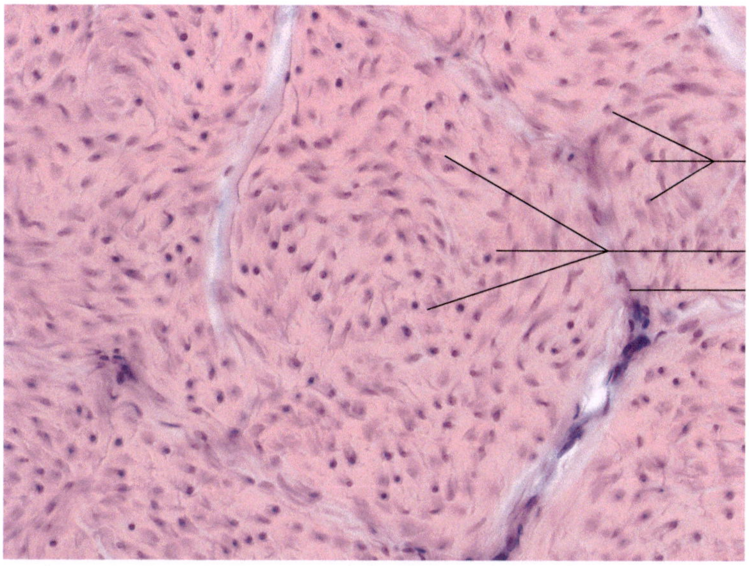

3.21 Transverse section of a tendon (pig). Dense regular connective tissue is composed of layers of collagen fibres bound together by connective tissue sheaths (endotendineum, peritendineum, epitendineum). Haematoxylin and eosin stain (x300).

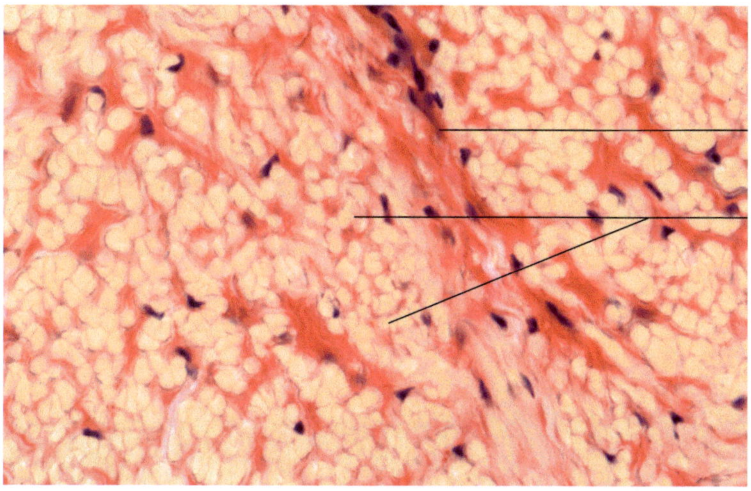

3.22 Nuchal ligament (ox). In transverse section, elastic fibres appear as isolated, yellowish clumps, surrounded by a delicate network of reddish-staining fibres. van Gieson stain (x480).

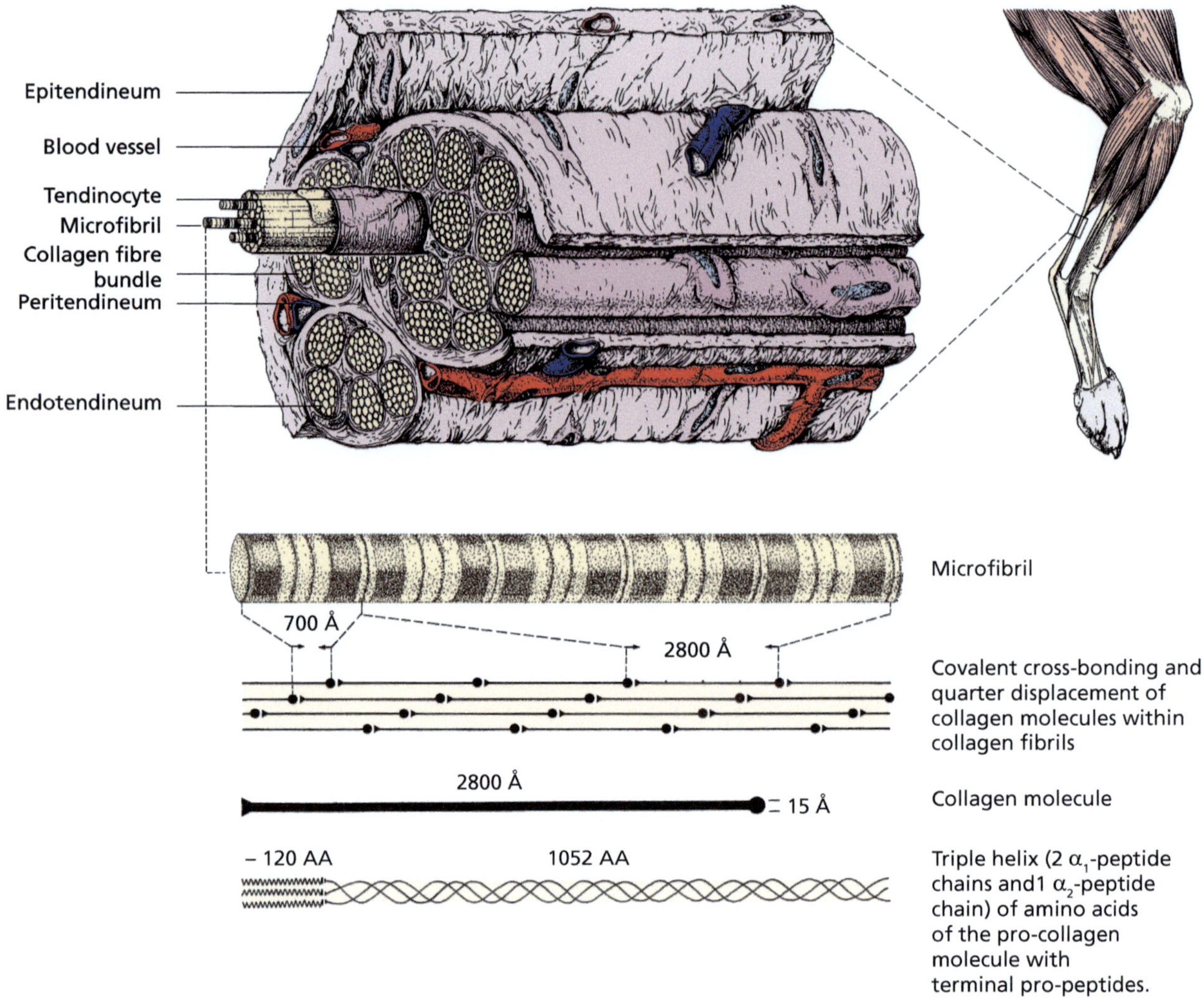

3.23 Light microscopic, ultrastructural and molecular composition of collagen fibres and fibrils (microfibrils), and their associated sheaths, in dense connective tissue (schematic).

The basic structure of **elastic ligaments** (**fibrae elasticae**) is similar to that of tendons, though the fibres are mainly elastic. Large individual elastic fibres (30 μm) are surrounded by a fine network of collagen and reticular fibres. This displaceable layer contains small fibroblasts and fibrocytes. Elastic ligaments are poorly vascularised. Due to the high proportion of elastic fibres, they are typically yellow in colour (Figure 3.22).

Types of supportive tissue

The main components of supportive tissue are cartilage and bone, both of which are derived from mesenchyme. Mesenchymal stem cells differentiate into cartilage- or bone-forming cells (chondro- or osteoblasts) that produce collagen fibres and ground substance rich in glycosaminoglycans. These synthetically active cells differentiate into mature cartilage and bone cells (chondro- and osteocytes). The structural and functional differences between cartilage and bone are attributable primarily to variation in the chemical composition of the ground substance and in collagen fibre content.

Cartilage (textus cartilagineus)

Cartilage is distinguished by a **high degree of compressive elasticity**. It is partially deformable, has shock-absorbing properties and yet is firm in consistency. Cartilage is the primary supportive tissue in the developing embryo and forms the framework from which most of the skeleton develops. The diversity of its predominantly mechanical functions arises from the highly specialised structure of the extracellular matrix. The arcade-like arrangement of collagen fibres, together with the abundance of glycosaminoglycans in the amorphous ground substance, provides cartilage with its structural integrity. Moreover, the hydrophilic nature of the proteoglycans in the ground substance contributes substantially to its elasticity and pliability.

Without exception, cartilage is **avascular** and contains **no nerves**. It receives its nutritional supply by diffusion from the surrounding connective tissue, from the fluid within synovial joint cavities and from the medullary vessels of underlying bone. In this respect, the ground substance again plays a significant role; through their extensive capacity for binding water molecules, proteoglycans facilitate the intra-chondral transport of substances involved in metabolism.

Cartilage formation (**chondrogenesis**) begins in the mesenchymal connective tissue, which condenses to form a layer that surrounds the cartilage throughout the life of the organism (**perichondrium**). Mesenchymal cells (perichondral fibroblasts) differentiate into **chondroblasts** (Figure 3.24). These begin to produce cartilage matrix consisting primarily of water (70%), collagen or elastic fibres and glycosaminoglycans. As synthesis of the matrix progresses, the cells move further apart. Eventually, the flattened peripherally distributed chondroblasts differentiate into chondrocytes. These cells are surrounded by cartilage and are typically large and vesicular in shape.

Chondrocytes have an ovoid to spherical nucleus, surrounded by cytoplasm rich in organelles. Large numbers of expanded cisternae of the rough endoplasmic reticulum and a prominent Golgi apparatus are morphological indicators of active protein and carbohydrate synthesis (production of collagen fibres and glycosaminoglycans).

Metabolism within chondrocytes is anaerobic. Energy is derived from abundant intracellular glycogen and lipid droplets. Chondrocytes occupy cavities, or lacunae, within the **cartilage matrix**. The wall of the lacuna is referred to as the **capsule**.

Chondrocytes are responsible for **synthesis** and **maintenance** of the extracellular matrix. Pro-collagen formed within chondrocytes is released into the extracellular space. As is the case in fibrocytic fibrogenesis, pro-collagen chains combine to form collagen fibres (see 'Connective tissue fibres'). Under certain circumstances, chondrocytes and their precursors, chondroblasts, also synthesise elastic fibres. Based on its fibre content, cartilage is categorised as **hyaline cartilage, elastic cartilage** and **fibrocartilage** (Figures 3.25 to 3.28).

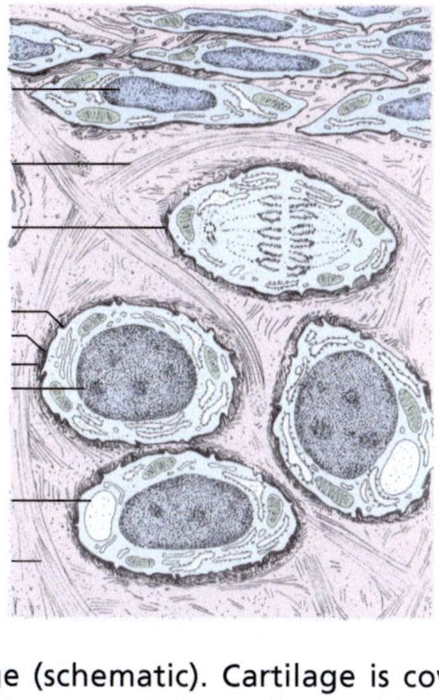

3.24 Hyaline cartilage (schematic). Cartilage is covered with perichondrium containing cells capable of differentiating into chondroblasts.

Chondrocytes are enclosed by a dense fibrillar collagen network, giving rise to a thin region (1–2 μm) termed the **capsular** (**pericellular**) **matrix**. Cellular products are released, via finger-like cytoplasmic processes, into the narrow space between the cell surface and the capsular matrix. The extracellular phase of fibre synthesis and the interweaving of fibres with proteoglycans occurs in this region. Under the light microscope this area usually appears as artificially expanded, as the cell surface shrinks away from the wall of the lacuna.

Chondrocytes also synthesise **amorphous ground substance**, consisting of glycosaminoglycans (hyaluronic acid and proteoglycans with numerous chondroitin-4-sulfate, keratin sulfate and chondroitin-6-sulfate side chains). The relationship between these molecules and the extent of their interconnection with collagen fibres determine the properties of the cartilage.

Functionally, chondrocytes and their associated capsular matrix are the key structural elements of cartilage. Together, they are referred to as **chondrons** or **territories**. These are separated by **interterritorial regions** (**interterritorial matrix**) (Figures 3.24, 3.26 and 3.28).

Cartilage grows in one of two ways. During **appositional** growth, perichondral chondroblasts multiply and differentiate, with cartilage formed at the surface of the tissue. This is the more common form of cartilage growth. **Interstitial** growth involves the replication of differentiated chondrocytes, primarily within incompletely formed matrix. These cells elaborate new ground substance, and thereby become increasingly isolated from each other. Chondrogenesis is promoted by vitamin A. Vitamin C stimulates synthesis and maintenance of collagen fibres and cartilage matrix. Growth hormone, thyroxin and reproductive hormones increase the secretory activity of chondrocytes, while ACTH and cortisol retard cartilage maturation.

Hyaline cartilage (cartilago hyalina)

Hyaline cartilage is the most widespread type of cartilage. It forms the basis of the embryonic cartilage template and constitutes the articular cartilage, costal and nasal cartilage, and the cartilage of the airways (Figures 3.24, 3.26 and 3.29).

Immature hyaline cartilage appears bluish-white, becoming yellowish with increasing age. The structure of hyaline cartilage is largely as described above. It consists of:

- chondrocytes,
- type II collagen fibres and
- homogeneous, largely amorphous matrix.

Peripherally located **chondrocytes** tend to occur in groups as flattened, spindle-shaped cells. Usually, each capsule contains only one cell. Due to cell division, however, several

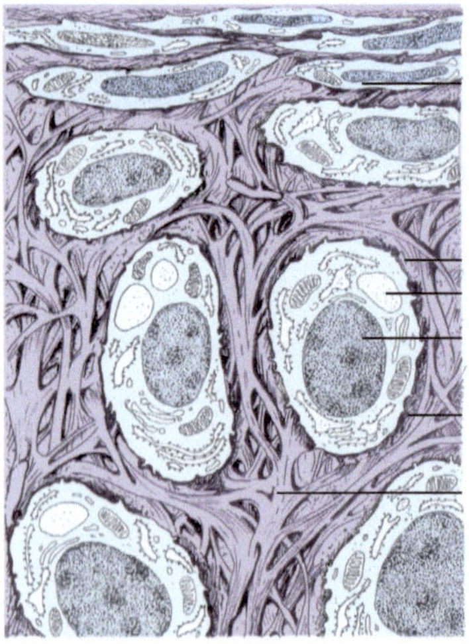

3.25 Elastic cartilage (schematic). The network of elastic fibres exhibits extensive branching.

cells may be present within the same lacuna (**isogenous cell group**). Mitosis is an indicator of interstitial cartilage growth. Mature cartilage is capable of only limited regeneration, with fibrous scar tissue occurring in its place.

The **collagen fibres** in hyaline cartilage are arranged along lines of mechanical pressure and tension. At the surface, the fibres are curved to form arcades, from which they transition into a more **oblique** orientation (Figure 3.24). The fibres within the cartilage are in contact with fibre bundles in the perichondrium. This arrangement results in even distribution of mechanical stresses across multiple chondrons. The **type II collagen fibres** cannot be identified under standard light microscopy, as these are **masked** by the homogeneous glassy (hyaline) matrix in which they are embedded. They can be identified using biochemical and immunocytochemical techniques, and with electron microscopy. Under polarised light they are **uniaxially birefringent**.

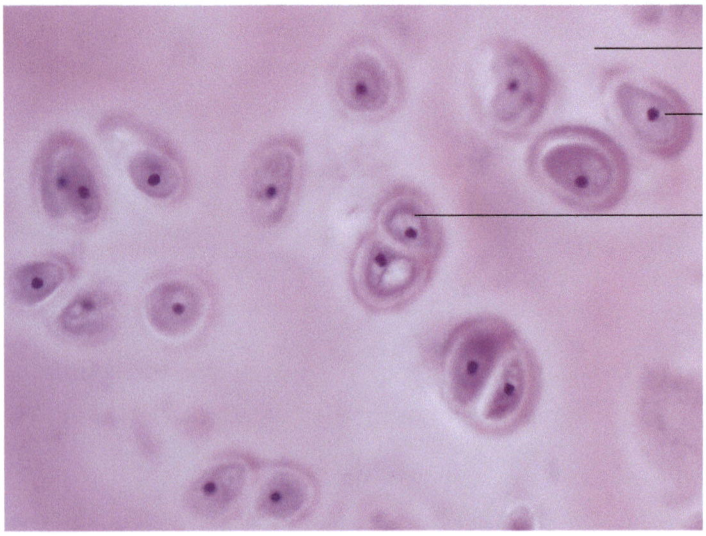

3.26 Features of hyaline cartilage include isogenous cell groups (formed primarily by superficial chondrocytes) and pale-staining, homogeneous interterritorial matrix. Collagen fibres are not discernible. The chondrocytes lie in lacunae. As a result of tissue preparation, the cells exhibit a varying degree of shrinkage. Hyaline cartilage of the third eyelid, horse. Haematoxylin and eosin stain (x480).

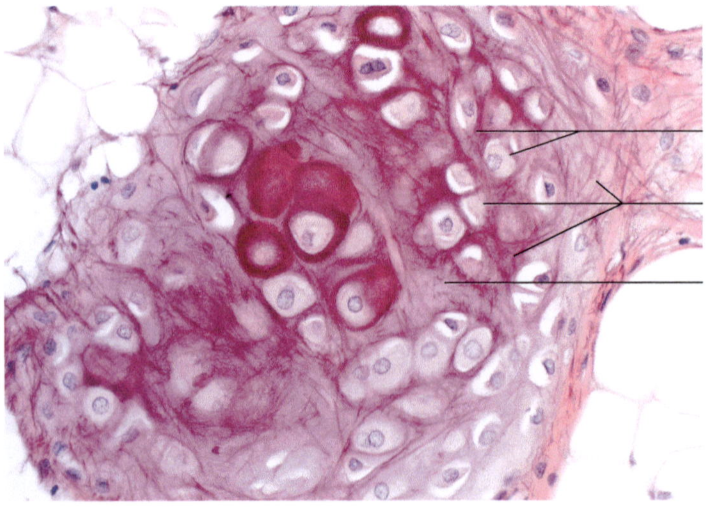

3.27 Epiglottis (dog). Elastic cartilage features a dense network of dark red-staining elastic fibres and paler ground substance. Chondrocytes are located between the branching fibres. Orcein-haemalaun stain (x480).

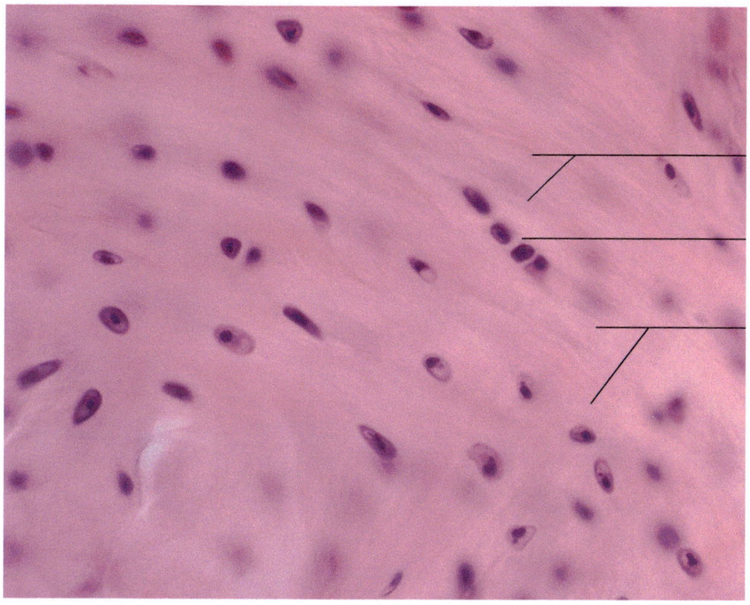

3.28 Meniscus (pig). Fibrocartilage contains bundles of collagen fibres that are visible under the light microscope. The chondrocytes are arranged parallel to the direction of the collagen fibres. The ground substance is sparse and homogeneous. Haematoxylin and eosin stain (x300).

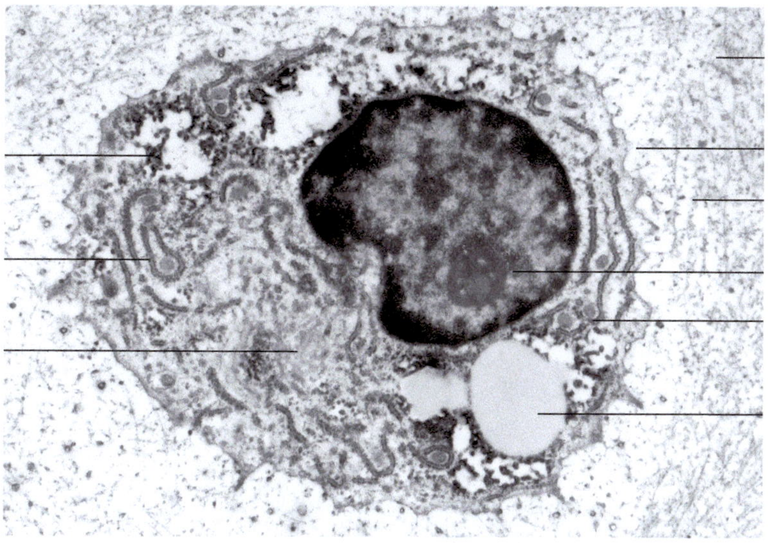

3.29 Fine structure of a chondrocyte with ground substance and type II collagen fibrils (x5000).

Elastic cartilage (cartilago elastica)

The ground substance of elastic cartilage incorporates a strongly branching network of elastic fibres (Figures 3.25 and 3.27), allowing this tissue to adapt to varying types of bending forces. The elastic fibres, which impart a pale yellow colour to this type of cartilage, can be demonstrated with orcein and resorcin stain. Elastic cartilage is stabilised by collagen fibres that, as in hyaline cartilage, are hidden by the proteoglycans in the matrix. The chondrons are small and regularly arranged, with spherical to ovoid chondrocytes. In contrast to hyaline cartilage, age-related ossification does not occur in elastic cartilage.

Elastic cartilage is found in the pinna, parts of the external acoustic canal and in the epiglottis.

Fibrocartilage (cartilago fibrosa)

Fibrocartilage develops from dense connective tissue that is subjected to pressure as well as a certain degree of tension. As such, it can be regarded simply as dense connective tissue that has undergone chondrification. The cartilaginous nature of the tissue is indicated by the presence of a matrix rich in glycosaminoglycans. However, the matrix is so poorly developed that it incompletely masks the collagen fibres within it. The fibre bundles are visible under light microscopy, aligned in the direction of greatest ten-

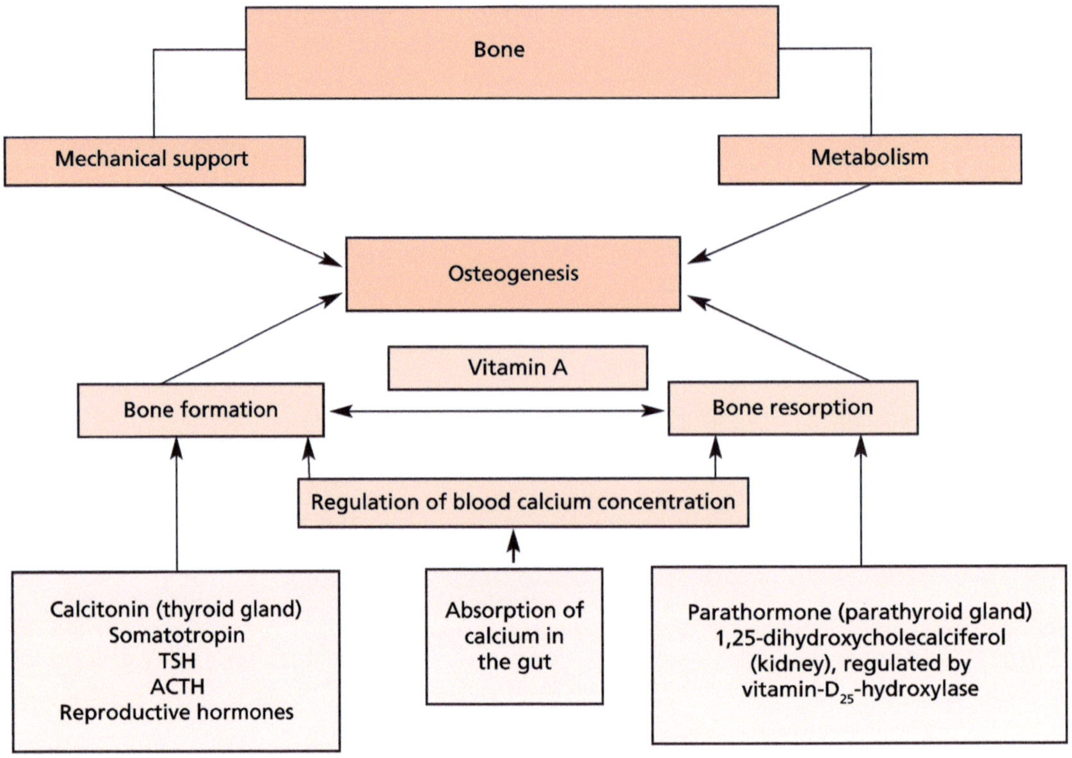

3.30 Mechanical and metabolic relationships of bone (schematic).

sion (Figure 3.28). Chondrocytes are typically oriented parallel to the fibres. They are scattered, often lying in rows between the fibre bundles. Near the chondrocytes, some masking of the fibre bundles may occur.

Fibrocartilage is a highly resilient tissue occurring in intervertebral discs (disci intervertebrales), the cartilage of the hoof, articular discs and menisci, and as cartilaginous inclusions in the m. biceps brachii of the horse.

Bone (textus osseus)

Bone has several **functions**. It forms the skeleton of the body, provides attachment sites for the muscles and constitutes the structural framework of the thoracic and abdominal cavities. Bone also houses haemopoietic tissue (bone marrow) and serves as a reservoir for various minerals.

These functions can be divided into two categories: **support** and **metabolism** (Figure 3.30). Interactions between these supportive and metabolic functions influence the structure of each individual bone, thus shaping the **framework of the whole body**. Through its capacity for metabolism, bone can adapt to particular mechanical requirements. Thus, both the outer **compact bone** (**substantia compacta**) and inner **spongy** or **trabecular bone** (**substantia spongiosa**) undergo continuous remodelling. Bones subjected to the greatest mechanical forces, such as those in the extremities and the bones of the vertebral column and pelvis, undergo more intensive structural modifications than others (e.g. bones of the skull). Under constant exposure to pressure and tension, the bone wall becomes markedly thickened, particularly in the mid-section, where the load is greatest. Towards the extremities of the bone, the thickness of the wall decreases. Any changes in the prevailing forces of pressure, tension and shear are quickly followed by additional remodelling.

In addition to its supportive role, compact bone encloses the spongy bone and bone marrow.

The function of bone is also influenced by its connective tissue sheath, the **periosteum**. This is composed of an outer fibrous layer (**stratum fibrosum**) and a more cellular, inner osteogenic layer (**stratum cambium**). Periosteum surrounds the bone, except at articular surfaces and at many sites of muscle attachment. It contains sensory nerve fibres and a dense network of blood and lymphatic vessels for maintenance of the underlying bone. The pluripotent osteogenic layer of the periosteum is capable of rapidly producing new bone tissue, for example during bone growth, normal remodelling processes and fracture repair.

The specific metabolic functions of bone include the storage of calcium and phosphate (Figure 3.30). Through constant production and resorption, bone serves as a calcium depot and thus as a means of maintaining blood calcium levels within a certain range. Calcium metabolism is regulated by endogenous and exogenous mechanisms. Under the influence of parathyroid hormone (produced by the parathyroid gland), bone is resorbed by osteoclasts, elevating blood calcium. This is supplemented by increased absorption of dietary calcium in the small intestine, driven by vitamin D_3 (1,25-dihydroxycholecalciferol), and inhibition of calcium excretion by the kidney.

The hormone **calcitonin**, secreted by the **C-cells of the thyroid gland**, stimulates bone production by osteoblasts, reduces the activity of osteoclasts and promotes the incorporation of calcium into the bone matrix.

Somatotropin (**growth hormone**), **adrenocorticotropic hormone** (ACTH), **thyroid-stimulating hormone** (**TSH**) and male and female **reproductive hormones** also have a stimulatory effect on bone growth. In addition, **vitamin C** promotes the synthesis of collagen fibres by osteoblasts. **Vitamin A** acts as a regulator in maintaining an equilibrium between bone production and resorption (Figure 3.30).

Bone is derived from mesenchymal connective tissue. It consists of **bone cells** and **bone matrix**.

Bone cells

Bone cells are comprised of:

- osteoprogenitor cells,
- osteoblasts,
- bone-lining cells,
- osteocytes and
- osteoclasts.

Except for osteoclasts, cells found in bone represent different functional phases of the same cell type. **Osteoprogenitor cells** differentiate into **osteoblasts** (bone-forming cells). Osteoblasts synthesise the organic components of the bone matrix. After mineralisation of the matrix (in which osteoblasts also participate), osteoblasts transform into **osteocytes**. **Osteoclasts** are responsible for bone resorption (Figures 3.31 to 3.33).

OSTEOPROGENITOR CELLS

Osteoprogenitor cells develop from mesenchymal stem cells. Typically, these are flattened cells with pale cytoplasm and an ovoid to oblong nucleus. Osteoprogenitor cells are present in the endosteum and periosteum. These mitotically active cells eventually differentiate into osteoblasts.

As precursors of osteoblasts, osteoprogenitor cells are found predominantly in the osteogenic layer of the periosteum and along vessels of the bone marrow.

OSTEOBLAST (OSTEOBLASTUS)

Unlike their predecessor, **osteoblasts** do not undergo mitosis. These cells participate in bone formation in the following ways:

- synthesis of type I collagen fibres and non-collagenous proteins,
- production of glycosaminoglycans/proteoglycans,
- participation in mineralisation of bone matrix and
- modulation of osteoclast function.

Analogous to the mechanism of collagen fibril synthesis by fibroblasts, production of **type I collagen fibres** by osteoblasts commences within the cell (rER, Golgi apparatus) and is completed in the extracellular space. Osteoblasts also synthesise ground substance (glycosaminoglycans/proteoglycans, other non-collagenous proteins). Together, the irregularly arranged collagen fibres and ground substance form the organic, unmineralised bone matrix (osteoid). The fibres are masked by the ground substance.

Non-collagenous proteins such as osteocalcin, osteonectin and osteopontin (bone sialoprotein I, BSP-1) regulate the process of mineralisation. These molecules have a high affinity for calcium ions and hydroxyapatite.

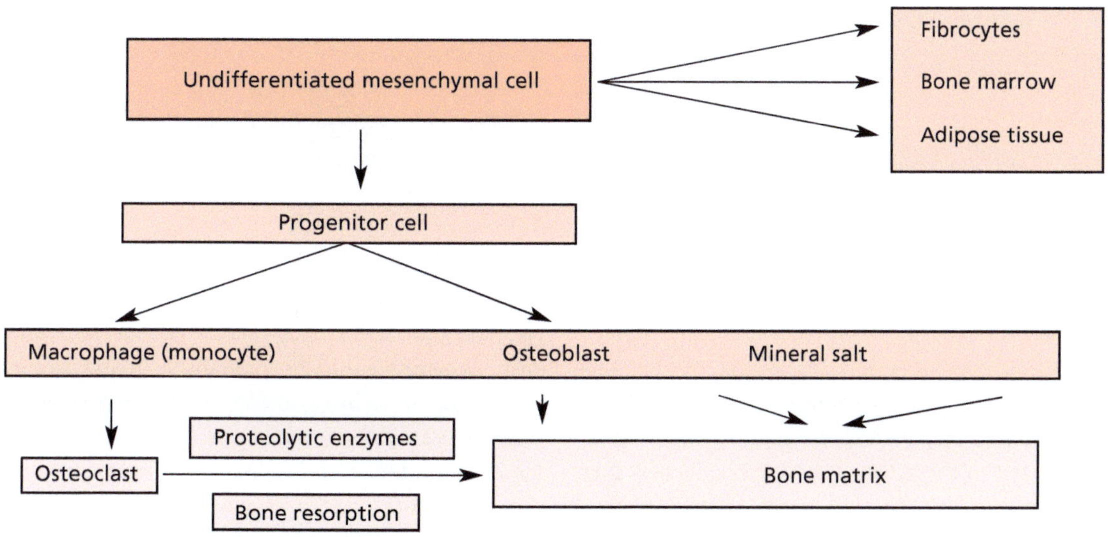

3.31 Cellular pathways in bone production and resorption (schematic).

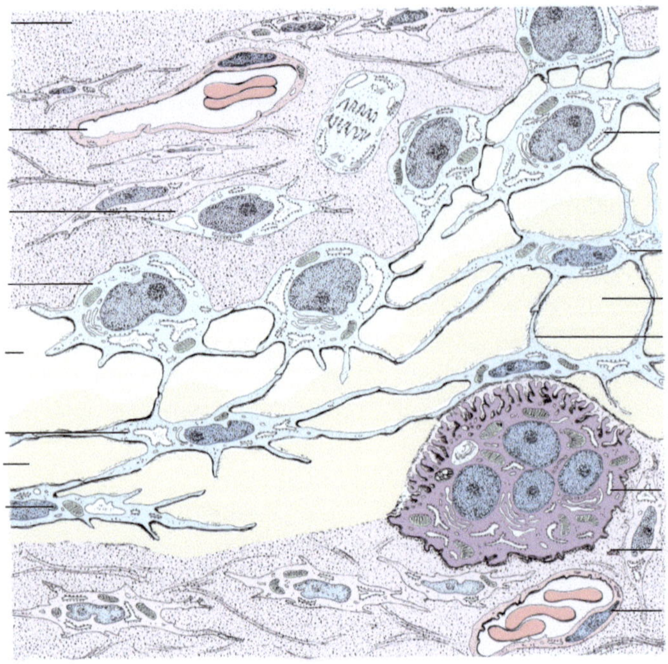

3.32 Intramembranous ossification. Osteoprogenitor cells differentiate into osteoblasts that produce, and become encased in, osteoid. As the osteoid becomes mineralised, the osteoblasts are transformed into osteocytes. Mineralised matrix is digested by osteoclasts.

Although it is a product of osteoblasts, osteopontin is involved in both formation and resorption of bone. The biosynthetic activity of mature osteoblasts can increase by up to a factor of two. The number of osteoblasts thus has a greater influence on bone production than their level of activity. Optimal therapeutic interventions for metabolic bone diseases involving reduced bone production are therefore targeted at promoting the proliferation of osteoblasts and their precursors.

Osteoblast-like cells have been found to regulate the proliferation of periosteal fibroblasts and the stimulatory effect of parathyroid hormone on osteoclast formation. Mature osteoblasts thereby play an important role in the autoregulation of bone cell precursors.

Osteoblasts regulate the formation of hydroxyapatite crystals (from calcium and phosphate) between the collagen fibrils in the bone matrix (mineralisation). Calcification begins within matrix vesicles (released by osteoblasts) and proceeds within the ground substance as well as on, and in, the collagen fibrils. Osteoblasts also exert an influence on osteoclast activity; release of neutral proteases and collagenases frees unmineralised matrix in preparation for resorption. Osteoblasts thus play a role in both deposition and resorption of bone. This regulatory function is directed by parathyroid hormone, calcitonin, steroid hormones and numerous cytokines (e.g. IL-1, IL-6, TNF-α, TNF-β, BDGF [bone-derived growth factor] and EGF [epidermal growth factor]).

Active osteoblasts (20–30 μm) form an epithelium-like sheet on the surface of bone spicules. They are basophilic, with a spherical nucleus and abundant secretory organelles (ER, Golgi cisternae, lysosomes) (Figure 3.32). Inactive osteoblasts are elongated and flattened (squamous). Osteoblasts contact one another via numerous cell processes extending from the osteoid-facing surface of the cell.

Osteoblasts produce approximately 1 μm of unmineralised osteoid per day, up to an average total thickness of 6 μm. Within 3–4 days, 70% of the osteoid becomes mineralised. Mineralisation of the remaining osteoid occurs over a period of 6 weeks.

Formation of new bone can occur:

- at the periosteum (periosteal bone formation),
- at the endosteum (endosteal bone formation),
- around blood vessels (perivascular) and
- by direct differentiation of bone cells from connective tissue.

BONE-LINING CELLS

Bone-lining cells, found on the surface of bone, are frequently referred to as **inactive** or **resting osteoblasts**. Neighbouring bone-lining cells are connected by gap junctions. Bone-lining cells are in direct contact with peripheral osteocytes via bone canaliculi. They are capable of replication and have osteogenic potential. They may return to the pool of **stem cells** or **osteoprogenitor cells**, or they may perish.

Bone-lining cells are also considered to serve as a **barrier** between fluid in the periosteocytic compartment and the extracellular fluid outside the bone. In this way, they perform an important role in **regulating mineralisation** and **bone metabolism**.

OSTEOCYTE (OSTEOCYTUS)

Osteocytes are mature bone cells that develop from osteoblasts (Figures 3.32 and 3.33). This transformation process, which occurs in only around 10–20% of the osteoblast population, takes approximately 3 days. Osteocytes have numerous slender cytoplasmic processes (see below).

Osteocytes are surrounded by **calcified bone matrix**. They are flattened cells, located in narrow lacunae between lamellar layers of bone. Once osteocytes are completely embedded in the matrix, their metabolic activity dramatically decreases due to a reduction in nutrient diffusion and gas exchange. Osteocytes are important components of all bones, making a vital contribution to bone maintenance. When osteocytes degenerate, the surrounding matrix becomes resorbed.

The long, finger-like processes of osteocytes extend into **canaliculi** (**canaliculi ossei**) within the bone matrix (Figure 3.33). These processes establish direct contact with nearby cells, chiefly other osteocytes, via gap junctions. They participate in intercellular transport of ions, low-molecular weight substances, nutrients and waste products. The dense network of cell processes also permits osteocytes to communicate with osteoblasts, stimulating these to undergo differentiation. Through induction, a pre-osteoblast subsequently develops into a mature osteoblast that takes the place of the initially stimulated cell. This system of cellular interconnections combines blood vessels, interstitial fluid, osteoblasts and osteocytes into a functional unit.

During the **development of osteoblasts into osteocytes**, the size of the cell decreases by up to 70% and the number of organelles, particularly the rER and Golgi cisternae, diminishes. At some point, the lacuna in which osteocytes are located is partially or wholly surrounded by matrix that has not yet mineralised. These young cells are referred to as 'immature osteocytes'.

Immature osteocytes are located relatively close to the surface of the bone, between the osteoblast layer and the calcified bone matrix. With advancing age and maturity, the cell becomes increasingly incorporated into calcified bone until, as a mature osteocyte, it is wholly surrounded by mineralised matrix.

Osteocytes have a large, typically ovoid nucleus and relatively few metabolically active organelles (Figures 3.32 and 3.33). Gap junctions connect osteocytes with each other, and with cells at the bone surface. Their cell processes contain microfilaments that may assist in the transport of small molecules. Repeated shortening and lengthening of the cell processes facilitates diffusion of nutrients and waste products into the extracellular compartment. This cellular transport system also plays an important role in bone metabolism by mediating uptake and release of calcium and phosphate, as well as intracellular transport of these ions. While osteoblasts and osteoclasts are responsible for most of the calcium and phosphate transport, osteocytes contribute to the fine-tuning of blood calcium homeostasis. Changes in the mechanical load on bone result in structural adaptations within the intercommunicating network of osteoblasts and osteocytes, with rapid adjustments in the metabolic activity of mature bone cells. These observations have led to the conclusion that osteocytes function as **mechanosensory cells** capable of repairing microscopic bone defects and revitalising dead tissue.

In this scenario, osteocytes are still able to synthesise bone matrix and liberate calcium, as required. If these cells are released from the matrix by osteoclasts, they can potentially transform into osteoblasts. The metabolic functions of osteocytes are regulated by calcitropic hormones.

OSTEOCLAST (OSTEOCLASTUS)

Osteoclasts are multinuclear giant cells (10–20, maximum 100, nuclei per cell) (Figures 3.32 and 3.33) derived from pluripotent haemopoietic stem cells of the granulocyte-monocyte line. The mononuclear precursor cells undergo fusion to produce mature, multinucleate osteoclasts. Osteoclasts appear to extend their life through repeated fusion with mononuclear precursors. Under experimental conditions, the lifespan of osteoclasts in the absence of ongoing fusion has been identified as approximately 6 weeks.

Osteoclasts lie directly on the surface of bone tissue within lacunae formed by the resorption of bone. Resting and active forms of osteoclasts are recognised.

Active osteoclasts are highly polarised cells that resorb bone. The basolateral cell surface is oriented towards the blood capillaries. At the apical surface of the cell, infolding of the plasmalemma gives rise to numerous finger-like structures that **increase the area of the cell surface** (**ruffled border**). These frequently branching projections specifically serve to resorb the bone.

At an ultrastructural level, the ruffled border exhibits hair-like projections (15–20 nm). Associated with these are numerous vesicles that secrete acid through the ruffled border into the extracellular space. The resulting low pH initiates dissolution of the mineral matrix. Digestion of the organic matrix occurs via lysosomal enzymes released from the osteoclast.

Adjacent to the ruffled border is the '**clear zone**' (**sealing zone**), a region in which the cell **adheres** to the bone matrix via specific **binding structures** (**podosomes**). This essentially delineates the micro-environment in which bone resorption takes place. The cytoplasm of the clear zone is free of organelles but contains cytoskeletal

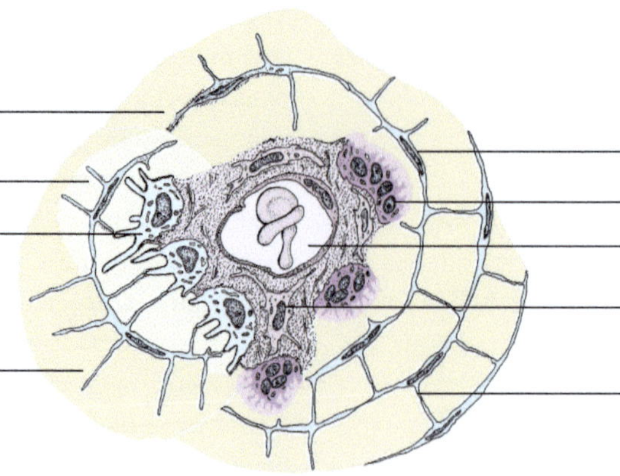

3.33 Transverse section of a Haversian system undergoing remodelling. Osteoclasts resorb bone tissue; osteoblasts differentiate from progenitor cells and initiate formation of new systems (schematic).

proteins. The capacity of osteoclasts to undergo polarisation, coordinate specific movements and bind to the extracellular matrix is largely attributable to this complex network of **protein filaments** (F-actin) and actin-binding proteins (e.g. vinculin). The circular alignment of F-actin in the clear zone is a morphological expression of increased cellular activity in an active osteoclast. It is regulated hormonally, by calcitonin and parathyroid hormone.

Active osteoclasts contain abundant mitochondria. Lying internal to the ruffled border, these organelles exhibit a high rate of aerobic metabolism. Due to the presence of large numbers of vacuoles and dense bodies, the cytoplasm of osteoclasts appears loosely structured. The vacuoles are associated with the endocytic, autophagocytic and exocytic functions of the cell.

The cell membrane of osteoclasts incorporates several classes and subclasses of **receptors** that aid in maintaining the seal between the cell and the bone matrix (integrin, vitronectin receptors), as well as myeloid antigens.

Bone resorption occurs in two ways: formation of lacunae (Howship's lacunae, resorption bays) by osteoclasts lying on the bone surface, or resorption of bone along vessels by one or more osteoclasts.

The **bone resorption process** consists of **two phases**. In the extracellular phase, the bone is degraded by acids and lytic enzymes released into the space between the osteoclast and the bone. In the intracellular phase, these degradation products are taken up at the ruffled border by endocytosis and further broken down in cytoplasmic vesicles (primarily lysosomes).

Osteoclasts are **highly mobile cells**. The texture of the bone matrix is an important determinant of the degree of their mobility. After resorbing bone in a particular area, osteoclasts detach themselves from the bone surface and migrate to another area before reattaching and resuming the bone degradation process.

The **activity of osteoclasts** is inhibited by calcitonin, and stimulated by 1,25-dihydroxycholecalciferol (vitamin D_3) and parathyroid hormone. Vitamin D_3 deficiency leads to accumulation of unmineralised bone matrix, resulting in the disease known as rickets. Bone resorption is further regulated by local paracrine and autocrine factors (cytokines, various interleukins, growth factors and prostaglandins, thyroid hormone). Per unit of time, osteoclasts resorb approximately three times as much bone matrix as that laid down by osteoblasts.

Structurally, osteoclasts are similar to chondroclasts and it has been proposed that these terms refer to the same cell type.

Bone matrix

Bone matrix is composed of:

- an organic component (collagen fibres and ground substance rich in glucosamine) and
- an inorganic component (minerals).

ORGANIC COMPONENT (COLLAGEN FIBRES AND GROUND SUBSTANCE)

Type I collagen fibres are the main component (approximately 90%) of the organic substance of bone. During bone mineralisation, these fibres provide a framework (crystallisation scaffold) for the deposition of hydroxyapatite crystals ($Ca_{10}[PO_4]_6[OH]_2$). Glycosaminoglycans and proteoglycans (chondroitin-4-sulfate, chondroitin-6-sulfate, keratin sulfate) make up 1–2% of the bone matrix. Together with lipids (5–10%), the structural proteins of the collagen fibres comprise around one third of the dry weight of bone tissue.

INORGANIC COMPONENT (MINERALS)

The inorganic component of bone matrix, which accounts for approximately two-thirds of the dry weight of bone, is composed predominantly of calcium phosphate (85–90%), calcium carbonate (8–10%), magnesium phosphate (1.5%) and calcium fluoride (0.3%). These minerals form a **crystal lattice** (consisting mostly of hydroxyapatite) alongside the collagen fibres, surrounded by proteoglycan rich ground substance.

Individual crystals are needle-shaped (20–40 nm long, 2–3 nm wide). The stability of bone results from the connection between the hydroxyapatite crystals and the collagen fibres.

Types of bone

Histologically, **bone tissue** can be divided into two types:

- woven bone (os membranaceum reticulofibrosum) and
- lamellar bone (os membranaceum lamellosum).

The same cell types are found in both types of bone, and both contain collagen and minerals. The principal differences between them are the organisation of the collagen fibres within the matrix and the proportion of cells and ground substance.

WOVEN BONE (OS MEMBRANACEUM RETICULOFIBROSUM)

Developmentally, woven bone is the simpler of the two forms. In a general sense, woven bone can be considered as ossified connective tissue that is found in locations subjected over extended periods to forces of pressure and tension. This type of bone is thus found wherever new bone is formed.

Woven bone is laid down during embryonic development. After birth, it is rapidly replaced with more highly differentiated lamellar bone. In certain locations, such as the osseous labyrinth of the inner ear, the external acoustic meatus and at the attachment sites of large tendons, woven bone is retained throughout the life of the animal.

Woven bone has a relatively high cell population, including osteocytes that are distributed randomly throughout the mineralised matrix. The ground substance is interspersed with an irregular network of collagen fibres comprising bundles of large and small fibrils that are not aligned in any particular direction. The mineral content of woven bone is lower than that of lamellar bone.

LAMELLAR BONE (OS MEMBRANACEUM LAMELLOSUM)

Lamellar bone (Figures 3.34 to 3.37) is distinguished by the arrangement of collagen fibres in accordance with the mechanical forces experienced by the bone.

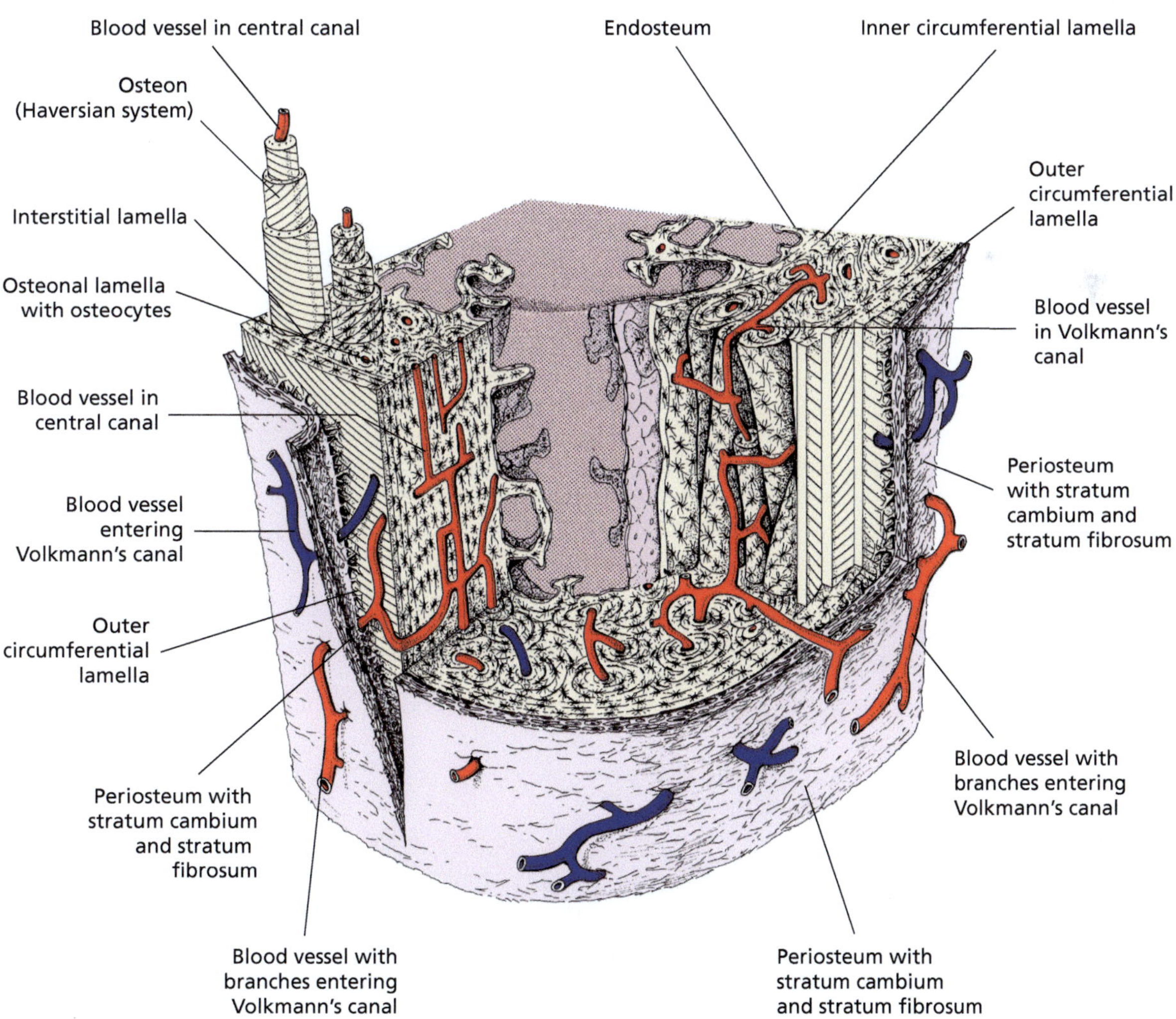

3.34 Section of compact bone from the diaphysis of a long bone (schematic).

The structural unit of compact lamellar bone is the osteon (**Haversian system**). Each osteon (diameter 20–100 µm) consists of a variable number (5–20) of concentric bone lamellae (Figures 3.34 and 3.35) surrounding a central canal (Haversian canal) containing mesenchymal connective tissue, a small blood vessel (e.g. capillary) and an autonomic nerve. Individual lamellae (width 4–10 µm) are composed of collagen fibres arranged in parallel and a mineralised bone

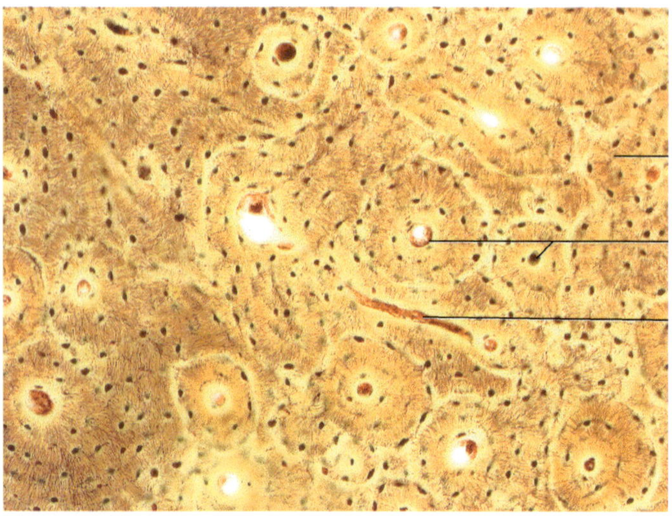

3.35 Transverse section of compact bone of a long bone including osteons and interstitial lamellae (dog). Schmorl's stain (x50).

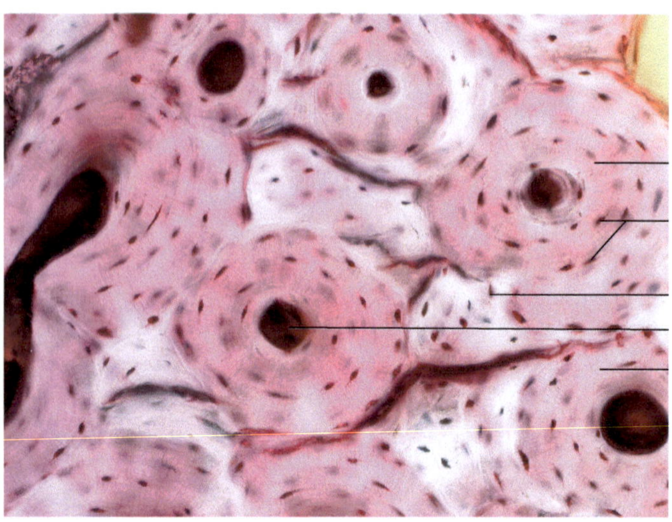

3.36 Ground bone: compact bone of a long bone with osteonal and interstitial lamellae (dog). Carmine stain (x250).

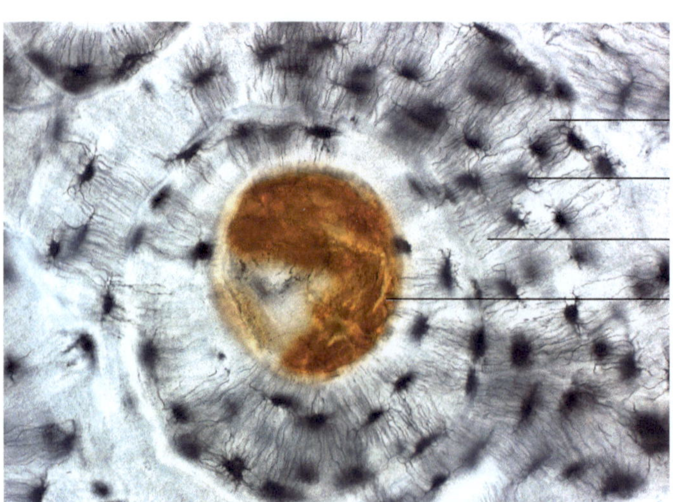

3.37 Ground bone (dog). High-power view of the wall of a Haversian system. The osteocytes are oriented parallel to the lamellae. The cytoplasmic processes of the osteocytes course transversely in the canaliculi ossei (x480).

matrix. The collagen fibres are arranged in spirals along the long axis of the central canal. In alternate lamellae, the spiral collagen fibres are oriented in different directions, forming a criss-crossing network. Cross-linkages are formed between adjacent lamellae. These features impart stability to the bone under forces of pressure and tension.

In additional to its structural role, lamellar bone – like all tissues derived from connective tissue – also plays a significant part in metabolism. This is enabled in large part by functional interactions between the bone cells, blood vessels and connective tissue within the osteon.

Osteocytes within lacunae are regularly arranged between the concentric lamellae around the central canal (Figures 3.34 to 3.37). Their long cytoplasmic processes radiate into interconnecting canaliculi (**canaliculi ossei**) extending from the lacunae. The cellular extensions establish contact with the processes of other osteocytes via gap junctions. This arrangement permits the transport of substances between the **blood vessel in the Haversian canal** and the bone matrix (both to and from the vessel). Channels running transversely through the bone (**perforating canals, Volkmann's canals**) connect central canals with each other, and with the endosteum and periosteum. Through this interconnecting network of blood vessels, bone is a well-vascularised tissue (Figure 3.34).

Lamellar bone serves as a metabolically active calcium depot. Under the influence of parathyroid hormone, activation of osteolytic **osteocytes** or, in larger areas of bone resorption, multinuclear **osteoclasts**, within bone lacunae and canaliculi results in rapid liberation of Ca^{2+} and PO_4^{3-} ions from the mineralised matrix. These ions are swiftly conveyed to the circulation by the intraosseous transport system.

Any change in the mechanical load on a bone results in dynamic adaptation of its internal structure. Non-functional osteons are broken down, leaving remnants referred to as **interstitial lamellae** (Figures 3.34 and 3.35). The structure of compact bone undergoes gradual alteration as part of lifelong bone remodelling. Loss of bone mass with advancing age is associated with a reduction in osteocytes and delayed mineralisation.

At the internal and external surfaces of the bone, the lamellae are arranged in circular sheets, forming the **internal circumferential lamellae** (adjacent to the endosteum) and **external circumferential lamellae** (lying against the internal surface of the periosteum). Collagen fibres that bind the periosteum to the bone (**fibrae perforantes, Sharpey's fibres**) are incorporated into the external circumferential lamellae. The endosteum, composed of osteoprogenitor cells and connective tissue, lines the internal circumferential lamellae and the trabeculae (Figure 3.34).

Trabecular (**spongy**) **bone** also contains lamellae, but these are not organised into osteonal systems. Remodelling processes occur at a particularly high rate in spongy bone.

New bone formation (osteogenesis)

The formation of new bone occurs in two ways. Development of bone directly from mesenchymal connective tissue without a cartilaginous precursor phase is referred to as **intramembranous ossification** (**primary** or **direct ossification**). This type of bone formation gives rise to certain flat bones of the skull and the bony collar of developing long bones. It is also observed in repairing bone fractures. Formation of bone based on a cartilaginous template is termed **endochondral ossification** (**secondary** or **indirect ossification**). This results first in (immature) woven bone that is gradually replaced by (mature) lamellar bone (sometimes referred to as replacement bone) (Figures 3.40 to 3.42).

INTRAMEMBRANOUS OSSIFICATION

In intramembranous ossification, osteoprogenitor cells differentiate into osteoblasts (Figures 3.38 and 3.39) that produce collagen fibres and osteoid. Through continued

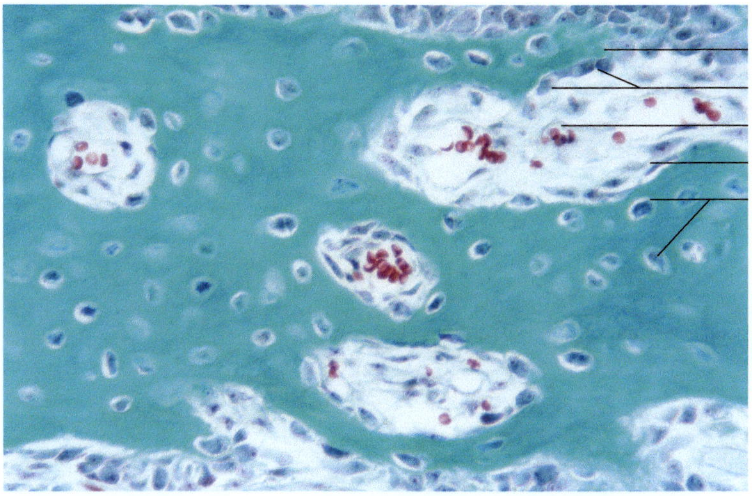

3.38 Intramembranous ossification: bone of cranium (juvenile dog). Near capillaries, osteoprogenitor cells within loose connective tissue differentiate into osteoblasts, which become arranged in sheets and liberate osteoid. As the bone matrix becomes mineralised, osteoblasts transform into osteocytes. Goldner's Masson trichrome stain (x480).

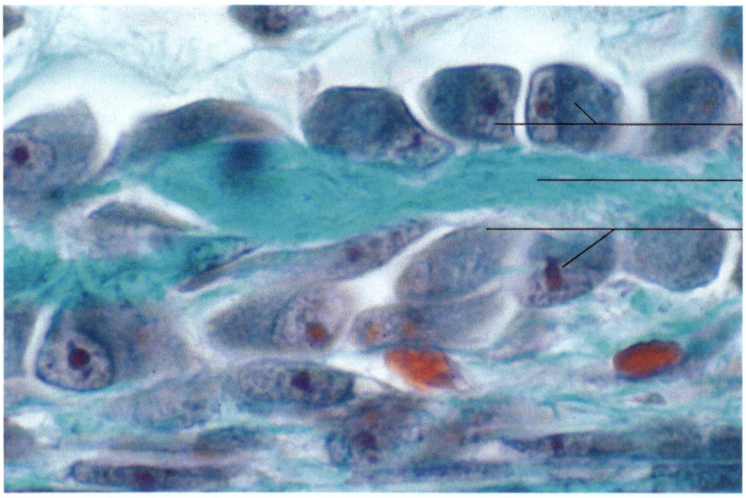

3.39 Intramembranous ossification: bone of cranium (juvenile dog). Active osteoblasts form a layer of cells immediately adjacent to the surface of ossifying spicules of osteoid. Their cytoplasm is strongly basophilic and their nuclei are typically spherical with nucleoli. Goldner's Masson trichrome stain (x720).

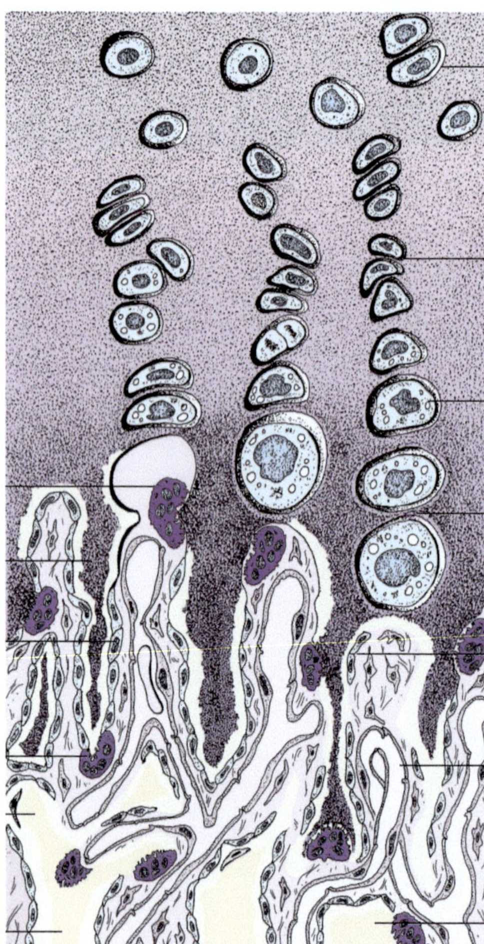

3.40 Processes involved in endochondral ossification in a long bone (schematic). Refer to text for elaboration upon the use of the term 'chondroclast'.

production of non-mineralised bone matrix, the osteoblasts gradually become walled off and the distance between them increases. They remain in contact, however, via their cellular processes. The ground substance gradually becomes mineralised and osteoblasts transform into osteocytes. The bone matrix contains predominantly irregularly arranged collagen fibres. At the beginning of the ossification process there is marked growth of blood capillaries into the connective tissue. These blood vessels are accompanied by additional mesenchymal connective tissue. Through this early vascularisation, the bone tissue establishes itself as a metabolically active **mineral depot**. The formation and resorption of the bone is closely regulated by various hormones (Figure 3.30).

ENDOCHONDRAL OSSIFICATION

Endochondral ossification involves the formation of bone from a **template** of hyaline cartilage (Figures 3.40 and 3.41). The cartilage also serves as the foundation for **lengthwise growth** of the bone. This function continues until the epiphyseal plate closes.

Endochondral ossification incorporates both perichondral ossification and endochondral (intracartilaginous) ossification.

Perichondral ossification proceeds according to the principles of intramembranous ossification. Chondroblasts in the perichondrium differentiate into osteoblasts. In long bones, transformation of connective into osseous tissue begins in the middle of the future diaphysis, forming a bony collar around the cartilage model. The perichondrium becomes the periosteum. Ossification of the diaphysis continues in the direction of the epiphyses.

As the bony collar develops, the chondrocytes hypertrophy and calcify the surrounding cartilage matrix. Calcification of the matrix impedes the supply of nutrition to the chondrocytes, resulting in their degeneration. At the same time, blood vessels penetrate the bony collar and enter the cartilage. It is considered by some authors that these blood vessels are accompanied by chondroclasts (possibly the same cell type as osteoclasts, see above), which break down the remaining cartilage. The space created by the degeneration of the cartilage is infiltrated by capillaries and mesenchymal connective tissue, and the process of endochondral ossification commences. After differentiating from mesenchymal stem cells, osteoprogenitor cells give rise to osteoblasts. These lay down osteoid on remaining spicules of calcified cartilage. A constant process of bone formation and breakdown results in formation of the medullary cavity. Mesenchymal connective tissue in the cavity transforms into haemoreticular tissue, filling the cavity with red bone marrow.

As ossification is taking place in the diaphysis, chondrocytes located at the end of the model become aligned in columns. At the same time, mitotic division of the chondrocytes results in lengthwise growth of the cartilage and thus, subsequently, of the bone.

The processes involved in endochondral ossification of the cartilage template, the eventual degradation of the cartilage and the formation of new bone from mesenchymal connective tissue can be particularly clearly observed at the **physeal–metaphyseal** region between the diaphysis and epiphyses. The following zones can be distinguished (from most to least distal to the diaphysis) (Figures 3.40 to 3.42):

- reserve zone,
- zone of proliferation,
- zone of hypertrophy,
- zone of ossification and
- zone of resorption.

In the reserve zone, the morphology and arrangement of the chondrocytes is typical of hyaline cartilage. The next zone towards the medullary cavity is the relatively wide **zone of proliferation**. Here the chondrocytes, arranged in columns, undergo division. Intercellular matrix is less plentiful in this zone and the cells are packed together more closely. In the **zone of hypertrophy**, the chondrocytes increase in size. The intercellular matrix becomes reduced to narrow spicules and begins to undergo calcification. Within the adjacent **zone of ossification**, calcification of the cartilage matrix is completed and the chondrocytes degenerate. At the same time, blood vessels and perivascular connective tissue invading from within the medullary cavity permit **chondroclasts** (possibly the same cells as osteoclasts, see above) to access the zone of ossification, where they engage in enzymatic digestion of calcified cartilage remnants (**zone of resorption**).

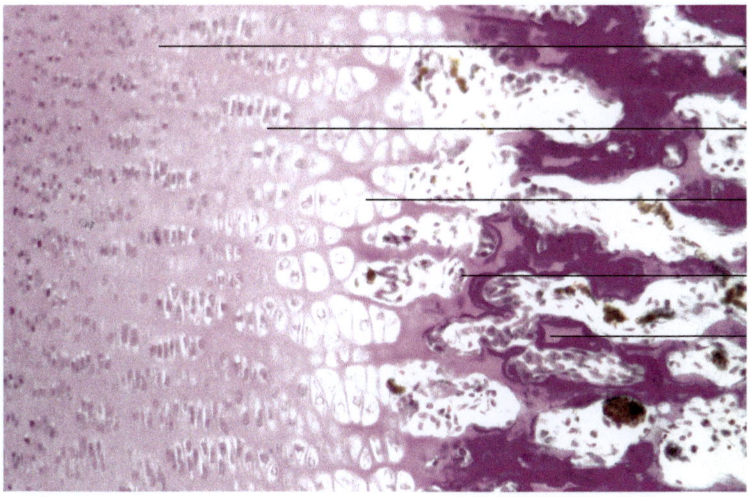

3.41 Section of the growth plate between the epiphysis and diaphysis of a long bone (dog). Haematoxylin and eosin stain (x100).

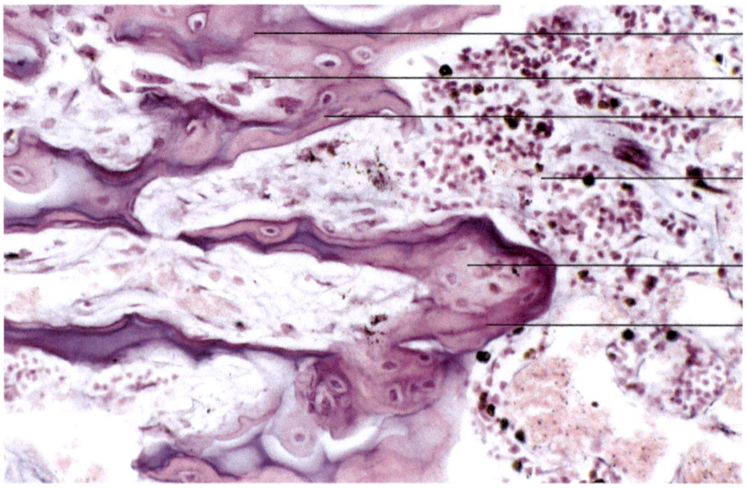

3.42 Section of the resorption zone of a long bone with calcified, deep violet-staining cartilage, osteoid, mineralised bone matrix and medullary cavity (dog). Haematoxylin and eosin stain (x300).

Osteoblasts accompanying these vessels enter the expanding spaces within the tissue, where they lay down new bone on remaining cartilage matrix. This marks the beginning of new bone formation. The woven bone that forms initially is gradually replaced by mature, lamellar bone.

4

Muscle tissue (textus muscularis)

All cells have the capacity for movement. Processes such as mitosis, phagocytosis and the amoeboid migration of white blood cells into extravascular tissue all involve some degree of mobility or contraction. In higher organisms, a specialised form of contractility is expressed by cells that constitute muscle tissue.

The primary distinguishing feature of muscle tissue is the transformation by muscle cells of **chemical energy** (**adenosine triphosphate**, **ATP**) into **mechanical energy** and **heat**. This functional specialisation necessitates the differentiation of specific structural features. Based on its physiological function, muscle tissue is divided into two types:

- smooth muscle and
- striated muscle.

Smooth muscle (textus muscularis nonstriatus)

As well as forming the muscular component of most internal organs, smooth muscle surrounds the secretory ducts of glands and forms part of the wall of blood and lymphatic vessels. Smooth muscle cells also perform important functions in the lung, genital apparatus and the skin.

Fine structure of smooth muscle cells (myocytus nonstriatus)

Smooth muscle tissue is composed primarily of spindle-shaped smooth muscle cells measuring 20–500 µm in length (Figures 4.1 to 4.5 and Table 4.1). The term 'smooth' is used for this muscle type because its myofilaments lack the ordered arrangement observed in striated muscle. The ovoid to oblong, usually slightly notched nucleus is typically located centrally, becoming shortened during muscle contraction. The cytoplasm (**sarcoplasm**) contains numerous mitochondria and a variably developed endoplasmic reticulum (**sarcoplasmic reticulum**). The functions of the endoplasmic reticulum include storage of Ca^{2+}. Micropinocytic vesicles (**caveolae**) are found along the cell membrane, predominantly at the ends of the cell (Figures 4.5 and 4.6). These are believed to be involved in transport of Ca^{2+}. An increase in sarcoplasmic Ca^{2+} and associated muscle contraction is triggered by various

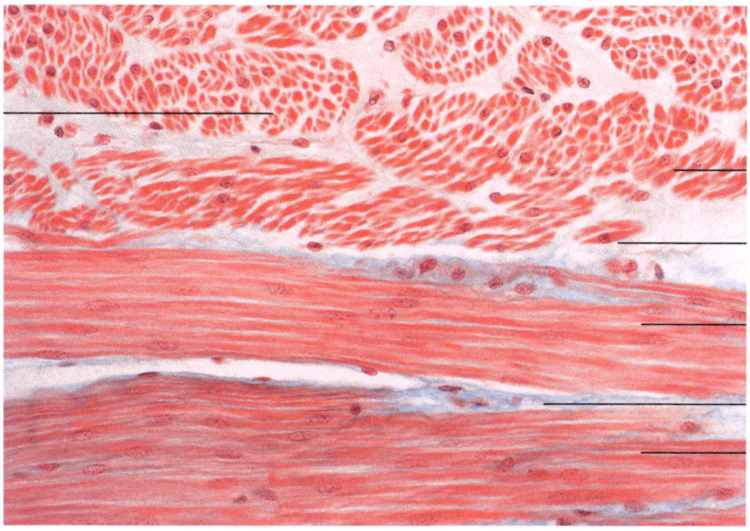

4.1 Smooth muscle of small intestine in longitudinal and transverse section (cat). Haematoxylin and eosin stain (x200).

factors, including depolarisation (via the neurotransmitters acetylcholine and noradrenaline), mechanical stretching and chemical stimuli.

In histological sections of smooth muscle, the **myofilaments** within the smooth muscle cells (**actin**-, **myosin**- and **intermediate filaments**) appear to be oriented in various directions, forming a network (Figure 4.5).

The **actin filaments** (1 µm in length) are anchored to each other and to the inner surface of the plasmalemma by **dense bodies** (**areae densae**). Dense bodies also serve as insertion sites for intermediate filaments, in which the contractile actin filaments are enmeshed (Figures 4.5 and 4.6).

Dense bodies are considered to be equivalent to the Z line of striated muscle. **Myosin filaments** are interspersed among the network of actin filaments. These are soluble, highly labile proteins that increase in number during contraction. They are not attached to dense bodies. **Intermediate filaments** (**desmin**) form the cytoskeleton of smooth muscle cells. They are not contractile.

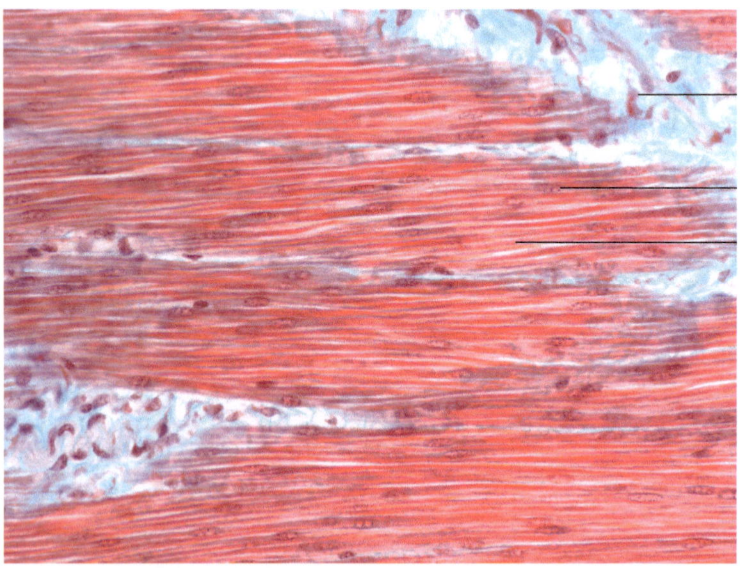

4.2 Longitudinal section of a bundle of smooth muscle fibres in the stomach (cat). The nucleus of smooth muscle cells is situated centrally. The surrounding sarcoplasm is drawn out, conforming to the fusiform shape of the cell. The surface of the smooth muscle cell is invested by connective tissue (endomysium). Goldner's Masson trichrome stain (x200).

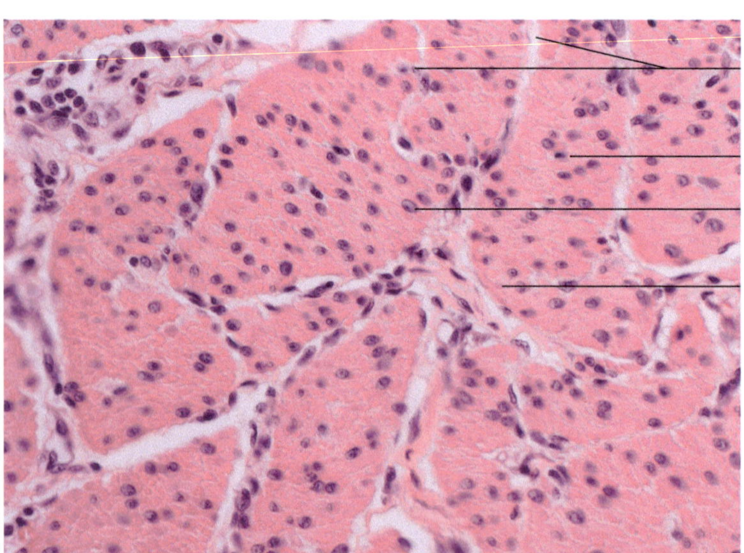

4.3 Transverse section of a bundle of smooth muscle fibres in the stomach (cat). The nucleus is located centrally. In some cases, the section has passed through a region of the sarcoplasm in which the nucleus is not present. Connective tissue surrounds individual cells (endomysium) and fibre bundles (perimysium). Haematoxylin and eosin stain (x480).

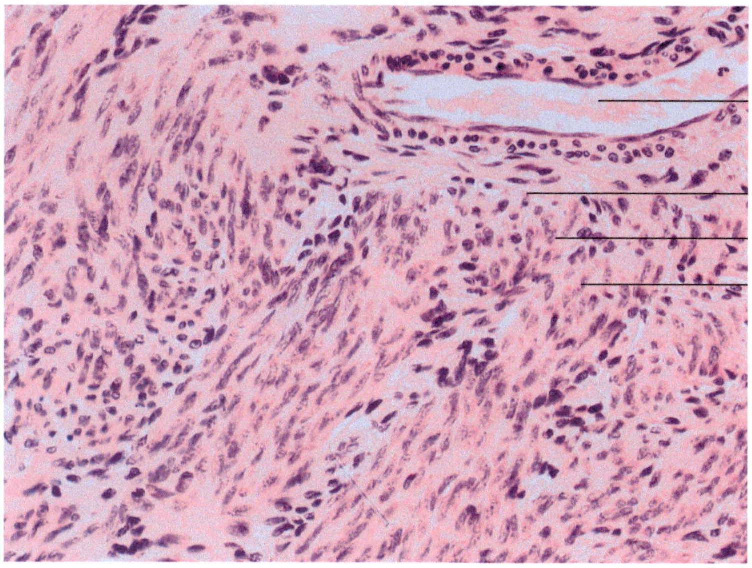

4.4 Bladder (dog). In the wall of the bladder, smooth muscle cells are arranged in oblique spirals in which vessels and autonomic nerve fibre bundles are interposed. Haematoxylin and eosin stain (x180).

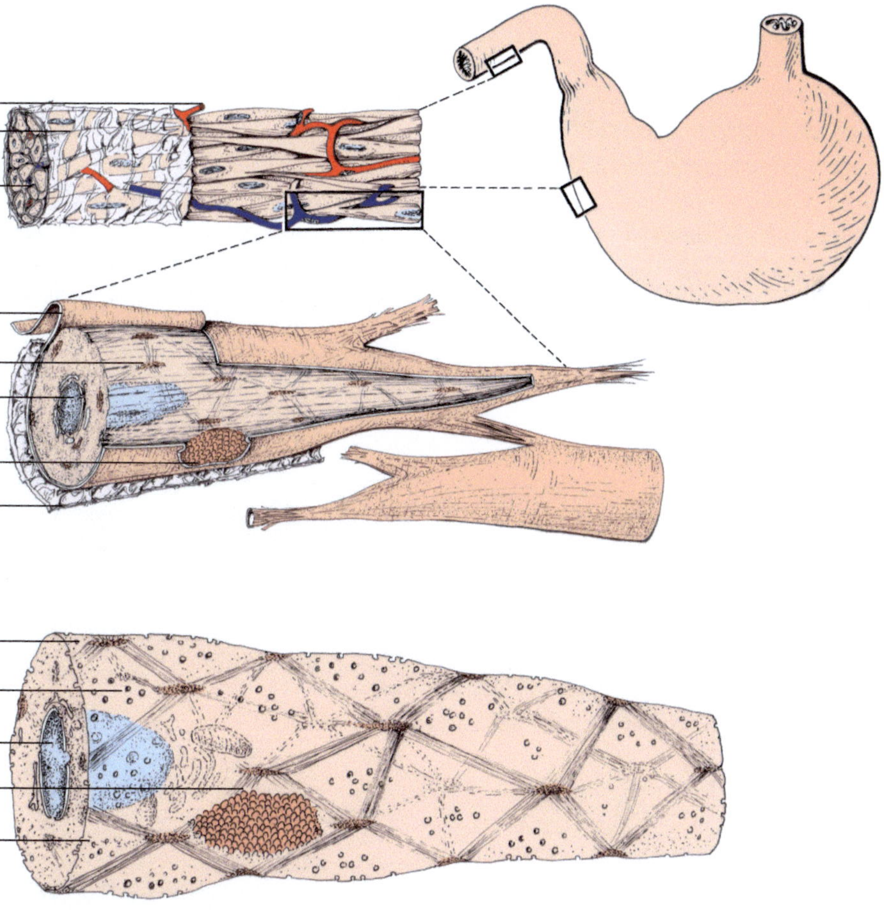

4.5 Light microscopic and fine structure of smooth muscle tissue (schematic).

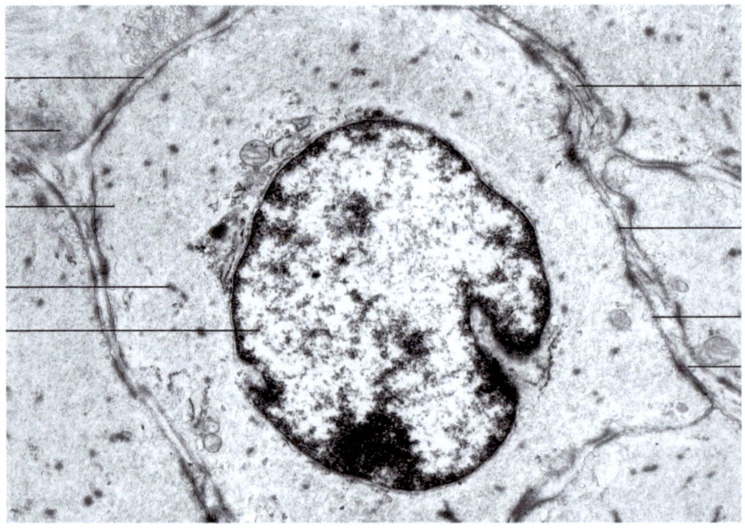

4.6 Fine structure of a smooth muscle cell (transverse section; x10,000).

During contraction, the myosin filaments undergo structural reorganisation resulting in movement of the actin over the myosin filaments. As the actin filaments are anchored to the dense bodies, the distance between the bodies decreases. The muscle cell contracts and increases in thickness.

Muscle contraction

The surface of smooth muscle cells is surrounded by a delicate mesh of collagen fibres, reticular fibres and in some cases elastic fibres (endomysium). In association with this connective tissue sheath, **autonomic nerves** extend close to or, less frequently, make contact with, the plasmalemma of the muscle cell. Nerve fibres generally pass to within 10–20 µm of the muscle fibre, forming numerous synaptic contacts referred to as **bouton en passant**. In contrast to striated muscle, the excitatory stimulus is not transmitted through a motor end plate. Instead, the surface of smooth muscle cells exhibits a large number of **adrenergic** α-, α_1-, β-, β_1- and **cholinergic receptors**.

Muscle contraction is controlled by Ca^{2+}. An increase in sarcoplasmic Ca^{2+} is produced either by opening of Ca^{2+} channels in the cell membrane (via membrane depolarisation) or second messenger-induced Ca^{2+} release from the sarcoplasmic reticulum (via binding of hormones with cell membrane receptors). Under the influence of complexes formed between Ca^{2+} and the intracellular protein calmodulin (**Ca^{2+}–calmodulin complexes**), the light chains of the myosin filaments undergo phosphorylation. The actin-binding site of the myosin head is thereby activated, allowing contraction to occur.

Smooth muscle of the gastrointestinal system is also innervated by the enteric division of the autonomic nervous system (see Chapter 16, 'Receptors and sense organs').

Based on the type of stimulus that brings about contraction, smooth muscle can be divided into two groups. As well as responding to neural and hormonal signals, the muscle of the walls of hollow organs (e.g. stomach, intestine, uterus, larger blood vessels) is capable of contracting spontaneously, under the influence of 'pacemaker' cells (**myogenic contraction**). The excitatory stimulus spreads quickly through the muscle via gap junctions, and the muscle contracts as a unit (**single-unit muscle**, **unitary smooth muscle**).

In contrast, smooth muscle cells in structures such as the smaller vessels, the airways and the ciliary body are individually innervated by autonomic nerve fibres. Nerve impulses reach the cells through the neurotransmitters noradrenaline and acetylcholine (**neurogenic contraction**). This is referred to as **multiunit muscle**.

Striated muscle (textus muscularis striatus)

Striated muscle is thus named because of the ordered arrangement of myofilaments in the cytoplasm of individual cells. This gives rise to regularly repeating cross-bands that are oriented perpendicular to the long axis of the cell. Striated muscle can be further divided into:

- skeletal muscle and
- cardiac muscle.

Skeletal muscle (textus muscularis striatus skeletalis)

Skeletal muscle forms the contractile component of the locomotor apparatus. It constitutes the tissue generally referred to by the lay term 'muscle'. Skeletal muscle is composed of parallel bundles of skeletal muscle cells (up to several centimetres long, 10–100 µm in diameter). It is extensively vascularised and is innervated by sensory and motor nerve fibres. Connective tissue surrounds the muscle cells, dividing skeletal muscle tissue into functional units of various size.

Fine structure of skeletal muscle cells (myocytus striatus skeletalis)

The striated muscle cell is a **syncytium** formed by the fusion of myogenic stem cells (myoblasts). An individual cell, also referred to as a muscle fibre, contains over 100 nuclei (Table 4.1). The nuclei are flattened and fusiform and are predominantly **located peripherally**, at the inner surface of the plasmalemma (subplasmalemmal).

Individual skeletal muscle cells are surrounded by a basal lamina and a meshwork of reticular fibres. This casing lies immediately adjacent to the plasmalemma of the muscle cell (**sarcolemma**) (Figures 4.7 and 4.8). A glycoprotein-dystrophin (400 kD) complex connects the sarcolemma to laminin within the basal lamina.

At regular intervals, tubular invaginations of the sarcolemma pass deep into the sarcoplasm forming the structural framework of the transverse tubular (T) system of striated muscle cells (see below).

SARCOPLASM

A substantial portion of the sarcoplasm is occupied by myofibrils. The organelles are displaced to the periphery, near the nuclei, and between the contractile filaments of the myofibrils.

Golgi apparatuses are located near the nuclei. They are usually relatively small. **Mitochondria** (**sarcosomes**) are arranged in parallel rows among the myofibrils. Enzymes associated with the electron transfer chain and oxidative phosphorylation (ATP–ADP cycle) are particularly abundant in the mitochondria of muscle cells. They include enzymes of the citric acid cycle and those associated with β-oxidation (in the mitochondrial matrix), cytochrome oxidase (inner mitochondrial membrane), adenylate kinase for synthesis of energy-rich phosphates (intermembrane space) and monoamine oxidase (outer membrane). The cells contain relatively little rough ER and few free ribosomes. The sarcoplasm contains glycoprotein as a source of energy, and the muscle pigment myoglobin for storage of O_2. Interspersed between the myofilaments are two structurally independent yet functionally coupled membrane systems, the sarcoplasmic reticulum and the T system.

SARCOPLASMIC RETICULUM

The **sarcoplasmic reticulum** forms a fenestrated system of membranes around individual myofibrils (Figure 4.7). It incorporates Ca^{2+}/Mg^{2+}-dependent ATPase and acts as an intracellular reservoir for free Ca^{2+}. The primary function of this network of cisternae is the intracellular transport of Ca^{2+} and thus regulation of muscle contraction. Where two adjacent networks meet, the sarcoplasmic reticulum expands into **terminal cisternae** (see below).

TRANSVERSE TUBULAR SYSTEM

The longitudinally oriented, variable calibre cisternae of the sarcoplasmic reticulum are interposed between tubular invaginations of the plasmalemma, the **transverse tubular system** (**T system**) (Figures 4.7, 4.11, 4.13 and 4.14). The interior of the T system is continuous with the extra-

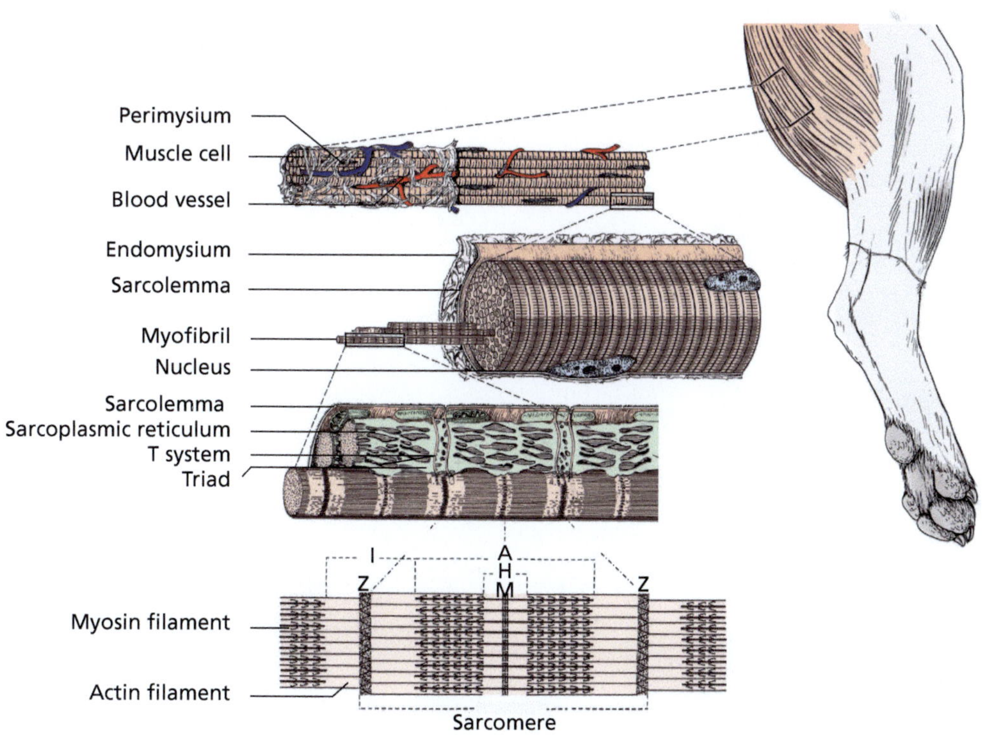

4.7 Light histological and fine structure of skeletal striated muscle (schematic). Refer to text for explanation of labelling of the sarcomere.

cellular compartment. The tubules of the T system form ring-like anastomoses yet are separated from the terminal cisternae of the sarcoplasmic reticulum by a space. The region in which two terminal cisternae of the sarcoplasmic reticulum lie adjacent to a tubule of the T system is referred to as a **triad** (Figure 4.7).

The T system enables rapid transmission of the nerve impulse (depolarisation with influx of sodium) from the cell membrane to the interior of the cell and facilitates coordinated contraction of the whole muscle fibre. At the triads, the impulse is transmitted to the sarcoplasmic reticulum, from which Ca^{2+} is released. Ca^{2+} thus acts as a mediator between electrical stimulation at the cell membrane and contraction of the myofibrils within the cell.

A single muscle fibre is estimated to contain around 1000 myofibrils. In longitudinal section, these exhibit a characteristic banding pattern (light and dark) arising from the ordered, parallel arrangement of their component myofilaments (Figures 4.7 to 4.14). The bands can be distinguished on the basis of their refractive properties:

- isotropic, monorefringent (= light) I bands and
- anisotropic, birefringent (= dark) A bands.

These bands are bisected by transverse bands of different density:

- The I band is bisected by a dense intermediate disc ('Zwischenscheibe') termed the Z line.
- The A band is bisected by a less dense region (H band) which in turn is bisected by the narrow, dense M line.

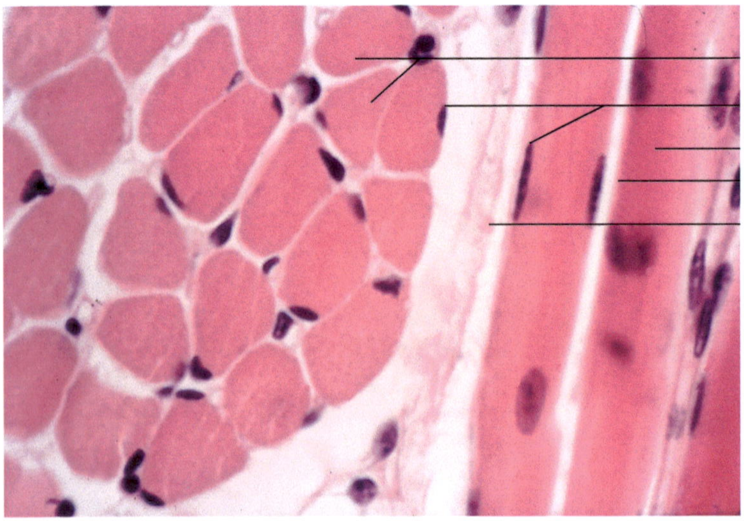

4.8 Skeletal muscle fibres in the tongue (dog). The nuclei are located peripherally (at the sarcoplasmic surface of the sarcolemma). In transverse section, the arrangement of myofibrils produces a faint mosaic-like effect (Cohnheim fields). Individual muscle cells are surrounded by endomysium, muscle fasciculi are invested by perimysium. Haematoxylin and eosin stain (x180).

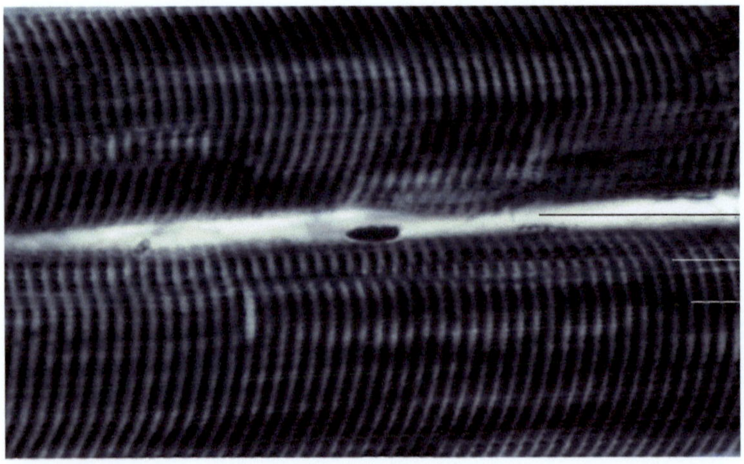

4.9 Skeletal muscle fibres in the tongue (dog). Longitudinal section with periodic isotropic and anisotropic cross-banding. Iron haematoxylin stain (x1000).

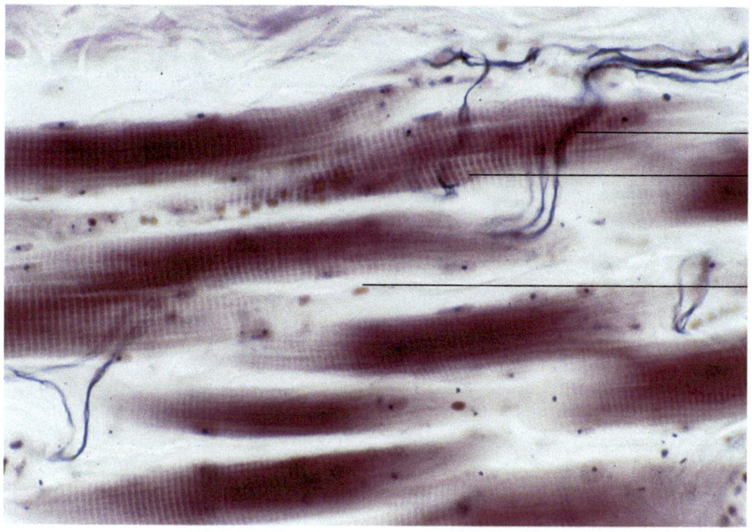

4.10 Skeletal muscle fibres in cutaneous muscle (cat). Longitudinal section with periodic isotropic and anisotropic banding and motor nerve fibres. Schefthaler–Mayet method (x200).

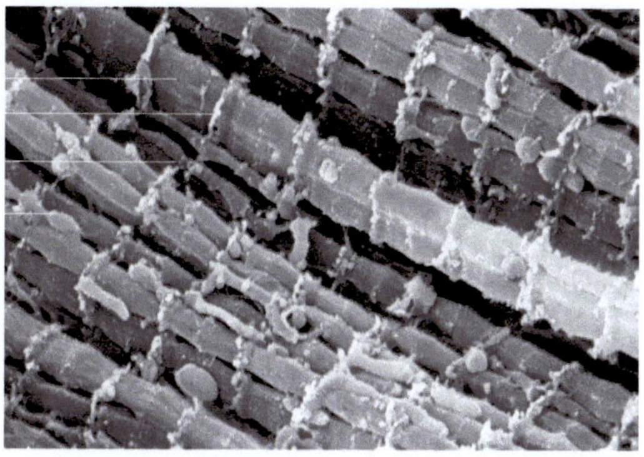

4.11 Scanning electron micrograph showing a surface view of a bundle of myofibrils in a skeletal muscle cell. Freeze-fracture method.

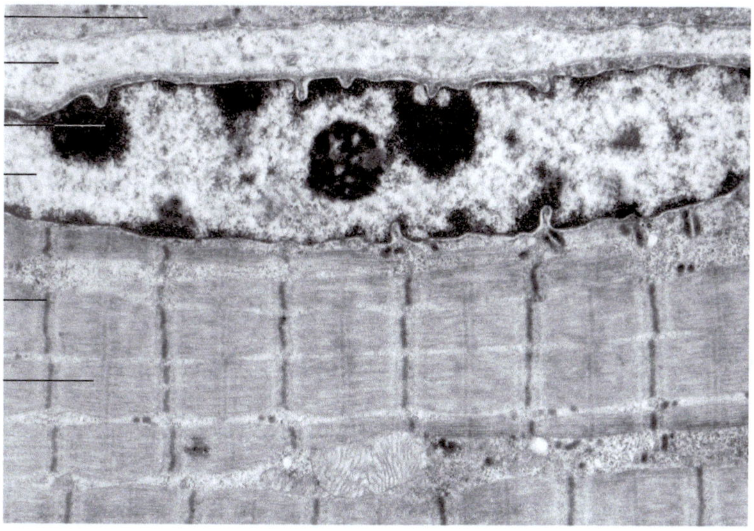

4.12 Fine structure of a skeletal muscle cell with peripherally located nucleus (x5000).

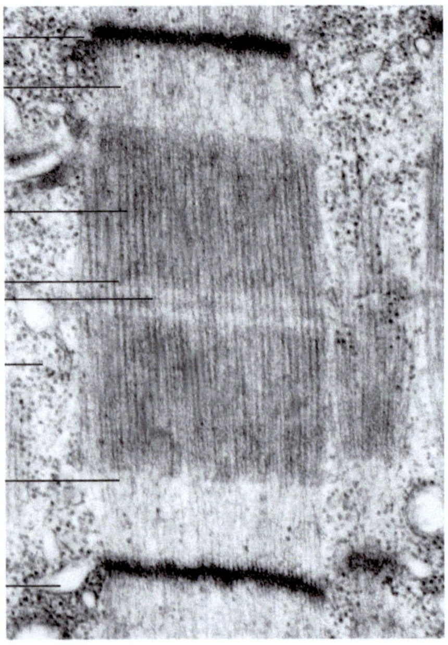

4.13 Fine structure of a sarcomere in the non-contracted state in a skeletal muscle cell (x12,000).

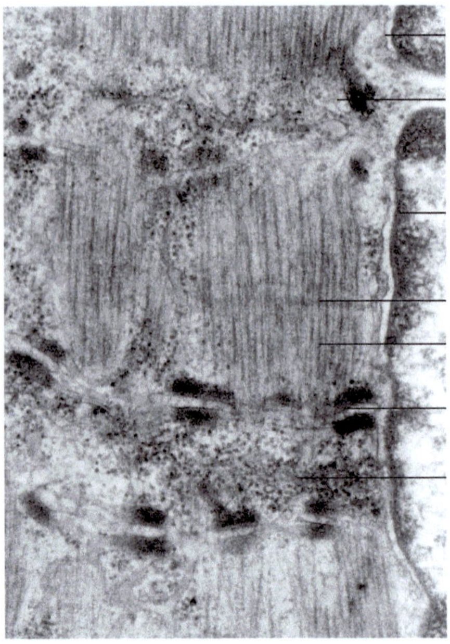

4.14 Fine structure of a contracted sarcomere with nearby triad in a skeletal muscle cell (x12,000).

Between the two Z lines lies the smallest functional unit of striated muscle myofibrils, the **sarcomere** (length 2 μm, width 1.5 μm) (Figure 4.7). Changes in the length of a group of sarcomeres results in lengthening or shortening of the muscle. Sarcomeres thus represent the **contractile units of the muscle**.

The cylindrical **myofibrils** are composed of parallel bundles of **thin actin** and **thick myosin filaments** (Figure 4.7). **Actin filaments** traverse the length of the I band and insert on the Z line. These filaments are 1 μm long and have a diameter of 6 nm. Actin filaments are composed of a **double helix** of **F actin**, a polymer of globular actin molecules. An elongated molecule, **tropomyosin,** is wound around the actin double helix, its periodicity corresponding to that of the actin molecule. Attached to each tropomyosin molecule is a globular troponin complex, comprising three subunits. During contraction, Ca^{2+} binds to troponin, which acts on tropomyosin to expose the binding site for myosin.

Myosin filaments (**myosin II**), which constitute the thick fibres of the A band, are approximately 15 nm wide and 1.6 μm long. They are composed of six protein chains. The myosin molecule is divided into the following components:

- a rod-like, double helical tail (**light meromyosin**) and
- two globular heads (**heavy meromyosin**).

Heavy meromyosin has ATPase activity. Light meromyosin is flexible, permitting coupling of myosin with actin (**actin–myosin complex**). Shortening of skeletal muscle is brought about by the sliding of actin and myosin filaments over one another (sliding filament theory, refer to biochemistry texts for further detail).

Muscle contraction

Contraction is initiated by release of Ca^{2+} **into the sarcoplasm**. Following depolarisation, Ca^{2+} ions penetrate the interior of myofibrils and activate the contractile mechanism. Calcium acts on the **troponin–tropomyosin system**. In the absence of free Ca^{2+} ions, troponin inhibits the interaction between actin, myosin and the magnesium–ATP complex. Binding of Ca^{2+} with troponin overcomes this blockage by causing tropomyosin to move away from the myosin binding site on the actin filament. The myosin heads, which act both as centres of enzymatic ATP hydrolysis and as actin-binding sites, contact the actin filaments.

Energy from ATP hydrolysis is used to reposition the myosin head, which then reattaches to the actin filament and returns to its original position causing the thin filament to move along the thick filament. This results in shortening of the sarcomere.

During repolarisation, the release of Ca^{2+} ceases and a Ca^{2+}-activated ATPase pump returns Ca^{2+} against a concentration gradient to the sarcoplasmic reticulum, resulting in muscle relaxation.

Fibre types

Skeletal muscle cells, or muscle fibres, can be divided into three types:

- **type I** (**slow oxidative**) **fibres** (red muscle):
  - ample sarcoplasm, relatively few myofibrils,
  - high myoglobin (muscle pigment) content (dark red in colour),
  - abundant mitochondria with high levels of enzymes involved in cellular respiration (cytochrome),
  - high density of adjacent capillaries and
  - contract slowly, suited to sustained effort.
- **type II** (**fast glycolytic**) **fibres** (white muscle):
  - little sarcoplasm, large numbers of myofibrils,
  - little myoglobin ('white' in colour),
  - relatively few mitochondria and
  - contract quickly, fibres fatigue rapidly.
- **intermediate** (**fast oxidative glycolytic**) **fibres**:
  - functional characteristics intermediate between those of type I and II fibres.

Satellite cells

Satellite cells are small cells with heterochromatic nuclei. They lie adjacent to skeletal muscle cells between the plasmalemma of the muscle fibre and the basal lamina. These cells can undergo mitotic division and are responsible for muscular regeneration.

Skeletal muscle is capable of only limited regeneration. Tissue that is damaged – for example due to injury or surgical intervention – is generally replaced by fibrous scar tissue. When the basal lamina surrounding the muscle cell is preserved and the blood supply and innervation remain intact, satellite cells undergo myogenic differentiation and new muscle fibres are formed.

Innervation

Nerve impulses are transmitted to skeletal muscle at the **neuromuscular junction** (**motor end plate**). Each skeletal muscle fibre is innervated by at least one axon of a **motor nerve** arising from the **spinal cord** or **brain stem**. The **neurotransmitter** (**acetylcholine**) released at the point of contact between the nerve fibre and the muscle cell (**synapse**) stimulates receptors on the muscle cell surface. This opens Na^+ channels in the sarcolemma, triggering an influx of sodium into the muscle cell. The cell membrane depolarises and the process of muscular contraction is initiated (see Chapter 5, 'Nervous tissue'). Skeletal muscle tissue also contains stretch receptors associated with proprioception (see Chapter 16, 'Receptors and sense organs').

Connective tissue associated with skeletal muscle

Each skeletal muscle is composed of numerous bundles of muscle fibres (fasciculi). The outer surface of the muscle is invested by a sheath of connective tissue, the **epimysium**. Primary, secondary and tertiary fasciculi are surrounded by connective tissue termed the **perimysium**. Like the epimysium, the perimysium is composed of dense connective tissue. It contains blood and lymphatic vessels as well as nerve fibres.

The smallest functional unit of the muscle, the individual muscle fibre, is enclosed by a delicate network of reticular fibres. Referred to as the **endomysium** (Figure 4.7), this layer contains fibroblasts, histiocytes and mast cells as well as capillaries and nerve fibres.

Microvasculature

At particular locations, blood vessels and nerves penetrate the connective tissue covering the muscle and ramify in the perimysium. Within the endomysium, they loop around the individual muscle fibre forming a network that can adapt in width, according to the degree of muscle contraction.

Cardiac muscle (textus muscularis striatus cardiacus)

Cardiac muscle (**musculus cardiacus**) is similar in structure to skeletal muscle (Figures 4.15 to 4.18). However, in accordance with the functional demands on the heart, the structure of the muscular walls is specialised and cardiac muscle tissue has the capacity for **spontaneous generation** and **independent intracardiac conduction of nerve stimuli**. This, together with other morphological features, distinguishes cardiac muscle from skeletal striated muscle.

Structure of cardiac muscle

Cardiac muscle comprises the contractile portion of the walls of the organ, the myocardium.

FINE STRUCTURE OF CARDIAC MUSCLE (MYOCYTUS STRIATUS CARDIACUS)

In contrast to skeletal muscle cells, **cardiac muscle fibres** reach lengths of only 50–100 μm (Table 4.1). They generally contain a **single**, **centrally located nucleus** although two nuclei are occasionally present. Cardiac muscle cells are connected end to end by tissue-specific regions known as **intercalated discs** (Figures 4.15 and 4.18). Some cells are connected with more than one other cell. This branching configuration forms the basis of the three-dimensional framework of the muscle of the heart.

SARCOPLASM

In accordance with their high metabolic rate, cardiac muscle cells are richly endowed with **metabolically active organelles** (Golgi apparatus, endoplasmic reticulum, ribosomes). **Mitochondria** are plentiful and large, reflecting their degree of activity. Abundant **glycogen granules** supply the cell with energy. In addition, lipid droplets and

Table 4.1 Distinguishing structural features of smooth, skeletal and cardiac muscle.

	Smooth muscle	Skeletal muscle	Cardiac muscle
Cell shape	Spindle-shaped	Polygonal	Branched
Length of individual cell	20–500 μm, up to 800 μm in the gravid uterus	Few mm to 10 cm	50–100 μm
Diameter of individual cell	3–10 μm	10–100 μm	10–30 μm
Nucleus number and location	Single nucleus, central location, elongate, fusiform	Many nuclei (up to several hundred, depending on length of cell; syncytium), peripherally located, flattened	Single nucleus, central location, spherical, ovoid
Fibres	Complex arrangement of myofilaments, no cross-banding	Cross-banding	Cross-banding
Special features	Spheroid caveolae (with Ca^{2+} pumps; association with sarcoplasmic reticulum), no T system	Narrow T tubules at the level of the A–I band junction, triads	Expanded T tubules at the level of the Z line, diads
Innervation	Autonomic	Somatic	Autonomous stimulus initiation and conduction, autonomic innervation
Neuromuscular relationship	Nerve fibres passing close to muscle cells, gap junctions	Neuromuscular junction (motor end plate)	Gap junctions
Occurrence	Walls of many organs	Locomotor apparatus	Myocardium
Regenerative capacity	Limited	Via satellite cells	Conditional
Special features	Dense bodies (areae densae)	Satellite cells (capable of forming new muscle cells)	Intercalated discs (disci intercalares), gap junctions, desmosomes, electrical coupling

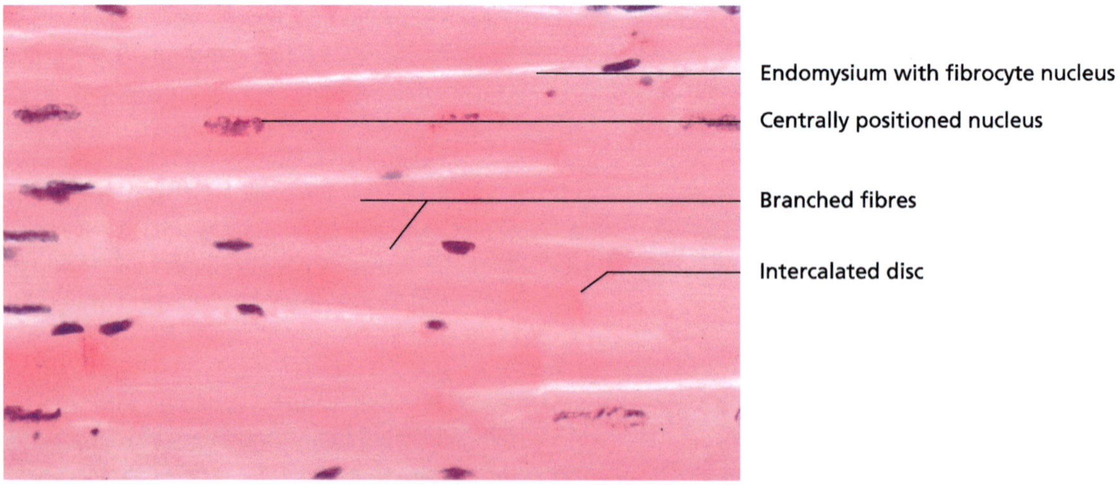

4.15 Longitudinal section of cardiac muscle (ox). This muscle type is characterised by a centrally located nucleus, striation of the myofibrils, branched muscle fibres and the interconnection of cells by intercalated discs. Haematoxylin and eosin stain (x480).

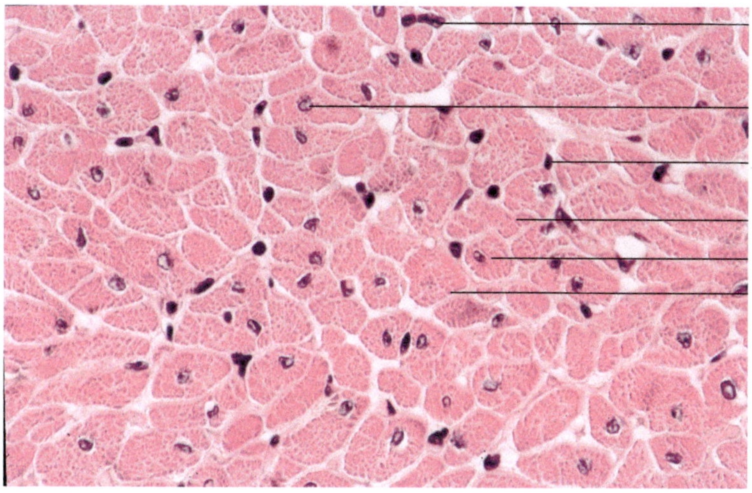

4.16 Transverse section of cardiac muscle (ox). The nucleus is located centrally. Individual muscle cells are surrounded by endomysium. Haematoxylin and eosin stain (x480).

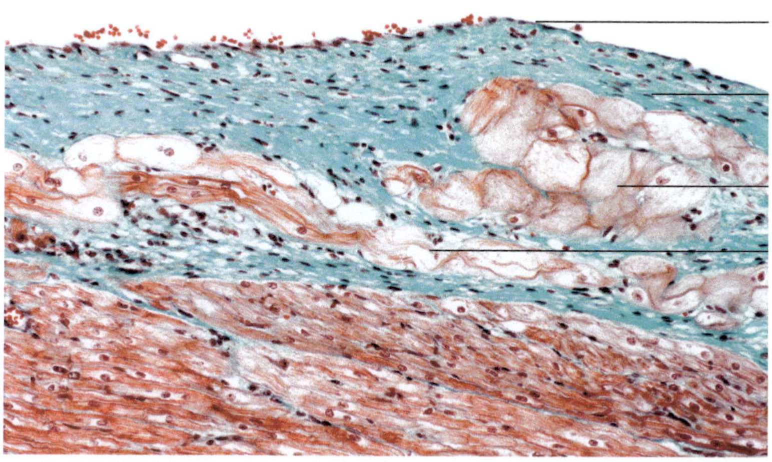

4.17 Purkinje fibres in the inner wall of the heart (ox). These are modified cardiac muscle cells that retain some marginally located myofilaments. The nuclei are pale, the cytoplasm is light staining. Goldner's Masson trichrome stain (x480).

brown **lipofuscin pigment** may be observed as paraplasmic inclusions between the myofibrils.

Cardiac muscle cells, particularly those of the atria and auricles, contain **secretory granules** enclosing **atrial natriuretic peptide** (**ANP** = **atriopeptin**). This hormone increases the glomerular filtration rate and regulates fluid balance in the central nervous system.

SARCOPLASMIC RETICULUM

Whereas the **T system** is more prominent in cardiac muscle than in skeletal muscle, the reverse is true of the **sarcoplasmic reticulum**. In place of a triad, a **diad** is formed by one-sided indirect contact between the tubules of the T system and the sarcoplasmic reticulum (Figure 4.18). Calcium-dependent contraction of cardiac muscle is further regulated by the autonomic nervous system, via adrenergic and cholinergic receptors on the cell membrane. The arrangement of actin–myosin complexes and the biochemical processes associated with muscle contraction are similar to those occurring in skeletal muscle.

The branched cardiac muscle fibres form a **network** in which fibres contract together as a unit ('all-or-none' contraction). This is facilitated by specialised sites of attachment between the muscle cells at which the cell membrane exhibits specific modifications. Using the light microscope, these **intercalated discs** (**disci intercalares**) appear as dense, transversely oriented bands (Figures 4.15 and 4.18).

At the site of the intercalated disc, the membranes of adjacent cells interdigitate (Figure 4.18). **Adhering junctions** (**fasciae adherentes**) serve to anchor the actin filaments within adjoining cells to the sarcolemma of the cell, allowing contractile forces to be transferred between adjacent cells. Additional structural support is provided

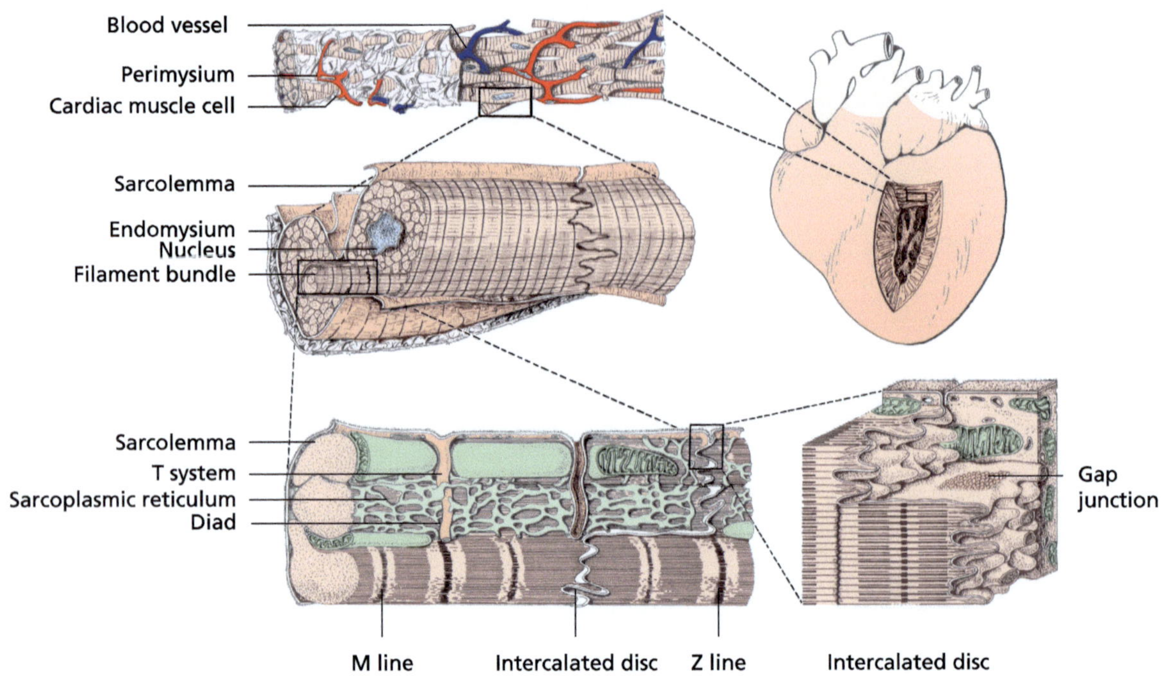

4.18 Light microscopic and fine structure of cardiac muscle and an intercalated disc (discus intercalaris) (schematic). The arrangement of the myofilaments actin and myosin is equivalent to that of skeletal muscle.

by **desmosomes** (**maculae adherentes**). **Gap junctions** enable the transmission of excitatory stimuli from one cell to the next, their pores providing passage for ions and low-molecular weight proteins. Due to the interconnected arrangement of cardiac muscle cells and the specialised structures of the intercalated disc, cardiac muscle constitutes an integrated structural and functional entity.

Impulse generation and conduction pathways

Stimulation and conduction of the excitatory stimulus in cardiac muscle is carried out by **modified cardiac cells** that transmit bioelectrical impulses. These include pacemaker cells, transitional cells and Purkinje fibres. Further information is provided in Chapter 6, 'Circulatory system'.

Nervous tissue (textus nervosus)

5

Excitability is one of the basic properties of living cells. Phylogenetic development has led to the differentiation of cells in which the capacity for excitability is particularly pronounced. These highly specialised **nerve** and **sensory cells** have the capacity to receive signals (stimuli), to direct these stimuli centrally, to process them and, with the input of higher centres or via reflexes, to initiate a response. The diverse functional capacity of these cells can be ascribed to their **neuro-ectodermal origin**.

During **embryonic development** the epithelial characteristics of this tissue are lost, but the deeper cell layers of the neuro-ectoderm remain in structural and functional contact through intimate interconnections and particularly long cell processes.

Nerve cells are so highly differentiated that they have lost the capacity for metabolic self-sufficiency. They require assistance in this regard from **supporting**, or **glial**, **cells**.

Nervous tissue is thus composed of two structural elements:

- nerve cells or neurons and
- glial cells, or neuroglia.

Nerve cells (neuron, neurocytus)

Nerve cells have elongated processes (**dendrites and axons**) that form complex connections (synapses) with other cells. **Dendrites** detect changes in their environment and transfer these signals to the cell body (**perikaryon**), from which the stimulus is transmitted along the **axon**.

While nerve cells exhibit exceptional variation in size and shape, they are consistent in their basic structure (perikaryon, and a number of variably branching cell processes [axons and dendrites]). The nerve cell inclusive of its processes represents a genetic, morphologic, functional and trophic unit referred to as a **neuron**.

The **perikaryon**, comprising the nucleus and surrounding cytoplasm, and the numerous dendrites constitute the **receptive portion** of the neuron. Dendrites (Gk *dendron* = tree) are extensively branched, elongated processes. At their extremities, they feature **specific sensory receptors** or form synapses with other neurons, from which they receive stimuli. Dendrites conduct impulses towards the perikaryon.

Each neuron has only one axon that transmits the signal away from the cell body. Axons may divide in the periphery, sending out collateral branches. At the target organ, axons typically exhibit terminal branching, forming the **telodendritic zone**. Individual free nerve endings, which vary in number and form, terminate in **end bulbs** (**boutons**). These represent the **effector component** of the neuron.

Classification of nerve cells

The diverse morphology of neuronal components is determined by the site of embryonic development of the nerve cell. Epithelial cells of the neural tube differentiate into bipotential progenitor cells, which give rise to neurons and glial cells. After the glial cell line has split off, neuroblasts eventually differentiate into mature neurons. These cells are not capable of division. Based on the number of cell processes, neurons are classified as:

- unipolar,
- bipolar,
- pseudo-unipolar or
- multipolar nerve cells (Figures 5.1 to 5.8).

Unipolar neurons

Unipolar neurons have a single cell process (axon). The existence of this type of neuron in differentiated nervous tissue is the subject of debate. The cells of the first neural layer of the retina (rods and cones) are frequently referred to as specialised unipolar neurons (Figure 5.6).

Bipolar neurons

In bipolar neurons, two processes (a dendrite and an axon) arise from opposite sides of the perikaryon. These are relatively uncommon, constituting the middle neural layer of the retina, the sensory cells of the olfactory mucosa and the cells of the spiral and vestibular ganglia of the inner ear.

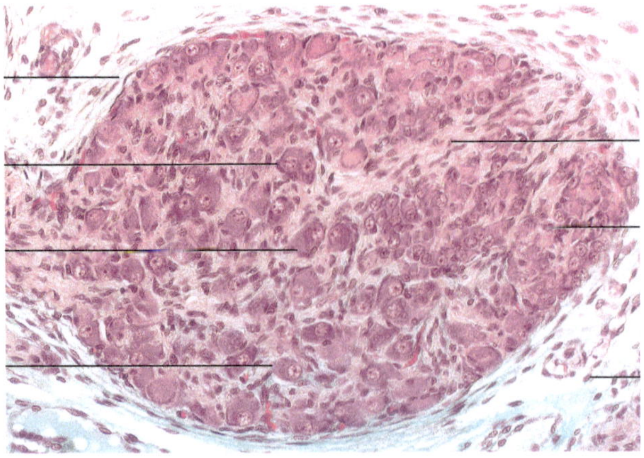

5.1 Peripheral (autonomic) ganglion with multipolar nerve cells in the urinary bladder (cat). Haematoxylin and eosin stain (x250).

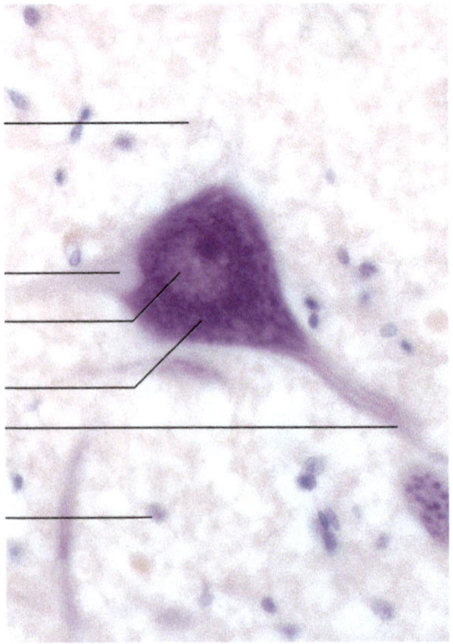

5.2 Multipolar neuron within the spinal cord (horse). Nissl method (x480). The term neuropil describes a network of neuronal and glial cell processes.

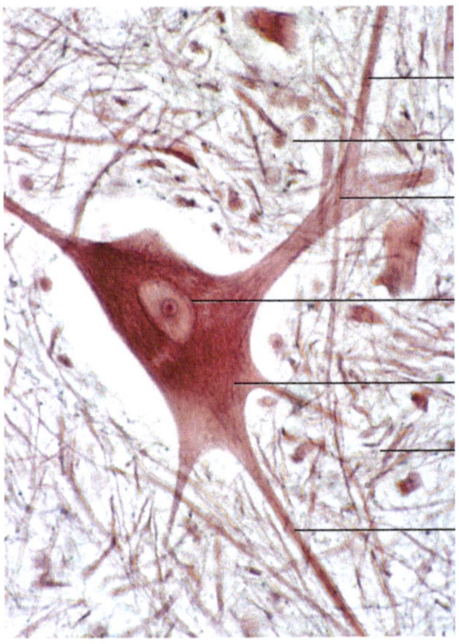

5.3 Multipolar neuron within the spinal cord (dog). Neurofibrils composed of neurofilaments and neurotubules are demonstrated using the Bodian method (x480).

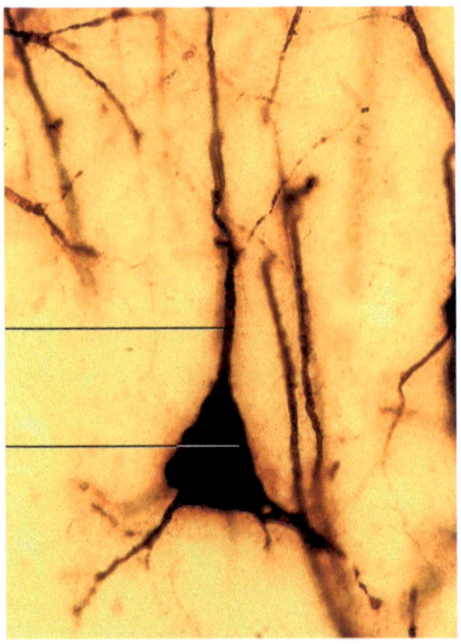

5.4 Pyramidal cells in the cerebrum (dog). Golgi silver impregnation method (x300).

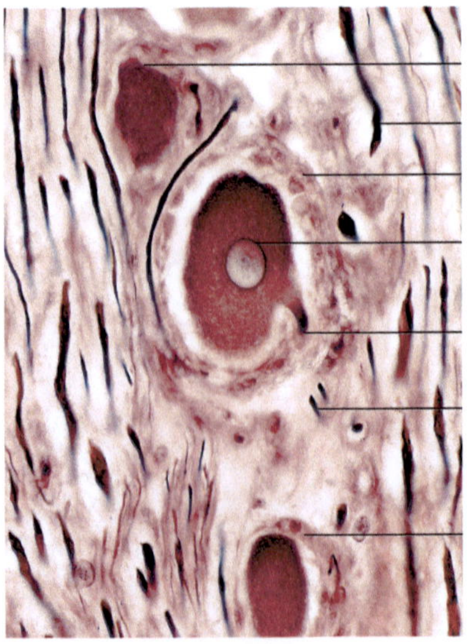

5.5 Pseudo-unipolar neuron in a spinal ganglion (ox). Haematoxylin and eosin stain (x400).

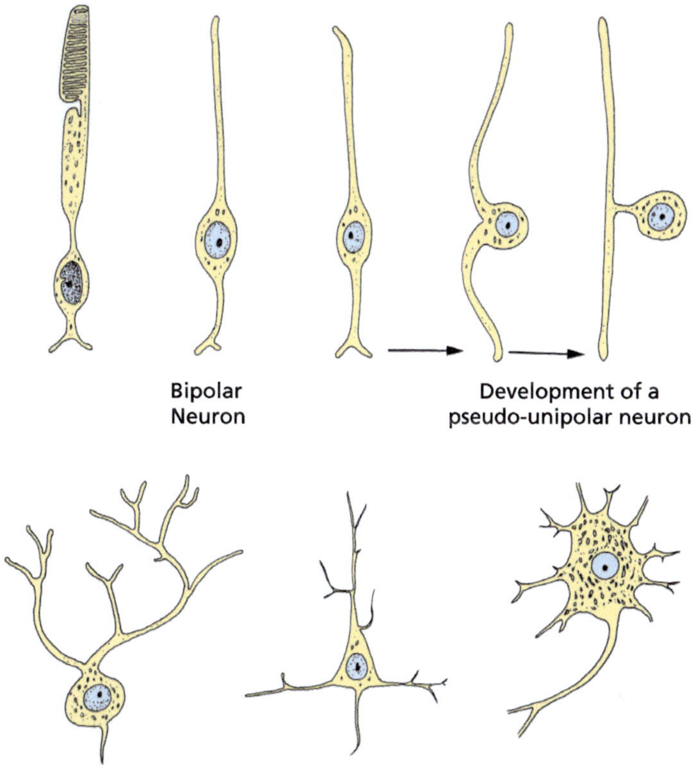

5.6 Types of nerve cell (schematic).

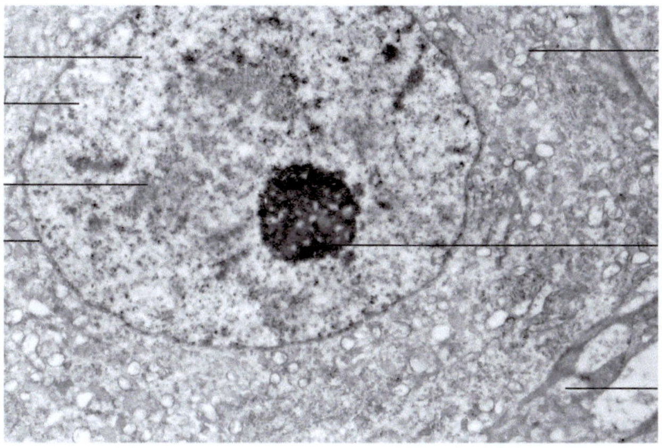

5.7 Fine structure of the perikaryon of a multipolar neuron within the cerebrum (x5000).

Pseudo-unipolar neurons

The cell bodies of pseudo-unipolar neurons are found in the sensory ganglia of spinal and cranial nerves (Figures 5.5 and 5.6). This type of nerve cell develops embryonically from a bipolar nerve cell. One of the two cell processes extends into the central nervous system as the axon, while the other passes with the anlage of the muscle and skin to the periphery to become the receptor portion of the cell.

During embryonic development, the two processes migrate to one side of the perikaryon and fuse, giving rise to a single origin. The process that extends to the periphery undergoes internal structural changes, coming to resemble an axon (dendritic axon). Both the axon and dendritic axon are part of the peripheral nervous system and both are myelinated.

Electrophysiologically, the sensory signal bypasses the perikaryon to pass directly into the dorsal root of the spinal cord. The cell body serves primarily as a potential means of regenerating nerve cell processes.

Multipolar neurons

Multipolar neurons are the most common type of nerve cell (Figures 5.1 to 5.3, 5.6 and 5.7). They develop, for example, from neuroblasts of the ventral and dorsal horns of the embryonic spinal cord. Several processes extend from the perikaryon of the neuroblast, beginning to branch at

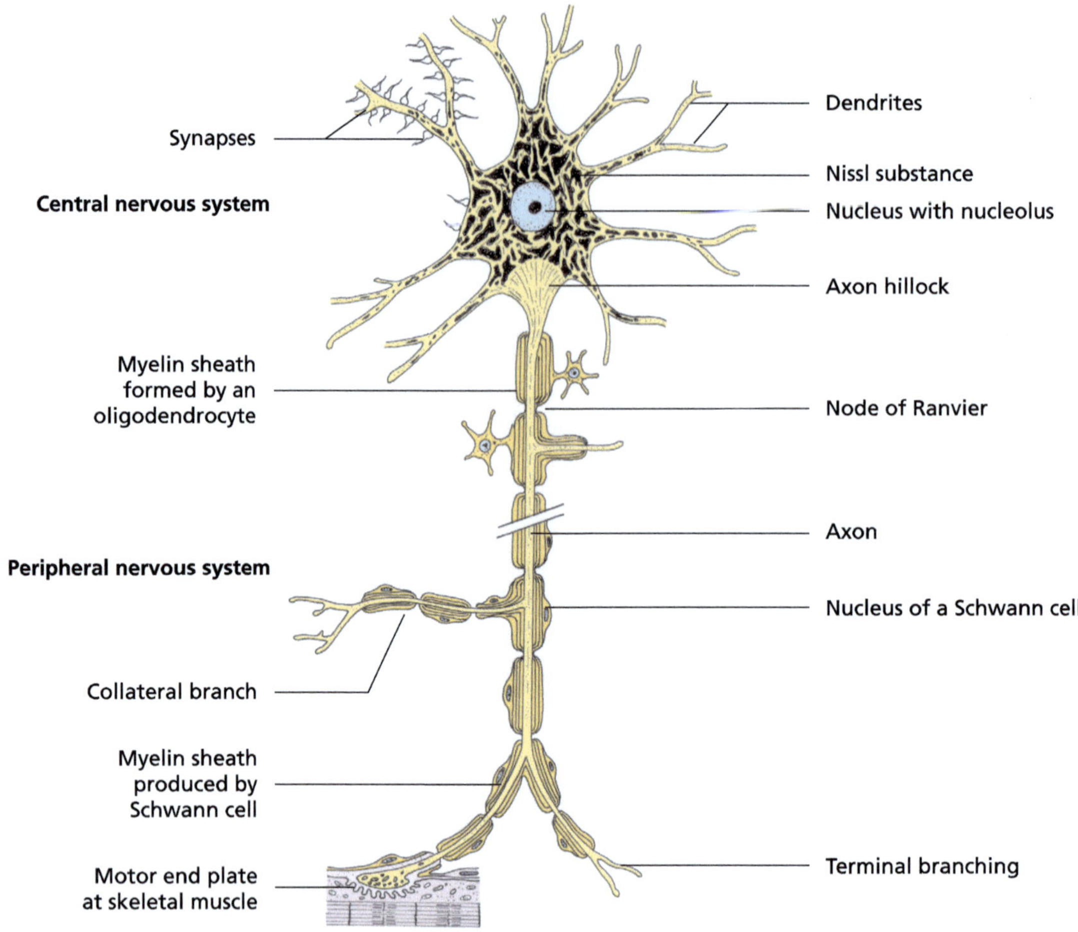

5.8 Central and peripheral components of a motor neuron (schematic).

their site of origin. The cells take on a stellate appearance with multiple dendrites and a single axon. Nerve impulses received by the dendrites from other multipolar neurons, via synapses, travel to the axon.

Multipolar neurons with a particularly dense network of dendrites and a long axon are referred to as **Golgi type I** neurons. These include lower motor neurons, **Purkinje cells** of the cerebellum and the **pyramidal cells** of the cerebrum. **Golgi type II** neurons are primarily relay cells (interneurons) within the central nervous system. Their cell processes are typically short but densely elaborated. Golgi type II cells are found mostly in the cerebral and cerebellar cortex, and in the olfactory bulb.

The neurons of the **autonomic ganglia** are also multipolar.

Neuronal structure

As described above, neurons have two basic structural components:

- the perikaryon – nucleus and perinuclear cytoplasm (Figure 5.7) and
- cell processes (dendrites, axon; Figure 5.8), frequently elongated.

Perikaryon

The cell body includes the nucleus and perinuclear cytoplasm (Figures 5.8 and 5.11). It is the site of metabolic processes associated with cell maintenance and function. The perikaryon continuously recycles cell components, including membrane proteins, and acts as a receptor for excitatory or inhibitory signalling substances that reach the cell body via synapses or dendrites. The cell body is usually round, oval or polygonal, and reaches 100 μm in size (only 4–5 μm in Golgi type II neurons).

The distinct **nucleus** is typically spherical and euchromatic. It contains a **nucleolus** and sparse heterochromatin. The predominance of loosely coiled euchromatin and the size of the nucleolus, as well as a prominent Golgi apparatus, endoplasmic reticulum and numerous lysosomes, indicate a high degree of metabolic activity in these cells.

The marked development of the **Golgi apparatus** reflects the synthesis and axonal transport of substances involved in neural transmission. The close association of cisternae of the Golgi apparatus in cerebellar neurons prompted the discoverer of this organelle, the Italian scientist Camillo Golgi, to describe it as an ***apparato reticulare interno***.

Lysosomes, multivesicular bodies and lipid droplets are found in close association with the Golgi apparatus.

Also well developed is the **rough endoplasmic reticulum**, which occupies a large proportion of the cytoplasm in synthetically active cells. As the ribosomes are basophilic, the rER can be seen under the light microscope using methylene blue or toluidine blue stains. Together, the ribosomes and associated rER are referred to as **Nissl substance**, after the German scientist Franz Nissl who first observed them (Figure 5.8). The typical staining of Nissl substance and the large nucleus aid in the histological identification of neurons.

The rER extends into the dendrites, but **not into the axon**. The ER-free site at which the axon arises from the cell body is termed the axon hillock (Figure 5.8).

Mitochondria are abundant in the body of active nerve cells. The endogenous pigment **lipofuscin** is usually also present, while **melanin** granules are occasionally observed. Accumulation of **lipofuscin** is common in senescent nerve cells.

Neurofilaments and **neurotubules** (**neuronal microtubules**) are characteristic features of nerve cells. Particularly in the perikaryon, these form the cytoskeleton of the cell and assemble the organelles into organised structures. Neurofilaments form aggregates (neurofibrils) that can be demonstrated using the **Bodian method** (Figure 5.3). Neurofilaments, neurotubules and mitochondria extend into the dendrites and the axon, where they serve to stabilise the cell and contribute to neuro-secretory processes.

Nerve cell processes

DENDRITES

Dendrites are arborising processes that extend from the perikaryon of most neurons (Figure 5.8). The organelles found in their primary stem and side branches are similar to those in the perikaryon (rER and free ribosomes, numerous neurofilaments and neurotubules), although the Golgi apparatus disappears with increased dendritic branching. The terminal dendritic branches contain numerous neurofilaments, neurotubules and mitochondria that facilitate dendritic transport. Distributed over the surface of the dendrites are numerous axodendritic synapses, at which the dendrites regulate control circuits between various neurons. Dendrites can also act as sense organs, taking up electrophysiological impulses directly from their environment. They convey neuronal impulses towards the cell body.

AXONS

Arising from the cell body at the axon hillock, the axon conducts neural impulses away from the cell body (Figure 5.8). Axons of different nerve cells vary in length. For a given type of nerve cell, however, the diameter of the axon (1–20 μm) is consistent along its length. The axonal cytoplasm (**axoplasm**) is contained within a membrane referred to as the **axolemma**. The axoplasm contains large numbers of neurofilaments and neurotubules, accompanied by relatively few elongated mitochondria, several smooth-walled vesicles and occasional multivesicular bodies. Ribosomes occur sporadically in the axoplasm and endoplasmic reticulum is sparse.

At isolated locations along their length, axons send out branches at right angles (**collaterals**). Axons end by arborising; the ends of the terminal branches have expanded tips (end bulbs) that synapse with other cell processes. Axons of motor nerve fibres and sensory dendritic axons of pseudo-unipolar neurons are surrounded by a sheath of myelin. The axons of postganglionic autonomic nerve fibres are not myelinated.

Energy supply and axonal transport

Mitochondria in the perikaryon, dendrites and axon are responsible for oxidative breakdown of glucose or ketones. The resulting ATP provides energy for synthesis of proteins and RNA (for ongoing cell renewal), for Na^+/K^+-ATPase in the axolemma (for signal conduction) and for axonal transport systems.

Enzymes and proteins required at nerve synapses must be transported to the terminals via axonal transport. Mitochondria and low-molecular weight substances, sometimes in the form of vesicles, are also transported within the axon. Dendrites and axons generally lack the full complement of organelles required for protein biosynthesis.

Axonal transport is categorised as fast (200–500 mm/day) or slow (2–5 mm/day). The process is ATP-dependent and utilises neurotubules and neurofilaments. Antegrade transport systems (fast and slow) carry substances from the perikaryon to the synapse. Concurrently, retrograde systems (fast) return metabolic end products in the opposite direction, to the cell body.

Synapse

Synapses are specialised intercellular junctions at which impulses are conducted by **electrical** or **chemical** mechanisms from one neuron to another, or from a neuron to an effector organ. **Electrical synapses** consist of **gap junctions** that permit rapid transmission of impulses across regions of reduced electrical resistance. While electrical synapses are common in invertebrates and fish, they occur only rarely between mature mammalian neurons (gap junctions between smooth muscle cells are functional equivalents).

Chemical synapses (Figure 5.9) are the main type of synapse, occurring predominantly at the **end of an axon**. They consist of:

- a presynaptic axonal component (synaptic end bulb),
- the synaptic cleft and
- a postsynaptic component (postsynaptic membrane).

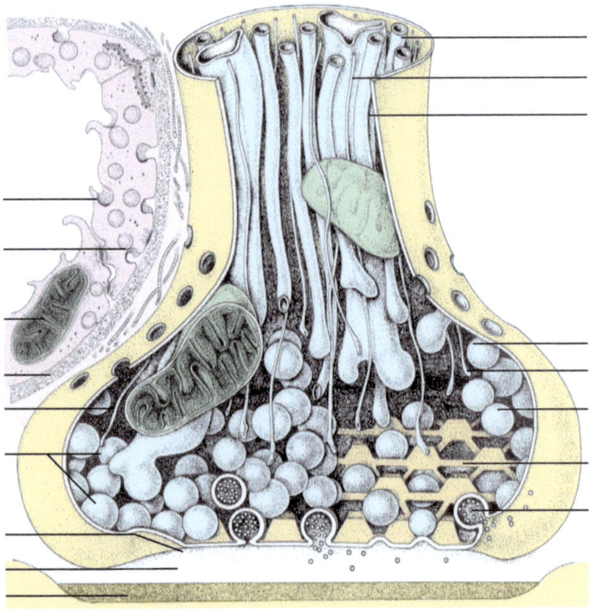

5.9 Chemical synapse with synaptic end bulb, synaptic cleft and adjacent capillary wall (schematic).

In some cases, axons form neurochemical junctions with other axons or dendrites along their length in the form of ovoid varicosities (e.g. nerve plexuses in smooth muscle).

Structure of a chemical synapse

Chemical synapses are largely consistent in their basic structure. The **presynaptic axonal component** (**synaptic end bulb, terminal bouton**) is a bulbous expansion containing mitochondria, smooth ER, neurotubules, neurofilaments and synaptic vesicles (Figures 5.9 and 5.10).

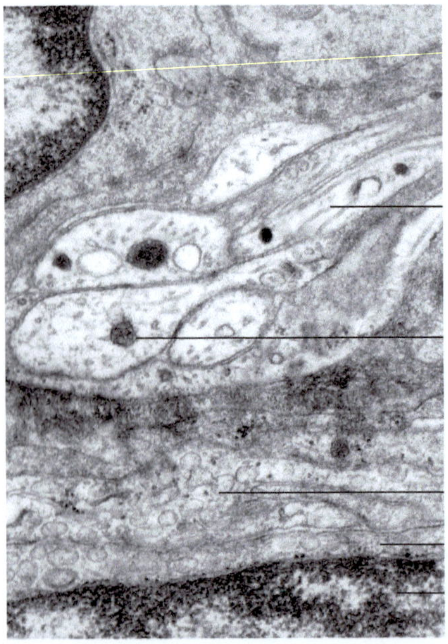

5.10 Fine structure of the club-like end bulb of a free nerve ending in the vicinity of a smooth muscle cell (x14,000).

The vesicles (20–60 nm) contain the chemical substances that transmit the nerve impulse across the synapse (**neurotransmitters**). The plasmalemma of the nerve terminal is termed the **presynaptic membrane**.

The **synaptic cleft** lies between the pre- and postsynaptic membranes. Typically 20 nm wide, the synaptic cleft encloses finely granular or, in places, fibrillar material.

The **postsynaptic component** is rich in mitochondria. The plasmalemma of this region of the receptor cell is termed the **postsynaptic membrane**. It is underlain by a region of dense material composed of a complex of proteins and associated cytoskeletal elements (postsynaptic density).

Chemical synapses are formed with different types of tissues through specifically **differentiated end bulbs**. On this basis, synapses can be categorised as:

- neurosensory synapses between neurons and sensory cells, e.g. in hearing and gustation,
- neuroglandular synapses between neurons and exocrine or endocrine glands,
- neuromuscular synapses between neurons and skeletal muscle (motor end plates),
- interneuronal synapses including:
  - axoaxonic synapses,
  - axodendritic synapses between axons and dendrites and
  - axosomatic synapses between axons and the perikaryon.

Function of the chemical synapse

Chemical transmission of neural impulses at the synapse is performed by **neurotransmitters**. These substances conduct the nerve impulse to other neurons or to effector cells. Neurotransmitters of the **peripheral nervous system** include **biogenic amines** (e.g. noradrenaline) and **carboxylic acid esters** (acetylcholine). In the **central nervous system**, impulses are transmitted by **biogenic amines** (noradrenaline, dopamine, serotonin and adrenaline), acetylcholine and other molecule classes (e.g. neuropeptides such as enkephalins, β-endorphins and substance P, amino acids including γ-aminobutyrate [GABA], glycine and glutamate). Small-molecule neurotransmitters are predominantly synthesised in the cytosol of the end bulbs, while neuropeptides are produced in the perikaryon.

Despite the wide variety of neurotransmitters, impulse transmission appears to proceed according to the same basic mechanism in all synapses. The sequence of events comprises:

- release of the neurotransmitter from the presynaptic nerve terminal into the synaptic cleft,
- interaction of the neurotransmitters with specific postsynaptic receptors,
- alteration of voltage across the postsynaptic membrane as a result of altered ion permeability and
- inactivation of the chemical signal by enzymatic cleavage of the neurotransmitter or reuptake of the neurotransmitter by the nerve terminal.

A nerve impulse arriving at a synaptic end bulb (**action potential**) leads to **transient depolarisation** of the presynaptic membrane. This promotes the influx of extracellular Ca^{2+}. Under the influence of the intracellular Ca^{2+} ions, synaptic vesicles are transported to the presynaptic membrane (possibly with the aid of neurotubules) and **neurotransmitters are released into the synaptic cleft**. The liberated neurotransmitter induces a **local voltage change** in the postsynaptic membrane.

The postsynaptic membrane contains specific receptors formed by membrane proteins. Upon binding with a neurotransmitter, the receptors undergo conformational alterations that result in opening of ion channels (e.g. for Na^+, K^+ and Cl^-). An increase in the passage of Na^+ ions into the cell results in depolarisation of the postsynaptic membrane.

There are two main types of postsynaptic membrane receptors. Ionotropic receptors contain ion channels, such that the conformational change induced by binding of the neurotransmitter leads directly to opening of the associated channel (e.g. nicotinic ACh receptors).

Metabotropic receptors do not incorporate an ion channel, rather their intracellular domain is linked to a G protein. Binding of the neurotransmitter alters the structure of the G protein, resulting in the formation of a second messenger molecule that opens ion channels located elsewhere in the membrane (e.g. adrenergic receptors).

Inactivation of the neurotransmitter occurs primarily through reuptake into the presynaptic membrane. This process is facilitated by high affinity of the transmitter for the membrane proteins. Reacquired neurotransmitters are recycled. In other cases, the neurotransmitter is broken down enzymatically into inactive molecules (e.g. acetylcholine is degraded by acetylcholinesterase into choline and acetate).

Neuromuscular synapse (motor end plate)

Motor end plates are specialised chemical synapses in which **motor nerve fibres** transmit neural impulses to skeletal muscle (Figure 5.13). They are also referred to as **neuromuscular** (or **myoneural**) **junctions.** Towards the end of the nerve fibre, the myelin sheath ends, and the axon divides into branches that come to lie in concavities in the muscle cell. Copious synaptic vesicles containing the neurotransmitter **acetylcholine** are located in the free ends of the axon. The postsynaptic membrane features multiple junctional folds. The synaptic cleft, including the spaces between the folds, contains the external lamina of the surrounding neurolemmocyte (see below). Mitochondria, ribosomes and glycogen granules are present under the thickened postsynaptic membrane.

The release of acetylcholine into the synaptic cleft results in depolarisation of the plasmalemma of the muscle cell. The action potential passes to the T system, from which it is transmitted to the sarcoplasmic reticulum (Chapter 4, 'Muscle tissue').

The transmission of sensory information from skeletal muscle involves specialised receptors termed neuromuscular and neurotendinous spindles. These are described further in Chapter 16, 'Receptors and sense organs'.

Nerve fibre (neurofibra)

The term nerve fibre refers to the **axon** of a neuron and its **outer covering**. The latter is formed by **glial cells** (oligodendrocytes in the central nervous system [forming the white matter]; Figures 5.11 and 5.12, Schwann cells [neurolemmocytes] in the peripheral nervous system). As well as being distinguished by the cells from which their sheaths originate, nerve fibres can be classified on the basis of function. Based on differentiation of neuronal pathways in the somatic and autonomic (vegetative) nervous system, nerve fibres are divided into:

- somatic afferent sensory nerve fibres: convey impulses from the periphery to the spinal cord or brain, and from some organs of special sense to the brain (e.g. the auditory and visual senses),

- somatic efferent motor nerve fibres: transmit impulses to the periphery (skeletal striated muscle),
- visceral afferent autonomic fibres and
- visceral efferent autonomic fibres: parasympathetic and sympathetic involuntary nerve fibres that regulate the function of the internal organs.

Glial cells accompany axons along their entire length, providing support and nutrition to the nerve fibre. They also perform an important role in the transmission of neural impulses, and thus it is functionally significant that the cells surround the nerve process completely. Nerve fibres that become invested in multiple concentric layers of glial cell cytoplasm are referred to as **myelinated fibres** (Figure 5.14). In **unmyelinated fibres**, the nerve fibre occupies an invagination in the glial cell cytoplasm.

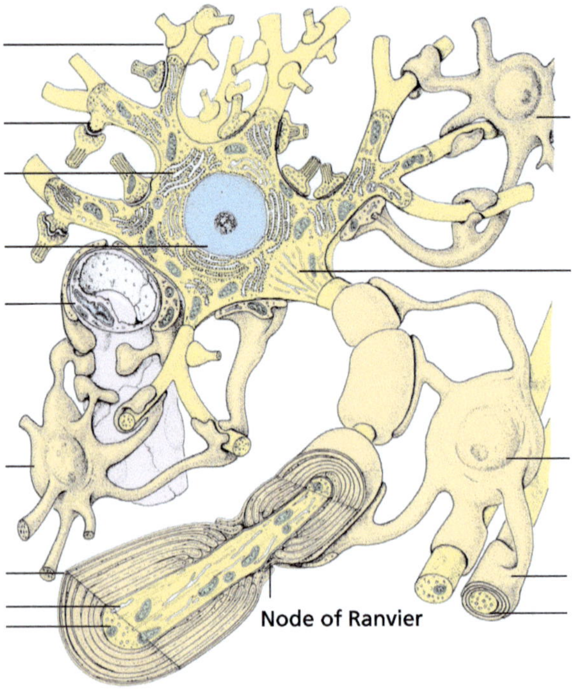

5.11 Multipolar neuron of the central nervous system with glial cells (astrocytes and an oligodendrocyte) (schematic).

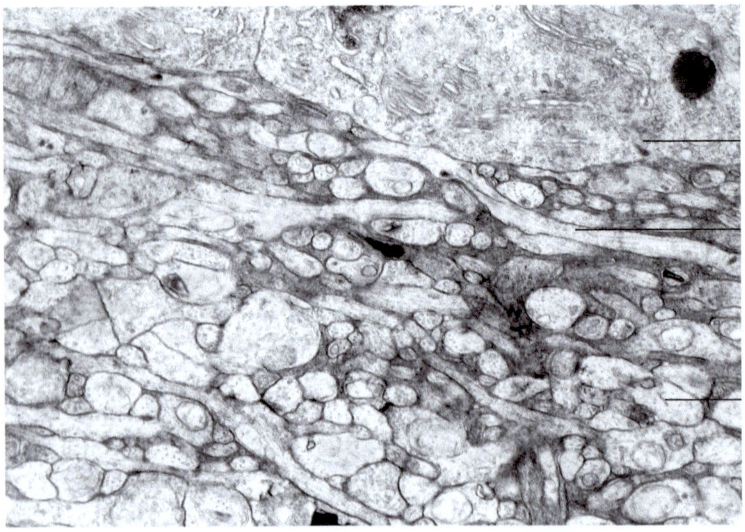

5.12 Portion of the perikaryon of a multipolar neuron (top right) with surrounding neuropil (network of neuronal and glial cell processes) (x9000).

Myelinated nerve fibres

A large proportion of the nerve fibres of the peripheral and central nervous systems are myelinated. The myelination process involves wrapping of the plasmalemma of the glial cell around the central axon in slender, yet often numerous, lamellae, forming the so-called **myelin sheath** (= **myelin**; Figure 5.14). The sheath is formed by **Schwann cells** in the peripheral nervous system and by **oligodendrocytes** in the central nervous system.

Depending on the number of lamellae, and thus the thickness of the myelin sheath, nerve fibres may be heavily or sparsely myelinated (Figures 5.15 and 5.16). A fibre is considered unmyelinated when lamellar layering is lacking.

The development of the myelin sheath is phylogenetically significant with respect to **differentiation of the nervous system**. Myelin sheaths increase the speed and distribution of the action potentials (depolarisation). The sheath thus serves to **isolate** the axon from its surroundings, reducing current leakage. The rate of **axonal conduction** increases with the thickness of the sheath: **heavily myelinated** fibres conduct nerve impulses faster than those that are **sparsely myelinated**. Furthermore, the velocity of action potential conduction is influenced by the diameter of the axon. A thick axon transmits signals faster than a thin axon.

FORMATION OF THE MYELIN SHEATH

The process of myelin sheath formation (**myelinisation**) occurs differently in the peripheral and central nervous systems.

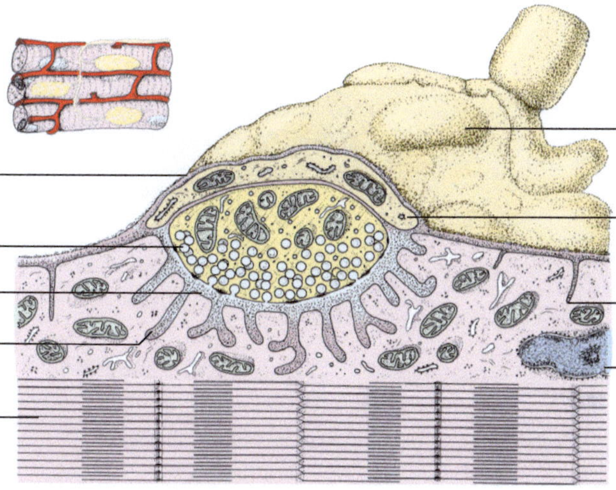

5.13 Neuromuscular junction (motor end plate) (schematic).

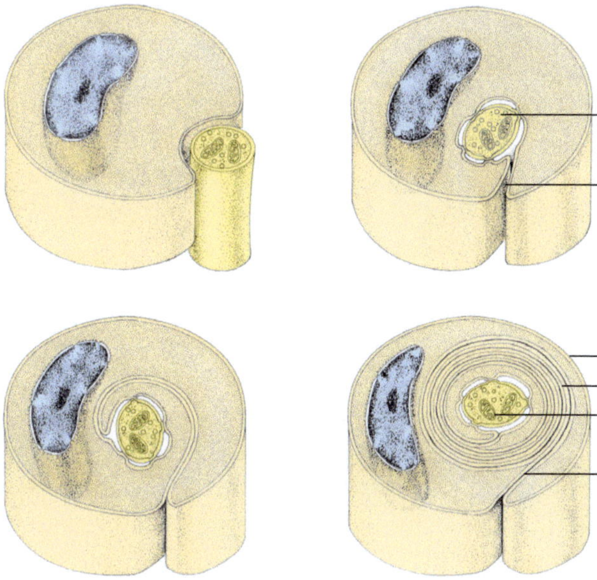

5.14 Formation of the myelin sheath of a peripheral nerve fibre (schematic).

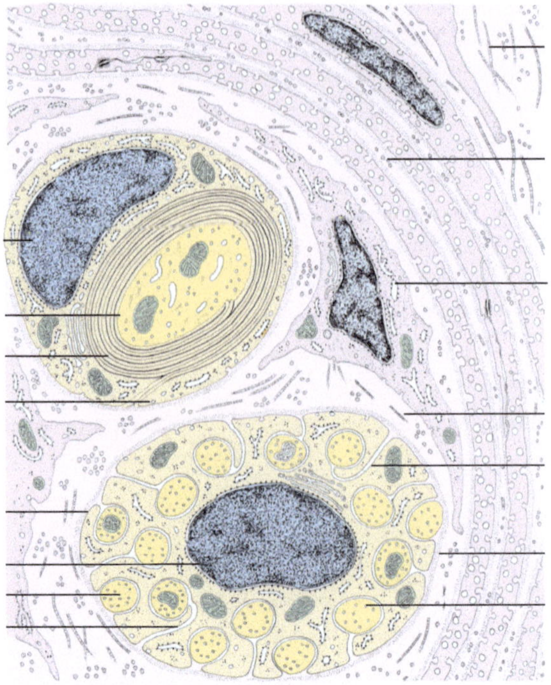

5.15 Structure of a myelinated and unmyelinated nerve fibre (schematic).

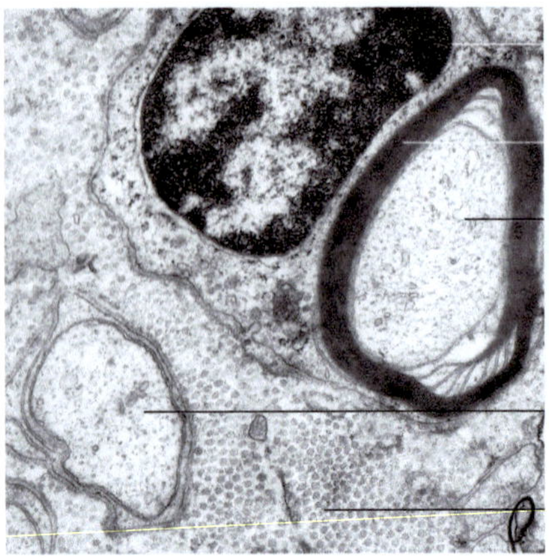

5.16 Fine structure of a myelinated and an unmyelinated nerve fibre (transverse section) with adjacent loose connective tissue (x6000).

MYELINATION OF PERIPHERAL NERVE FIBRES

Each **Schwann cell** is associated with only one axon. Initially, the Schwann cell lies adjacent to the axon, subsequently folding around it, displacing the axon to the centre. Opposing surfaces of the plasmalemma approach one another, eventually fusing to form a **mesaxon** (Figure 5.14). The mesaxon then extends around the axon to form **lamellae**. Initially the outer layers of plasmalemma become fused. As the mesaxon continues to extend, and the lamellae are formed, the inner layers also merge. The lamellae, in their entirety, constitute the **myelin sheath**.

The outer portion of the Schwann cell, containing cytoplasm and the nucleus, adjoins the myelin sheath. This layer is referred to as the **sheath of Schwann** (Figure 5.14).

MYELINATION OF CENTRAL NERVE FIBRES

Myelination of central nerve fibres differs primarily from that of peripheral nerve fibres in that one **oligodendrocyte** ensheathes **several axons** (Figure 5.11). Numerous trapezoid processes extend from the oligodendrocyte, their free edges becoming associated with, and wrapping around, multiple axons. These wrappings together constitute the **myelin sheath**.

COMPOSITION OF THE MYELIN SHEATH

The structure of the myelin sheath resembles that of two fused unit membranes. Electron micrographs reveal the presence of parallel, alternating **lipid** and **protein layers**. **Lipids**, mainly glycerine phosphatides, cholesterol and sphingolipids, make up around 70% of myelin. The **protein component** (30%) includes proteolipids, glycoproteins and myelin basic protein. Due to their high fat content, myelin sheaths can be demonstrated using **lipid staining techniques** (Figure 5.20).

Each Schwann cell or oligodendrocyte surrounds the axon over a distance of approximately 1 mm (Figures 5.8 and 5.11). Between two consecutive glial cells, the axon is exposed. This gap, 0.5 μm in width, is referred to as the **node of Ranvier** (Figures 5.8 and 5.11). The section of the myelin sheath between two consecutive nodes is the **internode**. Pockets of cytoplasm remain in the myelin sheath where fusion of the plasma membrane of the glial cell is incomplete. These conical compartments, known as **Schmidt–Lanterman clefts**, can be clearly seen in longitudinal sections of nerve fibres. It is thought they may facilitate deformation of the nerve within the tissue.

Unmyelinated nerve fibres

In unmyelinated nerve fibres, the Schwann cell surrounds the axon without subsequent **wrapping by the mesaxon**. In contrast to myelinated peripheral fibres, in which a Schwann cell is associated with only one axon, **several axons** are usually surrounded by the same Schwann cell in unmyelinated fibres (Figure 5.15). Neighbouring Schwann cells are closely apposed, such that nodes of Ranvier are not observed. In the central nervous system, unmyelinated axons often lie immediately adjacent to other neurons or glial cell processes.

Generation and conduction of nerve stimuli

The initiation and transmission of an electrical impulse occurs at the **plasmalemma** (**axolemma**) of the neuron. Central to this process is a change in the voltage across the membrane, resulting from the movement of particular inorganic ions (Na^+, K^+, Cl^- and Ca^{2+}) through specific channels within membrane proteins (ion channels).

Opening or closing of the ion channels alters the distribution of charge across the membrane and thus the membrane potential (voltage). An action potential is generated when Na^+ channels open in response to a depolarising stimulus, with a subsequent increase in membrane permeability to Na^+ and influx of Na^+ ions into the cell. This influx exceeds the efflux of K^+ ions, altering the resting potential to create an action potential.

In **myelinated fibres**, the alteration of membrane potential can only occur at the nodes of Ranvier. The majority of Na^+ channels are concentrated in these regions, with a density of several thousand channels per μm^2. The internode, the segment of the nerve fibre surrounded by the myelin sheath, is virtually devoid of Na^+ channels. The myelin sheath contributes significantly to nerve conduction by insulating the cell and preventing leakage of current. Consequently, the nerve impulses that give rise to the action potential 'jump' from one node of Ranvier to the next. This is referred to as **saltatory** (**discontinuous**) **conduction**.

The **speed of impulse conduction** within a neuron is constant and is related to the structure of the axon. This is accelerated by the myelin sheath, which enables the rapid spread of action potentials from one node of Ranvier to the next. Thus, saltatory impulse transmission through myelinated fibres is faster than the type of transmission that occurs in unmyelinated fibres. In addition, myelinated fibres require less energy as the processes involved in impulse conduction are limited to the nodes of Ranvier.

In unmyelinated fibres, the conduction of nerve impulses to the synapse occurs in a continuous wave over the surface of the axolemma. The spread of the impulse is slower due to the absence of nodes of Ranvier (and thus of saltatory conduction) and inferior conductivity of unmyelinated fibres.

In the Erlanger–Gasser system, nerve fibres are classified as A, B or C on the basis of diameter and conduction speed. **A fibres** are myelinated, rapidly conducting fibres that are predominantly associated with muscle fibres, muscle spindles or skin. They may be efferent or afferent. A fibres may be further subdivided into subgroups by their diameter and conduction speed.

Aα fibres (efferent and afferent innervation of muscle) are the thickest and fastest-conducting fibres (10–20 μm and 60–120 m/s). Below these in speed and diameter are the Aβ fibres (afferent fibres, touch and pressure) which measure 7–15 μm in diameter and conduct at 40–90 m/s. With a diameter of 4–8 μm, Aγ fibres (efferent to muscle spindles) are also relatively slow (30–45 m/s). Aδ fibres (3–5 μm) are slow-conducting fibres (5–25 m/s) involved in the monitoring of pain and temperature.

B fibres (1–3 μm) are myelinated fibres that conduct the action potentials of preganglionic autonomic fibres at a moderate speed of 3–15 m/s.

C fibres are thin, unmyelinated nerve fibres (0.3–1 μm) that conduct very slowly (0.5–2 m/s). They serve to convey impulses in postganglionic autonomic nerve fibres.

Nerves

The term 'nerve' applies to a **bundle of peripheral nerve fibres** that are combined by connective tissue into single, variably sized entities. Nerves containing fibres with varying characteristics are referred to as **mixed nerves**. In

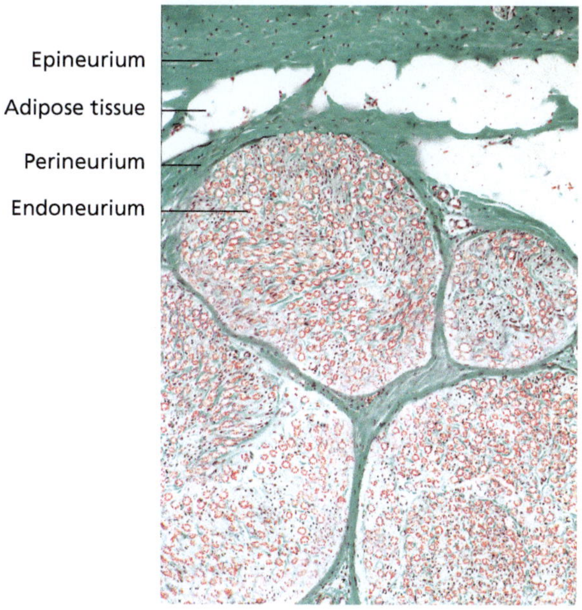

5.17 Mixed nerve fibre bundle with connective tissue investments (dog). Goldner's Masson trichrome stain (x120).

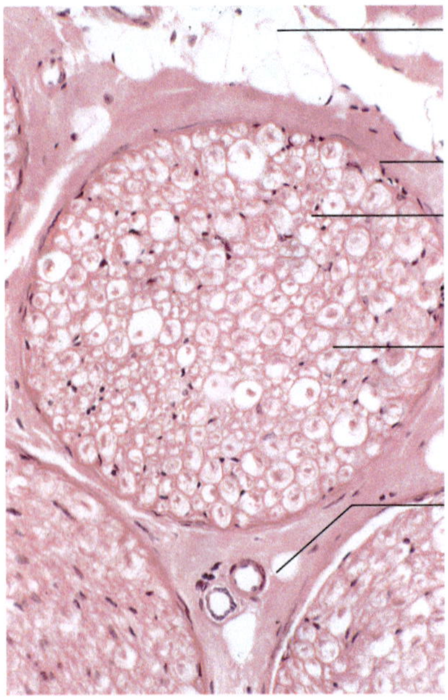

5.18 Mixed nerve fibre bundle (partial section) with perineurium, adipose tissue and smaller blood vessels (dog). Haematoxylin and eosin stain (x300).

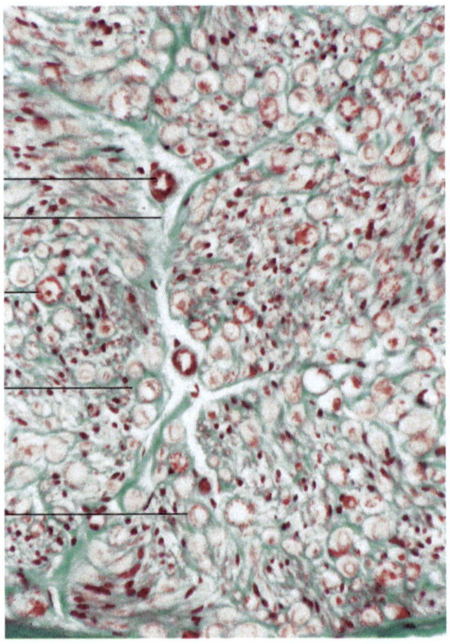

5.19 Section of a mixed nerve fibre bundle showing various degrees of myelination of axons (dog). Goldner's Masson trichrome stain (x360).

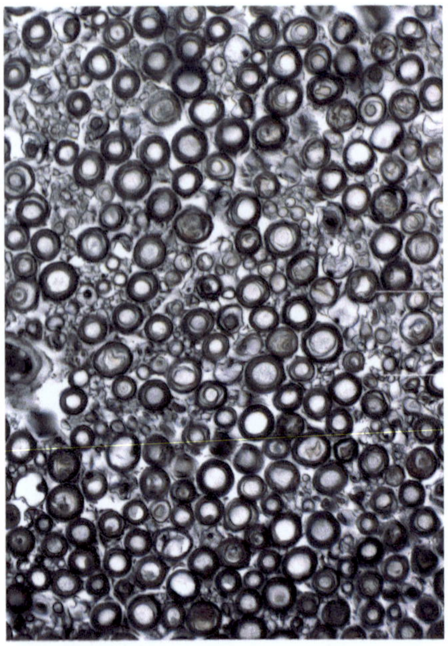

5.20 Section of a mixed nerve fibre bundle (heavily and poorly myelinated nerve fibres) (dog). Osmium impregnation technique (x480).

accordance with their function, the nerve fibres of the peripheral nervous system are predominantly myelinated. Each nerve fibre (**axon and associated supporting cells**) is invested by one or, usually, several **layers of connective tissue** (Figures 5.17 to 5.19).

Nervous tissue investments

Each nerve fibre is surrounded by a basement membrane, which is encircled by a fine network of loose connective tissue. Termed the **endoneurium**, this forms an incomplete casing around the nerve fibre. Together with the basement membrane, the endoneurium forms the endoneurial sheath. Groups of nerve fibres (fascicles) are enclosed in concentrically layered connective tissue septa (**perineurium, perineurial sheath**) (Figures 5.17 to 5.19). A dense, tough superficial connective tissue layer, the **epineurium**, encloses the whole nerve.

Regeneration of nervous tissue

Nerve cells cannot be replaced as they lose their ability to divide during the differentiation process. Under certain circumstances, however, peripheral nerves retain the capacity to regenerate through outgrowth of the axon. This is dependent on the integrity of the perikaryon and the supporting Schwann cells, which provide a scaffold for regeneration.

The regeneration of axons is a complex process. Initially, degenerating nerve fibres are degraded by phagocytosis. Concurrently, Schwann cells at the proximal and distal end of the nerve divide and arrange themselves in columns along the path of the original nerve fibre. New nerve processes (neurites) sprout from the regenerating axon, progressing along the columns at 1–2 mm per day. Within approximately 6 months, the axon regains its original morphology.

Glial cells (neuroglia, gliocytus)

Glial cells are essential components of nervous tissue. Without them, nerve cells are unable to function. As elaborated upon below, their functions include provision of nutrition and metabolic support to neurons and facilitation of the conduction of nerve impulses by the formation of neural sheaths. In some cases, glial cells contribute to innate immunity as specialised cells of the mononuclear phagocyte system.

Most nerve cells are closely related, both structurally and functionally, to **glial cells** (**neuroglia**), with which they share a **common embryonic origin**. Specific functions performed by glial cells include:

- physical support by occupying the spaces between perikarya, dendrites and axons, thus contributing to the organisation and spatial separation of neurons,
- metabolic support and exchange of substances between the nerve cells and capillaries,
- formation of the sheath of myelinated and unmyelinated nerve fibres, thus influencing the speed of nerve impulse conduction,
- neuronal regeneration, in which they act as a physical guide,
- contribution to the blood–brain barrier and other interfaces in the central nervous system and
- capacity for phagocytosis (certain cells).

Based on structural and functional criteria (Table 5.1), glial cells are divided into:

- glial cells of the central nervous system:
  - ependymal cells,
  - astrocytes,
  - oligodendrocytes and
  - microglia (Hortega cells) (Figures 5.21 to 5.25);
- glial cells of the peripheral nervous system:
  - Schwann cells (neurolemmocytes) and
  - satellite cells (amphicytes).

Table 5.1 Distinguishing microscopic features of neuroglia.

	Morphology	Occurrence	Function
Cells of the CNS			
Ependymal cells	Cuboidal to columnar epithelium with cilia, round to oval nucleus, basal cytoplasmic processes	Ventricles of the brain, central canal of spinal cord	Formation and circulation of cerebrospinal fluid in the ventricles of the brain and central canal of spinal cord, lining of ventricles and central canal
Astrocytes: protoplasmic	Numerous short, radiating, branching processes, prominent/abundant cytoplasm, large, oval euchromatic nucleus	Grey matter	Close association with capillaries, contribute to blood–brain barrier, surround nerve processes, maintain ion concentration, provide structural support
fibrous	Few, long, radiating, sparsely branched processes, small round nucleus with little euchromatin	White matter	Close association with capillaries, contribute to blood–brain barrier, contain numerous filaments, provide structural support
Oligodendrocytes	Few or no processes in routine light microscopic preparations, small, heterochromatic nucleus	Grey and white matter (oligodendroglia)	Formation of the myelin sheath (multiple neurons per oligodendrocyte) in the white matter
Microglia (Hortega cells)	Macrophage-like cells originating from bone marrow	Grey and white matter	Amoeboid phagocytes, well-developed lysosomal system, component of mononuclear phagocytic system
Cells of the PNS			
Neurolemmocytes (Schwann cells)	Elongated cell extension wrapped concentrically around an axon, flattened nucleus lying adjacent to axon	Myelin sheath of peripheral axons	Myelin sheath and nodes of Ranvier between consecutive Schwann cells facilitate propagation of nerve impulses
Satellite cells (amphicytes)	Compact, heterochromatic, round nucleus	Ganglia	Close contact with neurons, metabolic functions

Glial cells of the central nervous system

Ependymal cells (ependymocytus)

Ependymal cells are derived from the lining of the inner wall of the neural tube, remaining at their site of origin for the duration of their life. These cuboidal to columnar cells form the epithelial lining of the **ventricles of the central nervous system** (**CNS**) and the **central canal of the spinal cord.** Ependymal cells contribute to the circulation and cleansing of the cerebrospinal fluid (CSF) and participate in the transport of metabolites. These functions are facilitated by microvilli and cilia located on the apical cell surface.

At the basal cell surface, many cell processes of varying lengths lie adjacent to neurons and loose connective tissue. In its entirety, this epithelial layer serves as a **functional barrier** between the cavities of the nervous system and the neurons. Within the ventricles, ependymal cells have a specialised secretory function forming the epithelial lining of the **choroid plexi** which produce the cerebrospinal fluid. In addition to numerous cytoplasmic organelles, ependymal cells contain large numbers of osmophilic electron-dense bodies.

In several areas of the CNS, an elongated process extending from the base of ependymal cells makes contact with underlying capillaries. These ependymal cells are referred to as **tanycytes**. Tanycytes lack cilia on their apical surface, allowing them to be distinguished from other, ciliated ependymal cells. Numerous tanycytes are found in the wall of the third ventricle. These are well developed in the circumventricular organs, which lack a normal blood–brain barrier (e.g. median eminence, area postrema). Tanycytes are sometimes also located in the central canal of the spinal cord.

Occasionally axons come to lie on the surface of ependymal cells, covering the cells in a network of nerve cell processes.

Astrocytes (astrocytus)

Astrocytes are the **largest glial cells in the central nervous system**. Their processes make contact with other neurons and with the pia mater, and lie alongside blood capillaries (Figure 5.21). Terminal expansions of astrocyte processes (end feet) form the **glia limitans**, a barrier membrane that covers the surface of the brain and spinal cord (**membrana limitans gliae superficialis**) and separates **intracerebral blood vessels** from the brain (**membrana limitans gliae perivascularis**). Astrocytes are thus a component of the blood–brain barrier. Through this barrier function, astrocytes contribute to the establishment of neuronal microcompartments, which have considerable bearing on the function of nervous tissue.

Astrocytes play a prominent role in the **migration of neurons** during brain development and in regulation of **neurotransmitter activity**. They also transfer nutrients and serve as a buffer system within the CNS. Furthermore, astrocytes make an important contribution to repair and regeneration of damaged CNS tissue. In their capacity as antigen-presenting cells, astrocytes also participate in cell-mediated immunity within the CNS.

Through the connections between their cell processes and neurons, astrocytes facilitate the **transport of fluid** and **metabolites** between neurons and capillaries. Astrocytes regulate extracellular K^+ concentrations, thereby maintaining the conditions required for propagation of nerve impulses. Damage to this regulatory mechanism results in swelling (**oedema**) of the nervous tissue.

Based on their morphology, astrocytes can be classified as:

- protoplasmic astrocytes (astrocyti protoplasmatici) or
- fibrous astrocytes (astrocyti fibrosi).

PROTOPLASMIC ASTROCYTES (ASTROCYTUS PROTOPLASMATICUS)

Protoplasmic astrocytes are found predominantly in the grey matter of the central nervous system. They are characterised by a polygonal perinuclear region (15–25 µm) and many **extensively branched cell processes**. The generally short, thick processes terminate on neurons and form perivascular sheaths around capillaries (Figures 5.21 and 5.25).

FIBROUS ASTROCYTES (ASTROCYTUS FIBROSUS)

Fibrous astrocytes are located in the white matter of the brain and spinal cord (Figures 5.22 and 5.25). Measuring 10–12 µm near the nucleus, fibrous astrocytes exhibit long, sparsely branching processes that lie parallel to nerve fibres. They are reinforced by cytoplasmic glial filaments (also present to a lesser extent in protoplasmic astrocytes).

Oligodendrocytes (oligodendrocytus)

Oligodendrocytes are small glial cells (6–8 µm at the nucleus) occurring in the grey and white matter. The extent of their cell processes cannot always be demonstrated in routine light microscopic preparations, and thus they are sometimes incorrectly described as ‘unbranched cells’. The electron microscope reveals 10–50 extensively flattened sheet-like processes that are responsible for myelination of nerve fibres within the CNS. One oligodendrocyte can myelinate up to 50 axons (Figures 5.23 and 5.25).

Oligodendrocytes exhibit morphological and functional differences, based on the region of the CNS in which they are located:

- In white matter, oligodendrocytes are interfascicular cells, arranged in characteristic rows between nerve fibres.
- In grey matter, oligodendrocytes form satellites of neurons or blood vessels, their processes being closely associated with the perikaryon.

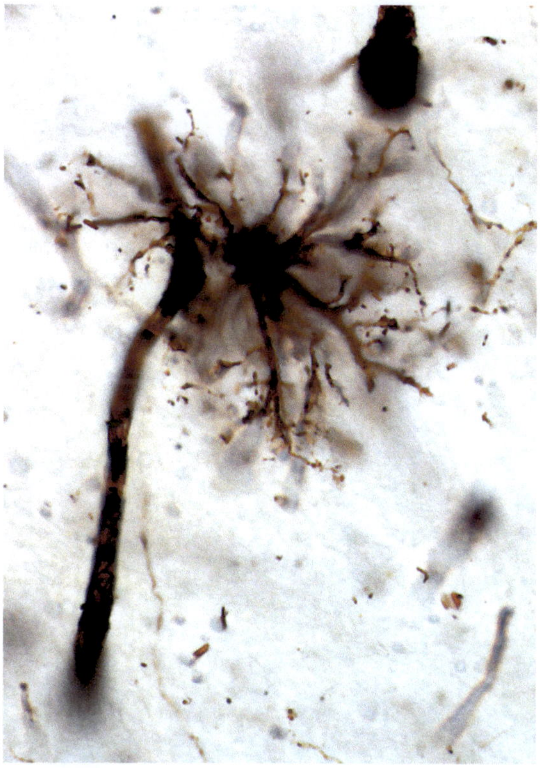

5.21 Protoplasmic astrocytes in the cerebrum (dog). Cajal silver stain (x1200).

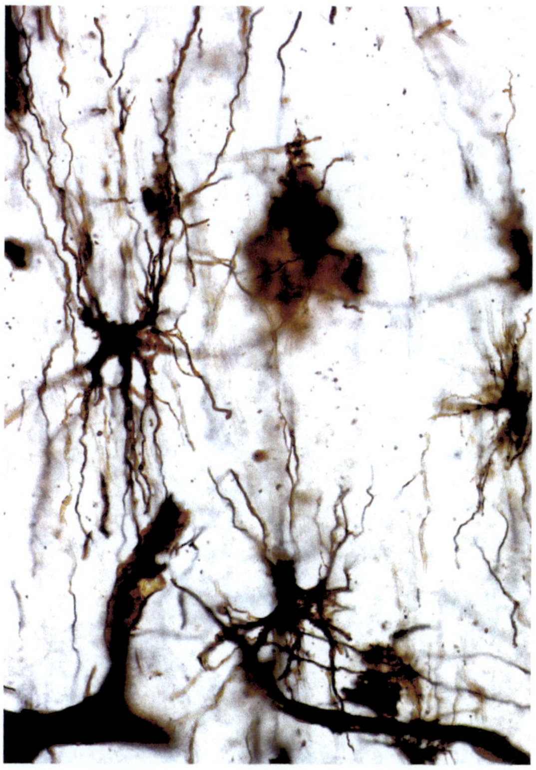

5.22 Fibrous astrocytes in the spinal cord (dog). Golgi silver stain (x480).

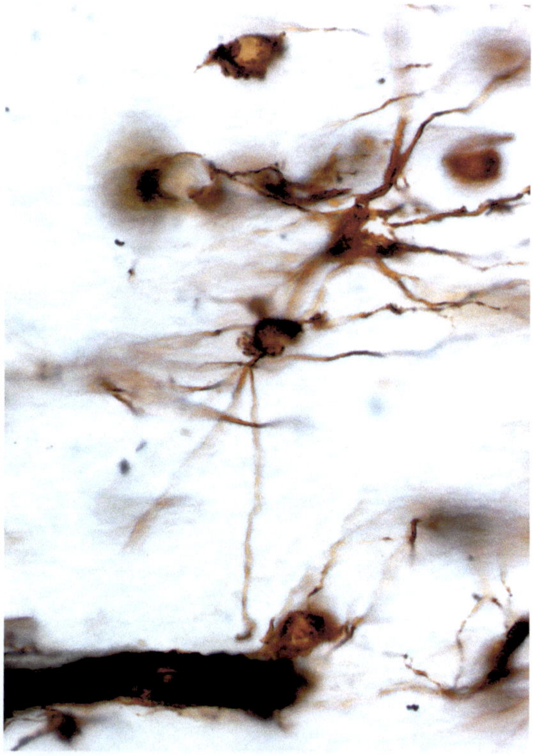

5.23 Oligodendroglia in the cerebellum (ox). Golgi silver stain (x480).

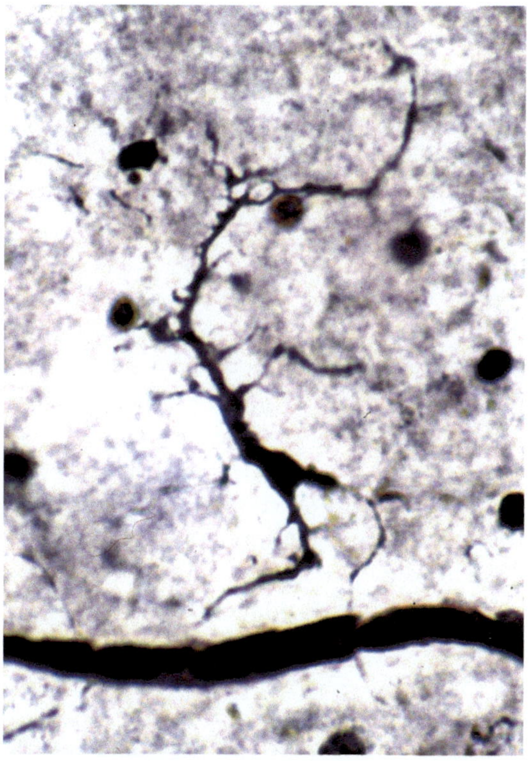

5.24 Microglia (Hortega cells) in the cerebellum (cat). Golgi silver stain (x480).

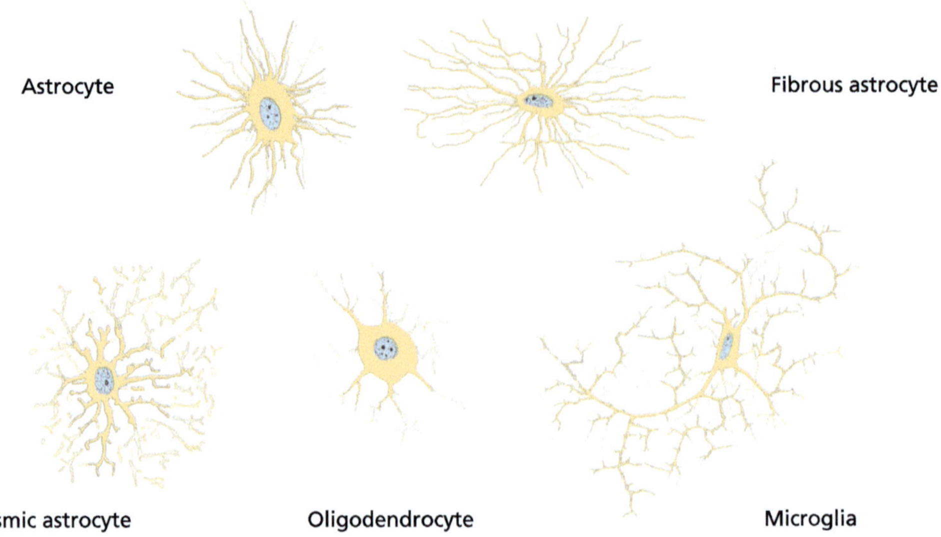

5.25 Glial cells of the central nervous system (schematic). The portions of the cell represented in the diagram as continuous lines can typically be demonstrated using silver staining methods. Subsequent branching of the cell processes can occasionally be shown with histological stains or with the aid of ultrastructural reconstructions.

Perivascular oligodendrocytes are numerous and are prominent around the blood vessels of the cerebral cortex. Interfascicular oligodendrocytes are by far the most common cell type in the white matter. Their processes run parallel to the nerve fibres, giving off branches that partially or completely surround the axon.

Based on their size and the length, arrangement and complexity of their processes, oligodendrocytes are subdivided into four types (Hortega types I–IV).

Oligodendrocytes have several functions. Interfascicular oligodendrocytes are responsible for the formation and maintenance of the myelin sheath of CNS nerve fibres, in which saltatory nerve conduction is an essential requirement. Oligodendrocytes also interact functionally with neurons and are a key component of iron metabolism in the CNS, requiring iron for synthesis of myelin. Oligodendrocytes inhibit the development of neurites.

Microglia (Hortega cells)

Microglia, also named Hortega cells after the neurophysiologist Pio Del Rio Hortega (1882–1945), are small, usually stellate glial cells, frequently located near blood vessels. They have an elongated nucleus and short, often bizarrely formed, processes. Microglia are found in both the grey and white matter. They frequently contain phagocytosed material originating from degenerating neurons. Their cytoplasm contains phagosomes.

The phagocytic capacity of microglia reflects their differentiation from migrating blood monocytes, macrophages, pericytes surrounding the walls of blood vessels or from the connective tissue of the meninges. In view of their mesodermal origin, they have also been referred to historically as **mesoglia** (Figures 5.24 and 5.25).

Glial cells of the peripheral nervous system

Schwann cell (neurolemmocyte)

Schwann cells form the **myelin sheath surrounding axons of peripheral nerves**. After coming to lie along an axon, the plasmalemma of the Schwann cell wraps around the axon and differentiates into the myelin sheath. Schwann cells surround peripheral axons over a distance of approximately 1 mm. The ends of consecutive Schwann cells are denoted by the node of Ranvier, where the myelin sheath is interrupted. The cytoplasm of the Schwann cell forms the sheath of Schwann, the outer surface of which is comprised of basal lamina.

Satellite cell (amphicyte, gliocytus ganglii)

Satellite cells surround the perikaryon of nerve cells in ganglia (autonomic, spinal, cranial nerves). They have dense, typically flattened nuclei. A basal lamina separates them from surrounding connective tissue. Satellite cells are functionally associated with capillaries and support the metabolic requirements of the ganglion cells.

6

Circulatory system (systema cardiovasculare et lymphovasculare)

The role of the circulatory system is to maintain uninterrupted flow of blood around the body, thus permitting constant exchange of oxygen and carbon dioxide, uptake of nutrients and elimination of waste. The circulatory system also serves to transport ions, hormones and enzymes, and contributes to thermoregulation. The **blood vascular** (**cardiovascular**) **system** is comprised of the heart, as its central organ, and the blood vessels (arteries, arterioles, capillaries, venules and veins). Together they form a **closed circulatory system**. Connected to the blood vascular system is a system of lymph vessels that drain lymph from the tissues.

The **heart** can be regarded as a highly differentiated segment of vessel wall with internal divisions that give rise to a smaller pulmonary and a larger systemic circulation. Rhythmic contraction of the muscular wall results in circulation of blood.

The vessels **travelling away from** the heart, the **arteries**, serve as the conduit for blood and its soluble contents to the peripheral tissues and organs. Arteries divide extensively into vessels with decreasing diameter. The smaller **arterioles** undergo multiple divisions before opening into dense networks of **capillaries**, in which gases and metabolic products are exchanged. Postcapillary segments converge to form **venules** (diameter 0.2–1 mm) which empty into vessels of increasing diameter – the small, medium and large **veins**. Venules and veins return the blood to the heart.

For **exchange of substances** to occur in the capillary bed, blood must flow at relatively slow speeds and low pressure. Thus, pressure in capillaries is reduced to 20–35 mmHg. The veins into which blood passes from the capillaries constitute a **low-pressure system** (5–10 mmHg). A **high-pressure system** exists near the heart and in the arterial circulation. Mean pressures in the high-pressure circulation vary considerably with species (65–140 mmHg).

The structure of the vessel walls varies to accommodate the requirements of this dynamic system. In particular, the flow of blood is influenced by differences in the degree of muscle development. The walls of the capillaries are devoid of muscle, while muscle tissue forms the bulk of the heart. Capillaries have the simplest wall structure and are therefore described first.

Cardiovascular system (systema cardiovasculare)

Capillaries (vas capillare)

Capillaries form a finely branched, metabolically active network between the smallest arterioles and the postcapillary venules. These thin-walled tubular vessels (average diameter 7–9 μm) permit the passage of blood cells and plasma as well as metabolic products into the connective tissue (interstitium). In addition, capillaries take up blood cells and interstitial fluid from the loose connective tissue, conveying these via postcapillary venules into the circulating blood (Figures 6.1 to 6.5). A capillary consists of:

- simple squamous epithelium (endothelium) that forms the inner lining of the tubular vessel and
- a basal lamina (complete or incomplete) externally adjacent to the endothelium; in certain capillaries this may be absent over segments of the capillary wall (sinusoids) (Figure 6.2).

Lying adjacent to the outer surface of most capillaries are perivascular cells called **pericytes**, that are partially enclosed by a basal lamina. These are undifferentiated mesenchymal cells that retain a significant capacity for transformation (e.g. into macrophages, fibroblasts).

The structure of the capillary wall is closely related to the **metabolic activity** of the tissue (see also Table 6.1). Passage of substances across the capillary wall can occur through **transcellular** or **intercellular** pathways. In the transcellular route, substances are transported through the cytoplasm in individual or aggregated pinocytotic vesicles (**transcytosis**, **cytopempsis**). This pathway is used for the transfer of water-soluble and larger molecules through the endothelium. New vesicles (up to 1000/mm^2) are continuously produced. After passing through the cytoplasm, they fuse with the plasmalemma of the endothelial cell and

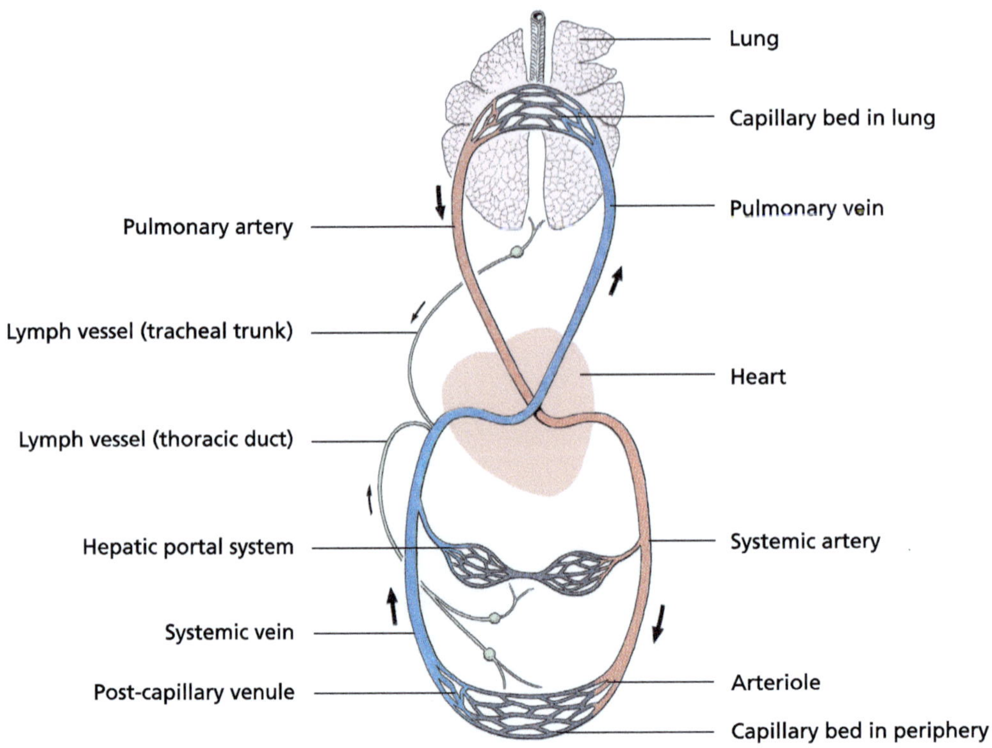

6.1 Schematic representation of the circulatory system with selected lymph vessels (König and Liebich, 2009).

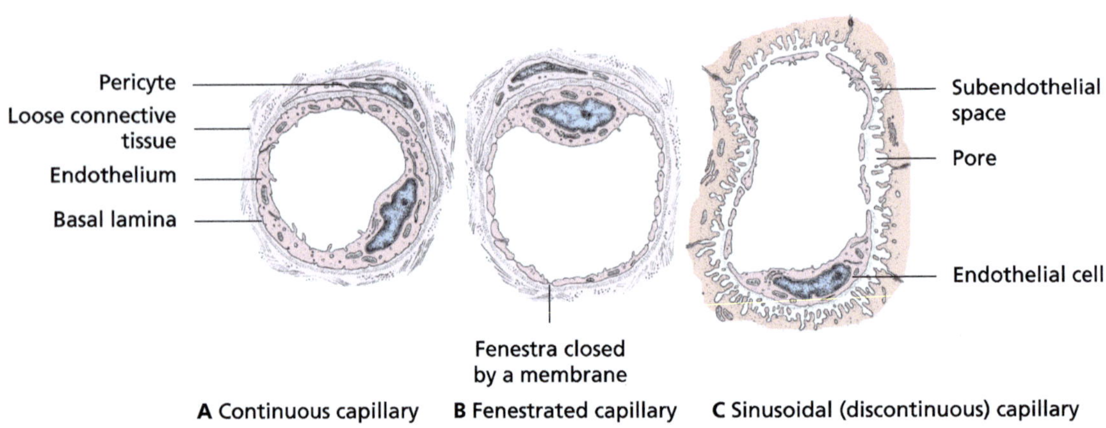

6.2 Types of capillary (schematic). A: continuous capillary, B: fenestrated capillary, C: sinusoidal capillary.

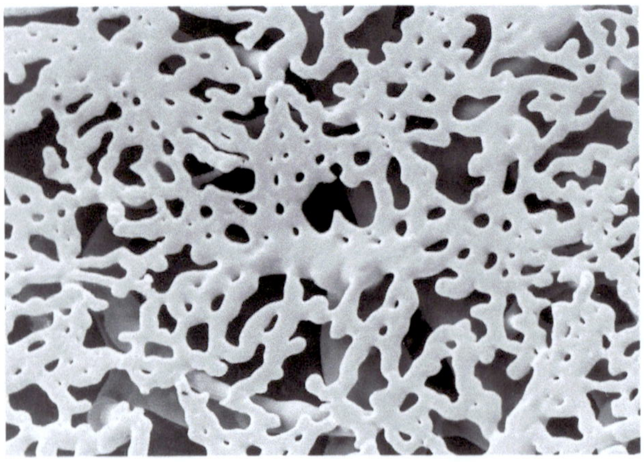

6.3 Scanning electron micrograph of a capillary bed in the vascular tunic of the eye (injected specimen, courtesy of Prof. König, Vienna).

open to the exterior. This process typically involves specific receptors for signalling molecules and proteins (**receptor-mediated transcytosis**).

Material endocytosed by the capillary endothelium may also be taken up by lysosomes.

The capillary wall plays a fundamental role in the uptake and exchange of O_2 and CO_2. These gases, as well as low-molecular weight substances and ions, pass through the endothelium by **diffusion** across a concentration

Table 6.1 Structural differences in the vessels of the blood vascular system.

Vessel type	Tunica intima	Tunica media	Tunica adventitia
Elastic artery (large artery)	Endothelium with basal lamina, thin subendothelial layer, thin internal elastic membrane	Numerous concentric elastic lamellae, smooth muscle cells between elastic lamellae, vasa vasorum and delicate nerve bundles, thin external elastic membrane	Thin
Muscular artery (small and medium arteries)	Endothelium with basal lamina, distinct internal elastic membrane	Variable number of layers of smooth muscle cells, external elastic membrane adjoining outer tunica media, few vasa vasorum and nerve fibres	Poorly developed
Arteriole (≤100 µm diameter)	Endothelium with basal lamina, thin subendothelial layer, internal elastic membrane lacking	1–3 layers of smooth muscle cells with delicate nerve fibres	Thin
Metarteriole	Endothelium with basal lamina	Smooth muscle cells forming precapillary sphincters	Poorly developed loose connective tissue
Capillary	Endothelium with variably developed basal lamina, pericytes present externally	No smooth muscle cells	Sparse, loose pericapillary connective tissue
Venule	Endothelium with basal lamina, pericytes present externally	Loose connective tissue with occasional smooth muscle cells	Poorly developed, loose connective tissue
Small and medium vein	Endothelium and basal lamina, valves	Loose connective tissue with smooth muscle	Distinct
Large vein	Endothelium and basal lamina, valves, occasional indistinct internal elastic membrane	Loose connective tissue with smooth muscle cells, thin-walled compared to accompanying artery	Well developed with isolated smooth muscle cells

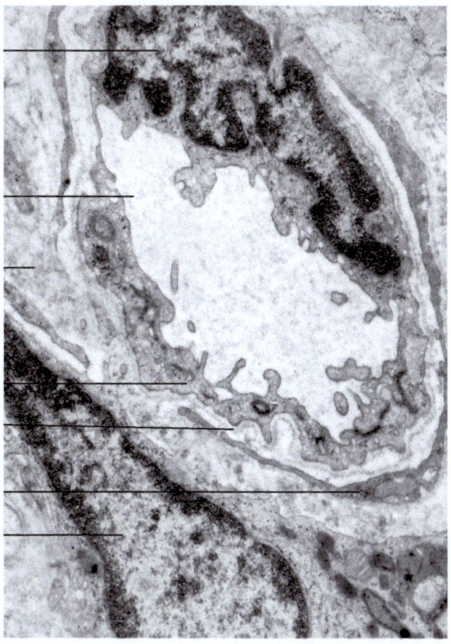

6.4 Fine structure of a capillary with adjacent pericyte (x6000).

gradient. Exchange of substances can also occur via the movement of water and solutes across pressure gradients (bulk flow). In the proximal portion of capillaries, hydrostatic pressure favours the movement of small molecules out of the capillaries (**filtration**). Towards the venules, colloid osmotic pressure causes dissolved substances to move into the capillary lumen (**absorption**).

The negative charge of the endothelial cell membrane is a significant factor in trans-endothelial transport. Negatively charged proteins are repelled by it and remain within the vessel. Proteins gain access to the extracellular space only via specific mechanisms, such as receptor-mediated transcytosis. Transcellular transport can be expedited by open endothelial pores and fenestrations (see below).

The intercellular pathway is used primarily by blood cells (erythrocytes, leucocytes, macrophages). The mechanism by which the cell accesses the extravascular compartment involves enzymatic digestion of intercellular junctions (zonulae occludentes). The movement of blood cells into the interstitial tissue is referred to as **diapedesis**.

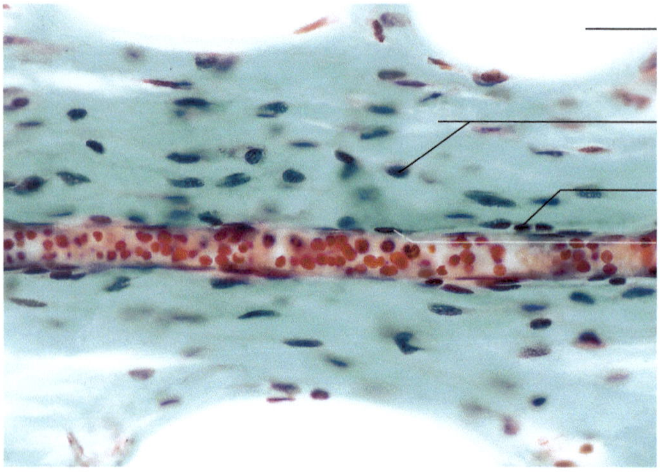

6.5 Capillary in greater omentum (dog). The capillary wall comprises a tube of squamous epithelial cells (endothelium). The nuclei of the endothelial cells protrude slightly into the lumen. Endothelial cells are often accompanied by pericytes, cells of mesodermal origin that lie on the outer surface of the endothelium. Goldner's Masson trichrome stain (x250).

Based on its multiple functions, the endothelium lining capillary walls is classified as a **transport epithelium** (see Chapter 2, 'Epithelial tissue').

Three types of capillary can be distinguished; their structure is related to the tissues and organs in which they are located (Figure 6.2).

Continuous capillaries

Capillaries lacking physical interruptions (non-fenestrated capillaries, endotheliocytus nonfenestratus) are by far the most common type of capillary found in the body. Their wall is relatively thick, limiting rapid trans-epithelial transport. They contain abundant pinocytotic vesicles. The barrier function of continuous capillaries is further reinforced by a layered basal lamina and numerous pericytes (e.g. in brain and muscle capillaries).

Fenestrated capillaries

This type of capillary is found mainly in tissues in which large volumes of fluid are exchanged at a rapid rate (e.g. capillaries involved in filtration in the glomerulus, absorption in the renal tubules, capillary loops in the intestinal mucosa, exocrine and endocrine organs). The endothelium (endotheliocytus fenestratus) is markedly flattened and is interrupted in a sieve-like fashion by numerous openings (fenestrae). The fenestrae are usually covered by a diaphragm. When the diaphragm is lacking, the openings are referred to as pores.

Sinusoidal capillaries (vas capillare sinusoideum)

Sinusoidal (discontinuous) capillaries, or sinusoids, are characterised by intercellular spaces, a typically discontinuous or absent basal lamina, numerous pores and an irregular shape. This type of capillary enables rapid exchange of metabolic substances (e.g. in the liver, spleen, adenohypophysis, adrenal cortex and bone marrow). Phagocytic cells of the mononuclear phagocytic system are often associated with the wall of the sinusoid.

Blood flow through the capillary bed is regulated by the contraction of smooth muscle in the wall of precapillary arterioles (**metarterioles**). These vessels provide temporary resistance to blood flow by way of **precapillary sphincters**. They are innervated by **adrenergic nerve fibres**. Changes in the diameter of these vessels alters vascular resistance and thus has a direct influence on blood pressure and blood flow through the capillary bed (Figure 6.12).

Capillary blood flow is also regulated by **arteriovenous anastomoses**. These specialised structures shunt blood directly from arteries to venules, bypassing the capillary bed (Figure 6.12, see also below).

The role of the capillary endothelium in the transfer of substances between the blood and the tissues has been described above. In addition, the vascular endothelium has several other important functions:

- synthesis of vasoconstrictors (endothelin) and vasodilators (nitrous oxide and prostacyclin),
- regulation of inflammation and immune responses (synthesis of IL-1, IL-6, IL-8, expression of adhesion molecules and histocompatibility antigens),
- synthesis of anticoagulants (thrombomodulin, heparin-like molecules) and
- regulation of cell growth by synthesis of growth factors and inhibitors.

Blood vessels

Structure

For functional reasons, the structure of larger vessels (arteries, arterioles, veins and venules) varies between the high- and low-pressure systems, and within individual organs. Nevertheless, the basic structure of the vascular wall is consistent (Figures 6.6 to 6.12 and Table 6.1), constituting three concentrically positioned tubes:

- tunica intima (interna) comprising the
  - endothelium,
  - stratum subendotheliale (subendothelial layer) and

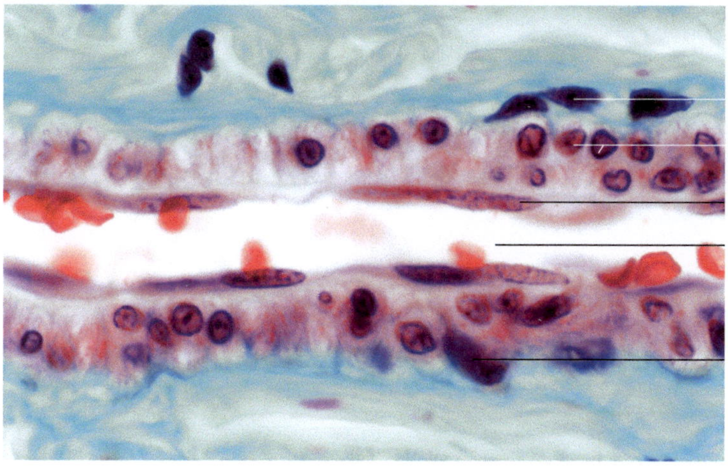

6.6 Arteriole in greater omentum (dog). Goldner's Masson trichrome stain (x1200).

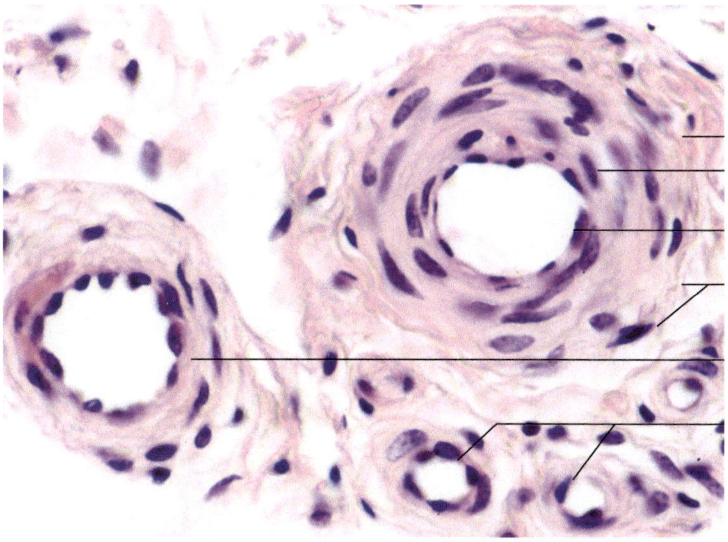

6.7 Small artery, venule and capillary in the skin (dog). Haematoxylin and eosin stain (x250).

- membrana elastica interna (internal elastic membrane);
- tunica media and
- tunica adventitia (externa).

The **tunica intima** constitutes the inner portion of the vessel wall (Figure 6.8). It consists of a single-layered endothelium and a continuous basal lamina, a subendothelial layer composed of connective tissue and an internal elastic membrane.

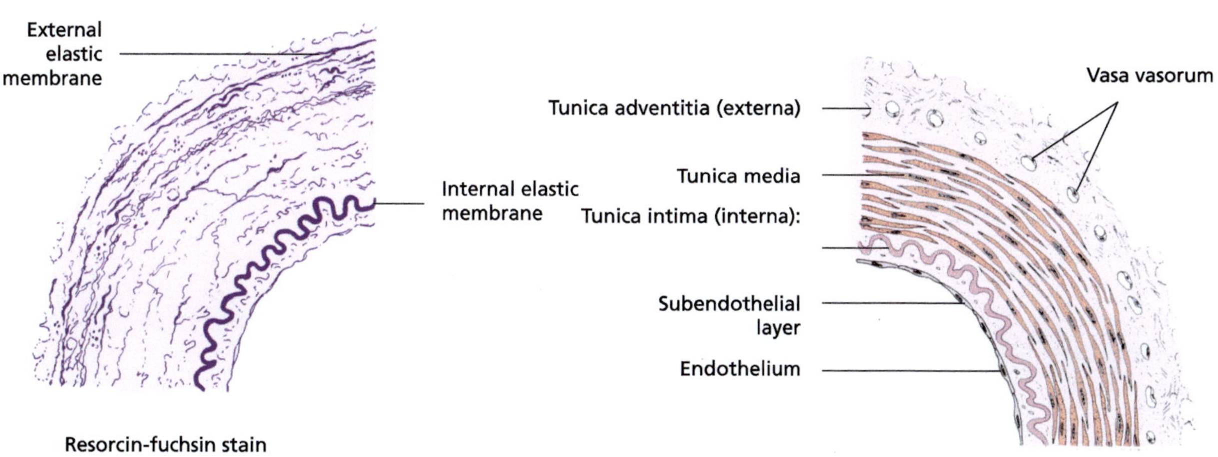

6.8 Structure of an artery (schematic).

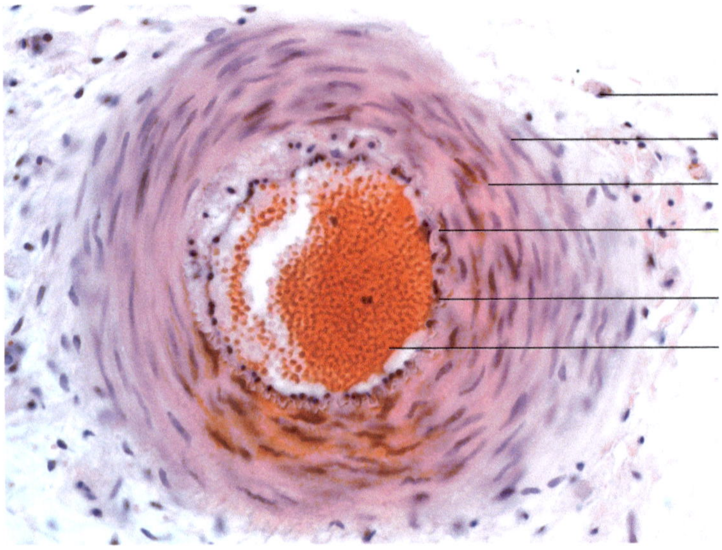

6.9 Relatively thick-walled artery in the subcutis (ox). Haematoxylin and eosin stain (x180).

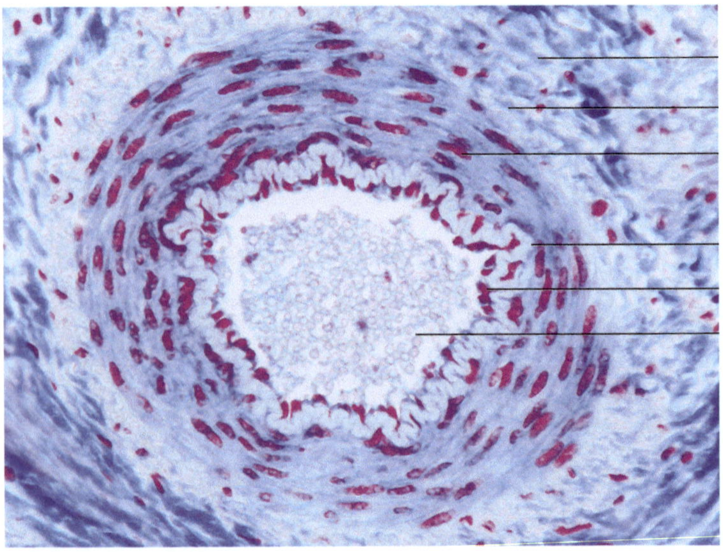

6.10 Thick-walled artery in the mesentery (dog). The muscle cells in the prominent tunica media are arranged in a predominantly circular, partly spiral orientation. Azan stain (x250).

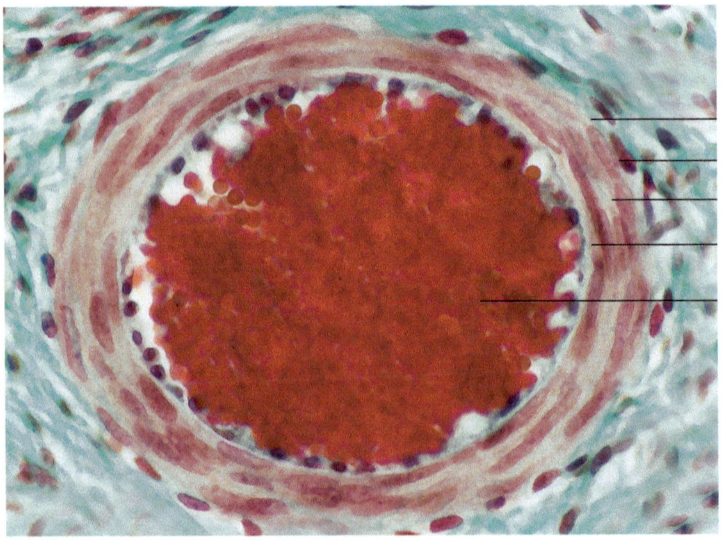

6.11 Thin-walled small artery in the subcutis (dog). Goldner's Masson trichrome stain (x270).

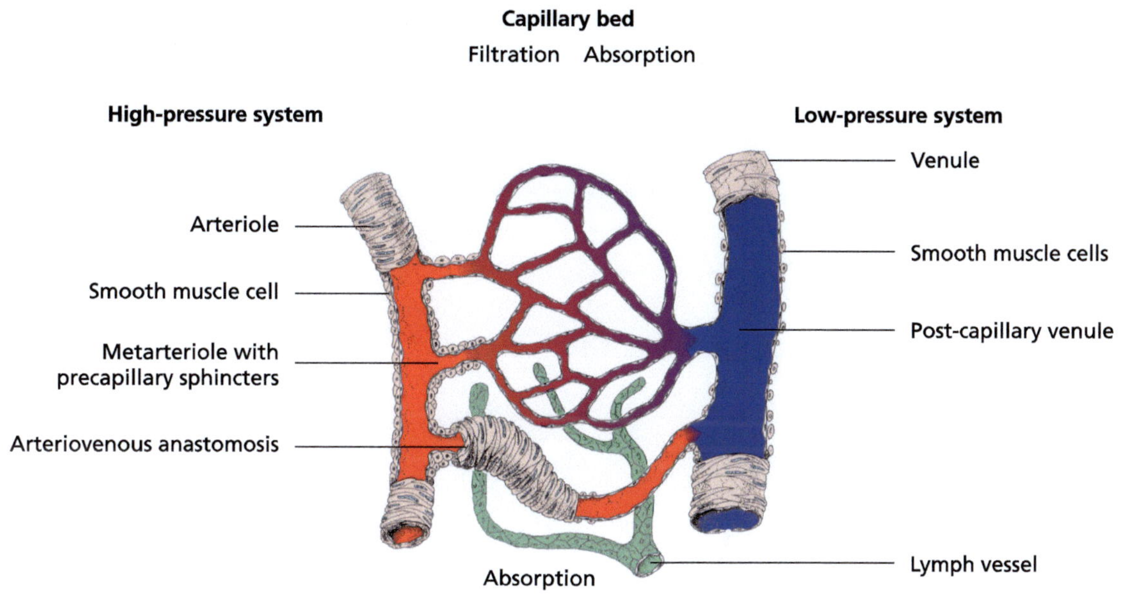

6.12 Capillary bed (schematic). A network of capillaries extends between an arteriole and a venule. Blood flow to the capillaries is regulated by contractile metarterioles and an arteriovenous anastomosis. When the autonomically controlled arteriovenous shunts close, blood flow to the capillary bed increases; when they open, less blood reaches the capillary bed. Lymph vessels drain metabolic by-products from the capillary bed.

The **endothelium** forms the inner lining of the vessel and participates in transvascular substance transport. It is also important for haemostasis. **Weibel–Palade bodies**, organelles specific to endothelial cells, contain **von Willebrand factor**, a substance important for thrombocyte aggregation. When a vessel wall is injured, von Willebrand factor induces binding of circulating platelets to exposed collagen fibres. Together with fibrin and erythrocytes, the platelets form a microthrombus that seals the vessel wall.

The subendothelial layer contains scattered elastic and collagen fibres, as well as fibrocytes, histiocytes and smooth muscle cells. The smooth muscle cells are relatively poorly differentiated, serving to synthesise fibres and phagocytose foreign materials.

The outermost layer of the tunica intima, the **internal elastic membrane**, is well developed in arteries, less so in the low-pressure components of the circulation.

The **tunica media** comprises several layers of **smooth muscle**, interspersed to varying degrees with elastic and collagen fibres. In large vessels, an **external elastic membrane** lies adjacent to the outer surface of the tunica media.

The **tunica adventitia** consists of a fibro-elastic (type I collagen) network. This loose, displaceable layer is in contact with the surrounding tissues.

Innervation

The walls of blood vessels are innervated by **poorly myelinated (sympathetic) autonomic nerve fibres**. These traverse the tunica adventitia to reach the tunica media, where they release adrenergic neurotransmitters at terminal synapses. Activation of α-receptors results in vasoconstriction, while stimulation of β-receptors causes vessels to dilate. Other substances, such as histamine, released by mast cells, and angiotensin also have vasoactive properties. Rhythmic neural stimulation of smooth muscle serves to maintain vascular tone.

Nutritional blood supply

Blood vessels receive their nutritional blood supply from vessels in the outer tunica media and tunica adventitia (vasa vasorum). Vessels are lacking in the tunica intima and inner layers of the tunica media. These layers are supplied via **diffusion** from the circulating blood. Nutrients pass through the endothelium and are distributed into the network of elastic fibres in the tunica media. The lining of the vessel walls is renewed through mitotic division of endothelial cells and by cells derived from the blood (e.g. monocytes).

Arteries (arteria)

Throughout the arterial tree, as far as the capillary bed, the arteries exert passive resistance to the pressure generated by the heart. Near the heart, the arteries also serve to transform the pulsatile ejection of blood from the heart into a continuous, even flow (elastic buffering, Windkessel effect). In accordance with these functions, the structure of the arteries exhibits considerable variation (Figures 6.8 to 6.14 and Table 6.1). The walls of the arteries of the lung, brain and meninges are relatively thin. In the peripheral high-pressure system, the arterial wall is noticeably thickened. Near highly mobile joints, such as the knee and shoulder, the arterial wall is particularly well developed. Arteries are categorised into two types:

- elastic arteries (arteria elastotypica) and
- muscular arteries (arteria myotypica).

ELASTIC ARTERIES (ARTERIA ELASTOTYPICA)

Arteries of the elastic type are **located close to the heart** and are characterised by a thick tunica media consisting predominantly of concentric fenestrated lamellae of elastic fibres (e.g. aorta, pulmonary artery) (Figure 6.13). The wide spaces evident between the lamellae contain delicate elastic fibre networks.

The **continuous endothelium** is underlaid by a **subendothelial layer** containing collagen fibres. An internal elastic membrane lies adjacent to the elastic layers of the tunica media.

The **elastic fibre bundles** are connected to individual smooth muscle cells, forming a muscular-elastic system. During systole, the numerous **elastic lamellae** become distended. In the subsequent diastole, recoil of the arterial wall results in smooth and uninterrupted onward transport of blood (**Windkessel effect**).

The proportion of smooth muscle cells in elastic arteries is much lower than in muscular arteries. As well as contributing to the muscular–elastic system, the contractile smooth muscle cells synthesise elastin, type I and III collagen and proteoglycans.

The outermost layer of elastic arteries, the **tunica adventitia**, is rich in collagen fibres that aid in preventing excessive stretching of the vessel wall.

MUSCULAR ARTERIES (ARTERIA MYOTYPICA)

Muscular arteries exhibit the typical three-layered arterial structure (Figures 6.8 to 6.11 and 6.14).

The outermost layer of the **tunica intima**, the **internal elastic membrane**, is well developed and easily distinguished in histological sections by its undulating appearance (artefactual contraction). The endothelium is connected by endothelial cell processes to the smooth muscle cells of the tunica media, which may also contribute to re-epithelialisation of the vessel wall.

Characteristic of muscular arteries are the well-developed, primarily circular or slightly spiralling smooth muscle cells (3–30 layers) in the **tunica media**. Individual muscle cells are connected by gap junctions and are surrounded by delicate bundles of collagen fibres, relatively few elastic fibres and proteoglycans. An indistinct outer layer of elastic fibres is also present.

The **tunica adventitia** contains collagen fibres and numerous, densely packed elastic fibres. The predominantly longitudinally oriented elastic fibres form an **external elastic membrane** adjacent to the tunica media. The tunica adventitia allows movement of the artery with respect to surrounding tissues. It is traversed by autonomic nerve fibres and smaller blood vessels that supply the arterial wall (vasa vasorum).

Most small to medium-sized arteries are muscular in type. The muscle layer maintains the pressure within the vessel and regulates the pulse wave in the high-pressure arterial system.

In certain **specialised arteries**, contractile cells embedded in the subendothelial layer can cause temporary constriction of the vessel, thus regulating blood flow through the tissue (referred to by some authors as 'barrier arteries' or 'polster arteries', see below). Such vessels are found in association with the bronchi and in the subcutis and penis.

Arterioles (arteriolae)

Arterioles are the smallest vessels (<100 μm) of the high-pressure system. Their flattened, continuous endothelium is surrounded by a thin subendothelial layer. A distinct internal

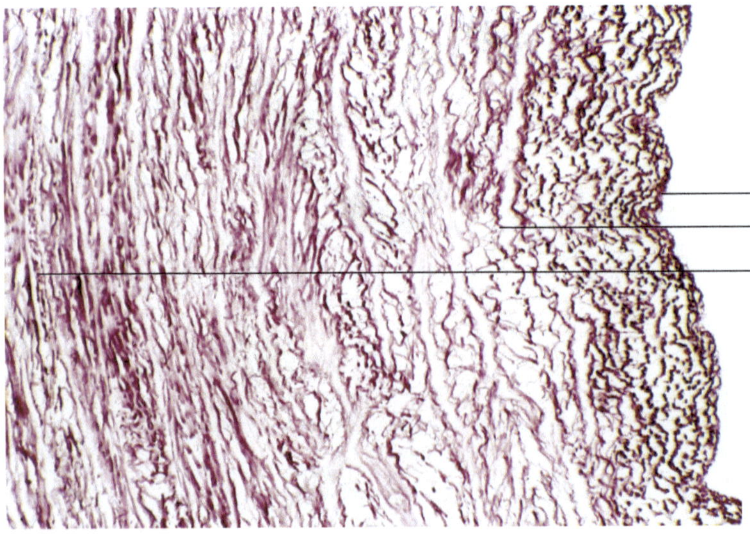

6.13 Elastic artery stained for elastic material (calf). Resorcin-fuchsin stain, nuclear-fast red (x300).

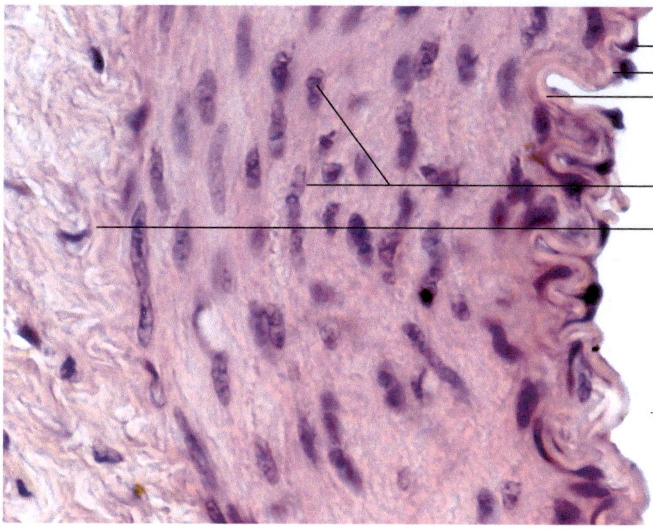

6.14 Muscular artery (pig). The endothelium is underlain by a thin subendothelial layer. The meandering internal elastic membrane is clearly demarcated. In the tunica media, the smooth muscle cells are arranged in a predominantly circular fashion with some obliquely running fibres. The large number of elastic fibres clearly distinguishes the connective tissue of the outer tunica adventitia. Haematoxylin and eosin stain (x480).

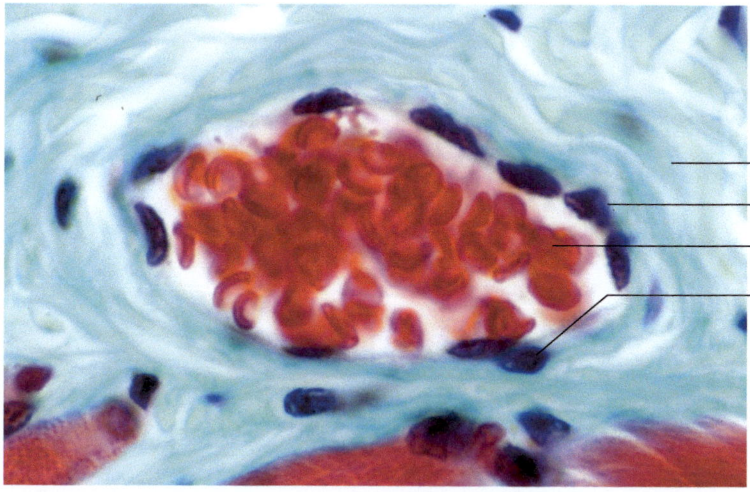

6.15 Postcapillary venule in the tongue (horse). The endothelium is surrounded by occasional pericytes and isolated smooth muscle cells. Expanded postcapillary venules can serve as a blood reservoir. Goldner's Masson trichrome stain (x200).

elastic membrane is usually lacking. The tunica media consists of **one to three layers of smooth muscle cells**. These join with endothelial cell processes to form a myoendothelial complex. Arterioles play a significant role in regulating peripheral blood pressure and, together with the precapillary sphincters, modify the flow of blood in capillary beds.

Veins (vena)

The low-pressure component of the circulatory system begins at the venous side of the capillary bed and extends to the right atrium of the heart. Its functions include:

- active metabolism (postcapillary venules),
- storage of blood and
- conduction of blood from the periphery to the heart.

The structure of veins is adapted to these roles (Figures 6.15 to 6.18 and Table 6.1). A key characteristic is the distensibility of the vessel wall, which is 200 times greater than that of arteries. Muscle tissue is poorly developed, while the tunica adventitia is distinctive and relatively thick (particularly in large veins).

The continuous **endothelium** is adjoined externally by a thin **subendothelial layer** supported by loose bundles of elastic and collagen fibres. Longitudinally oriented smooth muscle cells may be present. In place of a distinct **internal elastic membrane**, there is a thin network of elastic fibres (**rete elastica**).

Compared with corresponding arteries the **tunica media** is thin, containing mainly fibres of collagen and elastin. The collagen fibres are arranged in a lattice while

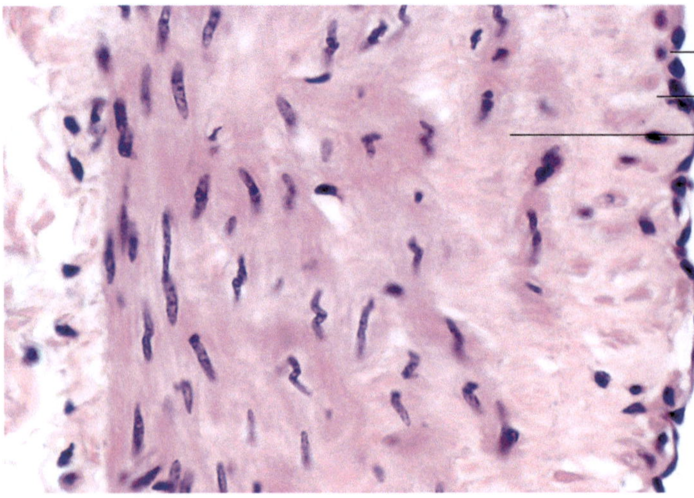

6.16 Vein (pig). The single-celled endothelium lining the internal vessel wall is adjoined externally by a narrow subendothelial layer. There is no distinct internal elastic membrane in the low-pressure venous system. In the tunica media, smooth muscle cells arranged in a predominantly circular orientation appear wavy due to contraction of the vessel wall. The adventitia incorporates elastic fibres. Haematoxylin and eosin stain (x480).

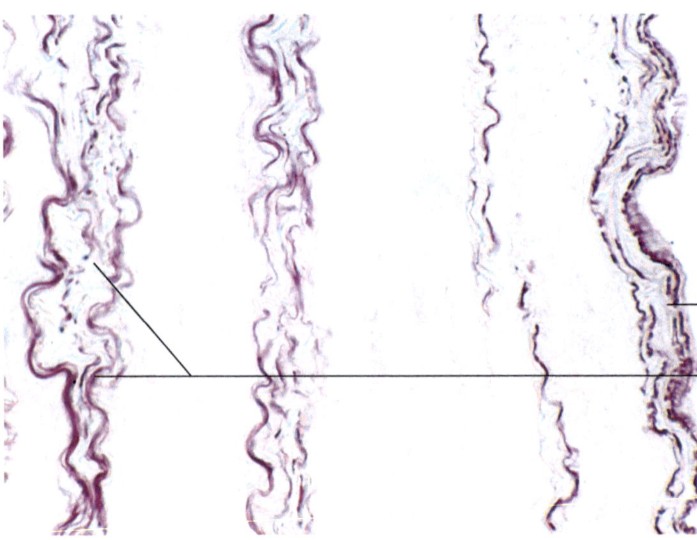

6.17 Vein stained for elastic tissue (dog). Resorcin-fuchsin stain (x480).

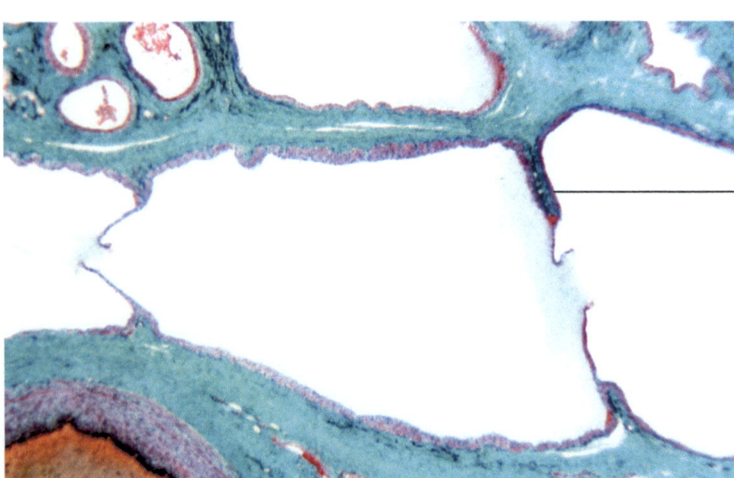

6.18 Valves in the venous component of the pampiniform plexus (bull). Goldner's Masson trichrome stain (x200).

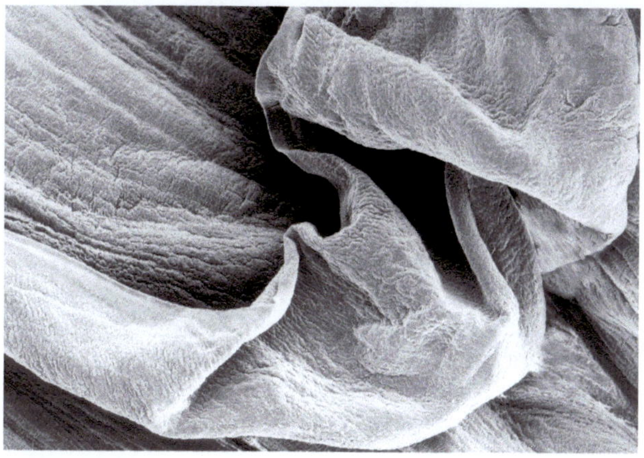

6.19 Scanning electron micrograph of a valve in a vein (pig; x1200).

the elastic fibres are longitudinally aligned. The relatively few smooth muscle cells are mostly arranged in a spiral configuration. This arrangement of fibromuscular elements imparts considerable distensibility to the wall of the vein.

The **tunica adventitia** establishes a fibrous connection to neighbouring tissues. An external elastic membrane is present. Due to the close spatial relationship between veins and skeletal muscle, the flow of blood through the low-pressure system is actively supported by skeletal muscle contraction. A feature of the low-pressure system is the presence, at regular intervals, of paired folds of the tunica intima referred to as **valves**. Structurally, valves consist of taut collagenous connective tissue, covered in a single layer of endothelium.

Valves facilitate the flow of blood towards the heart and prevent backflow (Figures 6.18 and 6.19).

In some veins, the tunica media is reinforced by distinct layering of smooth muscle. Referred to as **venae myotypicae**, these are found in locations such as the teat.

Venules (venula)

Venules are thin-walled postcapillary vessels (**venulae postcapillares**; Figure 6.15). In the lymph nodes and tonsils, because the endothelium of these vessels is almost cuboidal, these are referred to as high endothelial venules. The endothelium of high endothelial venules contains specific receptors for recognition of lymphocytes. These molecules are essential for the migration of circulating lymphocytes into the surrounding connective tissue.

Further along the returning venous network, smooth muscle cells appear in increasing numbers, eventually forming a thicker muscle layer. These vessels are termed **muscular venules** (**venulae musculares**). Initially, transport of substances across the walls of venules is still possible. As the vessels increase in diameter, they serve primarily as reservoirs of blood.

Arteriovenous specialisations

Structures involved in regulating blood flow are present in most organs of the body. These are associated with arterioles and venules, particularly at sites of vessel branching, and in pre- and postcapillary segments. They include:

- barrier arteries ('polster arteries'),
- throttle veins ('sphincter veins'),
- arteriovenous anastomoses
  - bridge form
  - coiled (glomus) form.

In **barrier arteries**, longitudinally oriented smooth muscle cells in the tunica intima partially or completely surround the lumen of the vessel. Through maximal contraction of these muscle cells and the smooth muscle of the tunica media, the artery can be almost completely closed off. The tunica intima of **throttle veins** (sphincter veins) contains circular or spirally arranged smooth muscle. These reinforce the vessel wall and, when contracting, restrict the vessel lumen. In contrast to barrier arteries, closure of the vessel is partial, manifesting simply as a bulge in the vessel wall. Functionally, contraction of these smooth muscle cell populations results in slowing of blood flow within the vessel with an increase in blood pressure.

Arteriovenous anastomoses constitute direct connections between arterioles and venules. As a result, a 'short-circuit' is formed with a portion of the local circulation bypassing the capillary bed. Arterial blood is thus diverted to the low-pressure venous system without the exchange of nutrients or metabolites.

Anastomoses may take the form of a short, curved or S-shaped **bridge**, in which the arterial component is recognisable by the thickness of its wall. These are characterised by circular and longitudinal muscle fibre bundles, reinforced by elastic fibres and in some cases by epithelioid cells. These anastomoses are found in the wall of the gastrointestinal tract, the respiratory tract, skin, uterus, ovary, penis and in several endocrine organs. They contribute to circulatory haemodynamics and peripheral thermoregulation (extremities, ear lobe, nose and skin).

The **coiled** form of arteriovenous anastomosis (**glomus**) is composed of heavily convoluted and often branched vessels that are richly endowed with unmyelinated nerve fibres. They occur in the tips of the phalanges and in the skin.

Heart (cor)

The heart can be viewed as a hollow muscle, its structure resembling a modified vessel wall. The heart comprises the following layers:

- endocardium (inner layer),
- myocardium (middle layer) and
- epicardium (outer layer).

The **endocardium** is similar to the tunica intima of blood vessels. Its innermost layer consists of a thin endothelium and loose subendothelial connective tissue. Adjoining this is a meshwork of collagen and elastic fibres in which smooth muscle cells are embedded (**stratum myoelasticum**). The endocardium is joined to the myocardium by a vascularised **tela subendocardialis**. This subendocardial layer contains the **fibres of the autonomic conduction system** (myofibra conducens cardiaca), known as Purkinje fibres (see Figure 4.17).

The **heart valves** are endocardial outfoldings with a tough 'skeleton' of **collagen fibres**. They are avascular, yet richly supplied with autonomic nerve fibres. The chordae tendinae attach the ventricular side of the atrioventricular valves to the papillary muscles.

The **myocardium** is composed of cardiac muscle cells (see Chapter 4, 'Muscle tissue') and a modestly developed connective tissue meshwork incorporating a dense network of capillaries. Arterioles supplying the myocardium exhibit several physiological specialisations that aid in meeting the oxygen requirements of this tissue. The myocardium also contains autonomic nerve fibres and numerous lymph vessels.

The heart muscle is attached to the fibrous cardiac skeleton, consisting of the annular rings (**annuli fibrosis**) surrounding the valves, the fibrous trigones that connect the rings, and the membranous part of the interventricular septum. Variation in the orientation of fibres in the ventricles gives rise to an outer layer of longitudinally oriented muscle fibres, a circular middle layer and an inner layer in which the muscle cells are arranged in spirals. The inner layer is continuous with the papillary muscles.

The **epicardium** is the visceral leaf of the pericardium, also constituting the pericardial subserosa. It consists of a simple epithelium overlying a thin connective tissue layer.

In contrast to the muscle of the blood vessels, the myocardium is composed of a specialised form of **striated muscle** (see Chapter 4, 'Muscle tissue'). Moreover, the heart is capable of generating and conducting electrical impulses, giving rise to rhythmic cardiac contractions without input from the central nervous system.

The conducting system of the heart

A feature of the cardiac muscle is its capacity for autonomous generation and propagation of rhythmic electrical activity (bioelectric impulses). This so-called conducting system of the heart is composed not of nerve fibres, but of **modified cardiac muscle cells**.

The impulse is initiated at the **sinoatrial node** (**nodus sinuatrialis**), referred to as the pacemaker of the heart. The impulse spreads smoothly and rapidly via the **atrioventricular node** (nodus atrioventricularis, Aschoff–Tawara node) and the **atrioventricular bundle** (truncus fasciculi atrioventricularis, bundle of His) to the bundle branches and the walls of the ventricles. The sinoatrial and atrioventricular nodes are interconnected by the atrial myocardium and are particularly well vascularised. The conducting system is composed of three cell types:

- nodal cells (pacemaker cells),
- transitional cells and
- Purkinje cells (myofibra conducens cardiaca).

Nodal (**pacemaker**) **cells** are found, together with transitional cells, in the sinoatrial and atrioventricular nodes, and in the conduction pathways. These pacemaker cells are characterised by lightly staining cytoplasm rich in mitochondria, a high density of glycogen granules and numerous pinocytotic vesicles. Myofibrils are sparse and are distributed diffusely within the cytoplasm.

Transitional cells appear to be localised at the final branches of the conduction pathway, between the Purkinje cells and the myocardium. They contain few mitochondria and little glycogen. The cells are arranged in longitudinal spirals.

The conducting system terminates in the ventricles as bundles of **Purkinje cells**. Transmission of impulses by the Purkinje cells results in myocardial contraction. Measuring up to 100 μm, Purkinje cells have pale cytoplasm with few, longitudinally aligned myofibrils, and are high in glycogen. Purkinje fibres travel beneath the endocardium, eventually ramifying in the myocardium. They are connected by gap junctions with ordinary myocardial cells, either directly or via transitional cells.

In addition to the conducting system, the heart contains a dense network of **sympathetic nerve fibres** that secrete adrenergic agonists (acting primarily on β-receptors). **Vagal** (**parasympathetic**) **fibre bundles** primarily innervate the atria. Atrial cells synthesise the peptide hormone ANP (atrial natriuretic peptide), which promotes diuresis (see Chapter 9, 'Endocrine system').

Lymph vessels (systema lymphovasculare)

Lymph vessels are the drainage system for the **extracellular fluid of the connective tissue**, serving to convey lymph to the blood vascular system (Figures 6.20 to 6.24). The system of lymph vessels begins as a network of anastomosing lymph capillaries that merge to form larger vessels. Lymph vessels typically pass via lymph nodes as they conduct lymph to the venous system, which they join near the thoracic inlet.

Lymph is composed of cells (particularly lymphocytes) and lymph plasma. The lymph plasma, a colourless to pale yellow fluid, contains proteins including albumin, prothrombin, fibrinogen and globulins. The fat content is determined largely by short-chain fatty acids absorbed from the intestine. These join with phospholipids, cholesterol and cholesterol esters to form droplets called **chylomicrons**. High fat diets cause the lymph to take on a milky appearance. Lymph also contains ions, hormones, enzymes, antibodies and metabolites.

Lymph capillaries (vas lymphocapillare)

Lymph capillaries consist of an irregularly expanded **endothelial tube**. Their diameter (10–50 µm) is markedly greater than that of blood capillaries. Lymph capillaries are **blind-ended channels** that take up fluid from the interstitium. The cells of the thin endothelium are connected by interdigitations and overlapping areas, occasionally only by zonulae occludentes. Spaces are often present between cells, and the **basal lamina** is usually absent or interrupted by large gaps. The exterior of the endothelium is connected by delicate anchoring filaments to the collagen fibres of the surrounding connective tissue. These appear to regulate the movement of fluid into the lymph capillaries (Figures 6.23 and 6.24). A **subepithelial network** of lymph capillaries is found in the connective tissue of the inner and outer surfaces of the body, and in the interstitial connective tissue of many organs. Lymph capillaries are absent from the central nervous system, bone marrow, red pulp of the spleen and hyaline cartilage.

Leading away from the lymph capillary network is a system of small, then medium and eventually large, lymph vessels. Their basic structure comprises a tubular endothelium and a sleeve of loose connective tissue. Depending upon species and body region, fibromuscular reinforcement of the vessel wall may be present. Like lymph capillaries, these vessels are located within connective tissue.

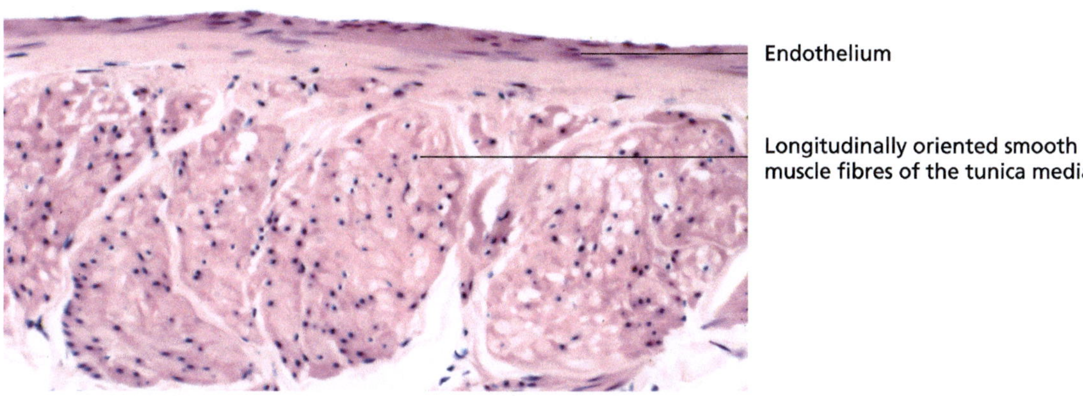

6.20 Transverse section of the wall of a collecting duct (thoracic duct; sheep). The flattened endothelium is surrounded by a broad subendothelial layer and a tunica media with longitudinally oriented smooth muscle cells. Haematoxylin and eosin stain (x300).

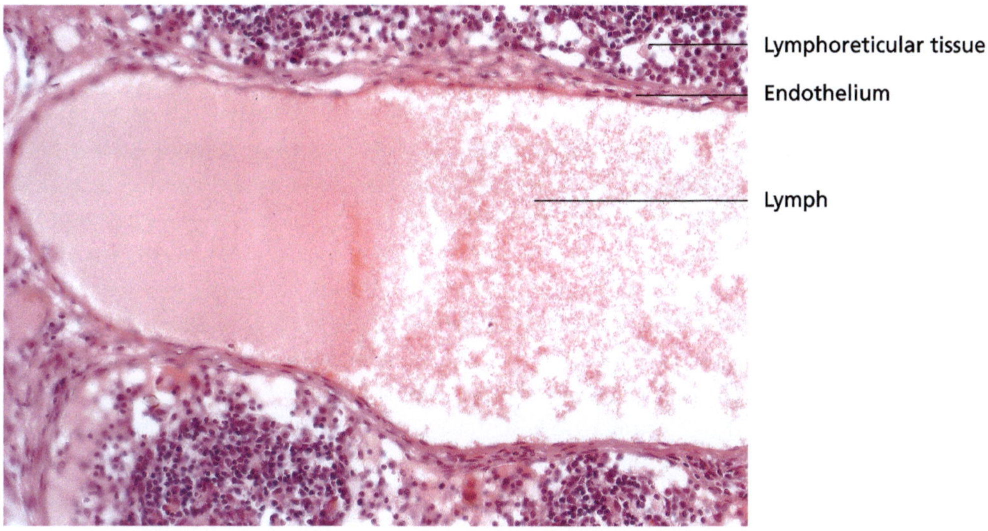

6.21 Partial section of the wall of a lymph vessel in the medulla of a lymph node (pig). Haematoxylin and eosin stain (x300).

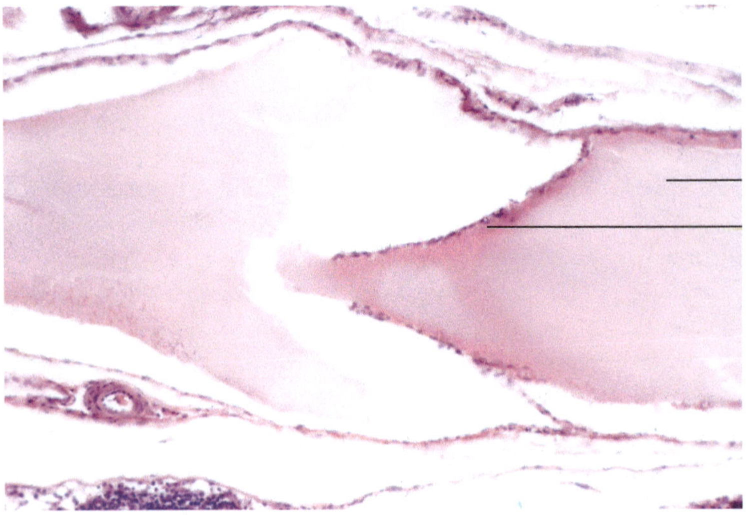

6.22 Longitudinal section of a lymph vessel, including a valve (hilus of a lymph node, sheep). The direction of flow of lymph is from right to left. Haematoxylin and eosin stain (x120).

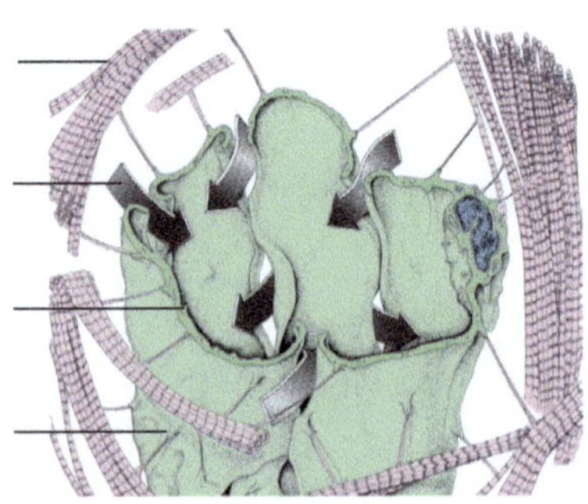

6.23 Schematic representation of the wall of a lymph capillary with slit-like spaces between adjacent endothelial cells. Anchoring filaments connect the endothelium with bundles of collagen fibres. At high interstitial pressures, the anchoring filaments cause the intercellular spaces to widen.

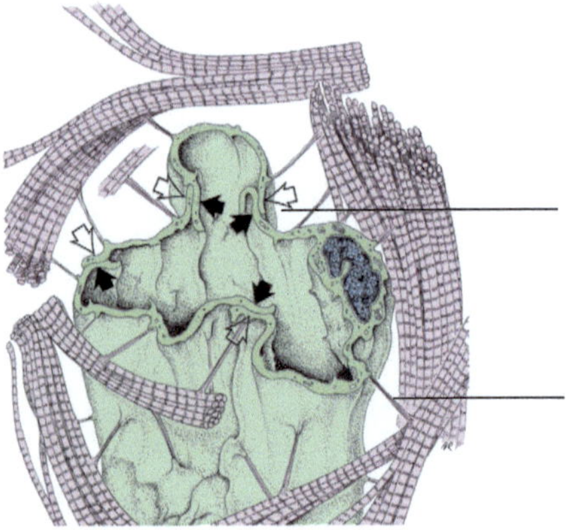

6.24 Schematic representation of the wall of a lymph capillary in which the intercellular spaces are closed off by overlapping of the endothelial cells. The anchoring filaments are shortened. Under low pressure, the interstitial space is condensed.

Collecting ducts (vas lymphaticum myotypicum)

The structure of the collecting ducts of the lymphatic system (**thoracic duct** and **tracheal trunk**) is similar to that of blood vessels (Figures 6.20 to 6.22). An inner tunica intima, composed of endothelium, is surrounded by mainly longitudinally oriented connective tissue fibres and isolated smooth muscle cells. The tunica media contains smooth muscle cells and a fibro-elastic connective tissue network. Adjoining the tunica media is a tunica adventitia containing smooth muscle cells arranged in a longitudinal or spiral fashion. The prominence and orientation of muscle fibres varies considerably with species.

Lymph vessels other than lymph capillaries routinely contain **valves**. These are similar in structure to valves occurring in veins. In addition, smooth muscle cells may be present.

Lymph heart of birds (cor lymphaticum)

The lymph hearts of birds are located outside the body cavity, at the caudal end of the synsacrum and dorsal to the transverse process of the first free caudal vertebra. The **wall of the lymph heart** consists of an endothelium-lined **endocardium** (with a connective tissue sheath incorporating smooth muscle) and a myocardium. Its outer layer comprises an adventitia of loose connective tissue with multilocular white adipocytes. The cells of the myocardium exhibit characteristics of skeletal, cardiac and smooth muscles.

The function of the lymph heart is age- and species-dependent. In avian species with a well-developed copulatory organ and a protrusible phallus, such as ratites and waterfowl, the lymph heart is wholly or predominantly integrated into the specialised lymphatic system of the copulatory organ.

Following erection, the lymph heart pumps lymph from the phallus and directs it to the venous system. As a secondary function, the lymph heart contributes to the regulation of blood pressure in the vertebral sinus durae matris and in the renal portal system.

Lymphoreticular formations of birds

The term formationes lymphoreticulares parenchymatosae describes diffuse, poorly demarcated lymphoreticular formations that may or may not have germinal centres. These occur mainly in parenchymatous organs such as endocrine glands, the liver and spleen.

Mural lymphoreticular formations are spindle-shaped thickenings of the walls of lymph vessels (Figures 6.25 and 6.26). They occur in all larger lymph vessels in the chicken and have yet to be found lacking in bird species studied to date. Mural lymphoreticular formations are just visible to the naked eye and can be considered as a **modified** and **smaller version of the avian lymph node**. They occur as both internal variants within the intima (interna) of the lymphatic vessel (formatio lymphoreticularis muralis interna), and as external variants in the thickened adventitia (formatio lymphoreticularis muralis externa). Lymph sinuses, originating from the lymphatic vessel, are only found in external formations (Figure 6.25).

Lymphoreticular cords within mural formations contain areas of T and B lymphocytes as well as postcapillary venules for lymphocyte recirculation. Mural formations are stimulated by the presence of antigens within their drainage area, potentially becoming so enlarged that they are distinguishable from lymph nodes only by the presence of the media in the lymph vessel wall. Collectively, mural formations have considerable immune potential and fulfil the role of lymph nodes.

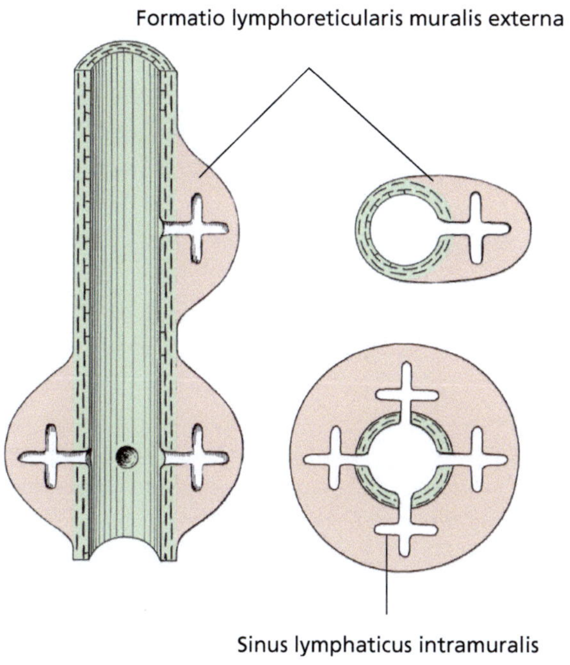

6.25 Wall of the initial segment of an avian lymphatic collector vessel (vas lymphaticum myotypicum) with external lymphoreticular formations (schematic; left – longitudinal section, right – transverse section).

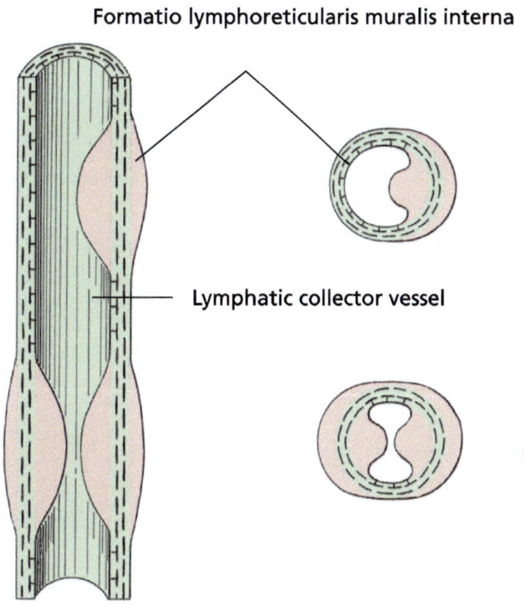

6.26 Wall of the terminal segment of an avian lymphatic collector vessel (vas lymphaticum myotypicum) with internal mural reticular formations (schematic; left – longitudinal section, right – transverse section).

Blood and haemopoiesis (sanguis et haemocytopoesis)

7

Blood, the essential functional element of the circulatory system, is distributed evenly throughout the body. It serves to maintain internal biological equilibrium, without which life cannot be sustained.

The composition of blood is correspondingly complex. It consists of **fluid** and **cellular** components, both of which have important functions. Blood has three fundamental roles: transport, homeostasis and immune defence.

Blood acts as a **vehicle** for the **transport** of oxygen and carbon dioxide, nutrients, intermediate and end products of metabolism and waste materials. It provides a means of distributing heat, and carries endogenous regulatory molecules (hormones), enzymes and vitamins.

In conjunction with organs such as the liver, kidney and lung, blood **supports homeostasis** by regulating tissue fluid levels, osmotic pressure, ion concentration and pH.

By way of its white blood cell population (granulocytes, lymphocytes, monocytes), blood contributes to **innate** and **adaptive immunity**. Substances produced by white cells (e.g. complement, leukotrienes, lymphokines, antibodies) circulate in the blood, reaching all tissues of the body.

The ability of blood to perform these functions is dependent upon additional physiological processes that maintain a balance between the **coagulation** of blood, for haemostasis, and lysis of blood clots. Platelets are the cellular component of the coagulation mechanism. In addition, plasma contains the soluble protein **fibrinogen** which, when clotting is activated by damage to a vessel wall, is converted to **fibrin**. The platelets and fibrin, together with red blood cells, form a blood clot. The term **serum** refers to plasma from which clotting factors have been removed.

In domestic mammals, the **blood cells** constitute between 32 and 45% of the blood volume. The blood cells are comprised of:

- red blood cells (erythrocytes),
- white blood cells (leucocytes):
  - granulocytes,
  - lymphocytes,
  - monocytes and
- platelets (thrombocytes).

Formation of blood cells (haemopoiesis)

The differentiation of blood cells begins during embryonic development, commencing in the wall of the **yolk sac** (**megaloblastic phase**). The second phase takes place in the liver and spleen (**hepatosplenic phase**). In the latter stages of foetal development, the **red bone marrow** (**textus haemopoeticus**) takes over the role of haemopoiesis (**medullary phase**). Blood cell formation in the liver and spleen gradually declines but can be reactivated in the presence of bone marrow disease. For the life of the animal, blood cells differentiate from **haemopoietic stem cells** (**HPCs**) and progenitor cells in the bone marrow (Figures 7.1 and 7.2).

Regulation of blood formation

Cytokines play a major role in regulating the differentiation of cells during haemopoiesis. These highly potent soluble signalling chemicals are produced by numerous haemopoietic and non-haemopoietic cells. Cytokines act via surface receptors on target cells. They exhibit autocrine, paracrine and endocrine activity. As intercellular mediators, they regulate the division, proliferation, differentiation, mobility and activity of haemopoietic cells. Cytokine expression, usually low, increases dramatically in response to tissue damage or infection. Physical strain also influences the homeostatic activity of cytokines.

The various cytokines are classified into partially overlapping categories. Haemopoietic cytokines include chemokines, growth factors and transcription factors (e.g. c-Myb, E2A). Of major importance are the **colony-stimulating factors** (**CSF**) (e.g. granulocyte-macrophage-colony-stimulating factor [GM-CSF]) and **interleukins** (**IL**). Among the interleukins, IL-3, IL-5 and IL-15 have a particular influence on cell differentiation.

The later stages of differentiation are stimulated in a targeted fashion by specific factors. **Thrombopoietin** produced by the liver and kidney regulates the development of platelets. A lack of oxygen or a fall in intravascular erythrocyte numbers triggers production of the sialoglycoprotein **erythropoietin** (**EPO**) by interstitial connective tissue cells located in the peri-tubular region of the nephrons, between the renal cortex and medulla. Erythropoietin

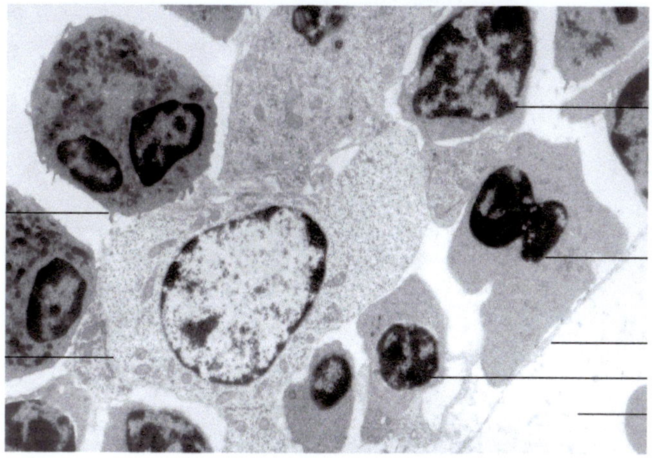

7.1 Fine structure of a reticular cell in the bone marrow, surrounded by unipotent haemopoietic progenitor cells (dog; x4000).

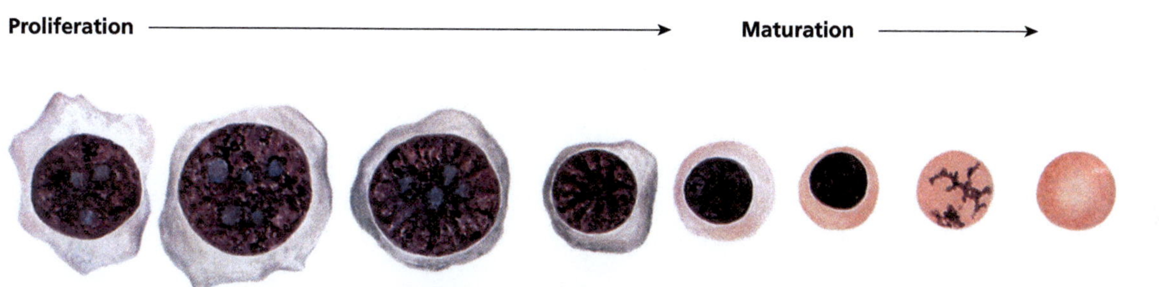

7.2 Erythropoiesis (schematic).

stimulates development of erythrocyte precursors in the bone marrow (erythroid colony-forming unit = CFU-E).

Cytokines that have a negative regulatory effect on haemopoiesis include interferons and tumour necrosis factor.

Bone marrow

Blood cells are produced by **red bone marrow**, which occupies the spaces between the spongy bone of the vertebral bodies, ribs, sternum, ilium and the proximal ends of the large long bones. In addition to the cellular components of haemopoiesis, the bone marrow contains reticular fibres (type III collagen), fibroblast-like reticular cells, adipocytes, macrophages and numerous, predominantly expanded, sinusoids (Figure 7.1).

The aforementioned **growth factors** and **cytokines** are produced by the endothelium of the sinusoidal capillaries, fibroblast-like cells and macrophages. The reticular matrix binds glycosaminoglycans and adhesion molecules, which also contribute to blood cell development. The wall of the **sinusoidal capillaries** is thin and lacks a continuous basal lamina. Blood cells from the reticular compartment enter the capillaries through transient **migration pores**.

Blood cell differentiation

Red bone marrow contains blood cells in wide-ranging stages of development. These may be arranged in clusters around central progenitor cells (e.g. erythroblastic nests) or may lie adjacent to the wall of a sinusoid (e.g. megakaryocyte).

Haemopoietic stem cells

All blood cells are derived from an **undifferentiated, pluripotent stem cell**, the **haemopoietic stem cell** (**haemocytoblast**). These cells form only around 0.01% of the cell population of the bone marrow. They can enter the blood circulation via the trans-endothelial route. Most haemopoietic stem cells exist in a quiescent state (G_0). Only an extremely small proportion undergoes division, according to demand. The daughter cell enters the pathway towards differentiation, while the other remains a stem cell. Stem cells are small, inconspicuous, dense round cells (ca. 12 µm) with a narrow rim of basophilic cytoplasm.

Progenitor cells

After undergoing division, haemopoietic stem cells develop and differentiate into progenitors of the cells of the lymphoid (lymphocyte) and myeloid (granulocyte/monocyte, erythrocyte/megakaryocyte) cell lines.

Progenitor cells are morphologically similar to one another, being relatively small and strongly basophilic with a round nucleus.

In vitro stimulation of progenitor cells using cytokines or other growth factors results in the formation of **clusters** or **colonies** of cells. These clonogenic cells are thus referred to as a 'colony-forming unit'.

Progenitor cells differentiate in the bone marrow into mature blood cells that are found in the circulation. These cells (and their differentiation) are termed:

- erythrocytes (erythropoiesis),
- granulocytes (granulopoiesis),
- lymphocytes (lymphopoiesis),
- monocytes (monopoiesis) and
- platelets (thrombocytes) (thrombopoiesis).

Red blood cells (erythrocytes)

A major function of the blood is the transport of O_2 and CO_2, bound to the pigment **haemoglobin**. This globular chromoprotein with a prosthetic haem group is concentrated in red blood cells, constituting over 30% of the **cytoplasm** (95% of dry weight). The high, reversible binding capacity of haemoglobin enables erythrocytes to take up oxygen in the lungs and deliver it to the peripheral tissues, and to transport carbon dioxide in the opposite direction. The bright red colour of arterial blood is derived from its content of oxyhaemoglobin. Venous blood contains haemoglobin in its reduced state and is thus dark red in colour.

Development of red blood cells (erythropoiesis)

In the initial stage of erythropoiesis, haemopoietic stem cells differentiate into precursor cells referred to as **proerythroblasts** (Figure 7.2). This process is driven by hormonal factors, particularly by **erythropoietin**, a sialoglycoprotein produced by the kidney in response to low blood oxygen levels (anaemia or hypoxia). Steroid hormones, peptides and Vitamin B_{12} also act as regulators of erythrocyte development.

Proerythroblasts are basophilic cells measuring 20–25 μm in size. They undergo rapid replication, during which the size of the nucleus decreases. Accumulation of haemoglobin in the cytoplasm begins in this early stage of differentiation. Further mitotic division gives rise to the **basophilic erythroblast** (**erythroblastus basophilicus**) (Figure 7.2). By this stage the nucleus has become noticeably smaller and heterochromatic. The cytoplasm is basophilic. Through endocytosis, basophilic erythroblasts acquire increasing amounts of ferritin from surrounding macrophages and reticular cells to support increased haemoglobin synthesis.

The basophilic erythroblast undergoes further differentiation to become the **polychromatophilic erythroblast** (**erythroblastus polychromatophilicus**). Due to the high haemoglobin content, the cytoplasm of polychromatophilic erythroblasts gradually becomes acidophilic with little remaining basophilia (Figure 7.2). With continued maturation and increasing haemoglobin concentration, the proportion of basophilic organelles (ribosomes, rER) declines, giving rise to the **orthochromatophilic** (**oxyphilic** or **acidophilic**) **erythroblast** (**normoblast, erythroblastus acidophilicus**) (Figure 7.2).

Species variation

Mammals: Following an increase in the density and compaction of the nuclear chromatin (pyknosis), the nucleus is ejected (enucleation). Loss of the nucleus during erythropoiesis is characteristic of mammals, including humans. The remaining organelles (Golgi vesicles, polyribosomes, ER) become clumped together in the cytoplasm. The enucleated cell is referred to as a **reticulocyte** (proerythrocyte). Within 24 hours, reticulocytes lose their internal organelles, becoming the haemoglobin-carrying cells known as **erythrocytes** (Figure 7.2).

Birds, reptiles, amphibians and fish (except cyclostomes): Enucleation does not take place. In these species, erythrocytes are nucleated and larger than those of mammals.

The morphological changes occurring during erythropoiesis can be summarised as follows:

- reduction in cell volume,
- decrease in basophilia,
- reduction and loss of nucleoli and cellular organelles,
- alteration of nuclear structure,
- increase in acidophilia and
- loss of the nucleus (mammals).

Erythrocytes

In most mammals, the **red blood cell**, or erythrocyte, is a **non-nucleated, biconcave, round disc** (Figure 7.3). The size of erythrocytes varies considerably with species, ranging in diameter from 4.1 μm in the goat to 7.3 μm in the dog (Table 7.1). In camels and dromedaries, the erythrocyte is oval. The number of circulating erythrocytes is related to their species-dependent variation in size. The smaller the cells, the greater their unit volume, as seen particularly in the goat.

Circulating erythrocyte numbers are further influenced by muscular effort, training, condition (horses), housing (pigs), altitude (e.g. alpine cattle) and sex (greater in males than females). Lacking a nucleus, erythrocytes exhibit a high degree of plasticity and elasticity and undergo continuous, reversible modifications of their shape. This facilitates their passage through even the smallest capillaries. In hypotonic solution, erythrocytes absorb fluid, resulting in swelling and possible disintegration. Under

Table 7.1 Physiological values for the number, diameter and lifespan of mature erythrocytes and haematocrit in various domestic mammal species.

Species	Number ($10^6/\mu l$)	Diameter (µm)	Lifespan (days)	Haematocrit
Horse	7.5 (6–9)	5.5	140–150	42
Ox	6 (5–7)	5.7	50–60	35–40
Sheep	10 (8–13)	5.1	110–120	32–38
Goat	14 (13–17)	4.1	125	34
Pig	6.5 (5–8)	6.1	65	41.5
Dog	6.8 (5.5–8)	7.3	107–122	45.5
Cat	7.5 (7.2–10)	5.7	68–77	37–40

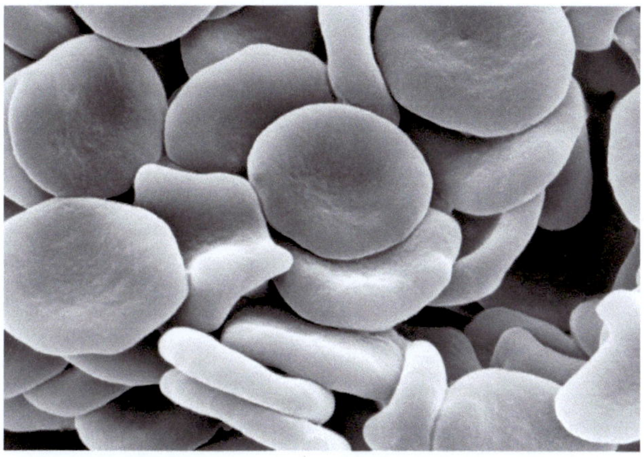

7.3 Scanning electron micrograph of canine erythrocytes.

hypertonic conditions, they release fluid, becoming thorny in appearance (crenated).

The lifespan of erythrocytes also exhibits species variation (Table 7.1). Breakdown of erythrocytes occurs primarily in the spleen. There, red blood cells pass from vessels known as terminal capillaries into expanded sinuses (red pulp). Changes in the surface membrane of senescent erythrocytes allow these cells to be recognised by cells of the mononuclear phagocyte system (MPS). Aged erythrocytes are digested by macrophages. The porphyrin scaffold of the haem molecule, from which iron has been released, is converted into biliverdin and bilirubin. Ferritin (24–36% iron) liberated from the haem molecule is stored as haemosiderin in macrophages and is used in the bone marrow for haemoglobin synthesis. Erythrocyte degradation also takes place to a limited extent at other sites such as the liver (Kupffer cells) and bone marrow.

White blood cells (leucocytes)

Leucocytes perform multiple roles in defending the body against foreign substances. Upon gaining access to the body, foreign materials can be eliminated by either non-specific processes (phagocytosis) or targeted immune responses carried out by lymphoid cells.

The complexity of these defence mechanisms is reflected in the morphology of the white blood cells. Leucocytes can be divided into two broad categories, **granulocytes** and **agranulocytes** (**mononuclear leucocytes**). Based on the staining properties of their granules, granulocytes are further divided into neutrophils, eosinophils and basophils. Agranulocytes include lymphocytes and monocytes.

Based on their principal functions, leucocytes can be categorised broadly as those involved in innate immunity (phagocytosis, inflammation, allergy; neutrophils, eosinophils, basophils, monocytes/macrophages) and those involved in adaptive immune responses (lymphocytes, monocytes/macrophages).

Specific surface molecules of different leucocytes form the basis of a further means of classification, referred to as the cluster of differentiation (CD) system of nomenclature.

Granulocytes (granulocytus)

In contrast to lymphocytes and monocytes, granulocytes are polymorphonuclear cells (though this term is sometimes reserved for neutrophils). In functional terms, these can be considered as **microphages**. They exhibit amoeboid motility and the capacity to move actively from the circulating blood through the wall of blood vessels (**diapedesis**). By releasing lytic enzymes, these cells can contribute to **innate defence** both within the circulatory system and in the interstitial tissue. They play a significant role in inflammatory processes. Granulocytes are also released from the bone marrow to participate in localised cell-mediated responses.

Granulocyte formation (granulopoiesis)

Granulopoiesis (**myelopoiesis**, **granulocytopoiesis**) refers to the formation and differentiation of polymorphonuclear leucocytes (granulocytes) (Figure 7.4). The pluripotent stem cells of the bone marrow, the **haemopoietic stem cells**, divide repeatedly to give rise to **myeloblasts** which serve as the common progenitor cell of all types of granulocyte. Myeloblasts (diameter 15 µm) have a round, euchromatic nucleus. The wide rim of cytoplasm contains numerous organelles, particularly

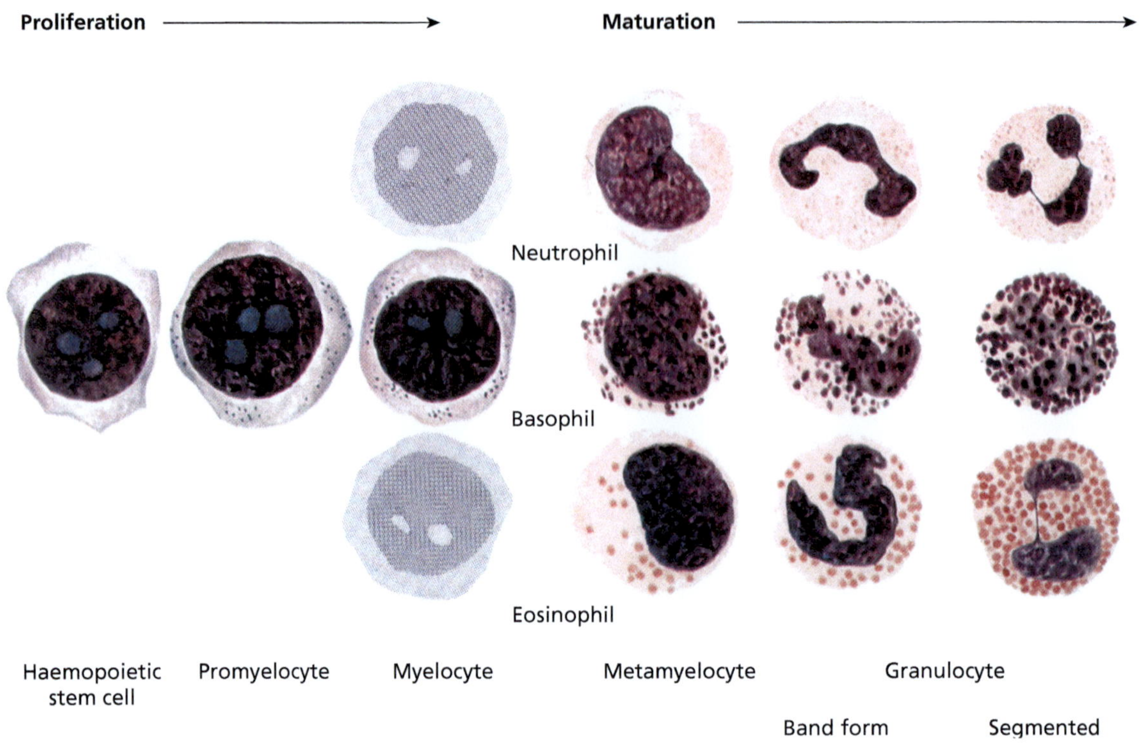

7.4 Granulopoiesis (schematic).

ribosomes, polyribosomes and ER, and is therefore strongly basophilic. With the development of membrane-bound azurophilic granules (diameter 0.25– 0.50 μm), myeloblasts become **promyelocytes** which undergo further mitotic division.

Promyelocytes are the largest cells in the granulopoietic pathway (18–25 μm). The nucleus is euchromatic. The cytoplasm contains numerous energy-supplying mitochondria and secretory dictyosomes (stacks of Golgi cisternae). Numerous protein biosynthetic organelles (ribosomes, polyribosomes, ER) indicate a high rate of metabolic activity. Within a week, the azurophilic granules differentiate into specific granules. As of this stage, (**myelocyte**), recognition of neutrophils, eosinophils and basophils becomes possible (Figure 7.4).

The main changes occurring during granulopoiesis include:

- shrinkage of the nucleus,
- development of non-specific (azurophilic) granules and
- development of specific granules.

Further differentiation gives rise to the **metamyelocyte**, which usually undergoes one additional division. A further week of maturation eventually results in formation of the **polymorphonuclear neutrophil**, **eosinophil and basophil**. During this latter stage of granulopoiesis, the nucleus condenses and becomes indented (kidney-shaped) (metamyelocyte). Subsequently, particularly in neutrophils, the nucleus becomes band-shaped (band form stage) and then segmented (Figure 7.4). A gradual reduction in the size of the cells occurs over the course of granulopoiesis.

Movement of mature granulocytes from the bone marrow into the circulating blood is controlled by a feedback mechanism driven by the availability of differentiated granulocytes.

Neutrophils (granulocytus neutrophilicus)

Neutrophils are polymorphonuclear granulocytes with an average diameter of 10–14 μm (Figure 7.5). In the horse, dog and cat they are the most abundant white cell type (55–70%) while in other species, lymphocytes predominate (Table 7.2). In younger neutrophils, the nucleus is elongated and unsegmented (**stab** or **band neutrophils**). The nucleus of mature neutrophils has two to five lobes, or segments, connected by a narrow chromatin bridge (**segmented neutrophil**).

The vast majority of the total neutrophil population is stored in the bone marrow, with only 10% occurring in the circulating blood and tissues. In acute infectious disease, immature band neutrophils pass from the bone marrow into the blood in greater numbers ('left shift').

The cytoplasm contains abundant granules of two types. **Azurophilic** (**primary**) **granules** (Figure 7.5) are **lysosomes** that contain enzymes including phosphatases, 5-nucleotidase, D-amino acid oxidase and peroxidase. They also enclose polypeptides that have marked antimicrobial activity against bacteria, fungi and certain coated viruses.

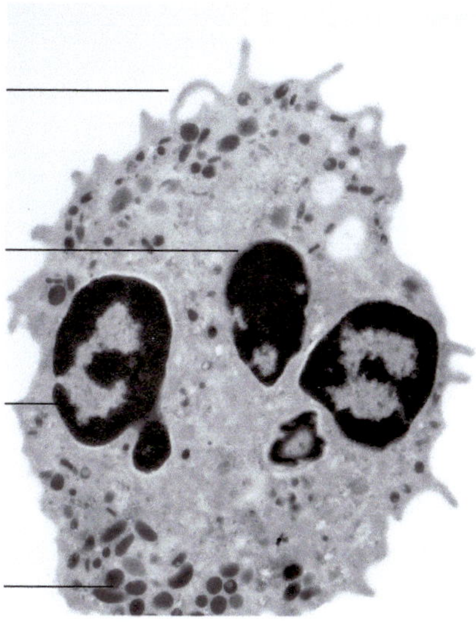

7.5 Fine structure of a neutrophil (dog; x10,000).

Following phagocytosis, these granules are transformed into phagolytic vacuoles. Lysozyme is also found in primary granules.

The abundant **specific (secondary) granules** are neutral-staining and contain substances including lactoferrin, alkaline phosphatase, NADPH-oxidase, histaminase and laminin receptors for attachment of the cell to the endothelium.

Contact between the neutrophil and the endothelium is established by **specific surface receptors** located on the neutrophil and on the endothelial cell (**selectins**). Binding is strengthened by integrins (on the neutrophil) and endothelial adhesion molecules, after which the neutrophil passes between the cells of the endothelium.

Neutrophils that are closely associated with the endothelium, and are thus available for extravasation, are referred to as the **marginal pool**. They are stimulated by physical or chemical factors (**chemotaxis**) to pass from the blood vessel to the tissues and release the contents of their granules (degranulation). This triggers a cascade of cellular responses that leads to the attraction of additional neutrophils.

The responding neutrophils phagocytose cell debris and foreign material, perishing in the process. Lysosomal enzymes are released into the interstitial tissue and cellular components become incorporated into the process of disintegration (**pus formation**). Thus, neutrophils (in particular, among the granulocytes) are referred to as **microphages**, as distinct from tissue macrophages.

Eosinophils (granulocytus eosinophilicus)

Eosinophils (Figure 7.6) are characterised by intensely acidophilic (eosinophilic) granules. The size of the granules varies with species (0.5–1.5 μm). They are particularly large and prominent in the horse (Figure 7.13).

The granules are membrane-bound lysosomes containing numerous enzymes, particularly catalases, acid phosphatases, proteases, dehydrogenase and cathepsin. With the electron microscope, the canine and feline granules can be seen to contain an elongated lamellar crystalloid protein. This is lacking in horses, cattle and

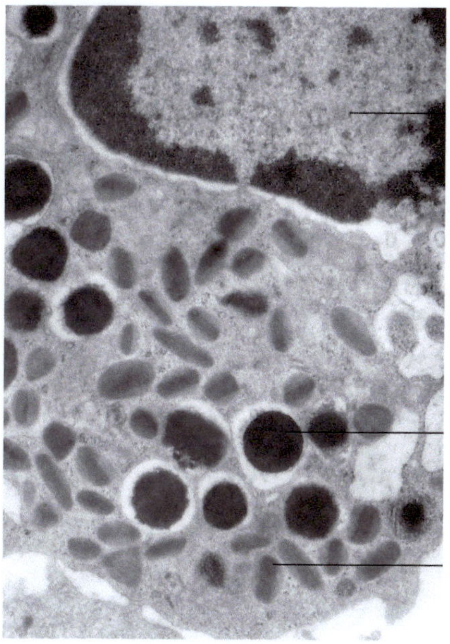

7.6 Fine structure of an eosinophil (dog; x10,000).

Table 7.2 Physiological values for the total number and relative proportions of circulating leucocytes in various domestic mammalian species.

Species	Leucocytes 1000/μl	Neutrophils (%)	Eosinophils (%)	Basophils (%)	Lymphocytes (%)	Monocytes (%)
Horse	9 (7–11)	52–60	2–4	<1	30–40	3–4
Ox	8 (5–10)	25–35	5–6	<1	55–65	5–10
Sheep	8 (6–12)	30–40	5–7	<1	45–70	2–5
Goat	10 (8–12)	40–45	3–5	<1	50–55	3–5
Pig	12 (8–16)	50–60	2–3	<1	35–50	2–6
Dog	12 (8–18)	55–75	3–10	<1	20–25	2–6
Cat	10 (9–24)	55–65	3–6	<1	30–35	2–5

pigs. Eosinophils form 2–10% of circulating leucocytes, a considerably lower proportion than neutrophils. Normal values vary with species (Table 7.2; chickens 2%).

Eosinophils measure 12–14 µm in diameter and have a segmented nucleus. They exhibit amoeboid motility and phagocytic activity, the latter being oriented particularly towards antigen–antibody complexes. Thus, an increase in circulating eosinophils (**eosinophilia**) is commonly observed in association with allergic responses (allergies, parasitism).

In these instances, eosinophils are activated by the release of chemical mediators (leukotrienes, histamine released by mast cells). Eosinophils also produce substances that inhibit the release of histamine, thus down-regulating the inflammatory response. Adrenocorticotropic (ACTH) hormone and cortisol have a negative effect on circulating eosinophil numbers, potentially causing **eosinopenia**.

Basophils (granulocytus basophilicus)

Circulating basophils are rare in mammals, representing 0.5% of the leucocyte count (Figure 7.7). The nucleus may be bilobed, irregular or segmented. The cytoplasm contains variably sized basophilic granules that frequently overlie the nucleus. These stain with basic and metachromatic dyes. The granules are water soluble and contain **histamine**, **heparin** and **leukotrienes**. As a source of heparin, basophils participate in regulation of coagulation. In their histamine and heparin content, basophils closely resemble mast cells, from which they can be distinguished by the presence of peroxidase positive granules.

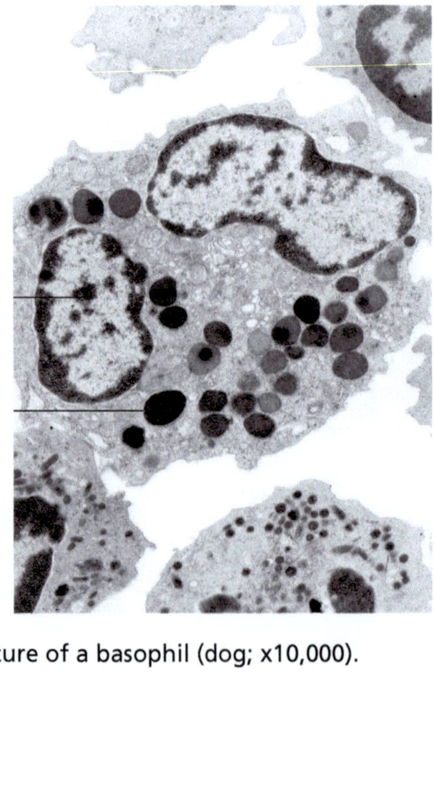

7.7 Fine structure of a basophil (dog; x10,000).

Agranulocytes

Agranulocytes lack distinctive granules. These cells include:

- lymphocytes and
- monocytes.

Lymphocytes

Lymphocytes are the most numerous agranulocytes (Figures 7.8 to 7.10). Only around 2% of these round, basophilic cells circulate in the blood, the majority being concentrated in lymphoid organs (for further detail see Chapter 8, 'Immune system and lymphatic organs').

The proportion of lymphocytes in the circulating leucocyte population varies with species (cattle, sheep, goats: 50–70%; horses and cats: 30–35%; dogs: 20–25%) (Table 7.2).

LYMPHOCYTE FORMATION (LYMPHOPOIESIS)

In common with other blood cells, lymphocytes originate from haemopoietic stem cells (**haemocytoblasts**) in the bone marrow. These pluripotent cells differentiate into **progenitor cells** bearing surface molecules that determine their subsequent differentiation into T or B lymphocytes. Mitotic division and cell differentiation result in a large reservoir of mature lymphocytes (Figure 7.8). Antigen receptors form on these cells early in the differentiation process, before they have reached functional maturity.

Lymphocytes undergo the final stages of differentiation and maturation in the **thymus** (**T lymphocytes**, **T cells**) or in the **spleen**, **lymph nodes**, **Peyer's patches** and **tonsils** (**B lymphocytes**, **B cells**). Following exposure to an antigen in circulating blood or in lymphatic organs, lymphocytes become actively involved in the cell-mediated or humoral immune response (see Chapter 8, 'Immune system and lymphatic organs'). Activated lymphocytes can also develop into **memory cells** that are available for future immune defence.

While lymphopoiesis always originates in the red bone marrow, most lymphocytes in the body arise from lymphocyte proliferation in the lymphatic organs. This applies particularly to T cells after the normal involution of the thymus at sexual maturity.

LYMPHOCYTE MORPHOLOGY AND FUNCTION

Lymphocytes are a morphologically and functionally heterogeneous group of cells (Figures 7.9 and 7.10). However, except for size, their distinguishing characteristics cannot be determined in a blood smear. Using immunological techniques, physical separation methods and the identification of specific surface receptors with fluorescence microscopy, lymphocytes can be identified as **immature** or **immunocompetent** T and B lymphocytes

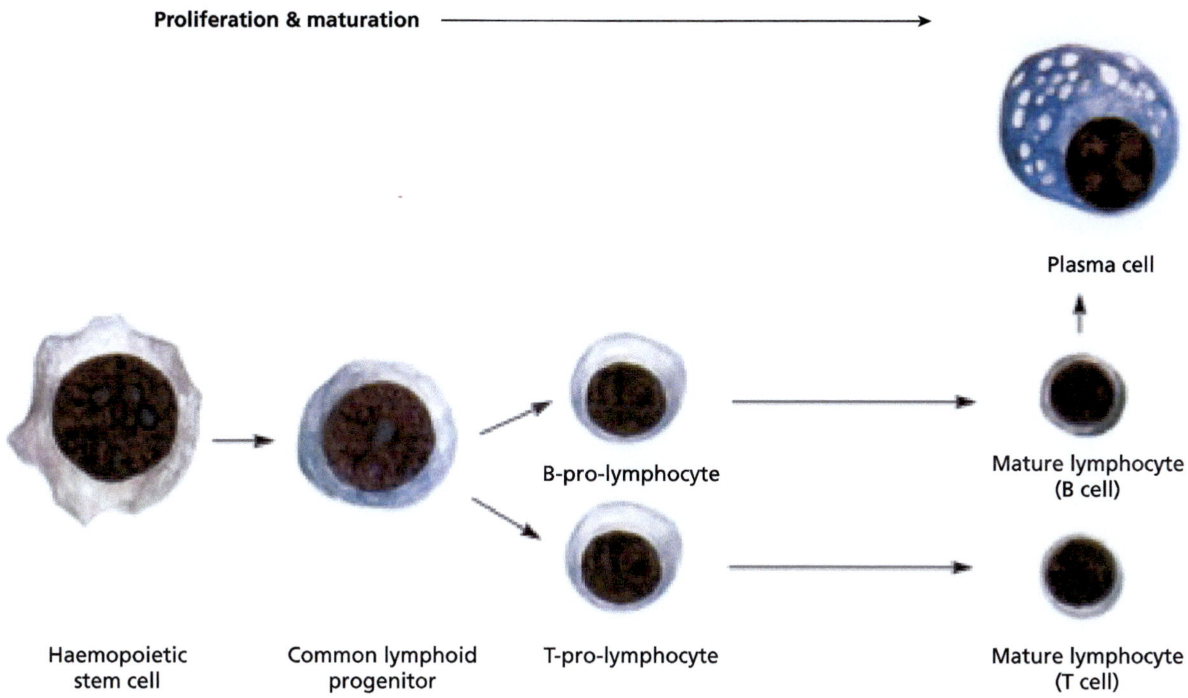

7.8 Lymphopoiesis (schematic).

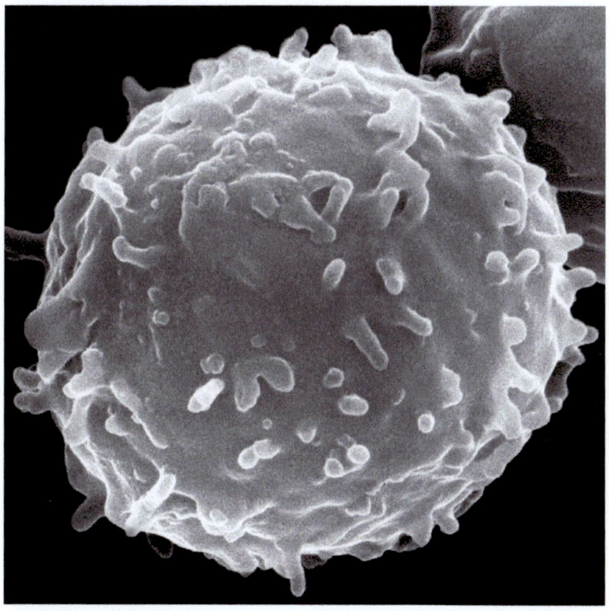

7.9 Scanning electron micrograph of a small lymphocyte (x9000).

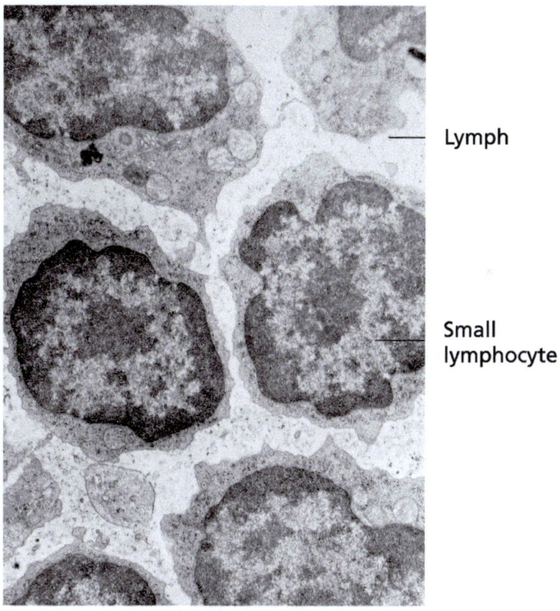

7.10 Fine structure of a small lymphocyte in the cortex of a lymph node (x4500).

and can be divided into subgroups based on function. Classification of lymphocytes based on size is of limited use as it provides no information about the specific function of the cell.

With the light microscope, lymphocytes can be categorised as:

- small lymphocytes (5–10 μm), representing the largest proportion of circulating lymphocytes,
- medium-sized lymphocytes (10–18 μm) or
- large lymphocytes (up to 25 μm), frequently considered to represent immunoblasts (activated lymphocytes) or natural killer (NK) cells.

Morphologically, lymphocytes are characterised by a round, heterochromatic nucleus (occasionally with a nucleolus), a narrow rim of cytoplasm and, typically, few organelles. Due to a high density of ribosomes, polyribosomes and rough ER, the cytoplasm is basophilic (Figure 7.8).

Lymphocytes exhibit a broad range of functional properties. Capable of amoeboid movement, they move from the blood and lymph vessels into the interstitial tissue and can reach the paracellular spaces between epithelial cells (intra-epithelial lymphocytes).

Lymphocytes have limited phagocytic activity but can influence the activity of other cells including phagocytes. **Lymphokines** (**chemical mediators**) produced by T lymphocytes are non-antigen-specific proteins that affect the biological activity of macrophages and granulocytes, as well as that of other T and B lymphocytes. Lymphokines can either inhibit or activate macrophage function.

Based on differences in their development and function, lymphocytes are divided into T lymphocytes (T cells), B lymphocytes (B cells) and natural killer cells (NK cells). Descriptions of T and B cells are provided below.

T LYMPHOCYTES (T CELLS)

T lymphocytes leave the bone marrow relatively early in their development from haemopoietic stem cells, passing to the cortex of the **thymus**. Under the influence of cellular and humoral factors, they mature into immunocompetent T cells and migrate from the medulla of the thymus to the peripheral lymphoid organs, where they become activated upon contact with antigens. T lymphocytes are involved in **cell-mediated immunity**. Following contact with an antigen, T cells are transformed into effector cells or memory cells. Based on function, T cells can be divided into:

- cytotoxic T cells,
- helper T cells,
- suppressor (regulatory) T cells,
- memory cells and
- natural killer T cells (NKT cells).

Based on differences in their surface molecules, T cells are classified as:

- $CD4^+$ T lymphocytes and
- $CD8^+$ T lymphocytes.

$CD4^+$ T lymphocytes: $CD4^+$ lymphocytes are helper T cells that recognise antigens bound to MHC II molecules and stimulate differentiation of B lymphocytes. This group can be further divided into two major subtypes:

- T_H1 cells and
- T_H2 cells.

T_H1 cells have an important role in infection, synthesising interferon, interleukin-2 and tumour necrosis factor-α. They promote activation of cytotoxic T cells and destruction of pathogens by macrophages.

T_H2 cells secrete numerous **immunomodulators** including interleukin-3, -4, -5 and -6. Their main functions include regulation of humoral immunity and activation of B lymphocytes, limitation of the inflammatory response and activation of allergic reactions. These cells regulate the transformation of B cells into plasma cells.

$CD8^+$ T lymphocytes: The role of these lymphocytes is primarily **cytotoxic**. They also produce cytokines and perform immunoregulatory functions.

Cytotoxic T lymphocytes destroy the target cell (e.g. cells containing bacteria or viruses) by secreting perforins, lytic enzymes and cytokines (e.g. interferon or tumour necrosis factor) that result in lysis of the plasmalemma. Cytotoxic lymphocytes may also be involved in lysis of antibody-coated cells through Fc receptor interactions, and apoptosis via proteases.

T-cell receptor (TCR): Found on the surface of T cells, the T-cell receptor (TCR) is a molecule that recognises antigens. It consists of an antigen-binding heterodimer comprising highly variable αβ (TCRab) or γδ (TCRgd) chains. TCRs regulate differentiation of T lymphocytes into $CD4^+$ or $CD8^+$ T cells. Cells that present antigens to T cells include interdigitating dendritic cells ('professional' antigen-presenting cells) and macrophages.

B LYMPHOCYTES

B lymphocytes are responsible for **humoral immune responses**. Induced particularly by foreign proteins, viruses or toxins, these result in the production of **specific protective products** (**immunoglobulins**, **antibodies**). In birds, B lymphocytes mature in the **bursa of Fabricius**, hence their designation as B cells. The bone marrow and gut (Peyer's patches) are considered the equivalent sites in mammals, though further differentiation also occurs in the secondary lymphoid organs. On their surface, B cells express many specific receptors (**membrane-bound immunoglobulins**) that function as the site of antigen binding. Antigen–antibody complexes are endocytosed by the B cell. Under the influence of activated helper T cells, activated B cells (**immunoblasts**) are transformed into plasmablasts (short-lived antibody-secreting cells), long-lived antibody-secreting plasma cells and memory B cells (Figures 7.8 and 7.11; see Figure 8.2). Memory B cells can generate antibodies more quickly when next exposed to the same antigen.

Follicular dendritic cells and **helper T cells** play an important part in antigen presentation during B-cell activation. Non-activated B cells have a lifespan of approximately 2 weeks (see also Chapter 8, 'Immune system and lymphatic organs').

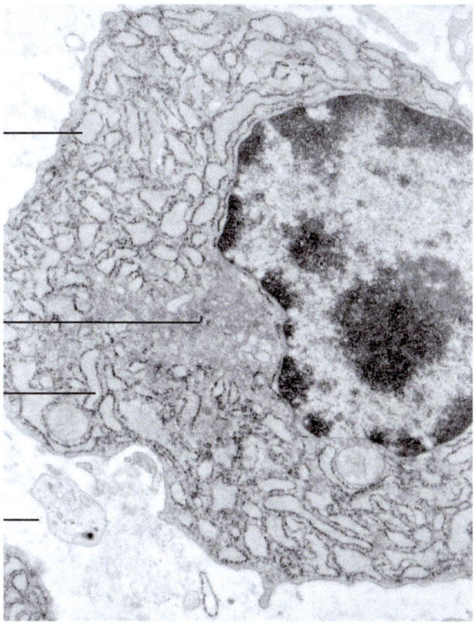

7.11 Fine structure of an active plasma cell in the medulla of a lymph node (x8000).

Monocytes

Monocytes have numerous functions, particularly in innate immunity and immunoregulation.

DEVELOPMENT OF MONOCYTES (MONOCYTOPOIESIS)

Division and differentiation of haemopoietic stem cells and progenitor cells in the bone marrow initially gives rise to **monoblasts** (Figure 7.12). These develop further into **promonocytes** (diameter 16–22 µm) containing azurophilic granules. After frequent mitotic divisions over the course of a few days, **mature monocytes** are formed (Figure 7.12). It appears that the early stages of development are shared with those of neutrophils, and that monocytes may arise from promyelocytes. The phagocytic potential of both cells may thus reflect a common origin.

Cellular changes occurring during monocytopoiesis include:

- appearance of azurophilic granules,
- alteration in the shape of the nucleus and
- decondensation of chromatin.

MONOCYTE MORPHOLOGY AND FUNCTION

Monocytes are classified as agranulocytes. In their mature form, these mononuclear cells are the largest leucocytes in the blood (12–20 µm) and represent 2–10% of circulating white blood cells. The shape of the nucleus is variable (often round, sometimes kidney-shaped or amoeboid) and the abundant cytoplasm is weakly basophilic with numerous mitochondria and clusters of Golgi cisternae. There are few ribosomes and the rER is poorly developed. Monocytes may contain **azurophilic granules**. These are lysosomes and thus contain numerous proteolytic enzymes. On the cell surface there are irregularly formed finger-like structures (**pseudopodia**) or individual microvilli that contribute to motility and phagocytic activity. Monocytes circulate (as 'blood macrophages') for a short period (2 days) before actively departing the blood vascular system and passing via amoeboid movement through the interstitial tissue. Their lifespan, once in the tissues, is unclear but is estimated at 60–90 days.

After leaving the blood circulation, monocytes transform into **tissue macrophages**. These include specific cell types such as Kupffer cells (liver), alveolar macrophages (lung), peritoneal macrophages, sinus endothelial cells (lymphoid organs), histiocytes (connective tissue) and osteoclasts. Macrophages are an important component of the **mononuclear phagocyte system**, sometimes referred to as the **reticuloendothelial system**.

Through their ability to phagocytose antigenic material, monocytes are involved in **innate immune responses**. They secrete complement and synthesise interferon. Monocytes also contribute to the destruction of aged red blood cells in the spleen, and to iron and fat metabolism. They also have a role in the adaptive immune response.

Figure 7.13 shows a blood smear from a horse with many types of blood cell visible.

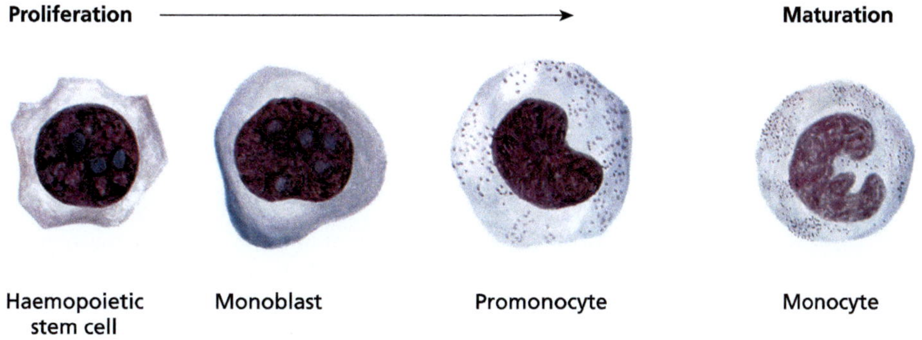

7.12 Monocytopoiesis (schematic).

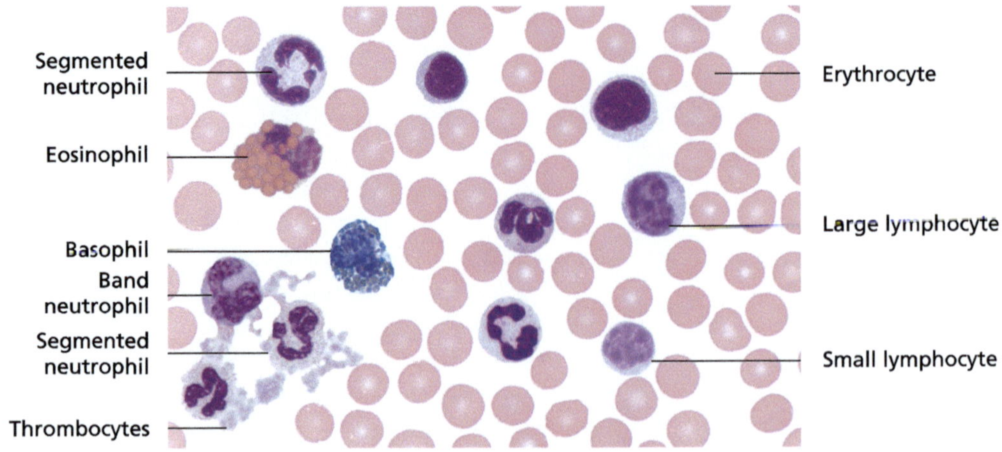

7.13 Blood cells of a horse. Pappenheim stain (oil immersion, x1000).

Platelets (thrombocytes)

For blood to act as a transport medium, it is necessary for a precise balance to be maintained between blood coagulation and fibrinolysis. These regulatory mechanisms have an important role in guarding against disruption of haemodynamics. Lesions of the blood vessel walls result in vasoconstriction, initiation of clot formation and activation of the coagulation cascade. Of primary importance in this process, in addition to plasma factors such as fibrinogen (Factor I), prothrombin (Factor II), tissue thromboplastin (Factor III) and calcium (Factor IV) are cellular elements of the blood referred to as **platelets** (**thrombocytes**).

Development of platelets (thrombopoiesis)

Thrombopoiesis is the formation of platelets in the red bone marrow (Figure 7.14). Differentiation of haemopoietic stem cells gives rise to the **megakaryoblast** (diameter 20–30 µm), which has a round, often indented, nucleus and several nucleoli. Multiple endomitoses (replication of chromosomes without nuclear division) occur within the megakaryoblast, forming a cell with a lobed, polyploid nucleus (**promegakaryocyte**).

These cells differentiate into **megakaryocytes** (diameter 50–70 µm). The nucleus is highly lobulated, and the cytoplasm contains numerous ribosomes and azurophilic granules. At maturity, **megakaryocytes** have abundant cytoplasm and a diameter of up to 100 µm, making them one of the largest individual cells in the body (Figure 7.14).

Megakaryocytes exhibit pseudopodial extensions and deep invaginations of the plasma membrane. The latter extend into the cell and make contact with a dense network of membranes of the smooth ER and with vesicular inclusions. A three-dimensional intracellular compartment is formed, enclosing areas of cytoplasm containing

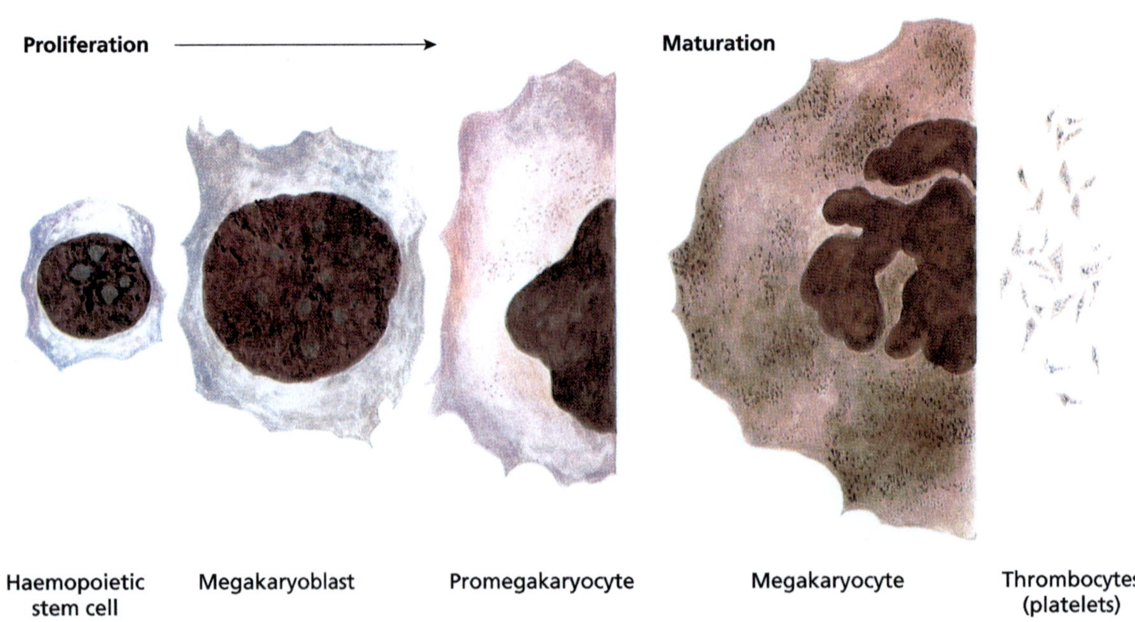

7.14 Thrombocytopoiesis (schematic).

azurophilic granules, vesicles, microtubules and microfilaments. These cytoplasmic components **become separated off** and undergo **fragmentation**. The membrane-bound fragmentation products constitute the **platelets**. The duration of platelet formation is considered to be 12 days.

Morphological changes associated with thrombopoiesis include:

- increase in cell volume,
- reduction in basophilia and
- appearance of azurophilic granules.

Platelet structure and function

In all domestic mammals, fully formed thrombocytes are non-nucleated fragments of cytoplasm derived within the bone marrow from **megakaryocytes** (Figures 7.15 and 7.16). **Platelets** (diameter 2–4 µm) are organised into zones:

- a central zone (granulomere), surrounded by
- a clear peripheral zone (hyalomere).

The **granulomere** (Figure 7.16) contains numerous azurophilic membrane-bound α-granules (diameter 0.2–0.3 µm) that contain thromboplastin, fibrinogen and platelet Factor IV. Other granules enclose ADP, calcium or serotonin (5-hydroxytryptamine). Also found in the granulomere are mitochondria, glycogen and ribosomes, as well as lysosomes containing endoglycosidase and heparin-cleaving enzymes. In addition, the granulomere includes a system of irregularly winding tubules.

The **hyalomere** (Figure 7.16) incorporates a system of vesicles and canaliculi that are formed by invagination of the plasmalemma. Microtubules and actin and myosin filaments form a network that maintains the shape of the platelet and enables contraction. The external surface of the cell membrane is covered with a glycocalyx. This incorporates fibrinogen and thromboplastin, which are important for formation of the **platelet plug** and adhesion of platelets to the vascular endothelium.

Blood clot formation

When a vessel wall is damaged, thrombocytes bind to collagen fibres in the endothelium that are not exposed under normal circumstances. Vasoconstrictors (e.g. serotonin) are released from granules within the platelets, the vascular lumen narrows and the rate of blood flow decreases. The platelets elaborate pseudopodia and aggregate with other platelets, forming a **plug** (**thrombus**).

The plug is reinforced by the action of coagulation factors. Platelet Factor III, a phospholipid released by platelets, activates thromboplastin. Under the influence of calcium, thromboplastin brings about the conversion of prothrombin to thrombin. Thrombin catalyses the conversion of fibrinogen into the thread-like fibrin. Fibrin rapidly forms a soluble mesh that subsequently becomes stabilised into a dense network of fibres. Circulating red blood cells become caught in this network, leading to the formation of a stable blood clot.

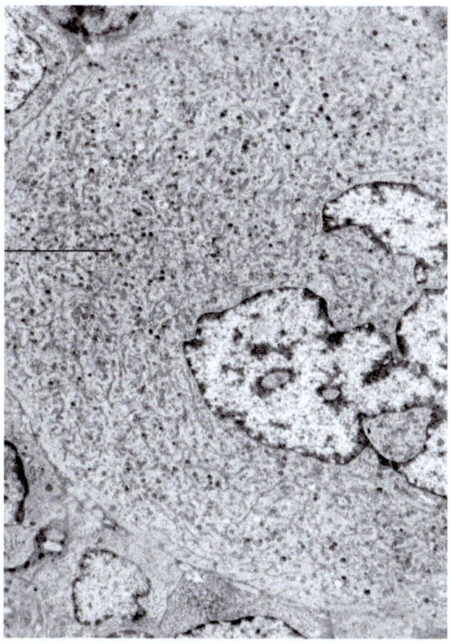

7.15 Fine structure of a mature megakaryocyte in the bone marrow (dog; x4500).

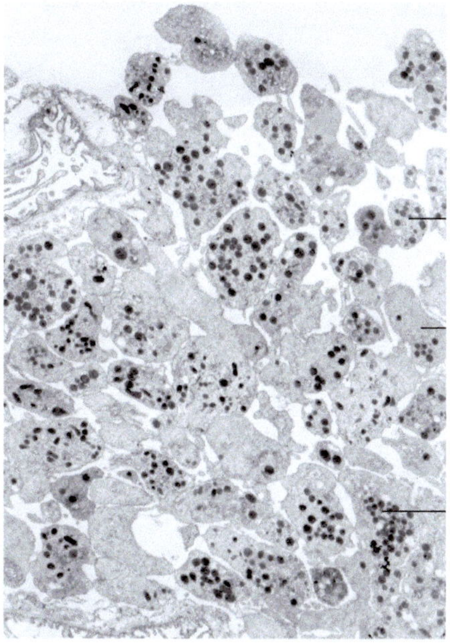

7.16 Fine structure of a platelet plug at a vessel wall (x9000).

8

Immune system and lymphatic organs (organa lymphopoetica)

Immune system

The immune system is a host defence mechanism that serves to protect the integrity of the organism. In addition to innate protective mechanisms (e.g. physical barriers, chemical factors, phagocytes), the immune system incorporates specific or adaptive defences that target particular antigens. Adaptive immune responses are carried out by the cells of the lymphatic system, via cell-mediated or humoral pathways.

Lymphocytes (Figure 8.1) play a key role in the adaptive immune response. During their differentiation, these cells attain the capacity to distinguish between 'self' and 'non-self'. With the aid of receptors on their cell membrane, lymphocytes can 'recognise' foreign substances (antigens) and initiate an immune response. This endogenous system of defence relies upon complex interactions between cell populations and the complement system.

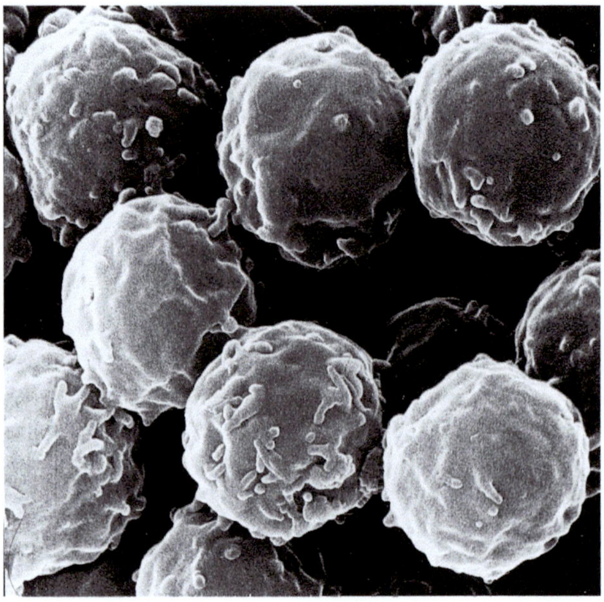

8.1 Lymphocytes as seen with the scanning electron microscope (x2000).

Principles of adaptive immunity

The cells of the adaptive immune system are comprised mainly of two groups (Figure 8.2) that arise from haemopoietic stem cells in the bone marrow:

- **lymphocytes**
  - T lymphocytes (T cells),
  - B lymphocytes (B cells),
- **antigen-presenting cells, including**
  - macrophages,
  - non-follicular dendritic cells and
  - follicular dendritic cells (FDCs).

An important characteristic of the immune response is the ability of the body to recognise the extremely large number of antigens to which an organism may be exposed during its lifetime. This function is performed by two groups of molecules, the **T-cell receptors** (TCR) and surface **immunoglobulins** on B cells.

During its differentiation, each lymphocyte develops a unique specificity (**theory of clonal selection**) that enables the cell to recognise one of the myriad possible invading antigens. Due to this selective differentiation, contact between a specific lymphocyte and corresponding antigen triggers the replication (**cloning**) of the lymphocyte over a period of just a few days. The number of different types of B-cell clones that can be produced is estimated at around 10^8.

The antigen receptors of the T cells (TCR) are membrane-associated immunoglobulin-like heterodimers consisting of $\alpha\beta$- or $\gamma\delta$-chains and an associated protein complex, CD3. Recognition of antigens by the TCR occurs in the presence of MHC molecules (see below). The antigen receptors found on B cells take the form of membrane-bound immunoglobulins (B-cell receptors).

Another key feature of T and B cells is their ability, once activated, to develop into **memory cells** that enable the body to detect a previously encountered antigen, and to mount a more rapid response.

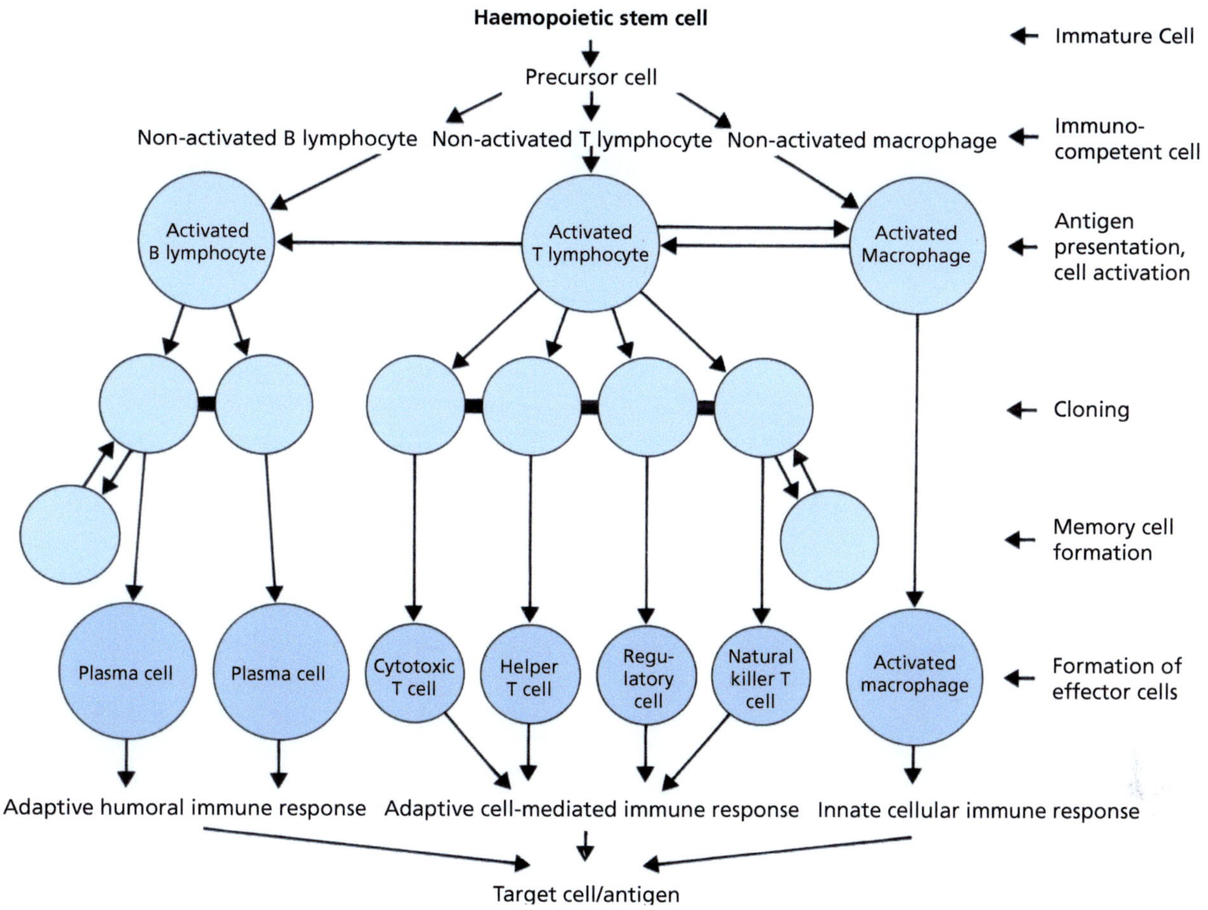

8.2 Schematic summary of immune cell differentiation and the sequence of events resulting from antigenic stimulation.

Cells of the adaptive immune response

T cells

T cells are involved in **cell-mediated immunity**. They serve to kill other cells through the action of cytokines, perforin and lytic enzymes including protease (**cytotoxic T lymphocytes**), or to mediate interactions between immunologically active cells.

Based on the structure of certain surface molecules, T cells are divided into $CD4^+$ and $CD8^+$ lymphocytes. $CD4^+$ lymphocytes are further subdivided into the groups T_H1 and T_H2 (see Chapter 7, 'Blood and haemopoiesis').

$CD4^+$ LYMPHOCYTES

This group of T lymphocytes incorporates the cells referred to as helper T cells. The functions and characteristics of helper T cells include:

- induction of B cell maturation,
- induction of proliferation of cytotoxic $CD8^+$ T cells,
- synthesis of cytokines,
- activation of phagocytic macrophages,
- stimulation of haemopoiesis and
- division into subgroups including T_H1 and T_H2.

Activated **helper T cells** have a **central role** in the elimination of antigens. They trigger the transformation of mature B cells into antigen-specific plasma cells and stimulate the activity of various cytotoxic cells. Some $CD4^+$ helper T cells (and some $CD8^+$ cells) influence the activity of other T cells (**suppressor** or **regulatory T cells**), resulting in down-regulation or termination of the immune response. Helper T cells also differentiate into memory cells that can respond more quickly to renewed antigen exposure. Clonal proliferation of T helper cells is prompted by a cascade of events, including production of interleukin 2.

$CD8^+$ LYMPHOCYTES

$CD8^+$ lymphocytes are primarily **cytotoxic effector cells**. Their functions include:

- synthesis of cytokines (interferon, tumour necrosis factor) and
- induction of cell death (e.g. via proteases).

As with $CD4^+$ lymphocytes, pools of memory $CD8^+$ lymphocytes are formed in response to antigenic stimulation.

B cells

B cells are responsible for producing antibodies (soluble, non-membrane-bound immunoglobulins). In most cases this requires interaction with T cells, though T-cell-independent activation may also occur. Upon encountering an antigen, the matching B cell (i.e. specific for that antigen) engulfs the foreign material and presents fragments of the antigen on its surface, bound to an MHC II molecule (see below). **Mature helper T cells** attach to the antigen–protein complex on the surface of B cells. The T cell then produces cytokines that stimulate B cell division and differentiation into plasma cells. Mature plasma cells release **antibodies** that attach to the antigen, targeting it for neutralisation or destruction. This is referred to as the **humoral immune response** (Figure 8.2).

Immune response to antigens

As part of the immune response, the foreign material induces mast cells to release histamine and promote bradykinin formation. Histamine and bradykinin increase the permeability of the vascular wall, facilitating the extravasation of lymphocytes, granulocytes and macrophages and the incorporation of these cells into the immune response. Cells-bearing antibody–antigen complexes are attacked and destroyed by macrophages and complement (Figure 8.2).

Concurrently, helper T cells stimulate **cytotoxic T lymphocytes** to attack antigen-carrying cells. Cells are killed by oxidising metabolites, penetration of cytotoxic substances (e.g. lymphotoxin) and by perforin-mediated mechanisms (**cell-mediated immunity**) (Figure 8.2). Some of the activated cytotoxic cells form a population of memory cells.

Activation of regulatory (suppressor) T cells by helper T cells limits the extent of the immune response. Debris resulting from the chain of cell-mediated and humoral immune reactions is phagocytosed by macrophages.

Major histocompatibility complex (MHC) proteins

Major histocompatibility complex proteins play an important part in adaptive immunity. With the aid of these molecules, the body can recognise genetically determined 'self-antigen' and thus tolerate its own cells. Cells of other organisms, or cells that are altered (e.g. by viruses), are recognised as foreign and are rejected. Acting as regulatory proteins, **MHC molecules** bind peptide fragments on the surface of cells and present them to T cells.

MHC molecules belong to the immunoglobulin superfamily of proteins and are divided into three classes.

MHC class I proteins

MHC class I proteins are glycoproteins found in almost all cells of the body. They present endogenous (cellular) antigens to **$CD8^+$ cytotoxic T cells**. If, for example, a cell has become infected with a virus, virally altered proteins are broken down into peptides by proteosomes in the cytoplasm, and the peptides are translocated to the cell surface in conjunction with an MHC I molecule. The antigen–MHC complex is recognised by a cytotoxic T cell and the cell is subsequently destroyed.

MHC class II proteins

MHC class II proteins are expressed on the surface of specialised **antigen-presenting cells** including macrophages, B cells and interdigitating dendritic cells. Under the influence of cytokines, they may also be expressed by endothelial cells, epithelial cells or fibroblasts, usually in association with inflammation. In this way, such cells may also become incorporated in the immune response.

Exogenous peptides that have been endocytosed by the antigen-presenting cell bind with MHC II proteins within the endosomal compartment of the cell. The antigen–MHC II complex is presented on the cell surface and is recognised by **$CD4^+$ T cells** (**helper T cells**), which initiate an immune response.

MHC class III proteins

MHC class III proteins are a component of the complement system which, with the assistance of plasma enzymes and effector proteins, attacks and destroys microorganisms. These factors also activate microphages (e.g. neutrophils) or macrophages to remove the resulting cell debris.

Antigen-presenting cells

Antigen-presenting cells (APCs) are an important component of the adaptive immune response. In principle, any cell expressing MHC I can present antigen to $CD8^+$ T cells if that cell has become altered (e.g. by a virus). Certain types of cells specialise in presenting foreign antigens to helper T cells ($CD4^+$). These include macrophages, dendritic cells and B cells. To a certain extent, endothelial cells lining the sinuses in lymphatic organs and reticular connective tissue also have a functional role in antigen presentation.

Fragments of antigenic material are loaded onto MHC II molecules on the surface of the processes of APC. The antigen–MHC II molecule complexes activate **$CD4^+$ helper T cells**, which then differentiate into T_H1 and T_H2 subtypes. B cells can bind with antigen directly, or recognise antigen presented by follicular dendritic cells.

Macrophages

Macrophages occur in various forms throughout the body. These cells **engulf antigens** by phagocytosis. Macrophages develop from monocytes, differentiating into carriers of cytolytic enzymes. Macrophages can also take up and destroy microorganisms (e.g. bacteria). In this capacity, they are considered part of the **innate cellular immune response**.

Macrophages are found in various locations including the lymph nodes and spleen, connective tissue and the lung (alveolar macrophages). They are components of the **mononuclear phagocyte system** (**MPS**).

In addition to their phagocytic function, macrophages are involved in the **presentation of antigens** to **T lymphocytes**. Molecules on the surface of the macrophage (e.g. MHC molecules, complement receptors, mannose receptors) mediate the recognition and internalisation of microorganisms. Fragments of the phagocytosed microorganism are bound to MHC II proteins and presented on the cell membrane. Binding of T cells to these antigen–MHC molecule complexes triggers the proliferation of T cells (**cloning**). The accumulation of T cells in turn stimulates the macrophages to release interleukin-1. The T cells differentiate into T_H1 lymphocytes, which promote the phagocytic activity of macrophages. Further T cell differentiation is also induced.

Non-follicular dendritic cells

Non-follicular dendritic cells are important first-line defence cells of the immune system. These bone marrow-derived cells are found in the mucosae, afferent lymph vessels, T-cell regions of lymphatic organs (**interdigitating dendritic cells**) and in the epidermis (Langerhans cells). Immature forms are also found in the heart, kidney and the blood.

Non-follicular dendritic cells serve particularly in presentation of peptide, allergenic and viral antigens. Antigen is presented to $CD4^+$ T cells. These differentiate into T_H1 cells that stimulate macrophages, cytotoxic T cells and B cells, and T_H2 cells that promote the production of antibodies by B cells, thus facilitating the **humoral immune response**.

Follicular dendritic cells (FDCs)

Follicular dendritic cells occur in the lymphoid follicles of secondary lymphatic organs, predominantly within the germinal centres, where they are involved in presenting antigen to B cells. They are markedly stellate cells with long processes. Surface molecules on follicular dendritic cells bind antigen–antibody complexes and complement. Follicular dendritic cells do not express MHC II molecules.

B cells

Through B-cell receptor-mediated endocytosis, B cells can process and present (via MHC II molecules) soluble or viral antigens to helper T cells.

Elimination of antigens

Elimination of antigens is a complex phenomenon involving various cell populations, including activated lymphocytes and APCs. Components of this system include:

- cytotoxic T cells,
- natural killer cells,
- specific antibodies produced by plasma cells, in conjunction with complement,
- macrophages and
- lymphokines (activation of leucocytes).

Lymphatic organs (organa lymphopoetica)

The lymphatic organs can be divided into:

- **primary lymphatic organs:**
  - thymus,
  - bone marrow,
- **secondary lymphatic organs:**
  - mucosa-associated lymphatic tissue (MALT), e.g.:
    - tonsils,
    - bronchus-associated lymphatic tissue (BALT),
    - gut associated lymphatic tissue (GALT),
  - lymph nodes and
  - spleen.

The **primary lymphatic organs** are the sites of lymphocyte production and maturation. All blood cells are derived from the bone marrow, where most become fully differentiated (haemopoiesis). However, T cells leave the bone marrow relatively early in their differentiation and travel to the thymus (hence 'T' lymphocytes). There, T lymphocytes undergo a process of 'education' that enables them to distinguish between 'self-' and 'non-self-antigens'.

B-cell precursors spend longer in the bone marrow where, as B lymphocytes, they obtain their first specific antigen receptors. Later, they pass to secondary lymphatic organs where they attain their definitive specificity.

Secondary lymphatic organs are populated by lymphocytes after their production in the thymus and bone marrow. The mucosa-associated lymphatic tissue (MALT) is localised on surfaces of the body, where it performs an important role in protection against invading antigens. In particular, these include the mucosa of the oral cavity, pharynx, intestine, airways and urogenital tract.

The lymph nodes and spleen constitute organised lymphatic tissue that is located deeper in the body, lacking contact with the body surfaces. These are surrounded by a capsule and have afferent (lymph nodes) and efferent lymph vessels (lymph nodes and spleen).

Thymus

The thymus is a **primary lymphatic organ** derived from two embryonic germ layers. Epithelial (endodermal) cells of the **third** and **fourth pharyngeal pouches** grow out into the underlying **mesoderm** in which they form a three-dimensional reticulum, hence their designation as epithelioreticular cells. During fetal development, this

Table 8.1 Structural features of lymphatic organs and tissues.

Organ	Stroma	Parenchyma	Vessels	Special features
Mucosa-associated lymphatic tissue	Non-encapsulated, network of reticular and collagen fibres	Localised lymphoid follicles with B-cell germinal centres and peripheral T-cell populations; common in the alimentary canal (gut-associated lymphatic tissue, GALT) and the lung (bronchus-associated lymphatic tissue, BALT)	Afferent and efferent blood vessels, efferent lymph vessels	Tonsils are surrounded by a capsule and are consistently located near glandular tissue
Thymus	Thin capsule, dense, irregular supportive network of trabeculae; epithelioreticular cells distributed through the cortex and medulla	Clear distinction between cortex and medulla; cortex contains large numbers of densely packed T cells as well as macrophages; epithelioreticular cells form a blood–thymus barrier; the medulla contains fewer T cells and appears less dense, with prominent epithelioreticular cells	Efferent lymph vessels, cortical capillaries drain into venules in the medulla	Site of T-cell production (early in development), T cells attain immunocompetence; concentrically layered epithelioreticular cells (Hassall's corpuscles) present in the medulla
Lymph nodes	Thin capsule, network of reticular cells and fibres	Divided into cortex, paracortex and medulla; cortex contains lymphatic follicles with B-cell germinal centres and lymphoid and reticular tissue; paracortex rich in T cells; medulla contains lymph sinuses and medullary cords containing lymphocytes, plasma cells and macrophages	Afferent lymph vessels enter the subcapsular sinus in the outer cortex; lymph drains into intermediate sinuses then medullary sinuses; efferent vessels leave the node at the hilus, together with venules	In the pig, the central portion resembles the cortex of other species, the outer portion resembles the medulla; afferent lymph vessels enter the node at the hilus and efferent vessels drain peripheral sinuses
Spleen	Thin capsule, supportive framework of loose connective tissue with smooth muscle, network of reticular cells and fibres	Divided into white and red pulp; white pulp consists of periarteriolar lymphatic sheaths with follicles; cells include lymphocytes and macrophages; red pulp consists of blood-filled sinuses and splenic cords	The splenic artery enters at the hilus, courses through trabeculae and divides in the parenchyma (surrounded by PALS); branches entering the red pulp deliver blood to the sinuses; blood drains into trabecular veins and leaves the spleen at the hilus via the splenic vein	The red pulp is well developed in domestic mammals, particularly in the horse and dog (storage spleen)

thymic anlage is seeded with **lymphocytes** originating from haemopoietic organs (liver, spleen, later bone marrow). These cells accumulate primarily in the periphery of the thymus. The thymus thus becomes a **lymphoepithelial organ** (Table 8.1).

The **central function** of the thymus is the differentiation of lymphocytes arriving from the bone marrow into mature (naïve) **T lymphocytes** (**T cells**). In this process, T cells attain the capacity to distinguish between 'self' and 'non-self'. They acquire immunocompetence, developing the capacity to initiate an immune response upon contact with an appropriately presented antigen.

The thymus is divided into lobes and incompletely separated lobules (Figures 8.3 and 8.4). Each lobule is com-

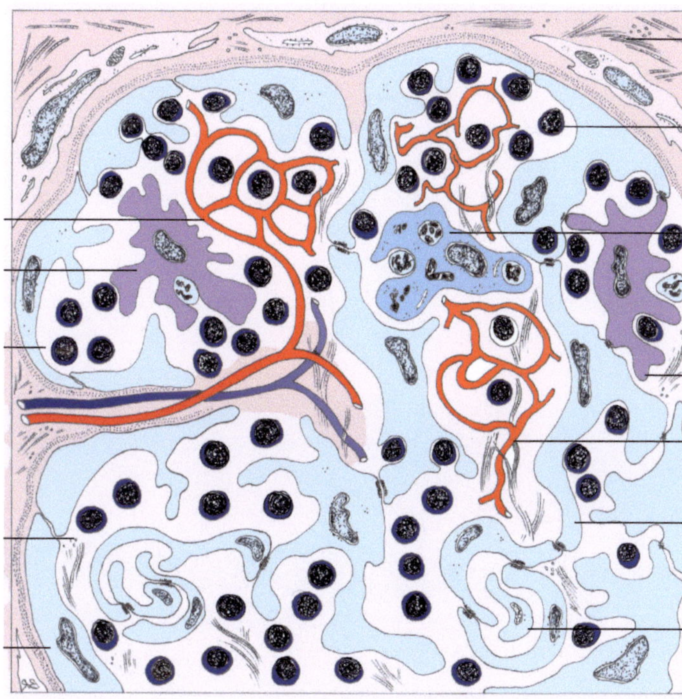

8.3 Thymus (schematic). Epithelioreticular cells form the structural foundation of the thymus. The spaces between these contain immature T lymphocytes that develop into $CD4^+$- and $CD8^+$-positive T cells as they move from the outer cortex to the medulla. The process of differentiation involves positive and negative selection (refer to text). Most immature T cells are eliminated by macrophages after undergoing apoptosis.

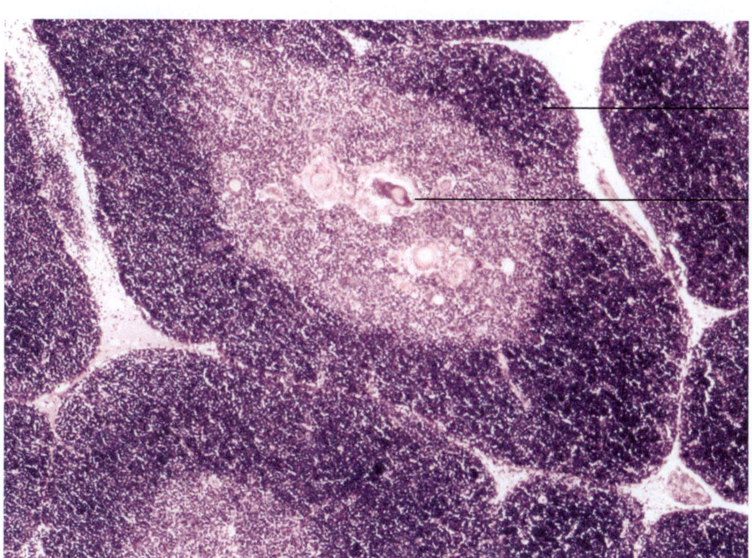

8.4 Thymic lobule (cat). The distinct lobules of the thymus are composed of a lymphocyte-rich cortex and a less cell-dense medulla. Haematoxylin and eosin stain (x80).

posed of an outer cortex that is densely populated with cells and a lighter, less cell-dense medulla. Maturing T cells are interspersed in a stromal network of epithelioreticular cells. Blood vessels, efferent lymph vessels and nerve fibres are also present. The surface of the thymus is covered in a connective tissue capsule. Septa arising from the capsule extend into the parenchyma, forming the lobules.

Cortex

The epithelioreticular cells divide the thymic cortex (Figure 8.4) into numerous, largely segregated, microcompartments in which lymphocytes divide and mature into immunocompetent T cells. This process is controlled by products of the epithelioreticular cells, including **thymopoietin I and II** and **thymosin**.

Long cell processes extending from epithelioreticular cells form a sheath around blood vessels, contributing to the **blood–thymus barrier**. This prevents exposure of T cells to antigens while they are undergoing maturation. (Figure 8.3). During fetal development, endogenous substances that may penetrate this barrier are tolerated by the immune system. Postnatally, this tolerance is lost. Structural support is provided by the epithelioreticular cells, capsule and septa. Numerous macrophages phagocytose dead lymphocytes.

Medulla

The medulla of the thymus is composed primarily of stellate epithelioreticular cells surrounding mature T cells ($CD4^+$ and $CD8^+$ T cells). The blood–thymus barrier is not present in this region.

A unique feature of the thymic medulla is the formation by epithelioreticular cells of concentrically layered structures referred to as **Hassall's corpuscles** (Figure 8.4). These may represent undeveloped thymic microcompartments. The cells comprising Hassall's corpuscles are subjected to hyaline or cystic degeneration and associated karyolysis, karyorrhexis, keratinisation or calcification. The number of corpuscles increases as the thymus undergoes **involution**. Development of Hassall's corpuscles can be induced experimentally by local introduction of antigens.

T cells that have differentiated in the cortex pass along the epithelioreticular cells in the medulla and leave the thymus via postcapillary venules. These cells populate the thymus-dependent zone of lymphatic organs (e.g. paracortex of lymph nodes, PALS of spleen). Further differentiation of T lymphocytes occurs in these organs. Due to the departure of T cells from the medulla, the density of lymphocytes in this region is lower than in the cortex.

DIFFERENTIATION OF T LYMPHOCYTES

The bone marrow-derived T cell precursors that arrive in the thymus and accumulate in the cortex lack specific antigen receptors. These cells are presented with self-peptides bound to MHC I and MHC II molecules expressed on the surface of epithelioreticular cells. T lymphocytes that interact with these MHC molecules continue to develop (positive selection), while others undergo apoptosis. In the next stage, lymphocytes binding to cells that express MHC I and II with self-peptide (dendritic cells, epithelioreticular cells) are eliminated by macrophages (negative selection). Cells that survive this selection process have the capacity to recognise foreign antigen but are tolerant of self-cells.

Thymic involution

Involution of the thymus begins at the onset of sexual maturity. T cells in the cortex are phagocytosed by activated macrophages and the cortex decreases dramatically in volume. Much of the epithelioreticular tissue is replaced by adipocytes and connective tissue. The thymus decreases in weight and the production of mature T cells declines. The distinction between the cortex and medulla is lost and the number of Hassall's corpuscles increases. These processes are accelerated by ACTH, cortisol and gonadotropins.

Bone marrow

The bone marrow is the site of blood cell formation (haemopoiesis). It is composed of stromal tissue in which the various blood cell lines (erythrocytes, leucocytes and thrombocytes) develop. As a primary lymphatic organ, the bone marrow is also the site of initial maturation of lymphocytes. This occurs under the influence of modified stromal cells, in the absence of antigenic contact (see Chapter 7, 'Blood and haemopoiesis').

Mucosa-associated lymphatic tissue (MALT)

Mucosa-associated lymphatic tissue (MALT) is located in the mucosa of the alimentary, respiratory and urogenital tracts. It serves primarily in the protection of the body against environmental antigens and pathogens. It is sometimes also referred to as lymphoepithelial tissue, as some components of MALT are integrated into the epithelium.

The functional elements of MALT include lymphocytes (T and B cells) and associated cells. These exhibit varying degrees of organisation, ranging from individual cells (e.g. intraepithelial cells, plasma cells) to lymphoid follicles (Table 8.1). Lymphoid follicles may occur as:

- solitary follicles (folliculi lymphatici solitarii) or
- aggregated follicles (folliculi lymphatici aggregati), as seen in tonsils and Peyer's patches.

Lymphoid follicles

Lymphoid follicles, also referred to as **lymphoid nodules**, are round to elliptical non-encapsulated accumulations of lymphocytes supported by a meshwork of reticular tissue. Solitary lymphoid nodules are found in various locations including the oesophagus, stomach and small intestine.

Based on structural and functional criteria, lymphoid follicles are categorised as either primary or secondary.

Primary follicles contain an accumulation of mature, yet incompletely differentiated (naïve), B lymphocytes that have not yet come into contact with an antigen. Upon antigenic stimulation, facilitated by reticular and dendritic cells, these become immunologically active B cells.

Secondary follicles develop following activation of primary follicles by contact with an antigen. They are characterised by the presence of a germinal centre where proliferation and differentiation of B cells takes place. Follicular dendritic cells, macrophages and helper T cells are also present in germinal centres; helper T cells play an important role in B-cell differentiation.

The germinal centre is composed of a **light zone** and an adjacent **dark zone**. A so-called mantle layer (corona) forms a thin layer around the light zone. After exposure to an antigen, B lymphocytes proliferate in the dark zone (usually located at one pole of the follicle). These proliferating B cells are referred to as **centroblasts**. Centroblasts differentiate into **centrocytes**, which give the germinal centre its relatively light appearance. Centrocytes present antigens on their surface. Those with a high affinity for antigen subsequently develop into plasma cells or memory cells. The remainder are eliminated by apoptosis.

Secondary follicles thus serve as centres of **proliferation** of B cells and their **active progeny**, **plasma cells**.

In addition to occurring as solitary structures, lymphoid follicles also manifest in aggregated forms – for example in lymph nodes, the white pulp of the spleen, the tonsils and Peyer's patches.

Tonsils and Peyer's patches

Tonsils are **aggregations** of individual lymphoid follicles, found particularly in the oropharyngeal region.

Tonsils are characterised by the following features:

- They are a component of the mucosa-associated lymphatic tissue and contain primary and secondary follicles.
- They are covered by epithelium; leucocytes are typically present between epithelial cells.
- Connective tissue surrounds (capsule) and subdivides the lymphoid tissue.
- They are located near primarily mucous (seromucous in carnivores) glands.
- They have only efferent lymphatic vessels; afferent vessels are absent.

Tonsils provide immune defence against antigens within the oral and pharyngeal cavities. Based on location, they are referred to as palatine tonsils, tonsils of the soft palate, pharyngeal tonsils, lingual tonsils, para-epiglottic tonsils or tubal (Eustachian) tonsils. **Structurally**, tonsils have either a smooth or invaginated surface.

Those with a smooth surface, the simplest form of tonsil, include the palatine tonsil of carnivores (Figure 8.5).

Other tonsils have deep fossules in their surface (fossula tonsillaris). These include the lingual tonsils of the horse, the tonsil of the soft palate of the horse and pig and the tubal tonsils of the pig. The invaginations of the palatine tonsil of ruminants are compound in nature, with the fossula opening into a branching tonsillar sinus (Figure 8.6).

Of particular note are the tonsil-like lymphatic organs of the gut, the **Peyer's patches**. These are found particularly in the ileum, but also in the duodenum and jejunum, and in

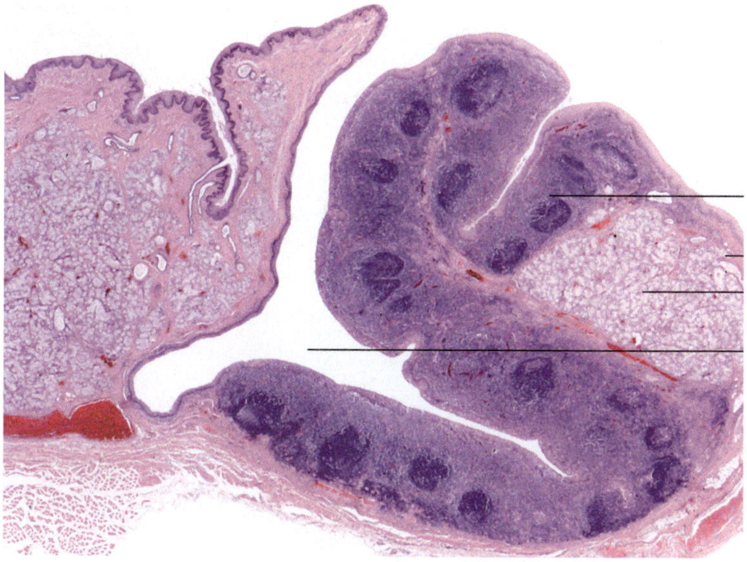

8.5 Palatine tonsil (dog). Tonsils are subepithelial accumulations of lymphoid follicles, enclosed in a capsule and located near glandular tissue. Haematoxylin and eosin stain (x8).

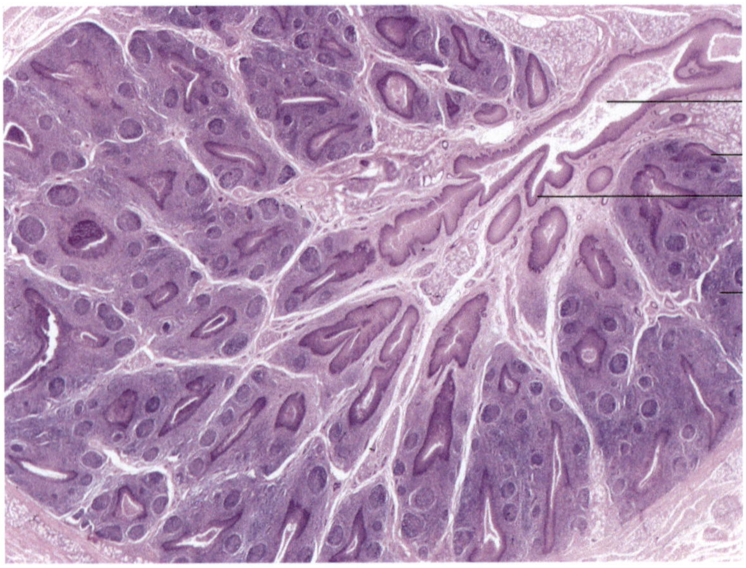

8.6 Palatine tonsil (ox). The lymphoid follicles surround a deep, branching tonsillar sinus into which fossula tonsillares open. Haematoxylin and eosin stain (x5).

the colon (pig). As 'intestinal tonsils', they are responsible for providing an immunological response to ingested antigens.

Peyer's patches have a smooth surface and are characterised by densely aggregated lymphoid follicles. The space-occupying follicles result in **plaque-like** elevation of the overlying epithelium. Leucocytes are interspersed in the epithelium. Specialised cells interposed between epithelial cells, referred to as **M cells**, facilitate the transport of antigens through the epithelium.

M cells are derived from intestinal stem cells. Together with immature dendritic cells, they take up antigens from the lumen of the gut and transcytose these into intraepithelial pockets. There they are brought into contact with B lymphocytes, which pass into the underlying follicles.

Antigen-stimulated B lymphocytes arriving in the lymphoid follicle activate plasma cell precursors, which migrate into the mucosa of the gut and other organs and produce IgA (secretory dimer).

Lymph nodes (nodi lymphatici)

Lymph nodes are composed of **lymphatic tissue** surrounded by a **capsule**. All lymph nodes have both **afferent** (**vasa afferentia**) and **efferent** (**vasa efferentia**) **lymph vessels** (Table 8.1). Lymph nodes are generally bean-shaped, featuring a hilus at which arteries, veins, lymph vessels and nerves enter and/or leave the interior of the organ (Figures 8.7 and 8.8). The connective tissue capsule is penetrated by numerous, usually afferent, lymph vessels. The pig is an exception, in which efferent lymph vessels pass through the capsule (Figure 8.9). Narrow **trabeculae** extend from the capsule into the parenchyma, providing structural support for the node. Between the trabeculae is a three-dimensional

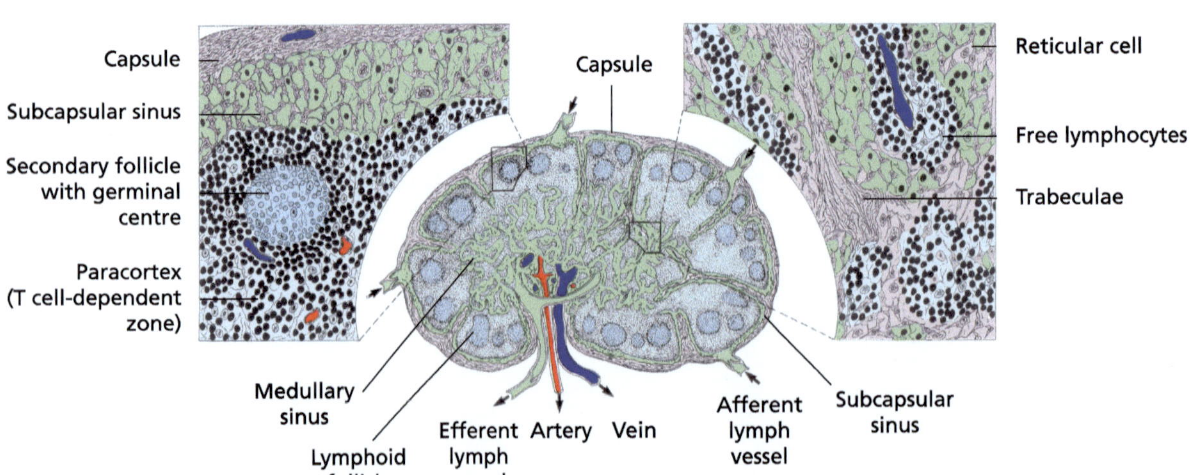

8.7 Structure of a lymph node with multiple afferent lymph vessels and a central efferent lymph vessel (schematic). The insets provide an enlarged view of the cortex and medulla.

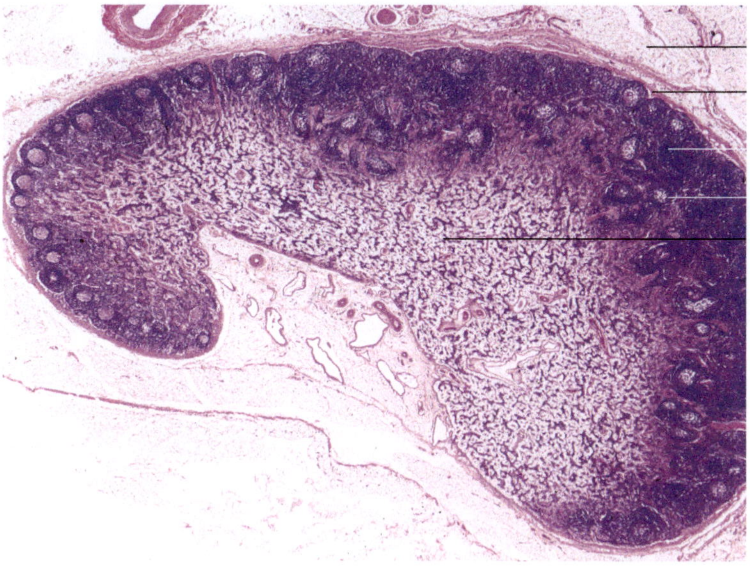

8.8 Lymph node (sheep). The cortex is heavily populated with lymphocytes. It contains primary and secondary follicles. The lighter medulla consists largely of a loose arrangement of reticular and lymphoid tissue. Lymph passes from afferent vessels into the node via the subcapsular sinus and leaves through efferent vessels at the hilus. Haematoxylin and eosin stain (x15).

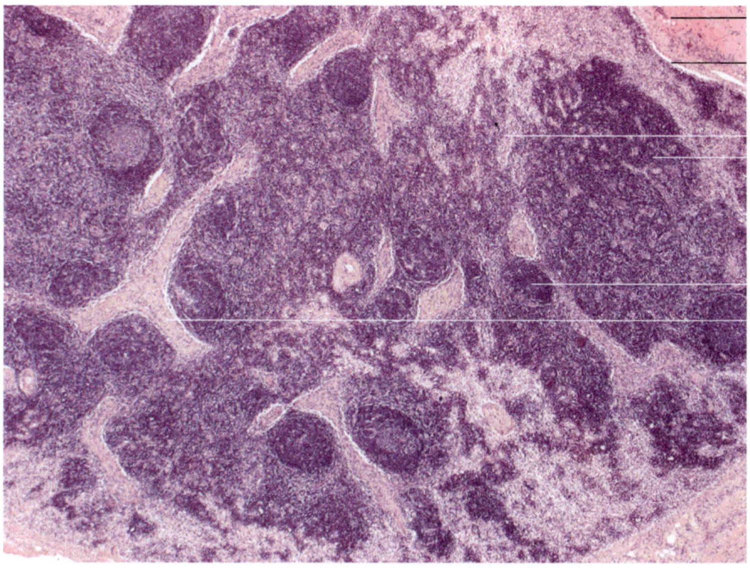

8.9 Lymph node (pig). In this species, afferent lymph vessels enter the node at the hilus and leave via the subcapsular sinus. Therefore, lymph follicles aggregate in the inner zone of the node, with only a few present in the outer cortical zone. Haematoxylin and eosin stain (x20).

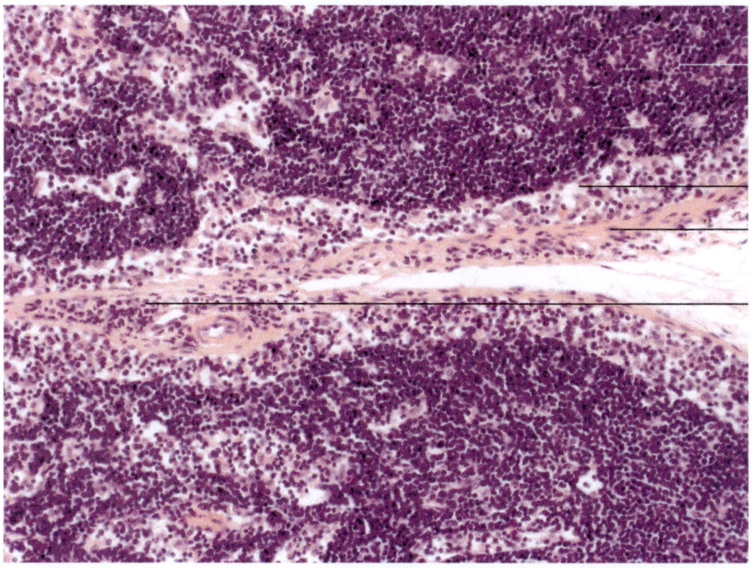

8.10 Detailed view of a section of the cortex of the lymph node (dog). Reticular cell processes, macrophages and lymphocytes are present within the subcapsular sinus, which continues into the intermediate sinus. Haematoxylin and eosin stain (x720).

meshwork of **reticular fibres** and **reticular cells**. The spaces within the meshwork are filled with **cells** including lymphocytes, plasma cells and macrophages (Figure 8.10).

Based on the differential distribution of these cells, lymph nodes are divided into regions designated as:

- an outer subcapsular cortex,
- the paracortex (thymus-dependent region) and
- the inner medulla, composed of lymphoid cells and reticular tissue (Figures 8.7 and 8.8).

The cortex consists largely of aggregations of primary and secondary follicles containing inactive and activated B lymphocytes (Figures 8.7 to 8.11). Lying between and deep to the lymphoid follicles is the **paracortex** (**parafollicular zone**), in which T cells are concentrated.

Within the paracortex, the evenly distributed T cells are surrounded by interdigitating dendritic cells and high endothelial venules. Introduction of an antigen to a lymph node initiates T- and B-cell cooperation and maturation. Activated B cells (along with some T cells) migrate to the follicles where they undergo further maturation before passing to the medulla as antigen-secreting cells.

The medulla contains connective tissue trabeculae through which numerous small blood vessels pass. The parenchyma consists of medullary cords (clusters of cells including lymphocytes, plasma cells and macrophages) separated by medullary lymph sinuses (see below). The cords are reinforced by a reticular meshwork.

Lymph nodes are involved in active filtration of lymph before it returns to the circulating blood. Cells of the immune system eliminate foreign and damaged endogenous cells via innate and adaptive mechanisms. Mononuclear phagocytes (macrophages) engulf cell debris, bacteria, viruses, toxins and exogenous pigments. T and B cells are responsible for cytotoxicity and specific antibody production.

Vessels and sinuses

The function of lymph nodes is closely related to the structure of the **lymph vessels** and their distribution in the **cortex** and **medulla**. After passing through the capsule, the **afferent lymph vessels** empty into an expanded **subcapsular sinus**. This gives rise to sinuses (oriented towards the centre of the node) that accompany connective tissue trabeculae through the cortex (**cortical** or **intermediate sinuses**). The cortical sinuses continue into an extensive interconnected network of chambers, the **medullary sinuses**. These converge to form **efferent lymph vessels** that leave the node at the hilus (Figure 8.7).

The **walls of the sinuses** are largely discontinuous, facilitating the passage of lymphoid cells into the parenchyma. The endothelial lining consists of modified reticular cells. Macrophages (**part of the MPS**) are present in the lumina of the sinuses. Antigens present in lymph can likewise traverse the sinus walls to reach the parenchyma, where they interact with antigen presenting cells, leading to T-cell and macrophage activation.

Activated T lymphocytes convey information to other lymphocytes within the follicles, triggering a cascade of cellular responses. In this process, the thymus-dependent paracortex becomes enlarged and the germinal centres develop through the activation of B cells and formation of plasma cells and memory cells. The lymph node increases in size. Activated plasma cells migrate into the medullary sinuses where they release specific antibodies into the lymph.

Species variation

Pig: The structure of the lymph nodes of the pig differs from that of other mammals (Figure 8.9), the main distinction being the arrangement of the lymph vessels. In porcine lymph nodes, the afferent lymph vessels enter at the hilus and the efferent vessels leave the node through the capsule.

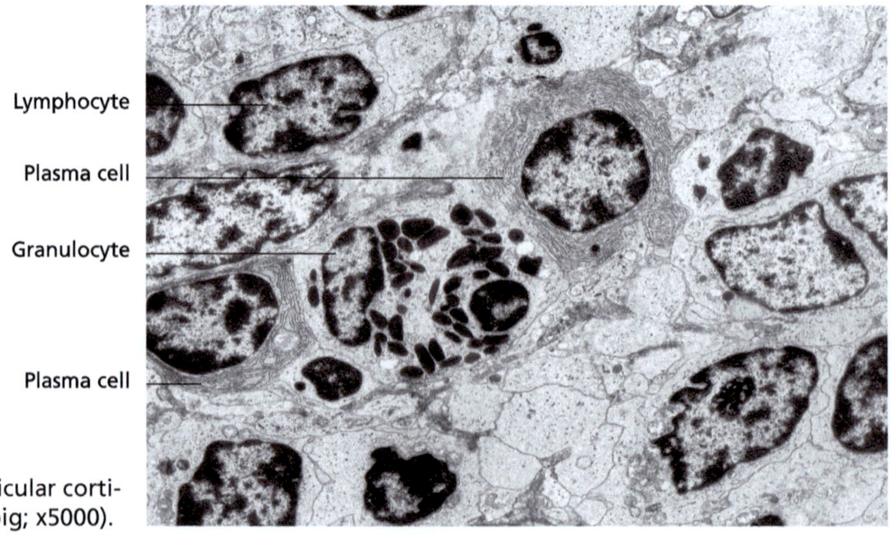

8.11 Fine structure of the follicular cortical zone of the lymph node (pig; x5000).

The flow of lymph is therefore opposite to that in other domestic mammalian species. Lymphoid follicles are grouped in the medullary region of the lymph node; the outer region contains mainly macrophages and plasma cells. The sinuses and cords are relatively poorly developed.

Spleen (lien)

In domestic mammals, the spleen is the largest organised form of lymphoid tissue in the body. In contrast to other lymphatic organs, it is interconnected with the **blood vascular** system. Accordingly, the spleen performs several specialised functions that 'cleanse' the circulating blood and its cellular components.

The principal functions of the spleen include **destruction** and **removal** of aging erythrocytes and **filtration of blood plasma** by activated macrophages. In domestic mammals, the spleen also serves as a **blood reservoir** (storage spleen), in contrast to the primary immunoprotective function performed by the spleen in rodents and humans (defence spleen). Storage of blood by the spleen is particularly pronounced in carnivores and horses. Up to a third of the circulating blood and platelets may accumulate here. Through its role in regulating **blood circulation**, the spleen contributes in a broad sense to **thermoregulation**.

During fetal development, the spleen is a site of **haemopoiesis**. This function is maintained for some weeks postnatally in the foal and calf. In adults, the spleen is a site of terminal erythrocyte differentiation.

The spleen also participates in immune responses. Splenic lymphoid **tissue** is involved in cell-mediated and humoral immunity. Monocytes are transformed into active macrophages in the spleen (part of the mononuclear phagocyte system).

The presence of the spleen is not essential for life. Following its removal (splenectomy), the functions of the spleen are taken over by the bone marrow, in particular, and by the liver and lymph nodes.

Structure of the spleen

The spleen is covered by a **capsule**, the outer layer of which (tunica serosa) forms part of the peritoneum (Figures 8.12 and 8.15). The subserosa consists of a vascular loose connective tissue layer interfused with elastic fibres and a dense connective tissue network with embedded smooth muscle fibres.

The amount and arrangement of smooth muscle varies with species. Flattened to rounded **trabeculae**, containing collagen fibres, elastic fibres and smooth muscle, extend from the inner layer of the capsule into the parenchyma (**splenic pulp**), incompletely subdividing the organ (Figure 8.15). Larger connective tissue septa provide passage for arteries and veins. The fibro-elastic and muscular elements of the spleen are important for the role of the spleen as a blood reservoir. Active contraction, induced by sympathetic nerve fibres, leads to the rapid ejection of blood.

Splenic parenchyma and blood vessels

The splenic parenchyma consists of a three-dimensional network of reticular cells and fibres enclosing lymphatic tissue within its spaces (Figures 8.12 to 8.15). It is divided into two components:

- white pulp (pulpa alba) and
- red pulp (pulpa rubra).

The **white pulp** comprises the lymphatic tissue of the spleen, including lymphoid follicles (Malpighian corpuscles) and **periarteriolar lymphoid sheaths** (**PALS**). These are arranged around arteries of the white pulp, also referred to as central arteries (Figure 8.15). Splenic follicles are spherical accumulations of lymphocytes and reticular tissue. Their structure and function are similar to those of other lymphoid follicles.

A particular feature of the spleen is the **marginal zone** located between the **white** and **red pulp**. In this region there is a close association between the peripheral blood vessels of the white pulp and the sinuses of the red pulp (and their associated macrophages and immunologically active marginal reticular cells). **Innate** and **adaptive immune responses** occur particularly in this region of the spleen.

The **red pulp** contains splenic cords composed of a loose meshwork of reticular cells and fibres enclosing

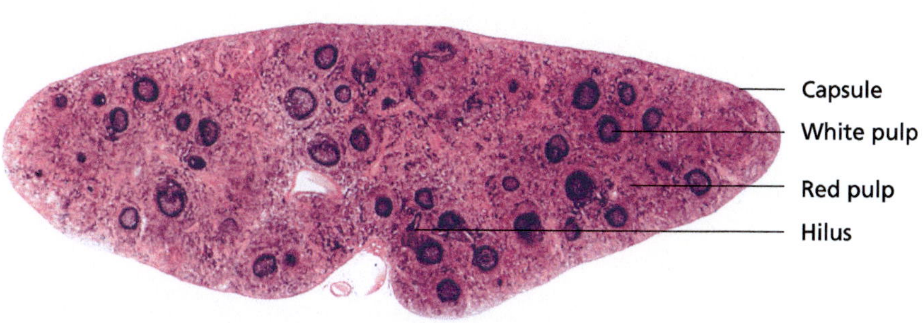

8.12 Spleen (young cat). Lymphoid follicles predominate in the white pulp of this specimen and are distributed throughout the spleen. The red pulp consists of splenic cords (reticular tissue, blood cells, macrophages) and blood sinuses. Haematoxylin and eosin stain (x10).

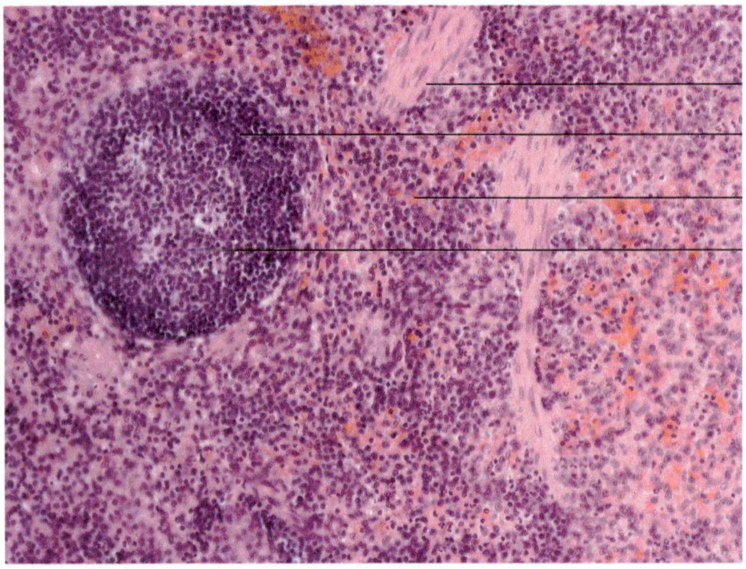

8.13 Detailed view of a secondary splenic follicle and adjacent red pulp in the spleen (cat). The sinuses of the red pulp are filled with blood. Haematoxylin and eosin stain (x80).

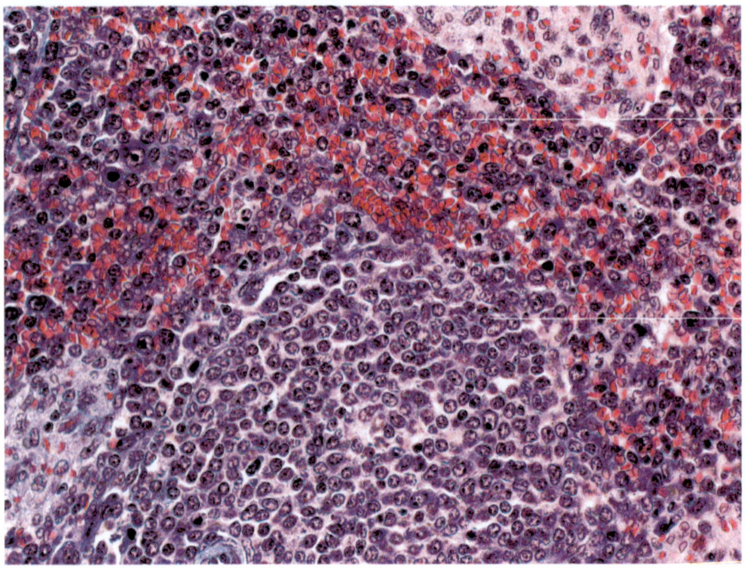

8.14 Detailed view of the marginal zone of a splenic follicle with sinuses and splenic cords (cat). Goldner's Masson trichrome stain (x300).

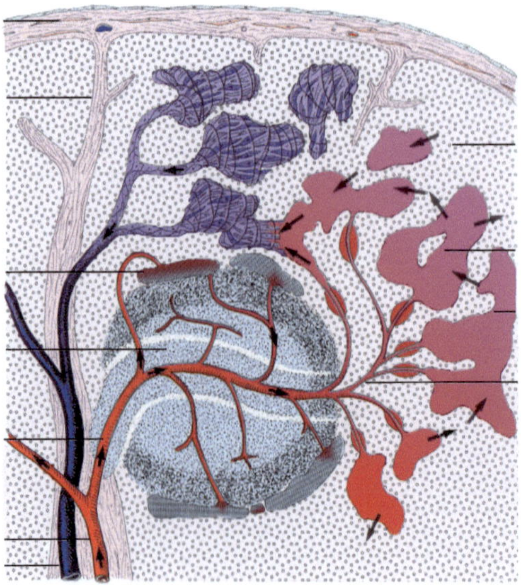

8.15 Blood circulation in the spleen (schematic).

erythrocytes, leucocytes, thrombocytes and macrophages (Fig 8.15). Distributed throughout the reticular meshwork are irregularly expanded anastomosing vascular spaces (diameter 12–50 μm) (**splenic sinuses**) (Figures 8.14 and 8.15). In some species these are not true sinuses, instead resembling venules ('non-sinusal spleens'). The walls of the sinuses are interrupted by longitudinally oriented spaces that permit the passage of blood cells. Actively phagocytosing macrophages tend to accumulate at these sites.

The distribution of blood vessels in the spleen is characteristic for this organ (Figure 8.15). Arteries entering at the hilus divide into **trabecular arteries**. These pass into the parenchyma as **arteries of the white pulp**, or **central arteries**. The central arteries are surrounded for some distance by a sleeve of lymphatic tissue, the periarteriolar lymphatic sheath (PALS). Branches of the arteries also enter the follicles. Some of these branches terminate in the marginal zone while others pass into the red pulp.

Upon entering the red pulp, the arteries exhibit tuft-like branching and are thus referred to as **penicillar arteries**, which are continued by capillaries. The walls of some of the capillaries become surrounded by a **pericapillary macrophage sheath** (**Schweigger–Seidel sheath**). The capillaries open into the cords of the red pulp (open circulation) or directly into the medullary sinuses/venules (closed circulation).

Blood leaving the sinusoids/venules passes into **red pulp veins** and then **trabecular veins**, exiting the spleen at the hilus via the **splenic veins**.

Lymphatic organs of birds

The lymphatic system of birds includes distinctive organs that differ, in some cases markedly, from those of mammals. Special features include:

- lymph heart (cor lymphaticum),
- mural lymphoreticular formations,
- a paucity of lymph nodes, limited to certain locations and
- the cloacal bursa (bursa Fabricii).

Lymph hearts and mural lymphoreticular formations are described in Chapter 6, 'Circulatory system'.

Lymph nodes

The relatively simple structure of avian lymph nodes resembles that of **mural lymphoreticular formations** (widely distributed specialisations of the walls of lymph vessels) and thus differs considerably from that of mammalian lymph nodes.

Lymph nodes are found only in water and marsh birds, occurring in the neck (cervicothoracic lymph nodes) and pelvic region (pelvic lymph nodes).

Avian lymph nodes are composed of a labyrinth of lymph sinuses interspersed with cords of lymphatic and reticular tissue (Figure 8.16). The sinuses, which branch from the afferent component of the lymphatic vessel, are lined with endothelium and contain valves. At the efferent end of the lymph node the sinuses drain into the lumen of the same lymphatic vessel. The sinuses are not subdivided into specific regions (e.g. marginal, intermediate, medullary), though a central sinus may be apparent (Figure 8.16).

The cords are composed of diffuse collections of T lymphocytes and areas (avian germinal centres) containing B lymphocytes. Reticular fibres (type III collagen) extend to the discontinuous basal membrane of the lymph sinus. Antigen processing takes place between the lumina of the sinuses (containing numerous lymphocytes, macrophages and occasional red blood cells and granulocytes) and the lymphoreticular cords.

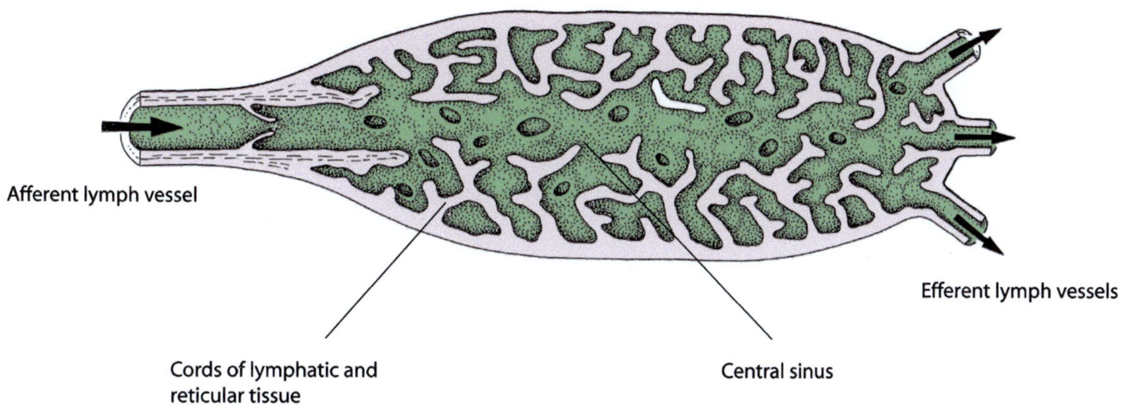

8.16 Schematic representation of the lymph node of a duck, adapted from Berens von Rautenfeld and Budras, 1983.

Lymphocytes **leave the lymph node** by the lympho-vascular route, after passing through inter-endothelial openings in the lymph sinus, and by the haemovascular route, via postcapillary venules.

Cloacal bursa (bursa cloacalis, bursa Fabricii)

The cloacal bursa is the site of B-lymphocyte maturation in birds.

Once mature, the B cells, which originated from the bone marrow, are responsible for the humoral immune response. The cloacal bursa is specific to the class Aves.

In most avian species the cloacal bursa is a pedunculated **dorsal appendage of the proctodeum**. In ratites, the non-pedunculated bursa is integrated into the dorsal wall of the proctodeum. The bursa is subdivided by **longitudinal primary folds** bearing secondary and tertiary folds. This gives rise to distinct lymphatic lobules, each consisting of a central pars lymphoepithelialis and a peripheral pars lymphoreticularis (in ratites this arrangement is reversed) (Figures 8.17 and 8.18).

Spleen

While the structure of the avian spleen does not differ significantly from that of mammals, the boundary between the red and white pulp is less distinct (Figures 8.19 and 8.20).

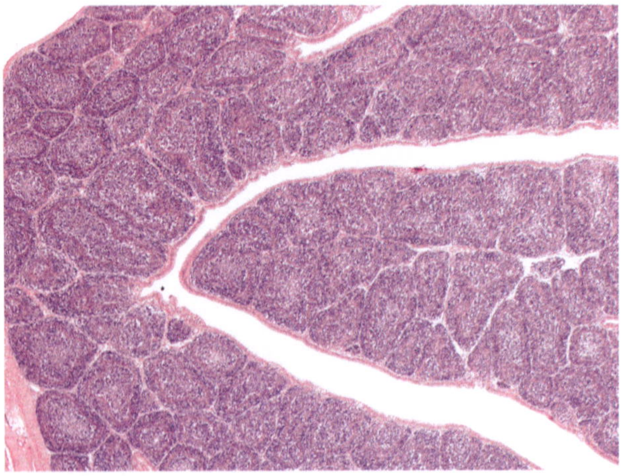

8.17 Cloacal bursa (chicken). The lobulation produced by primary, secondary and tertiary folds is evident. Haematoxylin and eosin stain (x20).

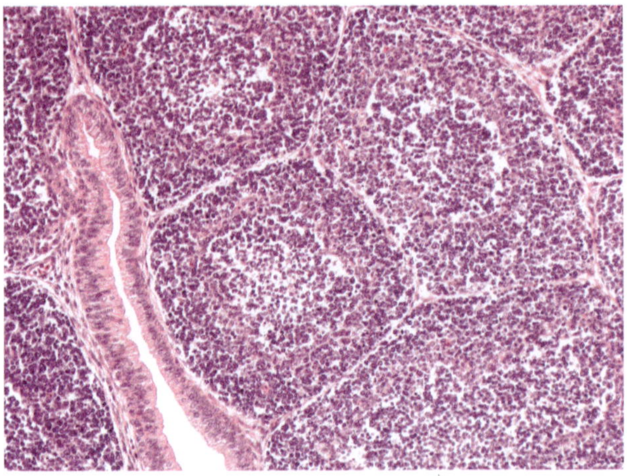

8.18 Cloacal bursa with individual lymphatic lobules comprising a central pars lymphoepithelialis and a peripheral pars lymphoreticularis (chicken). Haematoxylin and eosin stain (x80).

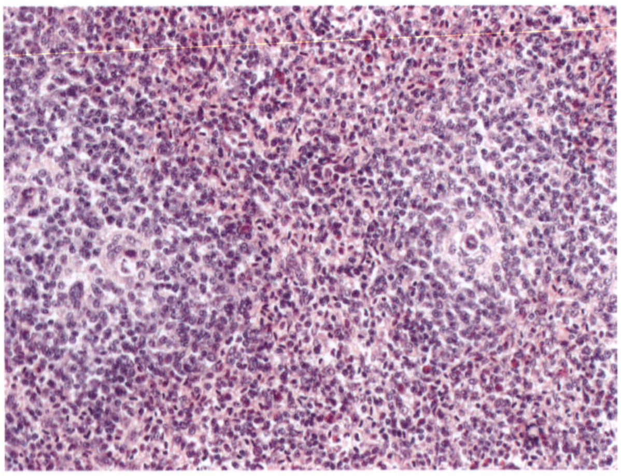

8.19 White pulp with central arteries and adjacent red pulp (chicken). Haematoxylin and eosin stain (x120).

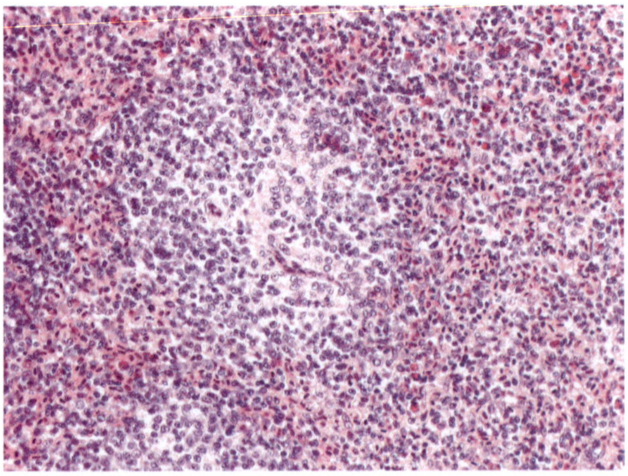

8.20 Splenic follicle with indistinct transition to red pulp (chicken). Haematoxylin and eosin stain (x240).

Endocrine system (systema endocrinum)

9

The activity of cells and organs is subject to constant control by higher-order regulatory mechanisms. The nervous, endocrine and immune systems exert a stimulatory, inhibitory or synergistic effect on target cells that carry specific surface receptors. These systems share the ability to secrete chemical messenger molecules that bind to the cell receptors, thereby initiating a chain of responses.

Chemical signals are transmitted in various ways.

- Nerve cells communicate with receptor cells at synapses, where they release specific molecules (neurotransmitters) that have a short duration of action.
- Endocrine cells secrete a range of chemical mediators comprising peptides, proteins and glycoproteins (hormones); these are either released into the bloodstream (endocrine signalling) to act on cells at a distant location, or they pass through the interstitial fluid to influence nearby cells (paracrine signalling).
- Tissue cells secrete signalling molecules that act as local chemical mediators (e.g. histamine, leukotrienes, prostaglandins, interleukins).

The nervous and endocrine systems are closely interconnected. Hypothalamic neurons release stimulatory and inhibitory peptides that influence the function of cells in the adenohypophysis. Furthermore, neurosecretory products pass via the hypothalamo-hypophyseal tract (tractus hypothalamohypophysialis) into the neurohypophysis where they are stored and released as required (neurosecretion). The hypothalamus also acts on the autonomic nervous system, thus influencing metabolic processes in peripheral tissues and organs.

The nervous and endocrine systems employ different mechanisms to convey their chemical signals to target cells. Neural transmission of information to effector cells occurs rapidly at special junctions (synapses). Neurotransmitters released from presynaptic axonal nerve terminals have a stimulatory or inhibitory effect on the postsynaptic target cell membrane. In contrast, the actions of the endocrine system are relatively slow and diffuse. Endocrine cells are typically, though not always, specialised to produce a single type of hormone. The effect of the hormone depends upon the number and affinity of corresponding receptors on the target cell. Hormones are transported by body fluids (blood, lymph, interstitial fluid). The transfer of information by the endocrine system can therefore take up to minutes or hours.

The endocrine system comprises three organisational forms:

- endocrine glands,
- groups or clusters of endocrine cells and
- individual endocrine cells.

Endocrine glands include the hypophysis, epiphysis, thyroid gland, parathyroid gland, adrenal gland and pancreatic islets. These organs are characterised by the absence of a secretory duct. They have a rich vascular supply and a fenestrated capillary endothelium. Endocrine glands are controlled primarily by feedback mechanisms.

Clusters of endocrine cells are organ components that act predominantly to regulate the function of that organ (e.g. follicular epithelial cells and corpus luteum of the ovary, Leydig cells of the testis). Endocrine cell clusters are also regulated by feedback loops.

Individual endocrine cells occur in surface and glandular epithelia (e.g. gastrointestinal and respiratory tracts). These are referred to as the diffuse neuroendocrine system (DNES) and include APUD (amine precursor uptake and decarboxylation) cells. In the gastrointestinal tract, intraepithelial DNES cells exert local regulatory effects via the paracrine mode of signalling (enteroendocrine system).

Hypothalamo-hypophyseal system

The hypothalamus and the two components of the hypophysis (**adenohypophysis**, **neurohypophysis**) have a **central regulatory role** within the endocrine system (Figures 9.1 and 9.2). **Releasing** and **inhibiting hormones** (**RH, IH**) synthesised by neurosecretory cells in the hypothalamus are transported to the adenohypophysis, where they influence the synthesis and release of hormones that regulate the function of other endocrine organs (tropic hormones). **Effector hormones** produced by neurons of the hypothalamus are conveyed by axonal transport to

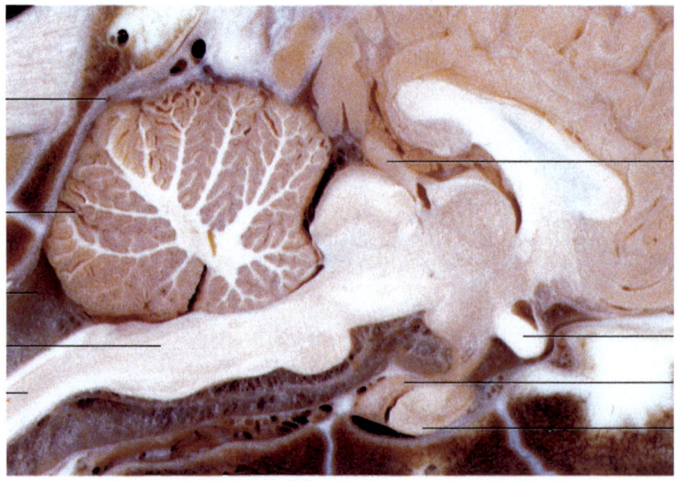

9.1 Paramedian section of the basal region of the brain showing the position of the hypophysis and epiphysis (calf) (König and Liebich, 2009).

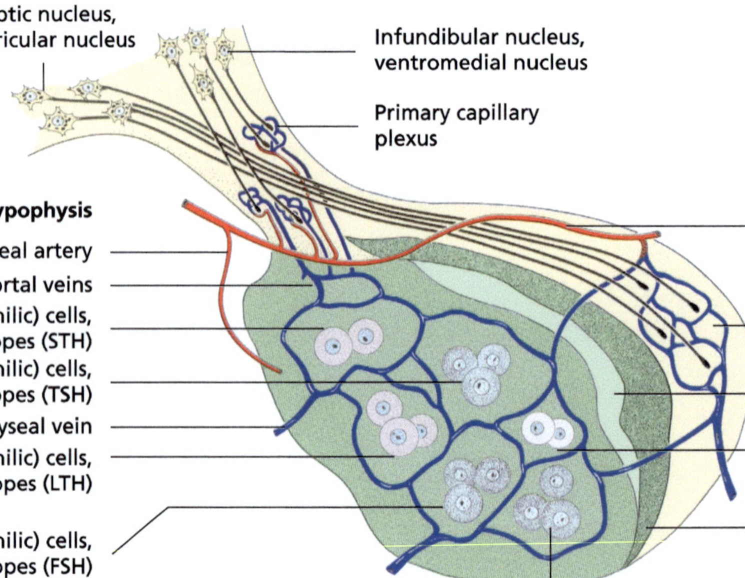

9.2 Hypothalamo-hypophyseal system (schematic).

the neurohypophysis for storage and release according to demand. These hormones act directly upon peripheral organs.

Hypothalamus

The neurons of the supraoptic and paraventricular nuclei (nucleus supraopticus, nucleus paraventricularis) synthesise the effector hormones oxytocin and vasopressin. Within the perikarya, the hormones are packaged in membrane-bound secretory granules. These neurosecretory granules are transported through the axons into the neurohypophysis. Accumulations of granules are visible with the light microscope (**Herring bodies**). Within the neurohypophysis, the granules are stored within the bulbous axon terminals. Upon membrane depolarisation, they are released by exocytosis into the fenestrated capillary network.

Neurons of the ventromedial and infundibular (arcuate) nuclei (nucleus ventromedialis, nucleus infundibularis) synthesise regulatory hormones (RH, IH) that are distributed by the hypothalamo-hypophyseal portal system to the adenohypophysis.

Hypophysis cerebri (pituitary gland)

The hypophysis consists of two functionally and embryologically distinct components, each of which is further subdivided:

- **adenohypophysis**, an ectodermal evagination from the roof of the stomodeum (Rathke's pouch), comprising the
  - pars distalis,
  - pars tuberalis and
  - pars intermedia;
- **neurohypophysis**, an extension of the floor of the diencephalon, consisting of the
  - infundibulum and
  - pars nervosa (neural lobe).

Both parts of the hypophysis (adeno- and neurohypophysis) are enclosed in a common connective tissue capsule which is continuous with the dura mater. In carnivores, ruminants and the pig, part of the lumen of Rathke's pouch remains as the **hypophyseal cavity** between the pars distalis and pars intermedia.

A particular feature of the hypophysis is its characteristic vasculature (Figure 9.2). The inferior hypophyseal artery primarily supplies the neurohypophysis. The superior hypophyseal artery provides blood to the capillary bed in the pars tuberalis of the adenohypophysis, from which capillary loops extend into the median eminence and infundibulum. This primary capillary bed receives the secretory products of the neurons of the ventromedial and infundibular nuclei (RH, IH).

Vessels draining the primary capillary plexus (**portal veins**) course through the pars tuberalis to the pars distalis where they expand into a secondary capillary plexus (Figure 9.2), downstream from the primary plexus. This enables the delivery of the hypothalamic regulatory hormones to the cells of the pars distalis. The vascular bed formed by the consecutive capillary beds and connecting portal veins are referred to as the **hypothalamo-hypophyseal portal system**.

The neurohypophyseal vascular bed supplied by the inferior hypophyseal artery is connected to that of the adenohypophysis by small vessels. The effector hormones vasopressin and oxytocin, originating from the supraoptic and paraventricular nuclei, are released into this vascular network. Hypophyseal veins drain into the sinus cavernosus.

Adenohypophysis

The adenohypophysis is larger than the neurohypophysis in the horse, ruminant and dog. In the cat and pig, the neurohypophysis is slightly bigger than the adenohypophysis.

The adenohypophysis serves as the overarching endocrine regulatory centre of the body, producing **tropic hormones** that influence the activity of almost all other endocrine glands. In addition, **effector hormones** produced by the adenohypophysis exert a direct influence on **peripheral tissues**.

PARS DISTALIS

The pars distalis is composed of cords or clusters of endocrine cells situated in close proximity to a dense network of sinusoidal capillaries with wide lumina. The endocrine cells are surrounded by reticular connective tissue containing occasional macrophages (cells of the **mononuclear phagocyte system**). Isolated small follicles featuring an outer, single-celled layer of endocrine cells may be found throughout the adenohypophysis.

The use of routine histological staining methods (haematoxylin and eosin, trichrome stains) allows endocrine cells to be divided into two categories, based on the staining properties of their secretory vesicles:

- chromophobic cells and
- chromophilic cells.

This classification is not indicative of the functional properties of the cells. Functional cell types can be identified using immunohistochemical techniques.

CHROMOPHOBIC CELLS (ENDOCRINOCYTUS CHROMOPHOBUS)

Chromophobic cells are those in which commonly used histological stains do not reveal the presence of secretory granules (Figure 9.2). They have relatively little, light-coloured homogeneous cytoplasm and a comparatively large nucleus. The electron microscope reveals that most of these cells do in fact contain endocrine granules.

Chromophobic cells are considered to be undifferentiated, **non-secretory stem cells** that transform into specific chromophilic cells when required. Conversely, chromophilic cells can degranulate and become chromophobic. This proposition is supported by the observation that, with the light microscope, many cells (around 50%) of the adenohypophysis appear chromophobic, while the electron microscope reveals that hardly any cells lack secretory granules. On this basis it has been suggested that chromophilic cells exhibit **cyclic secretory activity** incorporating stages of storage and synthesis.

CHROMOPHILIC CELLS (ENDOCRINOCYTUS CHROMOPHILUS)

According to the affinity of their secretory granules for acidic or basic dyes, chromophilic cells (Figures 9.2 to 9.4) are classified as:

- acidophilic cells and
- basophilic cells.

In both cell groups, protein hormones are synthesised in the rough endoplasmic reticulum, glycosylated in the Golgi apparatus and condensed and stored in membrane-bound secretory granules (endocrine granules). Once released by exocytosis, the contents of the granules pass through the fenestrated endothelium of the sinusoids to enter the bloodstream.

The number of chromophobic and different chromophilic cell types in the adenohypophysis varies considerably with species, age and sex. Generally, the highest proportion are chromophobes (50%), followed by acidophilic (40%) and basophilic (10%) cells.

Acidophilic cells (endocrinocytus acidophilicus) contain secretory granules that stain with eosin, orange G or azocarmine. They comprise two cell populations:

- somatotropes (STH or GH cells) and
- lactotropes (luteotropic cells).

The large, densely packed granules (diameter 300–350 nm) of the **somatotrope** (**STH cell**, **GH cell**, **endocrinocytus somatotropicus**) contain somatotropic hormone (somatotropin, STH; growth hormone, GH). Growth hormone

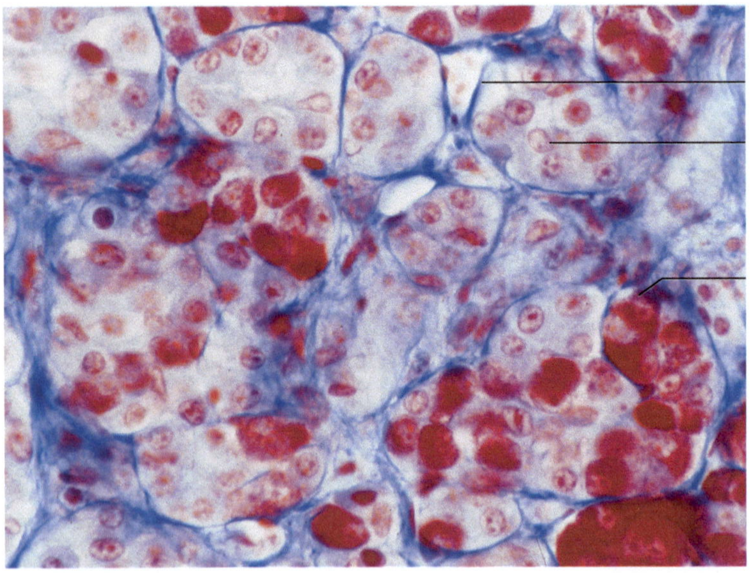

9.3 Adenohypophysis (ox). With the light microscope, chromophobic cells of the adenohypophysis are not seen to contain granules. In Azan-stained sections, the cytoplasm therefore appears pale and the nucleus stains red. Chromophobes are considered stem cells for other endocrine cells of the adenohypophysis, or as cells that are in an inactive phase following degranulation. Azan stain (x300).

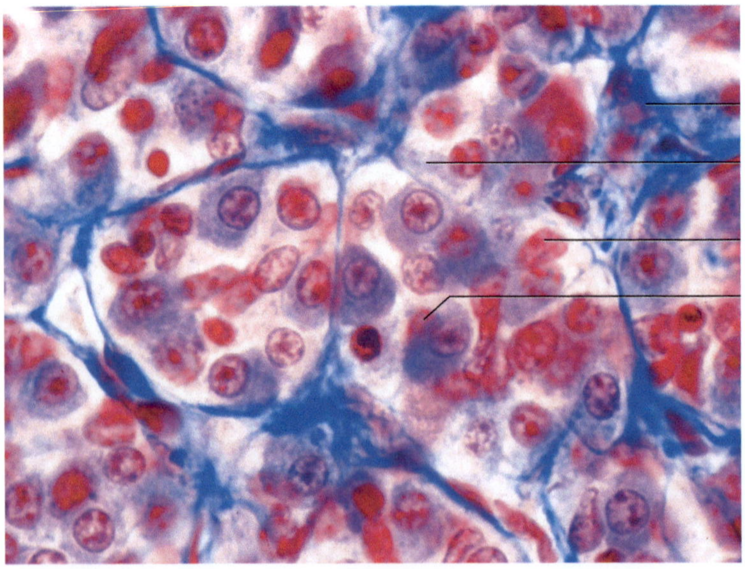

9.4 Adenohypophysis (ox). With the light microscope, chromophilic cells are distinguished by the presence of acidophilic or basophilic granules. Acidophils are somatotropes and lactotropes while basophils are gonadotropes, thyrotropes or corticotropes. Azan stain (x480).

stimulates protein synthesis, promotes the breakdown of fat and reduces glucose uptake. In addition, growth hormone induces the release of somatomedin, particularly by the liver, which stimulates the production of cartilage and bone and thereby contributes to body growth. The activity of somatotropes is controlled by the hypothalamic regulatory hormones GHRH (growth hormone-releasing hormone) and GHIH (growth hormone-inhibiting hormone = somatostatin). Within the acidophilic cell population, the somatotropes appear consistently as relatively small, round or oval cells lacking cytoplasmic processes.

Lactotropes (**endocrinocytus luteotropicus**) synthesise and store prolactin (PRL) in large, variably sized granules (diameter 500–900 nm). During gestation, prolactin stimulates development of the mammary gland. Lactation is inhibited prior to parturition by high levels of oestrogen and progesterone. As the levels of these hormones fall, lactation is initiated. Lactotropes often occur as single cells, are irregular in shape and appear as though they have been squeezed between other cell types. Secretion of prolactin is stimulated by oxytocin (released from the neurohypophysis). During gestation, the adenohypophysis almost doubles in size due to hypertrophy and hyperplasia of prolactin cells. At the end of the lactation period, the volume of the hypertrophied cells is reduced through autophagocytosis.

Basophilic cells (endocrinocytus basophilicus) are characterised by an affinity for basic dyes, particularly aniline blue in various trichrome stains. The tropic hormones produced by basophilic cells are heavily glycosylated (glycoproteins) and their secretory granules are therefore PAS-positive. Basophilic cells are larger than acidophils, though their secretory granules are typically smaller. Three types of basophilic cells are recognised:

- gonadotropes,
- thyrotropes (TSH cells) and
- corticotropes (ACTH cells).

Gonadotropes (**endocrinocytus gonadotropicus**) are relatively small, rounded cells containing PAS-positive granules (diameter 200–400 nm). Gonadotropes produce two types of gonadotropic hormone:

- follicle-stimulating hormone (FSH) and
- luteinising hormone (LH).

It has not yet been established definitively whether all gonadotropes secrete both hormones, or if particular gonadotrope cell populations secrete only one or the other.

In females, FSH stimulates cyclic maturation of ovarian follicles. Luteinising hormone directs ovulation and formation of the corpus luteum.

In males, FSH induces spermatogenesis at the onset of sexual maturity. Additionally, FSH promotes the production of androgen-binding protein by Sertoli cells. LH stimulates the activity of interstitial cells in the testis and has thus also been referred to as interstitial cell-stimulating hormone (ICSH).

The activity of gonadotropic cells is regulated by circulating levels of gonadal steroid hormones. An increase in the level of sex steroids inhibits the activity of gonadotropes (negative feedback). Accordingly, gonadotropic cells hypertrophy following castration.

Thyrotropes (**TSH cells**, **endocrinocytus thyrotropicus**) synthesise thyroid-stimulating hormone (TSH). Of the cells of the pars distalis, these have the smallest granules (diameter around 150 nm).

Corticotropes (**ACTH cells**, **endocrinocytus corticotropicus**) secrete adrenocorticotropic hormone (ACTH) and β-lipotropin (β-LPH). ACTH regulates the synthesis of mineralocorticoids, glucocorticoids and androgens in the cortex of the adrenal gland.

PARS TUBERALIS

The pars tuberalis is a projection of the adenohypophysis that incompletely surrounds the anterior portion of the infundibulum. This component contains dense capillary networks and is traversed by the portal veins of the hypothalamo-hypophyseal portal system. The cells of the pars tuberalis are arranged in clusters. They are largely chromophobic cells that may include small numbers of gonadotropes and thyrotropes.

PARS INTERMEDIA

The pars intermedia lies between the pars distalis and the neurohypophysis (Figure 9.2). Its parenchyma comprises basophils and chromophobes arranged in irregular clusters and follicles. The cells of the pars intermedia produce **melanocyte-stimulating hormone** (**MSH**), which regulates the distribution of melanin granules in amphibians and reptiles (resulting in darkening of the skin) and stimulates production of melanin by melanocytes in mammals. The large **prohormone** pro-opiomelanocortin, synthesised by cells of the pars intermedia, is cleaved to form β-endorphin and two types of MSH, α-MSH and β-MSH. Neurosecretory and aminergic axons extend from the neurohypophysis into the pars intermedia, and basophilic cells of the pars intermedia often migrate into the neurohypophysis (basophil invasion).

Neurohypophysis

The neurohypophysis is connected to the supraoptic and paraventricular nuclei of the hypothalamus by a bundle of non-myelinated axons (**hypothalamo-hypophyseal tract**). This connection is both structural and functional. The hormones of the neurohypophysis are synthesised in

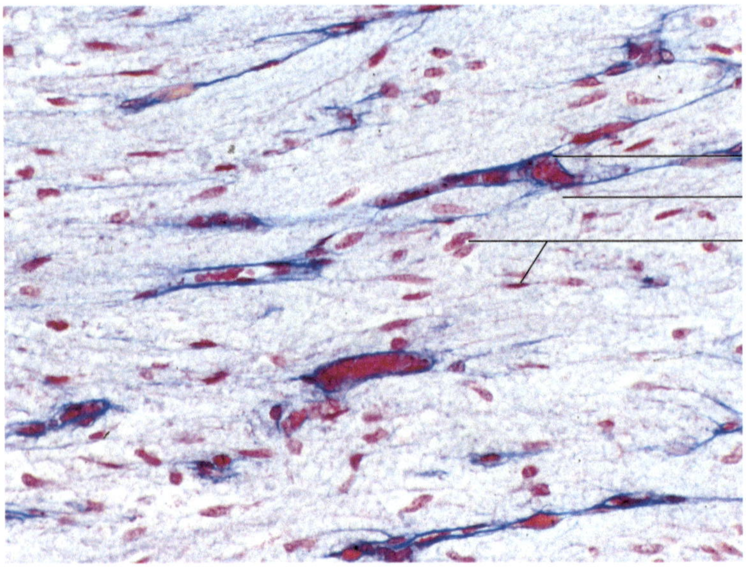

9.5 Neurohypophysis (ox). The neurohypophysis consists of neurosecretory nerve fibre bundles and their accompanying glial cells (pituicytes). Oxytocin and vasopressin are conveyed by neuroaxonal transport to axon terminals where they are released and taken up by capillaries. Azan stain (x300).

the perikarya of hypothalamic neurons and stored in **neurosecretory granules**. The granules are relayed by axonal transport through the hypothalamo-hypophyseal tract to the neurohypophysis, where they are stored in axon endings. They have a diameter of 120–200 nm and stain deep blue with chromalaun-haematoxylin; with the light microscope, groups of thus-stained granules are visible as **Herring bodies**.

The axon terminals within the neurohypophysis are surrounded by specifically differentiated glial cells termed **pituicytes**. These cells form a partial separation between the axon endings and adjacent blood vessels (Figure 9.5). Pituicytes possess complex, branching cell processes. Their cytoplasm contains many lipid droplets and light brown pigment.

The hormones of the neurohypophysis act directly upon peripheral organs. Vasopressin stimulates contraction of muscle cells within arterioles and small arteries. At the distal tubule of the nephron, vasopressin promotes reabsorption of water, thus regulating urine concentration, blood volume and osmotic pressure (hence its alternative name, antidiuretic hormone or ADH). Oxytocin stimulates contraction of uterine muscle cells and myoepithelial cells of the mammary glands (**oxytocin reflex**). Both hormones are synthesised as larger prohormones. No physiological function has yet been attributed to the molecules that are cleaved from the prohormone (**neurophysins**) during transit to the neurohypophysis.

Pineal gland (epiphysis cerebri)

The epiphysis cerebri is a dorsal projection of the diencephalon. It is surrounded by a delicate, highly vascular connective tissue layer (pia mater). From its surface, thin septa accompanied by blood vessels and nerve fibres extend into the parenchyma, partially subdividing the organ into lobules.

The principal components of the pineal gland (Figure 9.6) are:

- pineal cells (pinealocytes),
- interstitial cells (astrocytes),
- myelinated sympathetic nerve fibres,
- postganglionic, unmyelinated sympathetic nerve fibres and
- isolated nerve fibres.

The **pinealocyte** (**endocrinocytus pinealis**) is a polygonal cell. Its processes are in contact with fenestrated capillaries and adrenergic nerve fibres. The structure of pinealocytes is difficult to identify in routine histological preparations. Silver impregnation techniques reveal one or two extensive processes that end in terminal expansions on capillaries. Pinealocytes have oval, indented nuclei and an expansive endoplasmic reticulum. They are usually arranged in groups or clusters. The cytoplasmic processes are reinforced by microtubules and their distended terminals contain groups of synaptic vesicles.

A particular feature of the pinealocyte is the presence of **synaptic ribbons**. These are strips of electron-dense material, the surface of which is evenly lined with synaptic vesicles. Such structures are otherwise only found at synapses between sensory cells and afferent neurons. The number of synaptic ribbons in pinealocytes increases during the dark phase of the day–night cycle. Their function remains unclear.

The **interstitial cells** of the epiphysis are stellate modified glial cells (**pineal neuroglia**). They are in contact with

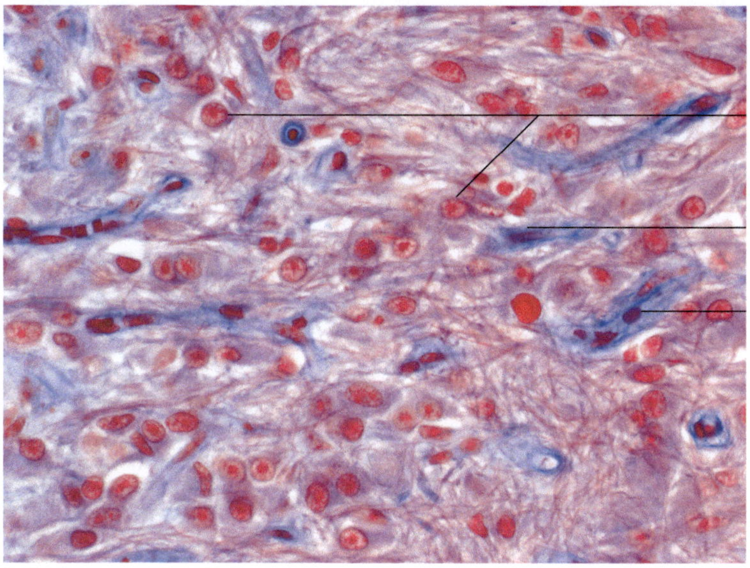

9.6 Epiphysis (horse). The epiphysis is subdivided by delicate connective tissue septa that surround pinealocytes, interstitial cells (astrocytes) and sympathetic nerve fibres. Azan stain (x480).

pineal cells, capillaries and paravascular channels. The chromatin of the oval nuclei of the interstitial cells is more dense than that of pinealocytes. Like the astrocytes of the brain, the interstitial cells exhibit extensively branching cytoplasmic processes containing bundles of intermediate filaments.

With increasing age, calcium deposits appear within the glial regions of the epiphysis and in spaces within the pia mater. These are referred to as **corpora arenacea** (**brain sand**).

The epiphysis is richly innervated with **sympathetic nerve fibres**. The perikarya of these nerve fibres are located in the cranial cervical ganglion. Within the terminals of sympathetic nerve axons are vesicles containing noradrenaline and neuropeptide Y.

The mammalian pineal gland is influenced by **daylight**, about which it receives information from the optic system: retina → suprachiasmatic nucleus → cerebrospinal tracts to intermediolateral nucleus in the first thoracic segments of the spinal cord → preganglionic fibres → cranial cervical ganglion → postganglionic sympathetic fibres to the epiphysis.

The synthetic activity of pinealocytes is regulated by noradrenaline released from the terminals of the sympathetic axons. Within the pinealocytes, **melatonin** is produced by methylation of serotonin. Epiphyseal activity is controlled by the day–night cycle: the concentration of melatonin in the blood increases during the dark phase, while light inhibits melatonin synthesis. The circadian melatonin rhythm regulates seasonal reproduction, providing information about changes in day length. In laboratory animals (golden hamster), the effects of photoperiod on gonadal function can be simulated by artificial manipulation of the day–night rhythm. These are measured by testicular weight, which can vary up to ten-fold under extreme conditions.

The significance of the epiphysis in non-seasonal breeders is incompletely understood. The onset of puberty is associated with a reduction in pineal activity.

Species variation

In lower vertebrates, rather than being a compact structure, the epiphysis of fish and amphibians is a saccular evagination referred to as the **intracranial epiphysis**. An additional component, the **parapineal organ** or **parietal organ**, manifests as a projection of the epiphyseal sac or as a separate, more rostrally located, projection from the roof of the third ventricle. The parietal organ comes to lie, at the end of a stalk, under the epidermis. In some animals (e.g. frogs) it can be visualised at the occiput with the naked eye. The ultrastructure of the cells of the parietal organ is similar to that of the photoreceptors of the retina, with a lamellated sensory process and a basal afferent synaptic connection (it has not been definitively established whether this 'parietal eye' is photoreceptive). It is assumed that these primitive photoreceptors are homologues of the photoreceptors of mammals.

Thyroid gland (glandula thyroidea)

The thyroid gland produces the hormones **tetraiodothyronine** (**thyroxin**, T_4), **tri-iodothyronine** (T_3) and **calcitonin**. Synthesis and secretion of thyroxin and tri-iodothyronine are controlled by thyroid-stimulating hormone (TSH) produced in the adenohypophysis. Calcitonin is regulated by a negative feedback loop, driven by plasma calcium concentrations.

Thyroxin and tri-iodothyronine bind to receptors in the cell nucleus and stimulate transcription. In this way, they regulate intracellular metabolism, stimulating protein synthesis and carbohydrate metabolism. In general, thyroid hormones increase basal metabolic rate, heat production and growth processes within the body.

Calcitonin reduces plasma calcium levels by stimulating osteoblasts, inhibiting the activity of osteoclasts and increasing urinary calcium excretion through decreased tubular reabsorption.

Structure of the thyroid gland

The thyroid gland is unique among endocrine glands in that it stores inactive hormones within vesicular structures termed **follicles**. It therefore serves as a glandular hormone reservoir.

The thyroid gland is enclosed within a thin connective tissue capsule. Delicate septa extend from the capsule into the interior of the organ, dividing the gland into lobes and lobules. Division of the gland is particularly prominent in ruminants and pigs. The thyroid follicles represent a structural and functional unit, bounded by a simple cuboidal epithelium. These are surrounded by a basal membrane and meshwork of reticular fibres, as well as a dense network of fenestrated capillaries (rete capillare) and lymph vessels (rete lymphocapillare).

The follicles constitute the parenchyma of the thyroid gland (Figures 9.7 to 9.10). The epithelial cells of the single-celled follicular wall exhibit polarity. The lumen of the follicle is filled with colloid, a gelatinous material produced by the follicle epithelium. Colloid may be viscous or thin, and is acidophilic and PAS positive. Depending upon the activity of the gland, the colloid becomes thickened by removal of water.

Thyroxin and tri-iodothyronine are stored within the large glycoprotein molecule **thyroglobulin**. When release of the active hormone is required, the thyroglobulin molecule is endocytosed and hydrolysed by lysosomes. According to the functional status of the gland, the follicles vary in shape (round to oval), size (diameter 50–500 µm) and height of the epithelium (Figures 9.7 to 9.9):

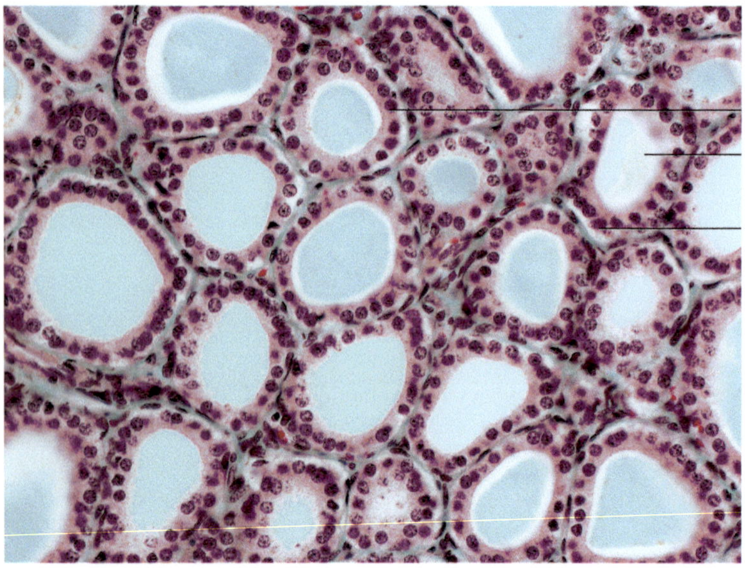

9.7 Thyroid gland (horse). During the secretory phase, the thyroid gland synthesises thyroglobulin which is stored within follicles. The follicle wall is composed of simple epithelium that varies in height according to the functional status of the gland (cuboidal in this image). Loose connective tissue surrounding the follicles contains vessels and autonomic nerve fibres. Goldner's Masson trichrome stain (x480).

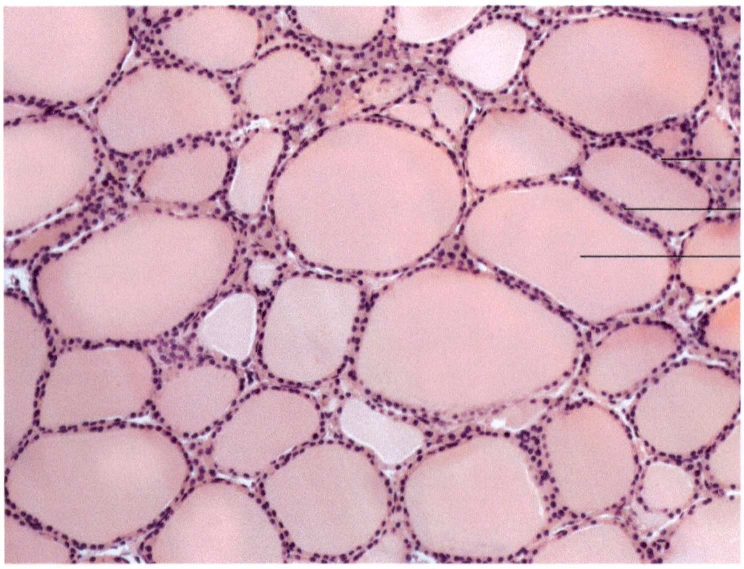

9.8 Thyroid gland (horse). In the storage phase, the follicles are enlarged with a flattened cuboidal epithelium. The follicles are round to oval in shape and therefore appear variably sized in histological section. Haematoxylin and eosin stain (x240).

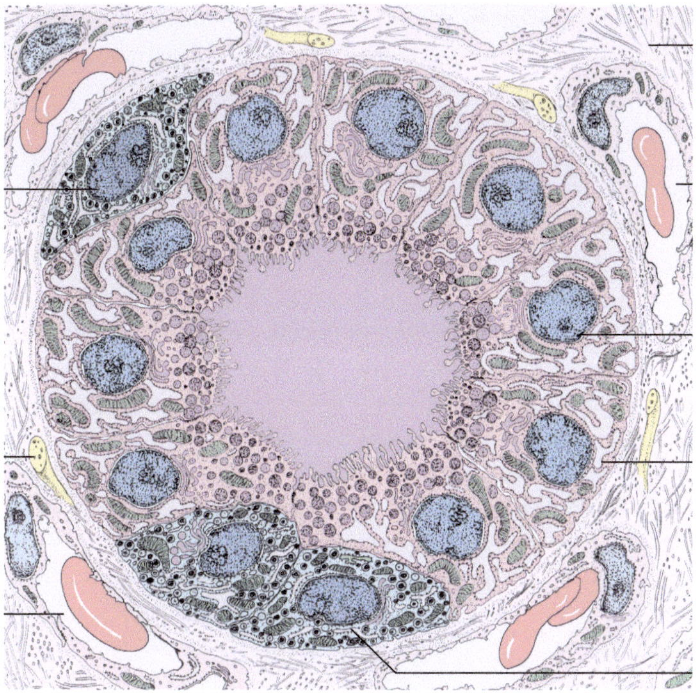

9.9 Thyroid follicle with adjacent capillaries and nerve fibres embedded in loose connective tissue (schematic).

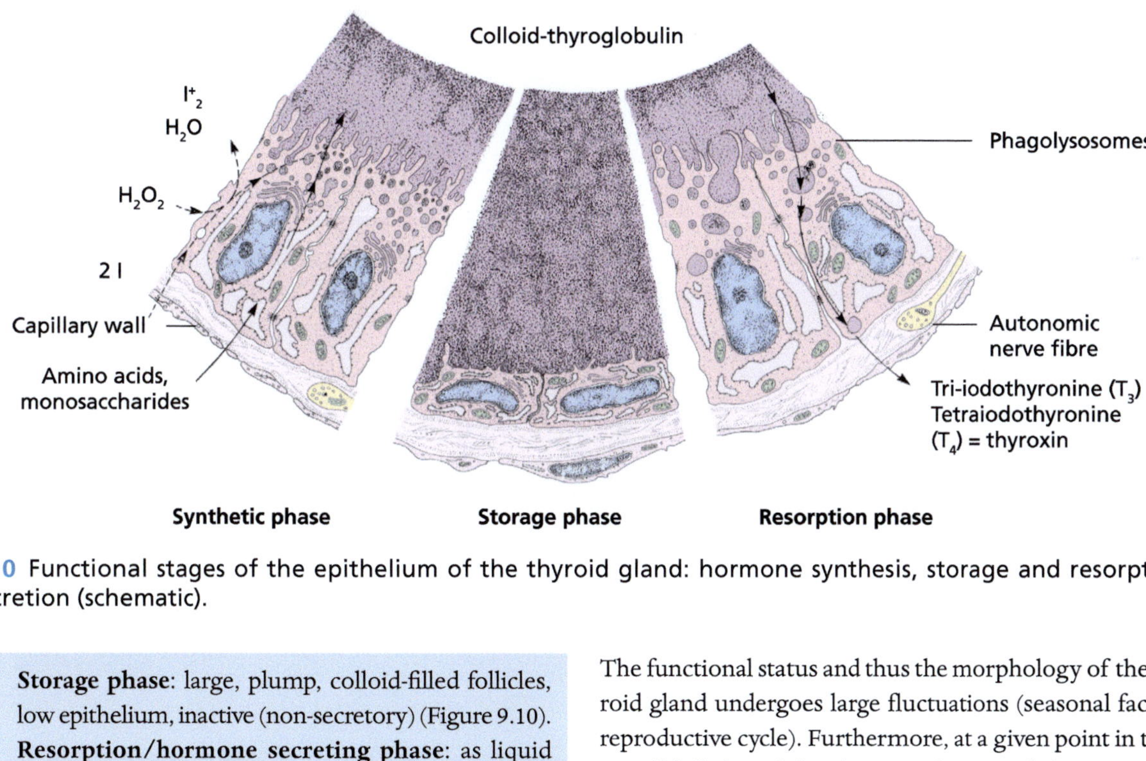

9.10 Functional stages of the epithelium of the thyroid gland: hormone synthesis, storage and resorption/secretion (schematic).

- **Storage phase**: large, plump, colloid-filled follicles, low epithelium, inactive (non-secretory) (Figure 9.10).
- **Resorption/hormone secreting phase**: as liquid colloid is taken up by follicular cells, the cells become taller, their nuclei occupy a basal position, colloidal resorption droplets appear in the apical cytoplasm and the adjacent colloid becomes interspersed with resorption vacuoles.
- **Synthetic phase**: the follicles are small due to a reduction in colloid volume, and the cuboidal to columnar epithelial cells release colloid into the follicular lumen.

The functional status and thus the morphology of the thyroid gland undergoes large fluctuations (seasonal factors, reproductive cycle). Furthermore, at a given point in time, not all follicles exhibit the same functional characteristics.

Follicular cells (endocrinocytus follicularis)

In follicular cells exhibiting a cuboidal morphology, the nucleus is round, centrally located and euchromatic. The supranuclear Golgi fields enclose small secretory granules (50–200 μm) associated with the early stages of colloid production. Lysosomes and phagolysosomes are present. The apical cell surface features microvilli and pseudopodium-like processes. A well-developed rough endoplasmic reticulum and abundant free ribosomes render the cytoplasm weakly basophilic. The epithelial cells are connected by junctional complexes, separating the follicle lumen from the interstitium. At their basolateral surface, epithelial cells take up amino acids, monosaccharides and iodide (via an iodine pump) from the surrounding capillaries. **Thyroglobulin** is synthesised in the rough endoplasmic reticulum (Figure 9.10), then glycosylated and packaged into secretory vesicles in the Golgi apparatus. The contents of the vesicles are released by exocytosis into the follicular lumen, where they are stored.

Within the colloid, iodide is oxidised to iodine (catalysed by membrane-bound thyroperoxidase). Iodine is complexed with free tyrosine group residues of thyroglobulin. Coupling of iodotyrosyl residues results in the formation of **tri-iodothyronine** and **tetraiodothyronine**. These are stored as inactive hormones within the thyroid follicle.

The follicular epithelial cells are activated by **thyroid-stimulating hormone** (**TSH**), produced by the adenohypophysis, and by autonomic nerves. Hormone synthesis, storage and release (Figure 9.10) are all under the influence of TSH. In response to a decrease in the plasma concentration of thyroxin, TSH stimulates the resorption of the thyroglobulin–hormone complex from the follicle into the follicular cells. This process is initiated by liquefaction of the colloid at the perimeter of the follicle. The colloid is then taken up by endocytosis into phagosomes which fuse with lysosomes to form phagolysosomes. Within the phagolysosomes, tri-iodothyronine and thyroxin are cleaved from thyroglobulin by hydrolysis. These hormones are released into the basal cytoplasm from which they pass into the capillaries.

C cells (cellula parafollicularis)

Parafollicular cells, or C cells, are found individually or in groups in the epithelium of thyroid follicles (Figure 9.9). These are located inside the basal lamina of the follicle but do not extend to the follicle lumen. C cells are argyrophilic and can be identified using immunohistochemical techniques. Their cytoplasm stains only weakly in routine preparations and thus appears pale; with electron microscopy, numerous endocrine granules are visible. The granules contain the peptide hormone **calcitonin** and, in smaller quantities, somatostatin, dopamine and serotonin. The release of calcitonin is controlled by plasma calcium concentrations.

> **Species variation**
>
> In birds, reptiles, amphibians and fish, C cells form a separate organ, the ultimobranchial body, that originates from the epithelium of the fifth pharyngeal pouch.

Parathyroid gland (glandula parathyroidea)

The small parathyroid glands lie near the thyroid gland. Septa comprising a lattice of fibres extend from the thin connective tissue capsule into the interior of the gland; in the ox and pig this results in distinct lobulation. In carnivores, the septa are so insubstantial that the gland consists essentially of parenchymal cells and capillaries. The capillaries have an irregularly expanded lumen and a fenestrated endothelium (**sinusoids**).

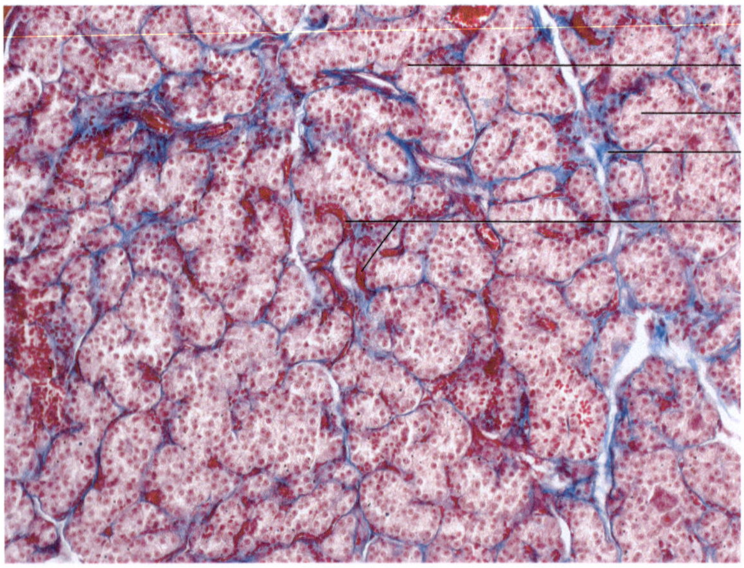

9.11 Parathyroid gland (horse). The parathyroid glands have a simple structure. Their functional cell population consists of small, polygonal principal cells with light or dark cytoplasm. Also present are oxyphilic cells, which have an acidophilic cytoplasm. A dense network of sinusoidal capillaries surrounds these cells. In most species, loose connective tissue results in limited lobulation of the gland. Azan stain (x150).

The parenchyma of the parathyroid gland consists of relatively small polygonal epithelial cells (Figure 9.11) arranged in **cords** or **clusters**. Two types of cells are recognised:

- **small principal** (**chief**) **cells** that occur in two functional stages exhibiting either light or dark cytoplasm, and
- **oxyphilic cells** – larger than principal cells, characterised by acidophilic cytoplasm with a fine granular substructure.

Light principal cells (**endocrinocyti principales lucidi**) have a round, centrally positioned nucleus. They contain few organelles and secretory granules (resting form) but store large amounts of glycogen. Most of the glycogen particles are dissolved during routine formol fixing, and thus these cells appear distinctly pale.

Dark principal cells (**endocrinocyti principales densi**) contain large quantities of electron-dense secretory granules (secretory form). Abundant rough endoplasmic reticulum and mitochondria are also present in the cytoplasm.

Oxyphilic cells (**endocrinocyti oxyphilici**) are larger than principal cells (22 µm in the ox, 27 µm in the horse). The chromatin of the centrally placed nucleus is often distinctly dense. The cells are filled almost exclusively with mitochondria and a little glycogen. The mitochondria are responsible for the granular light microscopic appearance of the cytoplasm. A **transitional cell type** exhibiting features of both principal and oxyphil cells may also be present. The function of oxyphilic cells is unclear; it has been proposed that these may be a degenerative form of cell as their numbers increase with age.

Species differences are observed in the arrangement of parenchymal cells, capillaries and perivascular connective tissue. In the dog, the cells of the parenchyma lie in cords along the usually wide capillaries. In transverse section, this arrangement resembles a rosette. In other domestic mammals, the parenchymal cells are predominantly organised in groups or clusters and the capillaries are narrower. In carnivores and in the ox, the histological appearance of the gland is dark as the cells are small, and the nuclei are close together. A greater volume of cytoplasm in the principal cells imparts a lighter appearance to the tissue in the pig and horse.

The parathyroid gland produces **parathyroid hormone** (**PTH**). The ribosomes of the rough endoplasmic reticulum of the principal cells produce the large pre-hormone pre-parathyroid hormone. This molecule is shortened by proteases during its passage through the endoplasmic reticulum, before being glycosylated in the Golgi apparatus and released by exocytosis into the capillaries. Parathyroid hormone increases calcium concentration in the blood and thus acts as an **antagonist of calcitonin** produced by the thyroid gland.

Parathyroid hormone acts rapidly upon bone, stimulating osteocytes to mobilise calcium from the surface of their lacunae (**osteocytic osteolysis**). It also exerts a long-acting effect by promoting the formation and activity of osteoclasts (**osteoclastic osteolysis**). In addition, parathyroid hormone inhibits calcium excretion in the kidney and stimulates absorption of calcium by the intestine through its regulatory effect on vitamin D metabolism.

Adrenal gland (glandula suprarenalis)

The adrenal gland is a vital, paired organ consisting of two embryologically and functionally distinct regions:

- adrenal cortex (cortex glandulae suprarenalis) and
- adrenal medulla (medulla glandulae suprarenalis) (Figures 9.12 to 9.14).

The adrenal cortex develops from the mesodermal coelomic epithelium, while the medulla is derived from the **neuroectoderm** (**neural crest**). The medulla thus constitutes a **sympathetic paraganglion** composed of neurosecretory cells that release transmitters into capillary networks.

The arrangement of the blood supply to the adrenal gland is related to the functional organisation of the gland (Figure 9.14). Beneath the capsule, an arterial plexus branches into **cortical sinusoids** that extend into the cortex along with delicate connective tissue septa. These fenestrated capillaries are accompanied by a narrow perivascular space containing macrophages of the mononuclear phagocyte system. At the junction between the cortex and medulla, the capillaries open into a network of venules located within the medulla. In addition, small non-branching arterioles pass through the cortex into the medulla (medullary arterioles) to supply the capillaries of the medulla directly with oxygenated blood.

The **venous vessels** of the medulla converge to form **central medullary veins** that leave the gland as the adrenal veins. The adventitia of the central medullary veins incorporates a longitudinal cushion of muscle which has a regulatory effect on blood flow. The medulla thus receives blood from two sources: an arterial supply, independent of the cortical vasculature, and blood from the cortical sinusoids, which is high in cortical hormones (corticosteroids). Corticosteroids regulate the synthesis of adrenaline in the chromaffin cells of the medulla.

Species variation

Lower vertebrates: In fish and amphibians, the adrenal cortex and medulla are separated into an **inter-renal organ** (homologous to the cortex) and an **adrenal organ** (chromaffin body, homologous to the medulla).

Adrenal cortex (cortex glandulae suprarenalis)

The parenchyma of the adrenal cortex comprises cords of epithelial cells, the surface of which is at least partially in contact with the fenestrated endothelium of cortical sinusoids. Based on the arrangement of these cellular chains, the adrenal cortex is divided into three, sometimes indistinctly demarcated, zones (Figures 9.12 to 9.14):

- zona arcuata (zona glomerulosa),
- zona fasciculata and
- zona reticularis.

Zona arcuata/glomerulosa

In the zona arcuata, the endocrine cells are predominantly arranged in **arcades** (Figure 9.13). The cells are weakly acidophilic with centrally positioned, heterochromatic and frequently irregularly shaped nuclei. The cytoplasm contains abundant smooth endoplasmic reticulum, mitochondria and small lipid droplets. The endocrine cells are surrounded by delicate reticular fibres and lie adjacent to fenestrated capillaries. The organisation of cells into arcades is observed in carnivores, pigs and horses. In ruminants, the cells are arranged in **clusters** or **tufts**; in these

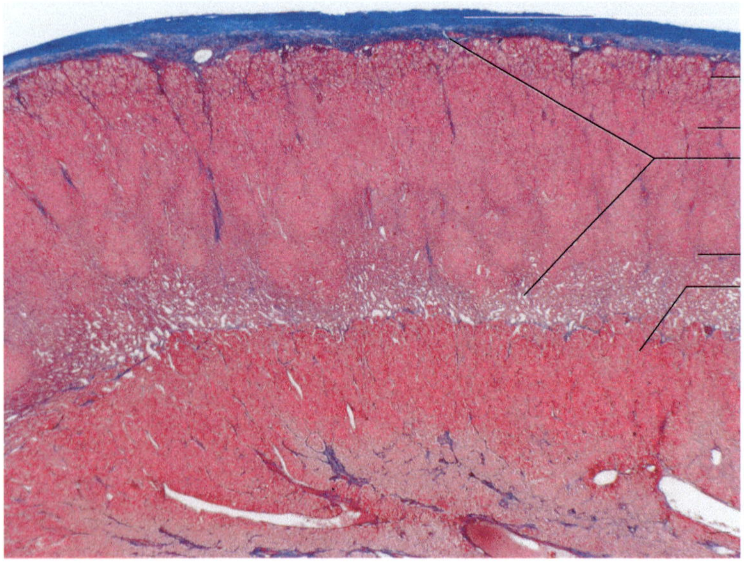

9.12 Adrenal gland (ox). The parenchyma of the adrenal gland has two embryonic origins. The cortex is derived from the mesoderm, the medulla from the neuroectoderm (sympathetic paraganglion). The cortex is divided into three zones: the zona glomerulosa, zona fasciculata and zona reticularis. Azan stain (x30).

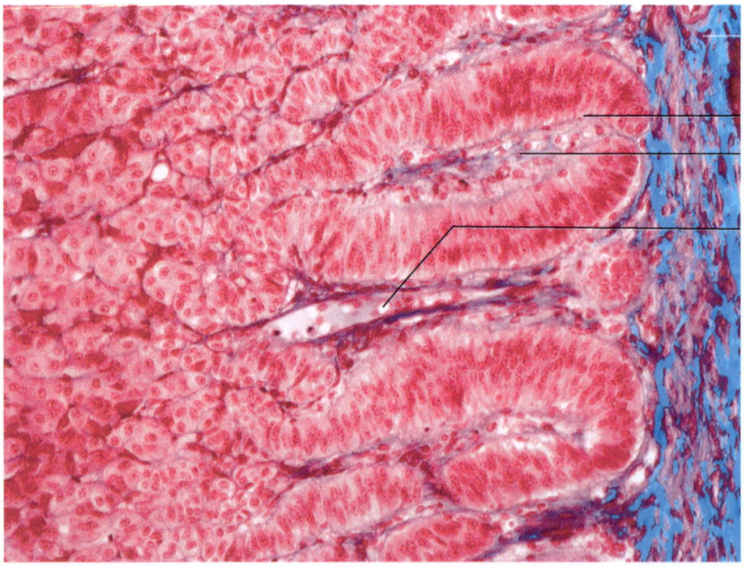

9.13 Zona arcuata of the adrenal cortex (horse). Beneath the connective tissue capsule, the endocrine cells are arranged in arcades. The mineralocorticoids produced in this region are released into a fine network of capillaries, which extends into the zona fasciculata. Azan stain (x360).

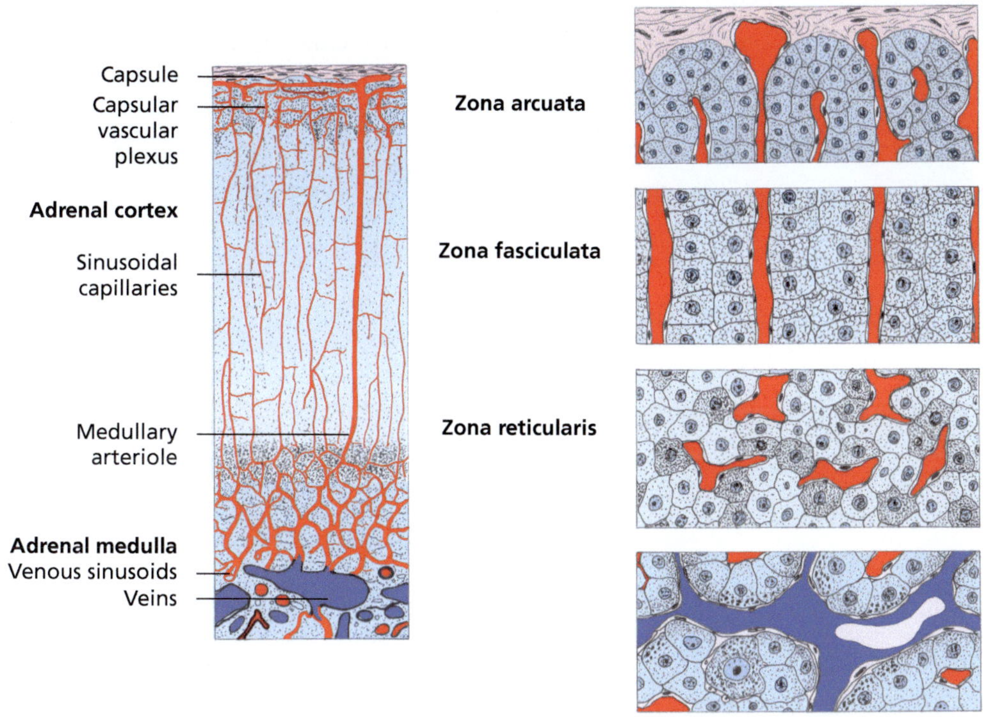

9.14 Structural organisation and vascular supply of the adrenal gland (schematic).

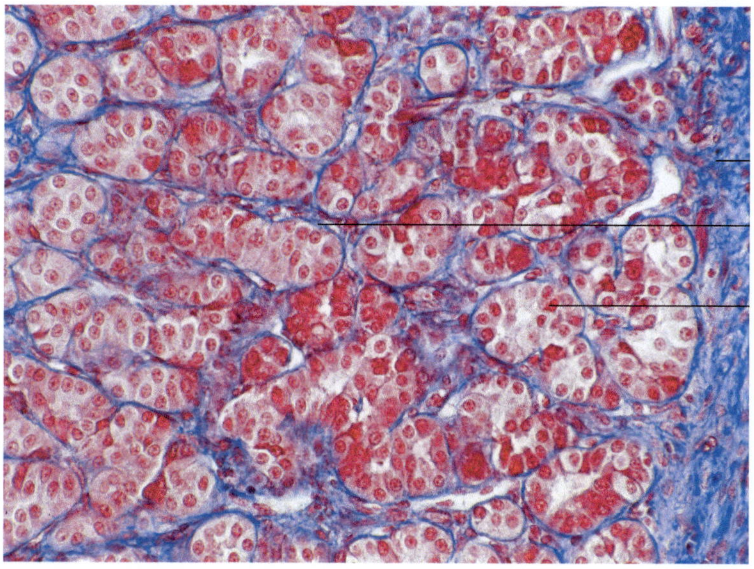

9.15 Zona glomerulosa of the adrenal cortex (ox.) Azan stain (x400).

species, the region is referred to as the **zona glomerulosa** (Figure 9.15).

The endocrine cells of the outer cortex secrete **mineralocorticoids**, particularly **aldosterone**. This hormone counters sodium loss, thus serving to regulate electrolyte and water homeostasis. In the distal renal tubules and collecting ducts, aldosterone promotes reabsorption of sodium (and thereby water) and excretion of potassium. The primary stimulus for release of aldosterone is angiotensin II (via the renin–angiotensin system), though ACTH and atrial natriuretic peptide also play a role.

Zona fasciculata

The broadest zone of the adrenal gland, the zona fasciculata, consists of **parallel cell columns** that are oriented radially, perpendicular to the capsule (Figures 9.12, 9.14 and 9.16). The cell columns are accompanied by connective tissue and fenestrated capillaries. The mildly eosinophilic cytoplasm of the polygonal cells encloses a centrally located nucleus, an extensive system of smooth endoplasmic reticulum and a conspicuous number of variably sized lipid vacuoles. At the electron microscope level, the mitochondria of the zona fasciculata are observed to be of the tubular (tubulovesicular) type.

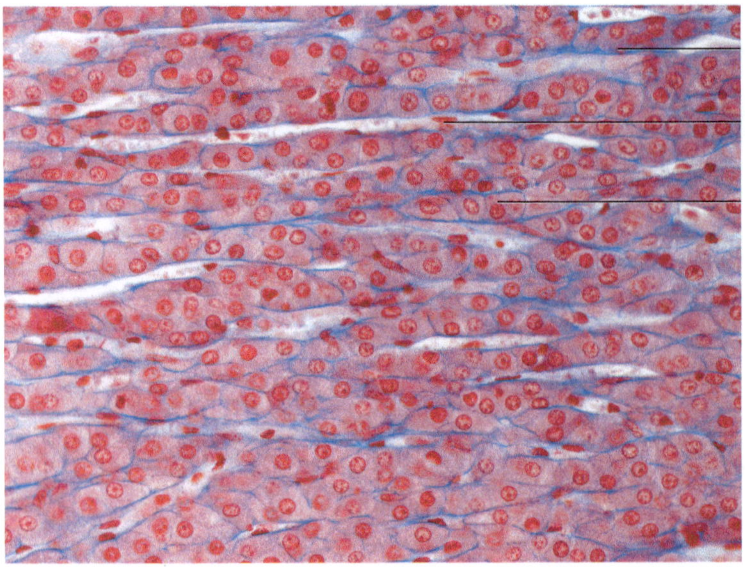

9.16 Zona fasciculata of the adrenal gland (ox). Azan stain (x440).

The cells of the zona fasciculata are regulated by **adrenocorticotropic hormone (ACTH)**, secreted by the adenohypophysis, which in turn is controlled by the hypothalamus (CRH) (negative feedback mechanism). They produce **glucocorticoids**, particularly cortisol and cortisone. These hormones influence carbohydrate, protein and fat metabolism; they inhibit protein synthesis, promote gluconeogenesis from amino acids and stimulate lipolysis within adipose tissue, through which they further contribute to gluconeogenesis. Additional important functions of glucocorticoids include reduction of inflammation and capillary permeability, and suppression of the immune response.

Zona reticularis

The zona reticularis is the **innermost layer of the adrenal cortex**. It consists of a **network of irregular cords of endocrine cells**. The cells are smaller and contain fewer lipid droplets than those of the zona fasciculata (Figures 9.12 and 9.14) and often enclose significant amounts of lipofuscin (zona fusca). As a result, this zone appears more dense and intensely stained, particularly at the boundary with the medulla. The acidophilic cytoplasm typically contains mitochondria with tubular cristae, smooth endoplasmic reticulum and lipofuscin granules. The cells of the zona reticularis produce small amounts of the androgenic hormone **dehydroepiandrosterone (DHEA)** and its sulfate.

Adrenal medulla (medulla glandulae suprarenalis)

The cells of the adrenal medulla contain catecholamine-filled granules that form a brown pigment when fixed with chromium salts (potassium chromate). Based on this so-called chromaffin reaction, they are referred to as **chromaffin cells**. These cells are arranged in clusters or cords that contact fenestrated capillaries with wide lumina (Figure 9.17). They are innervated by preganglionic sympathetic axons and are subdivided into two types: adrenaline secreting cells and noradrenaline secreting cells.

The adrenaline-containing granules of **adrenaline-secreting cells** are of low electron density. These cells form irregular clumps and cords located near the cortex. Adrenaline is formed from noradrenaline in a reaction catalysed by the enzyme phenylethanolamine N-methyl transferase (PNMT). This process is under the control of glucocorticoids, a phenomenon that is consistent with the proximity of these cells to the adrenal cortex.

Adrenaline promotes carbohydrate metabolism by increasing blood glucose concentration (via breakdown of glycogen in the liver and muscle), increases heart rate by stimulation of β_1 receptors and acts on β_2 receptors to bring about dilation of coronary vessels. Smooth muscle in the walls of blood vessels of the splanchnic bed, skin and lung contract under the influence of adrenaline. Lipolysis within adipose tissue is also triggered.

Noradrenaline-secreting cells contain numerous, poorly electron-dense granules filled with **noradrenaline**. These cells tend to be concentrated in the centre of the medulla.

Noradrenaline brings about generalised vascular constriction and thereby an increase in blood pressure.

The ratio of adrenaline- to noradrenaline-secreting cells varies between species. The latter predominate in cats while the reverse applies in herbivores and pigs. In addition to chromaffin cells, the adrenal medulla contains occasional sympathetic ganglion cells.

Innervation

The direct synaptic control of chromaffin cells is logical when viewed in terms of their embryological derivation

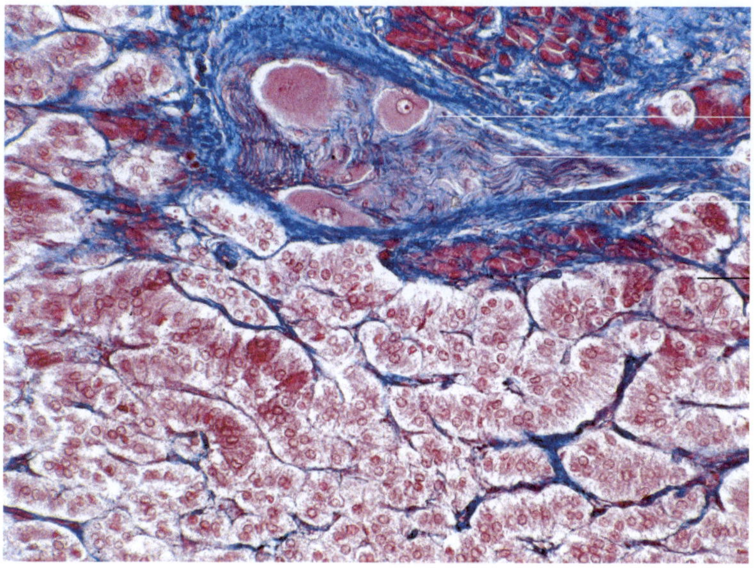

9.17 Adrenal medulla (ox). The adrenal medulla consists of cords of endocrine cells that stain with chromium salts. Located within these cells are granules containing catecholamines (adrenaline and noradrenaline). The medulla also contains sympathetic ganglion cells and nerve fibre bundles, and an abundance of blood vessels. Azan stain (x320).

from the **sympathetic anlage**, and when they are considered as modified sympathetic neurons. The adrenal medulla thus constitutes a **sympathetic paraganglion**. Preganglionic axons reach the adrenal gland via the splanchnic nerves and form synapses with the chromaffin cells. The neurotransmitter is acetylcholine. Neural impulses arriving at the synapse stimulate the chromaffin cells to secrete the catecholamines adrenaline and noradrenaline.

Paraganglia

Paraganglia are **collections of modified nerve cells** that originate from the neural crest and have an endocrine function. They occur as isolated cells or small clusters within or next to (para-) **sympathetic ganglia** or form small anatomically distinguishable organs:

- paraganglion aorticum abdominale (organ of Zuckerkandl) at the origin of the caudal mesenteric artery,
- paraganglion caroticum (carotid body) at the bifurcation of the common carotid artery and
- adrenal medulla (essentially comprises a paraganglion).

In the past, a distinction was made between chromaffin and non-chromaffin paraganglia based on whether the cells of the paraganglion underwent the chromaffin reaction. It was assumed that chromaffin paraganglia stored catecholamines (since these react with potassium chromate to produce the brown pigment), forming part of the sympathetic system. Non-chromaffin paraganglia were categorised as belonging to the parasympathetic system. Using improved immunohistochemical techniques, it was established that all paraganglion cells are capable of synthesising and storing **catecholamines**. The terms sympathetic and parasympathetic are still used to distinguish between paraganglia, based on their anatomical proximity to structures of the sympathetic or parasympathetic nervous systems. The main type of catecholamine (adrenaline, noradrenaline or dopamine) synthesised in paraganglion cells varies between species and individual paraganglia. The most frequently described paraganglion is the carotid body (paraganglion caroticum; Figures 9.18 and 9.20). The carotid body acts as a chemoreceptor, registering decreases in oxygen partial pressure, increases in the partial pressure of CO_2 and changes in pH (acidity). The parenchyma of paraganglia consists of **two cell types**:

- **Pale, oval principal cells** (**type I cells, chromaffin cells**). These have a euchromatic round nucleus and lightly staining cytoplasm; they contain variable quantities of small, dense granules (visible with electron microscope) filled with catecholamines that are released by exocytosis; they are innervated by sympathetic fibres.
- **Elongated support cells** (**type II cells**). These have a dense, elongated nucleus and long cytoplasmic processes that surround the principal cells; they are regarded as modified Schwann cells or, more generally, as peripheral glial cells.

Paraganglia are generously vascularised and are pervaded by numerous nerve fibres. In the case of the carotid body, the mechanisms of chemical signal processing and

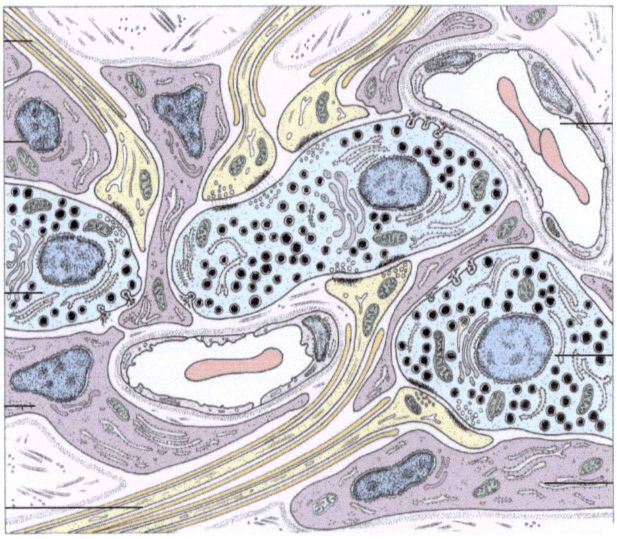

9.18 Carotid body with capillaries and autonomic nerve fibres (schematic).

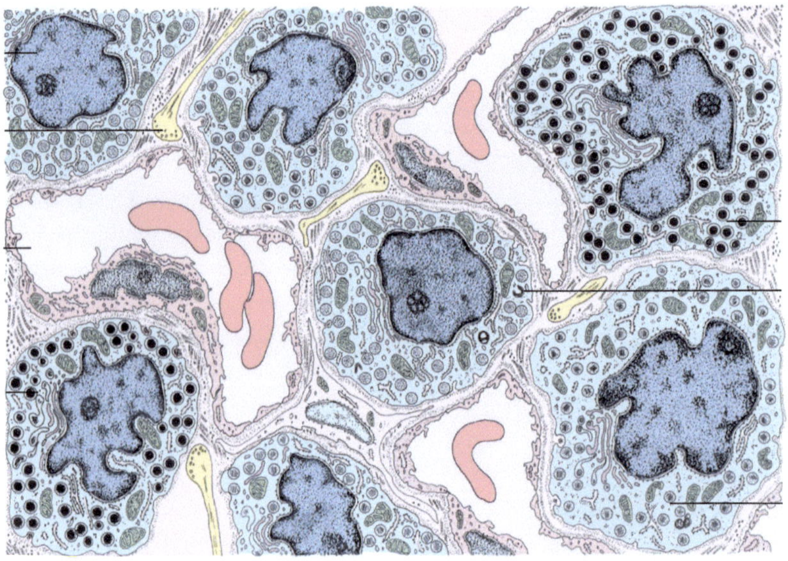

9.19 Pancreatic islet cells with capillaries and autonomic nerve fibres (schematic).

transmission by the cells and nerves of the paraganglion are the subject of ongoing research and are beyond the scope of this text.

Pancreatic islets (islets of Langerhans, insulae pancreaticae)

Endocrine tissue forms a small portion (1–2% of total volume) of the parenchyma of the pancreas, the remainder being exocrine. During embryonic development, epithelial cells bud off from the exocrine pancreatic anlage, forming isolated groups surrounded by capillaries. These are referred to as pancreatic islets (insulae pancreaticae) or islets of Langerhans. The cells within these variably sized (0.02–0.4 mm), predominantly spherical or ovoid clumps are arranged in irregular cords (Figures 9.19 and 9.21). Isolated endocrine cells are also found scattered throughout the exocrine pancreas. Within islets, the endocrine cells are polarised towards the numerous fenestrated capillaries. Unmyelinated (autonomic) axon endings are also found within islet tissue. Cell types found in pancreatic islets include:

- A(α) cells,
- B(β) cells,
- C cells,
- D(δ) cells and
- PP cells (F cells).

The individual cell types are differentiated by their structure and the content of their cell-specific (endocrine) granules. They cannot be distinguished in haematoxylin and eosin-stained sections.

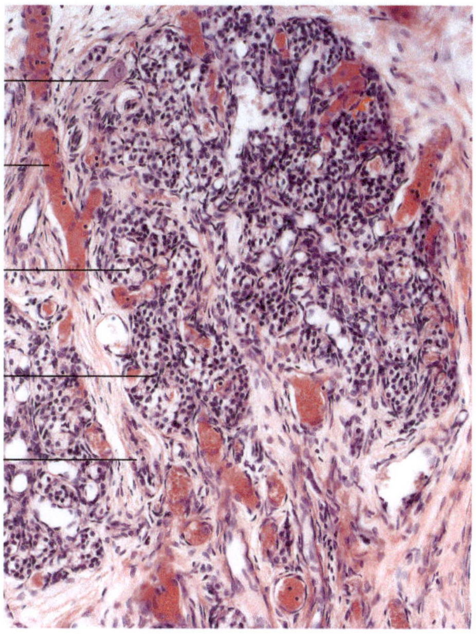

9.20 Carotid body (dog). The carotid body is a parasympathetic paraganglion composed of light chief cells, dense support cells, a capillary network and numerous nerve fibres. Haematoxylin and eosin stain (x225).

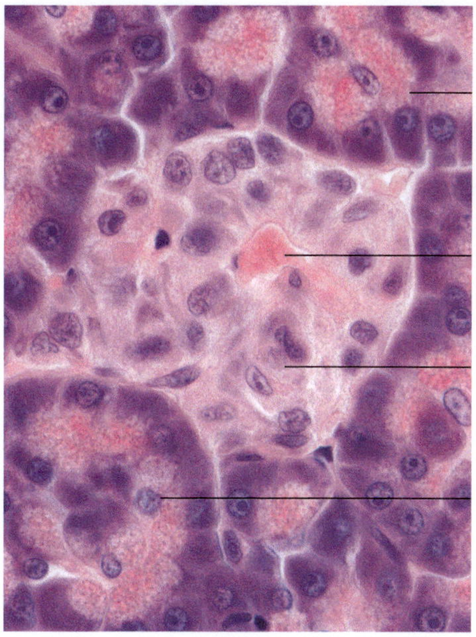

9.21 Pancreatic islet (cat). Pancreatic islets constitute the endocrine component of the pancreas. They contain α-, β, δ, C and PP cells and a delicate network of sinusoidal capillaries. Haematoxylin and eosin stain (x400).

A (α) cells contain dense, argyrophilic granules (200–300 nm). Their nucleus is usually distinctly indented. These cells comprise 5–30% of pancreatic islet cells. In the pig, their number decreases rapidly after birth (from 50 to 20%). In the horse, they accumulate in the centre of the islet; in the ox they are located peripherally. Their granules contain **glucagon**.

B (β) cells are larger than A cells and have an oval, loosely structured nucleus. They stain with Gomori's aldehyde fuchsin. At the electron microscope level, their granules are observed to have a distinctive, crystalline internal structure. The cytoplasm is rich in rough endoplasmic reticulum, mitochondria and Golgi fields. In most domestic mammals, B cells account for 60–80% of islet cells (up to 98% in the sheep). B cells tend to be located at the periphery of islets in the horse and more centrally in the ox. Their granules contain **insulin**.

Glucagon and insulin act antagonistically in regulating blood glucose concentration. Insulin secreted by B cells increases the uptake of blood glucose by the liver, muscle and fat. Triggered by an increase in plasma glucose concentration, the release of insulin causes the concentration of glucose in the blood to fall. Glucagon, the product of A cells, has the opposite effect, raising the **concentration of blood glucose** by activating glycogenolysis.

C cells have been proposed to represent undifferentiated stem cells. They may also be inactive forms of A or B cells.

D (δ) cells are relatively rare (5% in the dog). With the light microscope, they can be identified using Grimelius' silver stain. D cells give off slender cytoplasmic processes. The electron microscope reveals small endocrine granules (150–300 nm) of limited density. The granules contain **somatostatin**, a **growth-inhibiting factor** that inhibits the activity of A and B cells. Somatostatin is also produced in the D cells of the gastrointestinal tract, in the hypothalamus and in the C cells of the thyroid gland.

PP (F cells) constitute a very small group of heterogeneous endocrine cells that synthesise a variety of gastro-pancreatic polypeptide hormones (e.g. pancreatic polypeptide; vasoactive intestinal polypeptide, VIP; cholecystokinin/pancreozymin, CCK).

All pancreatic islet hormones are synthesised as precursors in the rough endoplasmic reticulum, packaged into secretory granules in the Golgi apparatus and transported as active hormone to the cell surface. Movement of the granules, along intracellular microtubules, is regulated by calcium. The hormones are released by exocytosis for uptake by the capillary network.

Enteroendocrine system

Located within the epithelium of the gastrointestinal system are numerous individual secretory cells that signal by the **paracrine mode**. Together, these are referred to as the enteroendocrine system. Cell types of the enteroendocrine system include the well-described **enterochromaffin cell**, which secretes serotonin, and a constantly growing list of cell types that synthesise peptide hormones. Currently, over 30 of such peptide hormones have been identified. They are stored, together with a **carrier pro-**

Table 9.1 Selected enteroendocrine cells of the gastrointestinal system.

Endocrine cell	Hormone	Location
EC cells	Serotonin	Entire gastrointestinal tract
ECL cells	Histamine	Gastric fundus
D cells	Somatostatin	Entire gastrointestinal tract and pancreas
G cells	Gastrin	Stomach and duodenum
I cells	Cholecystokinin (pancreozymin)	Small intestine
L cells	Glucagon-like peptide	Small intestine, large intestine
S cells	Secretin	Small intestine

tein, within membrane-bound endocrine granules. With the electron microscope, these granules are seen to vary in size, shape and density. The features of selected recognised enteroendocrine cells are summarised in Table 9.1.

Through **paracrine** signalling, these hormones regulate digestive processes by acting upon intestinal motility and perfusion of the intestinal mucosa.

Additional endocrine cells

The tunica media of the afferent arteriole of the glomeruli of the kidney contains epithelioid modified smooth muscle cells referred to as **juxtaglomerular cells**. These are polygonal cells characterised by euchromatic oval nuclei and distinctly pale cytoplasm. They are closely apposed (similar to epithelium), forming a collar around the lumen of the vessel. Electron microscope images show that the number of myofilaments in these specialised muscle cells is reduced. Within the cytoplasm are irregularly shaped dense secretory granules containing renin.

Using electron microscopy, endocrine granules containing **atrial natriuretic peptide** (**ANP**) are observed in the sarcoplasmic reticulum (particularly at the poles of the nucleus, near the Golgi apparatus) of certain atrial myocardial cells (**myoendocrine cells**). The stimulus for release of ANP is stretching of the muscle cells by high-volume filling of the atria. ANP promotes diuresis and sodium excretion.

10

Digestive system (apparatus digestorius)

The organs of the digestive system are responsible for decomposition of ingested nutrients into constituents that can subsequently be absorbed. The process of digestion begins with the mechanical breakdown of foodstuffs within the oral cavity, aided in some species by enzymes secreted by the salivary glands. After swallowing, digestion of carbohydrates continues in the intestine. Additional secretions (gastric and pancreatic secretions, bile) result in the breakdown of proteins and fats. The end products, including monosaccharides, amino acids, fatty acids and glycerides, are absorbed through the epithelium of the intestinal mucosa and are utilised as energy sources in cellular metabolism. In addition to these enzymatically derived molecules, water, electrolytes and vitamins are taken up across the intestinal wall.

The liver serves as an accessory organ to the intestinal tract, performing a central role in metabolism. As the largest gland in the body, the liver synthesises and stores endogenous substances and is responsible for producing bile.

End products of metabolism are excreted via the intestinal tract, kidneys, lungs and skin.

The digestive system of ruminants is characterised structurally and functionally by the multi-chambered forestomach. Microbial fermentation in the reticulum and rumen gives rise to volatile fatty acids, saturated and non-saturated fatty acids, ammonia, carbon dioxide, microbial proteins and lipids that are absorbed in the forestomach – particularly the rumen – and in the intestine (refer to veterinary physiology texts).

Macroscopically, the digestive system can be divided into a proximal portion associated with the head (oral cavity, salivary glands and pharynx), a distal portion (oesophagus, stomach, intestine and anal canal) and accessory glands of the intestine (liver and pancreas) (Figure 10.1; see *Veterinary Anatomy of Domestic Mammals: Textbook and Colour Atlas*). Minor modifications of this basic schema are observed in the avian digestive system.

Oral cavity (cavum oris)

The oral cavity serves to prepare ingested foodstuffs for enteral digestion. Food is prehended and directed into the oral cavity by the lips and tongue. In the oral cavity, it is reduced into smaller components by the teeth and mixed with secretions produced by the salivary glands. The food bolus is partially covered in mucus and prepared for swallowing. In pigs, and to a lesser extent in horses, digestion of carbohydrates commences within the oral cavity through exposure to enzyme-rich salivary gland secretions.

To withstand the mechanical impact of the predominantly solid diet of domestic mammals, the lining of the oral cavity is robust and has a high regenerative capacity. In addition, the underlying tissue is richly vascularised. The wall of the oral cavity exhibits the tri-layered structure characteristic of the intestinal tract, incorporating various special features:

- **Tunica mucosa:**
  - mucosal epithelium (epithelium mucosae):
    - stratified squamous,
    - pigmentation,
    - sensory receptors,
    - immune receptors,
    - regional specialisation: gums (gingiva),
  - lamina propria (lamina propria mucosae):
    - collagen and elastic fibres,
    - numerous vessels and nerves,
    - distinct papillae (interdigitations with epithelium),
- **Tela submucosa:**
  - glands (labial, buccal and lingual),
  - lymphatic tissue and
- **Tunica muscularis:**
  - skeletal muscle (lips, cheek, tongue).

The oral cavity is lined by **mucosa** composed of **stratified squamous epithelium** underlaid by a connective tissue layer (**lamina propria**).

The stratified squamous **epithelium** (thickness 200–500 μm) may be keratinised in places. Thickening of the epithelium occurs in areas subjected to greater mechanical strain. Heavy keratinisation is observed on the dorsum of the tongue and on the palate. In some breeds of cattle and dog, this epithelium may be strongly pigmented. Free nerve endings and Merkel cells in the epithelium serve as sensory receptors. Intra-epithelial Langerhans cells function as immune receptor cells in local immune responses.

Differentiation of the mucosa of the oral cavity is evident in the **gums** (**gingiva**). In this region, the mucosa covers the alveolar processes of the maxilla and mandible. The stratified squamous epithelium is keratinised to some extent and exhibits **rapid regeneration**. Taut bands of collagen fibres bind the tela submucosa tightly to the periosteum of the underlying bone.

The **lamina propria** is composed of loose connective tissue containing a network of collagen and elastic fibres. Abundant vessels and nerves are present. Papillae that interdigitate with the epithelium are particularly prominent in the palate and tongue, reflecting the mechanical load borne by these structures. This feature serves to anchor, and facilitate nourishment of, the overlying epithelium. The mucosa (epithelium and lamina propria) is **non-glandular** (**tunica mucosa non-glandularis**).

Lying deep to the non-glandular mucosa is a layer of connective tissue termed the **tela submucosa**. This layer contains blood vessels, a well-developed submucosal nerve plexus (Meissner's plexus, plexus nervorum submucosus), regionally distributed serous, mucous or mixed **glands** (e.g. labial, buccal and lingual glands) and aggregates of **lymphatic tissue** (lymphoid follicles and tonsils). In locations subjected to increased shear forces, the tela submucosa is particularly taut, relatively immobile and tightly bound to the underlying periosteum. Glands are absent in the tip and dorsum of the tongue, the hard palate and the gums. The wall of the oral cavity is extensively reinforced by the presence of **skeletal muscle** in the **tunica muscularis** (lips, cheeks and soft palate). Skeletal muscle also forms the structural foundation of the tongue (for further information regarding the layers of the wall of the digestive tract see 'Structure of tubular digestive organs').

Lip (labium)

The upper and lower lips surround the entrance to the oral cavity. They are used for sucking and prehension and may have a tactile function. The lips (Figure 10.2) are composed of the following layers:

- **outer layer of skin:**
  - modified epidermis,
  - sensory receptors and tactile corpuscles,
  - individually distinct surface patterns (planum nasolabiale),
  - subepithelial serous glands (planum nasolabiale, planum rostrale),
- **muscle layer**
  - m. orbicularis oris
- **internal mucosal layer:**
  - non-glandular mucosa and
  - papillae, glands

The **external surface** of the lips consists of **modified skin** (**integumentum commune**). Sinus hairs are present in carnivores, small ruminants and horses (see Chapter 15, 'Common integument'). Species-specific modifications of the skin of the upper lip include the planum rostrale of pigs, the planum nasolabiale of cattle and the philtrum of carnivores and small ruminants. The planum nasolabiale and planum rostrale lack sebaceous glands and hair (occasional hairs are found on the planum rostrale). Superficially, the lips are richly endowed with free sensory nerve endings. Particularly in pigs, the dermis contains numerous encapsulated tactile corpuscles. The stratified squamous epithelium of the outer surface of the lips interdigitates with pronounced connective tissue papillae. In cattle this results in grooves that form individually distinctive patterns on the planum nasolabiale (Figure 10.3).

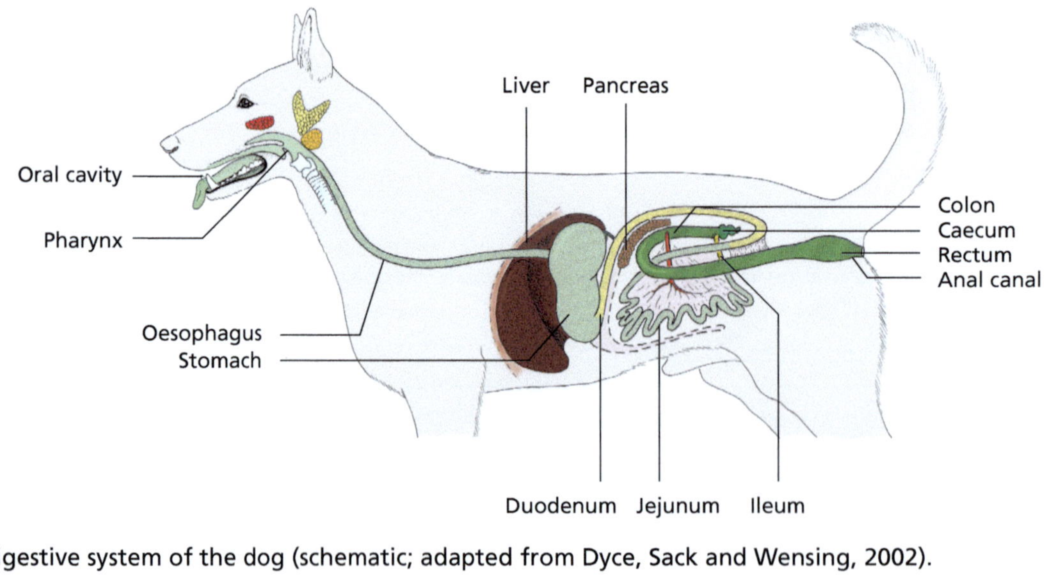

10.1 Digestive system of the dog (schematic; adapted from Dyce, Sack and Wensing, 2002).

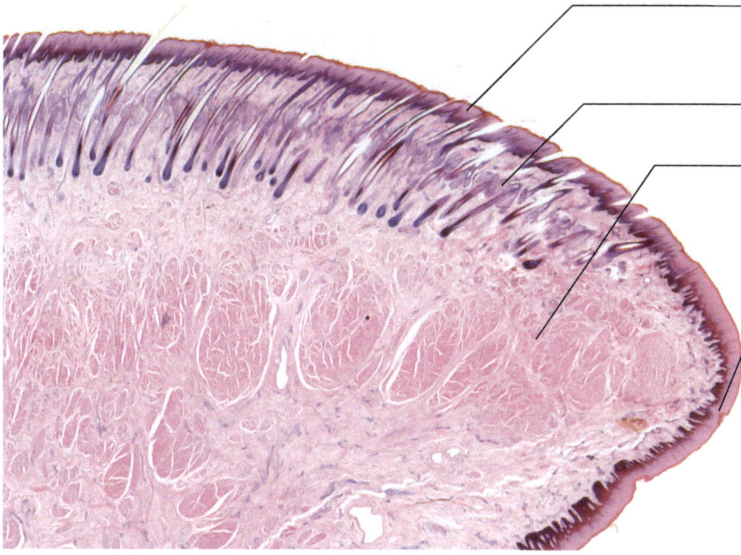

10.2 Lip (foal). The outer surface is lined with skin incorporating hair, sebaceous and sweat glands. The m. orbicularis oris forms the muscular core of the lip. The internal surface of the lip is composed of non-glandular mucosa, comprising stratified squamous epithelium and underlying lamina propria, and a tela submucosa. Haematoxylin and eosin stain (x20).

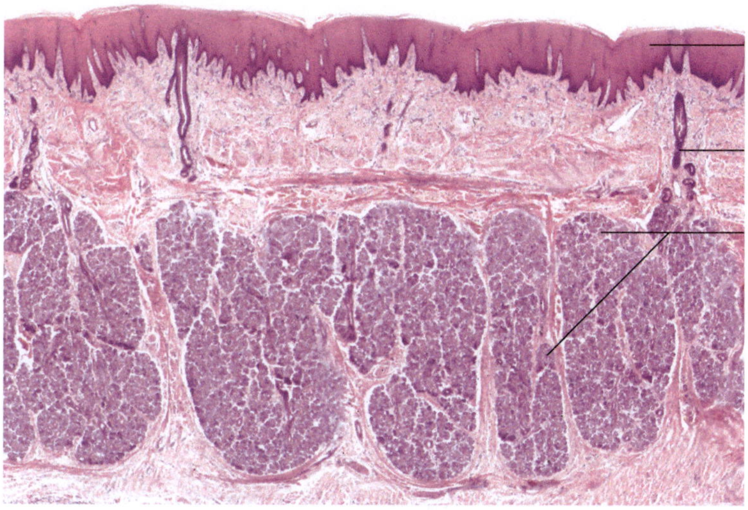

10.3 Nasolabial plate (ox). The surface exhibits the typical structure of skin, except for the absence of hair, sebaceous and sweat glands. Serous glands are embedded in the deeper layers. These empty into grooves at the skin surface. Haematoxylin and eosin stain (x36).

In cattle, substantial accumulations of **serous glands** (**glands of the planum nasolabiale**) beneath the epidermis produce a watery secretion that passes to the surface through excretory ducts and moistens the planum nasolabiale. The subepidermal connective tissue contains abundant collagen and elastic fibres (Figure 10.3). Merocrine sweat glands are present in the planum rostrale of pigs. The planum nasale of carnivores is moistened by nasal secretions.

The stratified **m. orbicularis oris** – together with tendons of the mimetic muscles – forms the structural core of the lip (Figure 10.2).

The **internal layer** of the lips is lined superficially by non-glandular mucosa. In ruminants the **stratified squamous epithelium** is keratinised and interdigitates with prominent connective tissue papillae. In carnivores and pigs, it is non-keratinised. Cornified conical papillae (**papillae conicae**) are present at the angle of the lips of cattle. These assist in the uptake of foodstuffs. The **tela submucosa** of the lips is extensively vascularised and, near the angle of the mouth, contains numerous **labial glands** (**glandulae labiales**). The labial glands are mucous in carnivores and small ruminants and mixed in other domestic species. They are extensively developed in horses and cattle. The tela submucosa is connected to the adjacent muscular layer by connective tissue septa.

Cheek (bucca)

The cheeks (Figure 10.4) are similar in structure to the lips, comprising the following layers:

- outer skin layer,
- middle muscle layer and
- inner mucosal layer.

Unlike the lips, the cheeks are covered externally by hair. The middle layer consists of the buccal musculature. The inner wall is composed of non-glandular mucosa lined by stratified squamous epithelium. In ruminants, buccal papillae (papillae conicae buccales) are present on the surface of the mucosa.

The tela submucosa contains extensive aggregates of **buccal glands** (**glandulae buccales**) that distribute their secretory product to the vestibulum oris through short ducts. The buccal glands are minor salivary glands. They extend deep into the buccal musculature, which aids in expressing the secretory product during chewing. The extent of the buccal glands and the composition of their secretions varies with species. Morphologically, they are classified as compound tubulo-acinar glands. Based on their secretory product, buccal glands are divided into:

- **serous glands**: ventral buccal glands of cattle,
- **mucous glands**: middle and dorsal buccal glands of cattle, ventral buccal glands of sheep, goats and carnivores and
- **mixed glands**: buccal glands of horses and pigs.

Palate (palatum)

The palate comprises the **hard palate** (palatum durum), which covers the bones of the roof of the oral cavity, and the **soft palate** (palatum molle, velum palatinum), which extends towards the pharynx.

Hard palate (palatum durum)

The lining of the hard palate comprises:

- keratinised stratified squamous epithelium that interdigitates with collagen-rich subepithelial connective tissue (papillation) and
- deeper connective tissue containing small vessels and a large venous plexus, as well as numerous fibrocytes, lymphocytes and macrophages (fuses with subepithelial connective tissue to form a propria-submucosa).

The mucosa of the hard palate is lined by stratified squamous epithelium. It is a mostly non-glandular, tough layer of tissue that is tightly bound to the periosteum of the underlying bone. The mucosa exhibits **transverse ridges** (**rugae palatinae**) that vary in number and prominence, depending upon species. The surface of the ridges is reinforced by thick sheets of non-glandular, heavily keratinised epithelium. Isolated mixed glands (**glandulae parapapillares**) occur between the caudal ridges in ruminants and in the dog, and more rostrally in the pig. The taut lamina propria blends without obvious demarcation with the tela submucosa, through which it is tightly fused to the periosteum. In carnivores and (particularly) in ungulates, the propria-submucosa contains an extensive branching venous network. In ruminants, the mucosa is

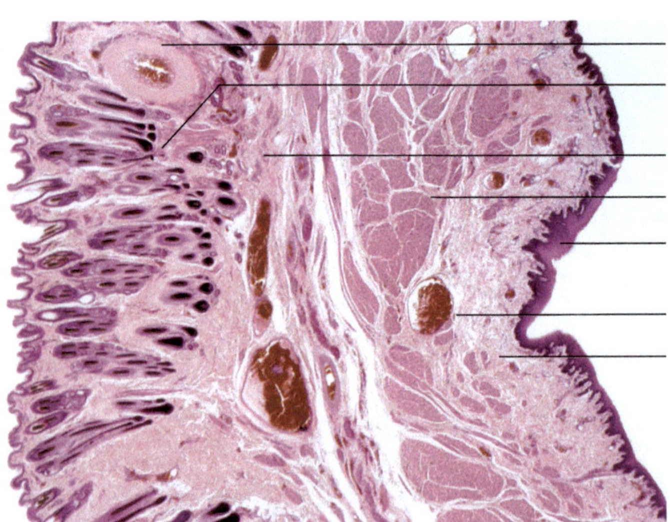

10.4 Cross-section of the cheek (dog). The outer surface is lined by skin in which numerous hairs and glands are present. A layer of muscle lies between the skin and the non-glandular mucosa of the oral cavity. Haematoxylin and eosin stain (x26).

thickened rostrally to form the dental pad (pulvinus dentale). The stratified squamous epithelium of the dental pad is heavily cornified.

Soft palate (palatum molle, velum palatinum)

The soft palate is a musculo-mucosal fold that separates the pharyngeal cavity into the ventral **oropharynx** and the dorsal **nasopharynx**. The mucosa is divided into the following regions:

- **facies oropharyngica**: ventral surface facing the oral cavity, lined by non-glandular mucosa (tunica mucosa oralis) – stratified squamous epithelium with distinct papillae,
- **arcus veli palatini**: free edge of the soft palate and
- **facies nasopharyngica**: dorsal surface facing the nasopharynx, lined by ciliated respiratory epithelium (tunica mucosa respiratoria); becomes stratified squamous epithelium caudally.

Aborally, the stratified squamous epithelium of the oropharyngeal surface becomes reduced in thickness and the papillation diminishes. Near the arcus veli palatini (location dependent on species) the epithelium transitions into pseudostratified respiratory epithelium.

On the facies oropharyngica, the **tela submucosa** houses a substantial repository of tubulo-acinar, mucous and seromucous palatine **glands** (**glandulae palatinae**) as well as diffuse lymphoid tissue. In the pig and horse, discrete **tonsils** (**tonsillae veli palatini**) are present. Glandular and lymphatic tissue is also located beneath the respiratory epithelium of the nasopharyngeal surface.

The structural core of the soft palate is formed by a muscular lamina (**lamina tendinomuscularis**) comprising longitudinally oriented sheets of collagen fibres and the skeletal **muscles of the soft palate** (m. palatinus, m. levator veli palatini and m. tensor veli palatini).

Species variation

Birds: The oral and pharyngeal cavities are combined to form a common oropharynx bounded dorsally and ventrally by the beak. The soft palate is absent (Figure 10.5). In granivores, the **beak** is lined externally by a **horny sheath** (**rhamphotheca**). In ducks and geese, the outer covering is soft and leathery (limited to the base of the upper beak in chickens) and the edges of the beak feature transversely oriented **lamellae**. The soft lining and lamellae contain numerous **sensory tactile corpuscles**. These are also found in large numbers in the **bill tip** of most avian species, where they are housed in so-called '**touch papillae**'. In the nail of the goose, these papillae have been observed at densities of up to 25 per mm^2. Each papilla contains up to 40 receptors. The cylindrical papillae are embedded within the keratinised tissue of the nail of the upper and lower beak, their tips extending to the free surface. The papillae consist of a dermal core, surrounded by a soft horny (epidermal) coat. Each papilla is innervated predominantly by myelinated, but also some unmyelinated, nerve fibres. The sensory receptors within the papilla include **Herbst corpuscles** and **Grandry corpuscles**. Together, these touch papillae comprise a sensory structure referred to as the **bill tip organ**. The bill tip organ is used for assessment of prehended foodstuffs and plays an important role in grooming of the feather coat. It is absent in pigeons and sparrows, which use their beaks primarily for picking at grain. In chickens, touch papillae are present only in the lower beak, though touch receptors are also found in the upper beak.

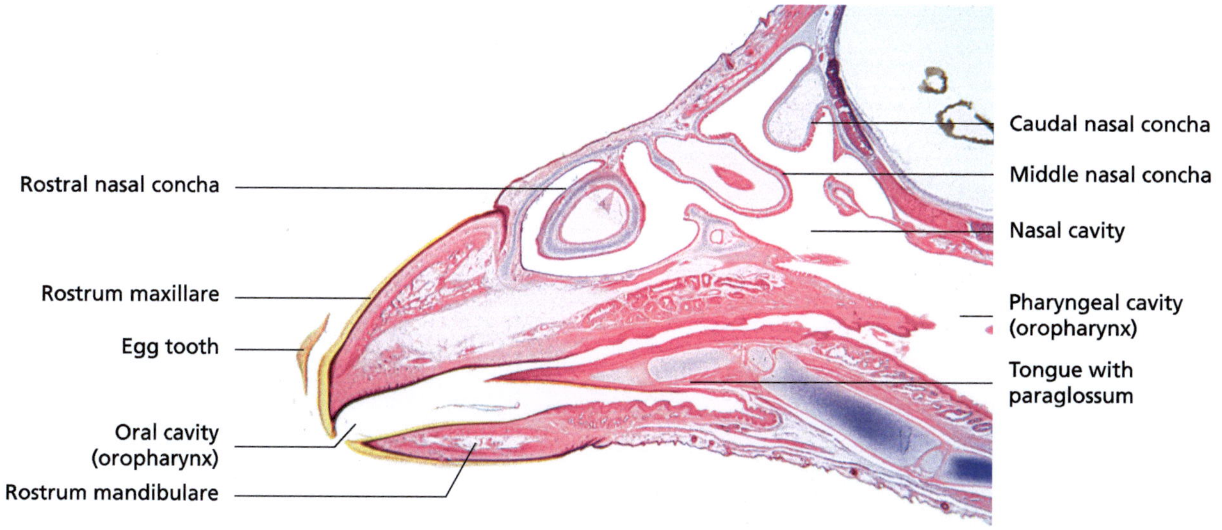

10.5 Paramedian section of the head of a chick with egg tooth. Haematoxylin and eosin stain (x2.5).

Tongue (lingua)

The **tongue of domestic mammals** is a highly mobile muscle. The **body** (**corpus linguae**) and **root** (**radix linguae**) project into the oral cavity and the **tip** (**apex linguae**) moves freely within the cavum oris. The tongue has several functions, including prehension of solid and liquid nutrients and detection of tactile and sensory stimuli. It is also used as an aid in grooming of the hair coat.

The non-glandular lingual mucosa is lined with **stratified squamous epithelium** of varying thickness. In keeping with the mechanical forces imposed by solid foodstuffs, the epithelium of the dorsum of the tongue is thick, heavily **keratinised** and strongly papillated, particularly in herbivores and cats. The margins and ventrum of the tongue are lined by a thin stratified squamous epithelium.

The considerable mobility of the tongue arises from the three-dimensional arrangement of the **striated muscle fibre bundles** within the m. lingualis proprius (Figure 10.6). The muscle fibres are oriented in three directions (longitudinal, vertical and transverse), crossing each other at right angles to form a regular lattice. The muscle bundles are separated by connective tissue septa. Depending on species, these may contain adipose tissue. Numerous blood vessels and nerves are also present. The tongue of the pig is particularly rich in unilocular adipose tissue.

The **lyssa** is an unpaired, rod-like support structure located ventrally at the apex of the tongue. It encloses adipose tissue, skeletal muscle and connective tissue. The lyssa is well developed in carnivores, predominantly filled with fat in pigs and rudimentary in horses.

Species variation

Horse: A fibro-elastic cord incorporating hyaline cartilage, muscle and adipose tissue (dorsal lingual cartilage) is embedded in the dorsum of the tongue.

Ruminants: A raised area with a thickened mucosa, the **torus linguae**, is present on the dorsal aspect of the caudal portion of the tongue.

Birds: The tongue of birds conforms to the shape of the lower beak. In the chicken, a transverse row of caudally directed papillae lies between the body and the root of the tongue. The body of the tongue is supported by a bone, the **paraglossum** (= entoglossum), the intrinsic musculature being only rudimentary. The shape and development of the avian tongue varies according to diet. The tongue of kolibris (hummingbirds) and insectivorous species is very long and highly protrusible. In most avian species, including the chicken, the tongue is pointed apically and slightly broadened at its base. The tongue is lined by **non-glandular mucosa**, in which the epithelium exhibits local areas of keratinisation. Ventrally, the tongue is supported by a keratinised plate (**cuticula cornea lingualis**). In ducks and geese, the edges of the tongue are lined with spiny keratinised bristles that are directed towards the pharynx. These assist with selective filtration during feeding on vegetable matter.

Lingual papillae

The surface of the tongue (mostly the dorsum) is covered with mucosal elevations that facilitate the uptake and sensory assessment of food. Termed **lingual papillae** (**papillae linguales**), these structures vary in their size, number and distribution over the surface of the tongue (Figures 10.6 to 10.9). A distinction is made between **mechanical papillae** (**papillae mechanicae**) and **gustatory papillae** (**papillae gustatoriae**), which are further subdivided as follows:

- **mechanical papillae (papillae mechanicae):**
  - filiform papillae (papillae filiformes),
  - conical papillae (papillae conicae),
  - marginal papillae (papillae marginales),

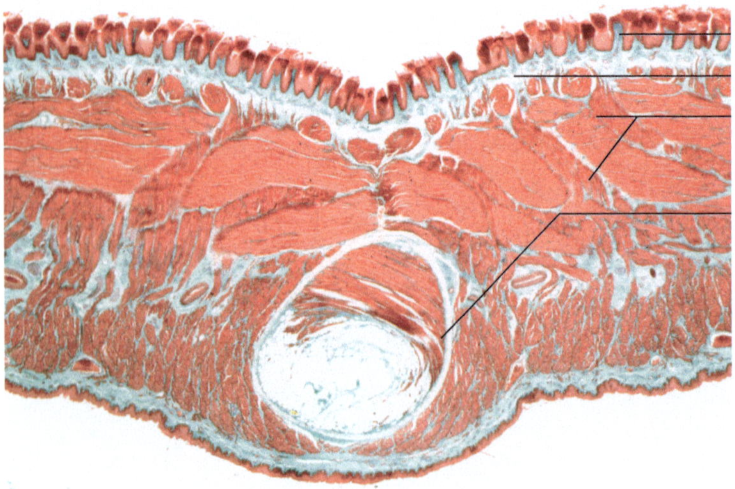

10.6 Cross-section of the tongue (dog). The dorsum of the tongue is covered with numerous mechanical papillae and is distinctly papillated. The orientation of the muscle fibres forms a three-dimensional lattice. The tongue of the dog is supported by the centrally located lyssa. Goldner's Masson trichrome stain (x20).

- **gustatory papillae (papillae gustatoriae):**
  - fungiform papillae (papillae fungiformes),
  - vallate papillae (papillae vallatae) and
  - foliate papillae (papillae foliatae).

MECHANICAL PAPILLAE

Mechanical papillae typically have a connective tissue core housing numerous nerve fibres and mechanoreceptors. Tactile stimuli are received by free nerve endings in the epithelium. The papillae are supplied by a dense vascular network.

The **filiform papillae** of horses, pigs and goats manifest as soft threads of epithelium that give the surface of the tongue a velvet-like smoothness. In cattle, sheep and cats, small keratinised spines project towards the pharynx from a connective tissue core. These are responsible for the characteristic roughness of the surface of the tongue in these species. In cats, the protruding spines are supported on their rostral aspect by an additional papilla (Figure 10.7).

Blunt **conical papillae** are found in carnivores, pigs, cattle and small ruminants. In neonatal carnivores and piglets, the margins of the tongue bear elongated **marginal papillae**. These form part of the lateral boundary of the oral fissure and facilitate sucking.

GUSTATORY PAPILLAE

In gustatory papillae, the stratified squamous epithelium contains specialised structures, termed **taste buds**, that are concerned with the perception of taste stimuli (see Chapter 16, 'Receptors and sense organs').

Fungiform papillae are distributed over the dorsum, margins and parts of the ventral surface of the tongue. They appear as small, mushroom-shaped elevations that protrude slightly above the tongue surface. Fungiform papillae are not as strongly keratinised as mechanical papillae. It is thought that fungiform papillae may contain **thermoreceptors**. Occasional taste buds are present in the epithelium in calves and horses; in carnivores they are abundant. Taste buds are more numerous in young animals during the suckling period.

Vallate papillae occur at the transition from the body to the root of the tongue. Horses and pigs have one pair of vallate papillae; two to three pairs are present in carnivores. Vallate papillae are most numerous in ruminants (up to 24 on each side in sheep) (Figures 10.8 and 10.9). Each papilla is surrounded by an annular sulcus, the outer boundary of which is slightly elevated. The papilla itself does not protrude beyond the surface of the tongue. The sulcus is lined by epithelium. On the papillary side, the epithelium contains numerous taste buds (number varies with species).

Tubulo-acinar serous glands (**Ebner's glands, gustatory glands**) lie deep to the vallate papillae, between the tela submucosa and muscle fibre bundles. Their secretory product passes through a branched system of ducts into the base of the sulcus. Continuous production of secretion ensures that dissolved nutrients within the saliva are constantly washed from the surface of the taste buds, allowing new gustatory sensations to be detected.

Foliate papillae are located laterally near the root of the tongue. They are well developed in the horse, less so in pigs and carnivores and absent in ruminants. These gustatory papillae consist of folds of mucous membrane separated by transverse furrows (Figure 10.9). The walls of the furrows house numerous **taste buds**. Dense accumulations of gustatory glands, similar in structure and

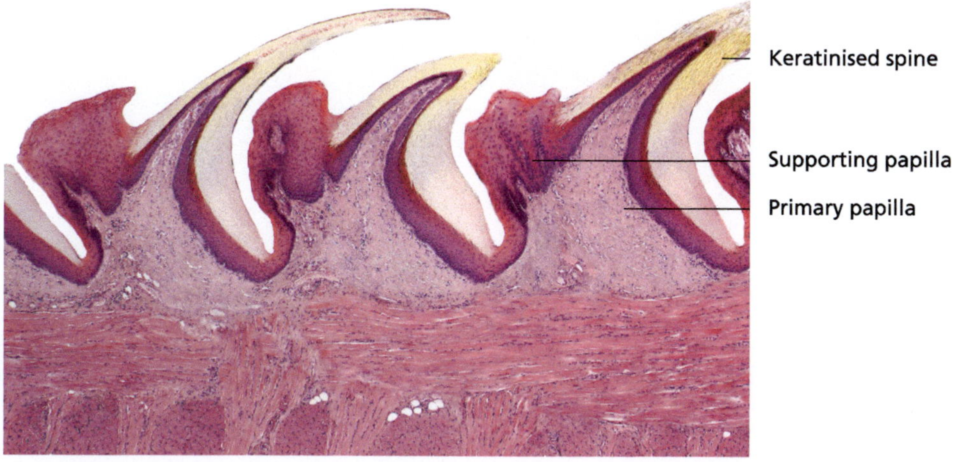

10.7 Filiform papilla (cat). This mechanical papilla is characterised by an aborally directed, conical spine arising from a primary papilla. An additional, supportive papilla lies on the oral aspect of the primary papilla. Haematoxylin and eosin stain (x32).

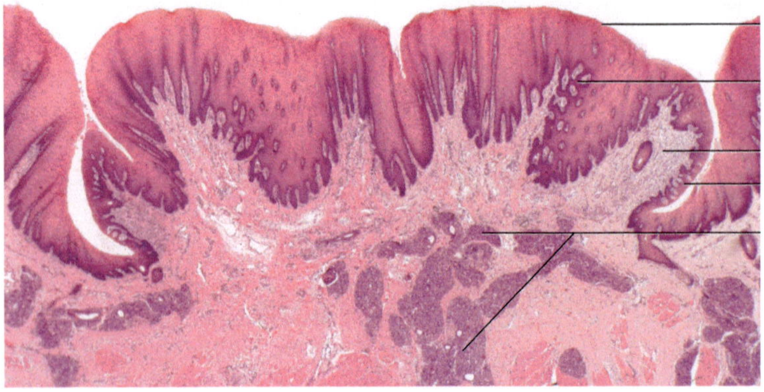

10.8 Vallate papilla (goat). These prominent papillae contain intra-epithelial taste buds and are underlaid by serous glands (Ebner's glands). Haematoxylin and eosin stain (x32).

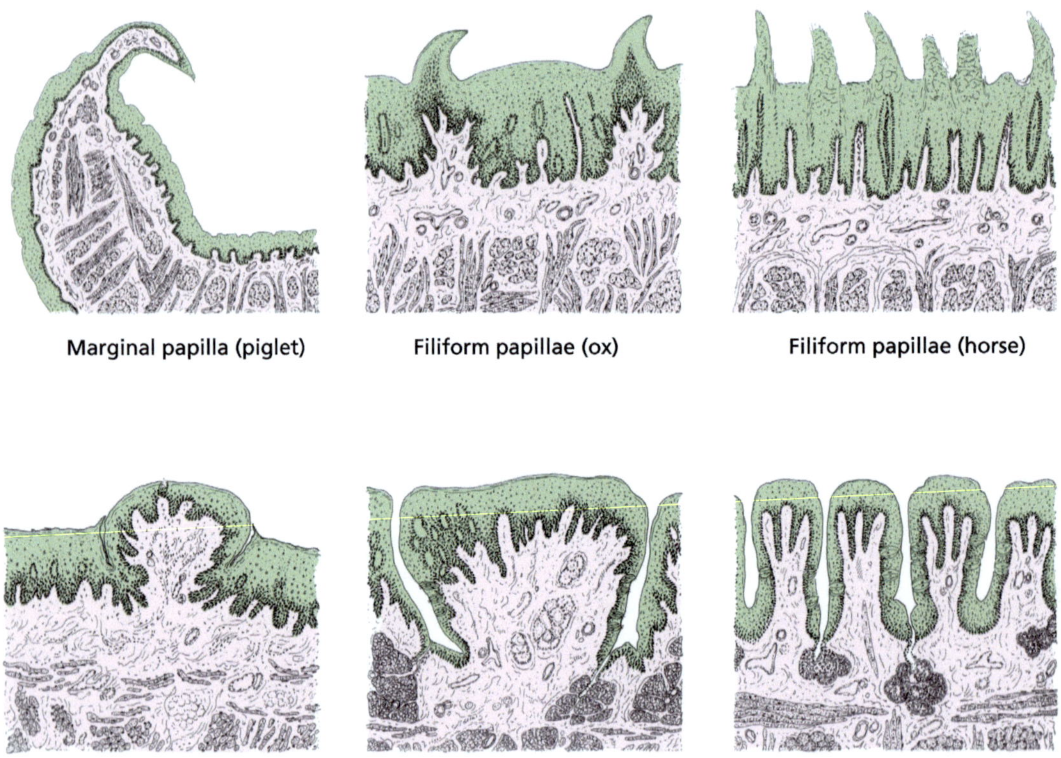

10.9 Lingual papillae (schematic).

function to those associated with vallate papillae, are present beneath the furrows.

The root of the tongue contains **lymphoid tissue** that contributes to cellular immune responses within the oral cavity. In horses and cattle, this tissue occurs in organised form as tonsils (**tonsillae lingualis**). Isolated lingual tonsils are also found in pigs. The lingual tonsils of small ruminants consist mainly of lymphoid tissue within the core of vallate papillae. In carnivores, only diffuse aggregates of lymphoid tissue and individual lymphoid nodules are observed.

Innervation and blood supply of the tongue

The hypoglossal nerve (XII) supplies motor **innervation** to the tongue. Mechanical, thermal and special sensory stimuli (touch, pain, temperature and taste) are conveyed by the mandibular branch of the trigeminal nerve (V) and the facial nerve (VII), glossopharyngeal nerve (IX) and vagus (X) nerve.

Blood supply to the tongue comprises dense capillary networks that tend to accumulate in subepithelial sheets. The margins of the tongue are particularly well vascularised. **Mixed glands** lie along the lateral margins of the tongue in horses and cattle.

Tooth (dens)

Working in concert with the lips, tongue, upper and lower jaw and masticatory muscles, the teeth serve in the prehension and breakdown of food. The dentition of the domestic mammals varies with species, the structure of the teeth being influenced by diet. Despite these differences, teeth are consistent in their basic structure (Figures 10.10 to 10.12), consisting of the:

- crown (corona dentis),
- neck (cervix dentis) and
- root (radix dentis).

The **crown** of the tooth is the visible (free, distal) portion that protrudes beyond the gingiva. The **neck** is surrounded by the gingiva. The **root** is the proximal portion of the tooth, which is embedded in the alveoli of the maxilla and mandible. These divisions are obvious in brachydont teeth. Hypsodont teeth (teeth of horses, cheek teeth of ruminants), in which the neck is hard to distinguish, may be described as consisting of a root and an elongated body.

The mineralised wall of the tooth surrounds the **pulp cavity** (**cavum dentis**), which encloses the central **dental pulp** (**pulpa dentis**). Towards the proximal end of the tooth, the pulp cavity narrows to become the **root canal** (**canalis radicis dentis**) that ends in the **apical foramen** (**foramen apicale dentis**) (Figure 10.12). The apical foramen is traversed by nerves and blood vessels entering and leaving the pulp.

In this region, odontoblasts (see below) produce predentin and contribute to the mineralisation of the **tooth root** (**root dentin**). External to the dentin is a bone-like substance, termed cementum, that is produced throughout life by cementoblasts.

The **crown** consists, from exterior to interior, of:

- enamel (enamelum),
- dentin (dentinum) and
- pulp (pulpa coronalis) within the pulp cavity (cavum coronalis dentis).

Enamel (enamelum)

Enamel is the hardest tissue within the body. It forms the outer layer of the crown of brachydont teeth and is located beneath a layer of cementum in hypsodont teeth (see *Veterinary Anatomy of Domestic Mammals: Textbook and Colour Atlas*).

Enamel is **acellular** and is composed of hexagonal to polygonal **enamel prisms** (**prismata enameli**) (Figures 10.10 and 10.11). It develops from an enamel matrix formed embryonically as the secretory product of **ectodermal ameloblasts** (**enameloblasts**). During embryonic development, ameloblasts are a component of the externally oriented enamel organ and spread to form a sheet of simple columnar epithelium. Their cytoplasm is eosinophilic, the nuclei strongly basophilic.

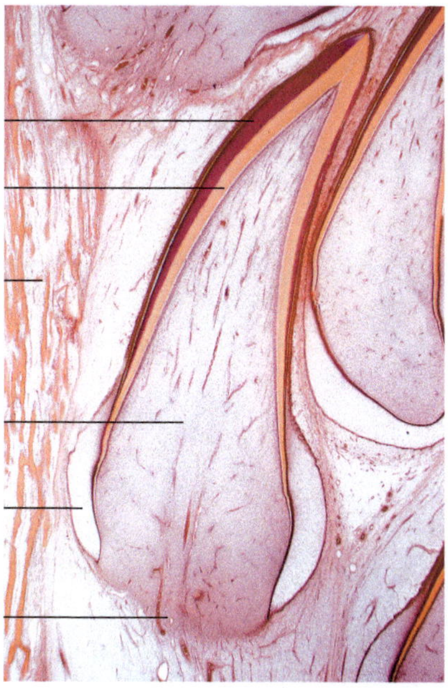

10.10 Tooth of a calf during embryonic development. Haematoxylin and eosin stain (x14).

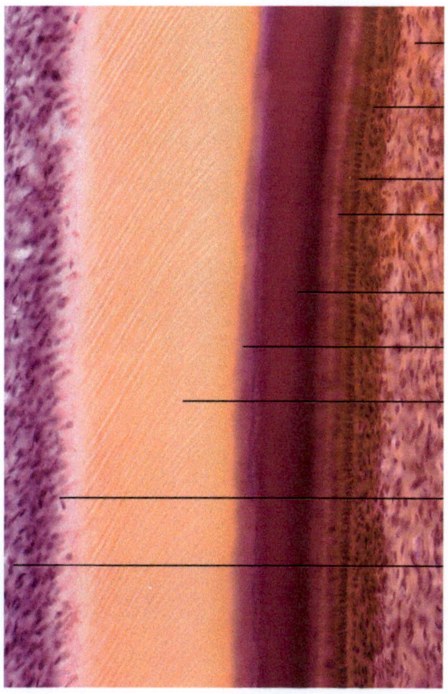

10.11 Wall of the tooth of a calf during embryonic development. Haematoxylin and eosin stain (x120).

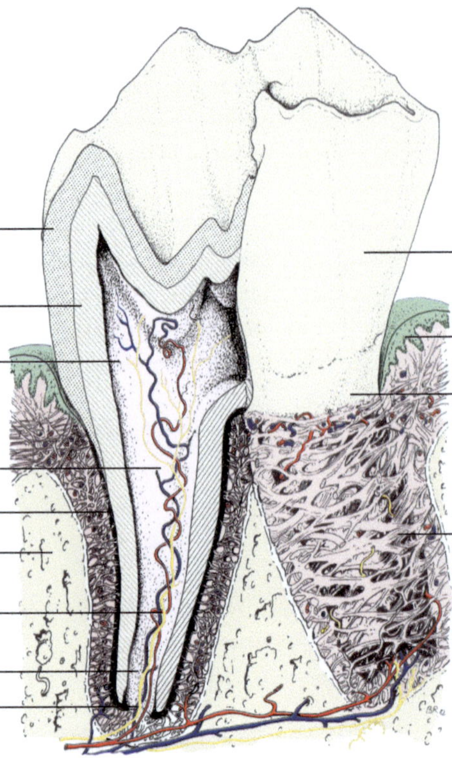

10.12 Structure of a tooth and supporting tissues (schematic).

The **enamel matrix** is composed of non-collagenous proteins (e.g. proline, glycine, leucine and histidine), glycoproteins and glycosaminoglycans. Through accumulation of inorganic substances (calcium and phosphates), together with processes performed by ameloblasts, the enamel matrix is transformed into **crystals** that form the structural foundation of the **enamel prisms**.

Enamel prisms (diameter 5–9 μm) are composed of up to 99% **hydroxyapatite crystals** (crystallum hydroxyapatiti), the remainder comprising an **organic matrix**. The prisms are arranged in groups that follow a spiral or curved course. Groups of prisms exhibit synchronous decussation on their path from the internal to the external surface of the enamel. This is demonstrated by the optical phenomenon known as Hunter–Schreger bands, observed when longitudinally sectioned enamel is visualised under reflected light.

Bands running parallel to the surface of the tooth (**striae of Retzius**) represent incremental growth of enamel during development. Enamel prisms exhibit a superficial groove. They are held together by enamel crystals.

Dentin (dentinum)

Dentin is harder than bone, but not as hard as enamel. It surrounds the pulp cavity, underlying the enamel in the crown, and the cementum in the root (Figure 10.12). At the occlusal surface of the cheek teeth and incisors of horses, and cheek teeth of ruminants, dentin is exposed between the enamel crests. Dentin is produced by a layer of **mesenchymal odontoblasts** located peripherally in the dental pulp (Figures 10.10 and 10.11). Pronounced, laterally branching **cytoplasmic processes** (**dentinal fibres**) extend from the odontoblasts. Odontoblasts produce **predentin**, comprising ground substance (including glycoproteins and glycosaminoglycans) and collagen. The mesodermal odontoblasts are arranged radially with respect to the ectodermal ameloblasts.

Through their processes, odontoblasts also secrete membrane-bound granules containing calcium and phosphate. In a process resembling ossification, the contents of the granules condense around collagen fibres as **apatite** crystals, leading to **mineralisation of the pre-dentin** to form **dentin.** Odontoblast processes lie within channels termed **dentinal tubules** (**tubuli dentinales**). The processes are immediately surrounded by mineralised dentin (**dentinum peritubulare**). Non-mineralised regions of predentin are referred to as **interglobular dentin** (refer to embryology texts).

In its final form, dentin consists of approximately 70% **inorganic substances** (hydroxyapatite crystals) and 30% **organic matter** (predominantly collagen and ground substance). The odontoblast processes enclosed in mineralised dentinal tubules permit the transfer of substances involved in metabolism to the inner portion of the dentin. Free nerve endings accompany odontoblast processes, gaining access to the dentin via dentinal tubules.

The dentin immediately surrounding dentinal tubules is the most highly mineralised. Intertubular dentin is less dense and is rich in collagen fibres. The outermost portion of dentin, known as **mantle dentin**, is separated from the overlying enamel by a basal lamina (formerly membrana praeformativa).

Dental pulp (pulpa coronalis)

The dental pulp lies within the pulp cavity. Its original mesenchymal characteristics are retained into adulthood (Figure 10.12). The constituents of dental pulp include loose connective tissue, blood vessels and nerve fibre bundles. Lymphatic vessels are absent. Myelinated and unmyelinated nerve fibres extend along the processes of odontoblasts into the dentinal tubules. The structural core of the dental pulp comprises a delicate network of type III collagen fibres in which fibroblasts and reticular cells are embedded. Odontoblasts form a layer at the periphery. Abundant amorphous ground substance is also present.

The odontoblasts in the outer dental pulp produce dentin throughout the life of the organism. The pulp cavity thus becomes smaller with age, with concomitant reduction in metabolic exchange.

Towards its proximal end, the pulp cavity narrows to form the **root canal** (**canalis radicis dentis**), which ends in the **apical foramen** (**foramen apicale dentis**) (Figure 10.12). Nerves and blood vessels enter and leave the pulp cavity through this opening.

Attachment apparatus of the teeth

The tissues involved in the attachment of the teeth are the:

- cementum,
- periodontal ligament and
- alveolar bone.

CEMENTUM

Cementum (Figure 10.12) forms by appositional growth on the outer surface of the root of brachydont teeth, and over the entire length of hypsodont teeth. Resembling bone in its structure, cementum is composed of **cementocytes** (**cementocyti**) and **mineralised organic matrix**. Near the enamel margin, the cementum is acellular. Collagen fibres extend from the alveolar bone into the cementum (Sharpey's fibres, see below).

PERIODONTAL LIGAMENT

The periodontal ligament consists predominantly of **collagen fibres** (**Sharpey's fibres**) that traverse the space between the alveolar bone and the cementum (Figure 10.12). The orientation of fibre bundles varies in different portions of the ligament. The fibres are firmly bound to the tooth, anchoring it to the alveolus and aiding in the absorption of compressive forces.

In addition to collagen fibres, the periodontal ligament contains fibroblasts that replenish its collagen content. Other cells present in the periodontal ligament include cementoblasts, cementocytes, osteoblasts and osteoclasts. The periodontal ligament is vascularised and contains free nerve endings that serve as pressure and pain sensors.

ALVEOLAR BONE

Alveolar bone, to which the tooth is connected by the periodontal ligament (Figure 10.12), is composed of lamellar bone that is perforated to facilitate the passage of blood vessels and nerves to and from the dental pulp.

Salivary glands (glandulae oris)

The salivary glands develop from cordlike down-growths of the epithelium of the oral mucosa into the underlying tela submucosa. Their ends branch to form compound tubulo-acinar secretory organs. Secondary lumen formation gives rise to the excretory system of ducts through which the secretions of the salivary glands are conveyed to the mucosal surface.

The secretory product, saliva, performs various functions including lubrication of the non-glandular oral mucosa and foodstuffs during mastication, thus aiding the swallowing of solids. Dissolution of water-soluble nutrients in saliva facilitates gustation and sensory investigation of food. The large volumes of alkaline saliva produced by ruminants (approximately 90–180 l per day in cattle) assist in neutralising short-chain fatty acids produced by microbial fermentation in the rumen. In the pig, the saliva is rich in amylase, an enzyme involved in the breakdown of carbohydrate.

Saliva contains immunoglobulin A and lactoperoxidase, and thus also has a role in immune defence.

Secretion of saliva is under neural (sympathetic, parasympathetic) and hormonal control. Sympathetic stimulation produces saliva rich in organic compounds, while the saliva secreted under parasympathetic stimulation (cranial nerves VII, IX and X) is watery and thin.

In addition, production of saliva is influenced by the smell, taste and composition of food, and by the process of swallowing. In the dog, dry food induces the synthesis of watery saliva whereas moist food promotes a more viscous secretion.

Salivary gland structure

Based on their size and location, the salivary glands are divided into the **minor salivary glands** (**glandulae salivariae minores**) and **major salivary glands** (**glandulae salivariae majores**). Located within the tela submucosa of the oral cavity, the minor salivary glands comprise the glands of the lips, cheeks, tongue and palate. These are included in the description of the individual components of the oral cavity.

The **major salivary glands** are connected to the oral cavity by a system of excretory ducts. They include the:

- parotid salivary gland (glandula parotis),
- mandibular salivary gland (glandula mandibularis),
- sublingual glands (glandulae sublinguales):
  - glandula sublingualis monostomatica and
  - glandula sublingualis polystomatica.

All salivary glands (Figures 10.13 to 10.17) are invested by a **connective tissue capsule** (**capsula glandularis**). Septa composed of collagen fibre bundles (septa interlobaria and septa interlobularia) extend into the gland tissue, giving rise to lobules of varying size. Vessels, autonomic nerves and portions of the duct system course within the connective tissue.

The **secretory product** is produced in **acinar or tubulo-acinar end pieces** and may be **mucous**, **serous** or **mixed** (Figures 10.14 and 10.15) (see Chapter 2, 'Epithelial tissue', 'Glandular epithelium'). Secretion occurs by the **merocrine** mode.

The glandular end pieces are surrounded by modified contractile epithelial cells, referred to as **myoepithelial cells** or **basket cells**. These cells lie within the basal lamina of the secretory epithelial cells. The product of the glandular epithelial cells passes into a **system of ducts** lined by cuboidal to columnar epithelium. Structural features common to the major salivary glands include:

- **acinar or tubulo-acinar end pieces:**
  - serous, mucous or mixed,
  - presence of myoepithelial cells,
  - merocrine mode of secretion,
- **intralobular ducts:**
  - located within a lobule,
  - intercalated duct (simple cuboidal) and striated duct (simple columnar),
- **interlobular, interlobar and main ducts:**
  - epithelium changes from simple to bi-layered columnar to stratified cuboidal to columnar; terminally the epithelium is stratified squamous,
  - smooth muscle cells and
  - goblet cells (main ducts).

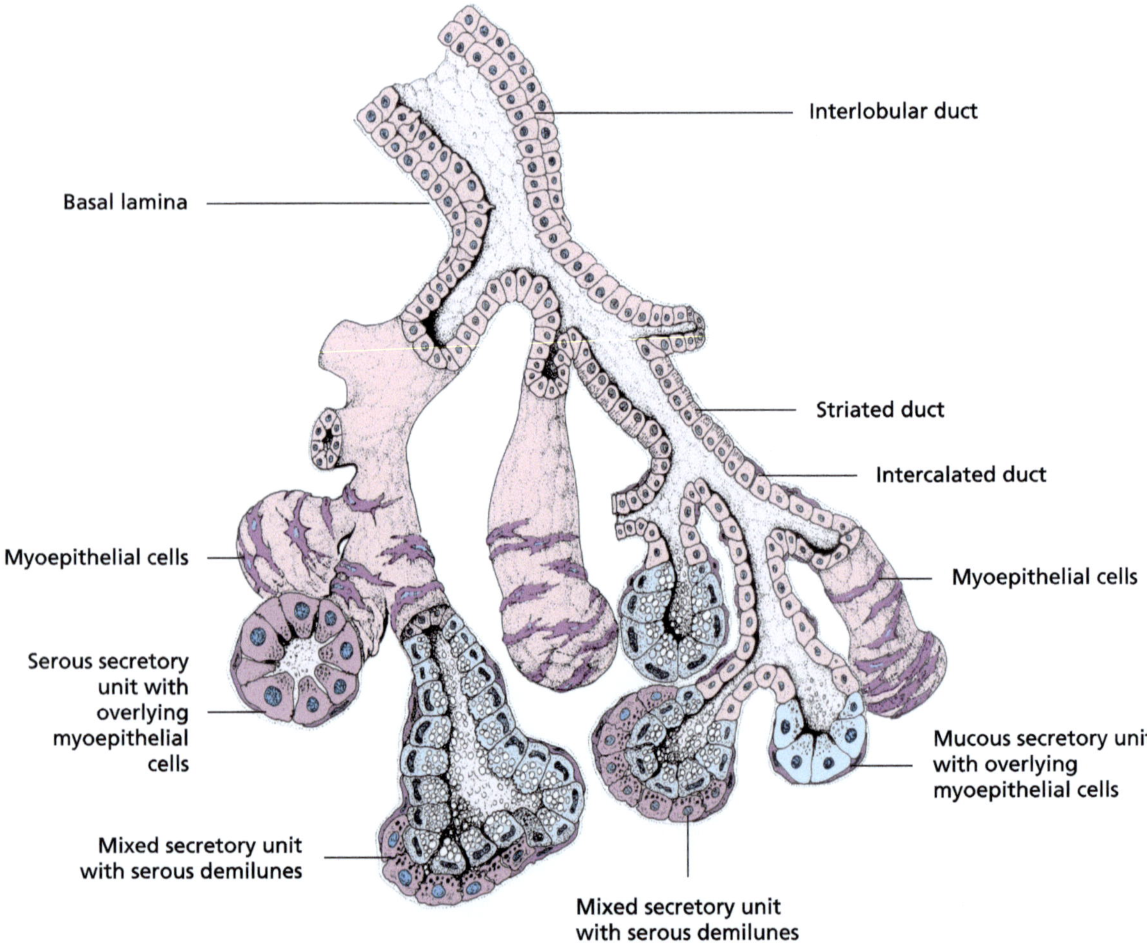

10.13 Structure of a tubulo-acinar compound salivary gland with serous, mucous and mixed end pieces (schematic).

The duct system begins at the **secretory end piece** with the **intralobular ducts**. These are composed of the **intercalated duct**, into which the secretory unit empties, and the **striated duct**, so named because of basal striations in the columnar epithelium (Figures 10.13 to 10.15 and 10.17).

Outside the small glandular lobules, intralobular ducts are continued by interlobular ducts (Figures 10.13 and 10.16), interlobar and main ducts. Smooth muscle cells are found outside the larger ducts. The stratified epithelium of main ducts contains occasional goblet cells. The size of the lumen gradually increases from the intercalated duct to the main duct (Figure 10.13).

Parotid salivary gland

The parotid gland is a compound acinar gland. In most domestic mammals it is a **serous gland**, though isolated mucous secretory units may occur peripherally in carnivores. The principal organelles within the acidophilic, granular cytoplasm of the secretory cells (see Figure 2.46) are mitochondria and organelles associated with protein synthesis (ribosomes and polyribosomes, rough ER). Apically, the area of the secretory cell surface is increased by numerous microvilli.

The low cuboidal epithelium of the **intercalated ducts** becomes columnar in the **striated duct**. The basal striations from which the ducts derive their name are visible with the light microscope. They are formed by regular infoldings of the plasmalemma enclosing stacks of mitochondria. The presence of an enlarged surface area

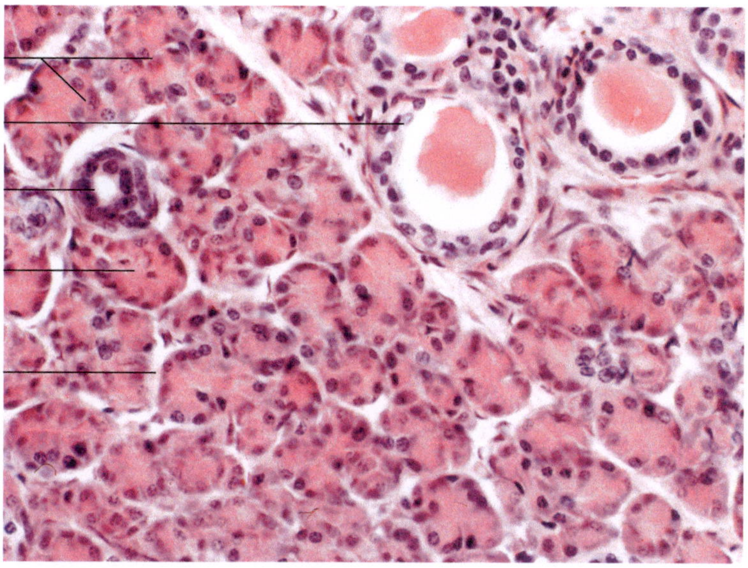

10.14 Parotid salivary gland (horse). Haematoxylin and eosin stain (x300).

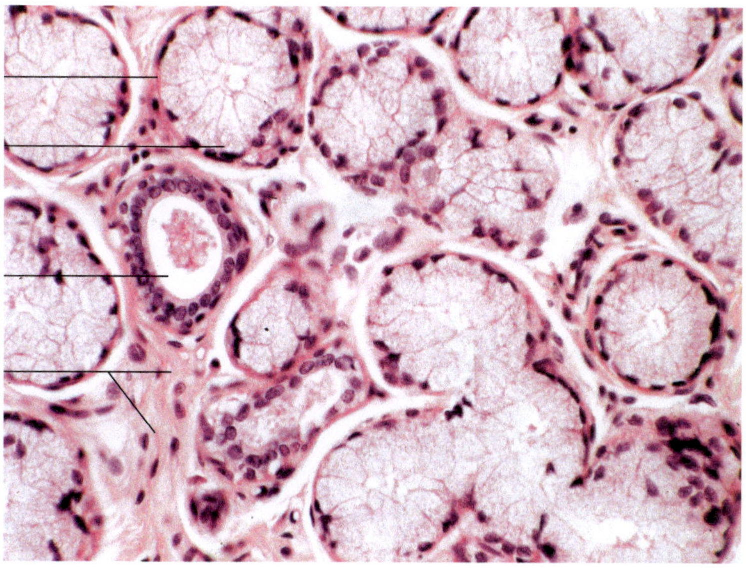

10.15 Predominantly mucous mandibular salivary gland in a dog. Haematoxylin and eosin stain (x300).

and energy-producing mitochondria facilitates **absorption of water and sodium ions**, and excretion of potassium into the duct lumen. Capillary networks surrounding the striated ducts participate in the reabsorption of fluid and ions from the saliva. Striated ducts thus serve to thicken the saliva and regulate its electrolyte content.

Mandibular salivary gland

In the horse, pig and ruminant, the tubulo-acinar mandibular gland is a **mixed gland** while in carnivores it is predominantly **mucous** (Figure 10.15). In the mixed form, serous and mucous cells frequently occur in the same secretory unit, though separate serous and mixed units may be present. In mixed units, mucous cells appear to be capped by **serous demilunes**. Recent findings suggest that these serous cells are in the same row as mucous cells, and that the 'demilune' shape is a fixation artefact. Mucus-secreting cells have a foamy basophilic cytoplasm and a basal nucleus. The lumen is relatively large. Mucous glands contain fewer intercalated ducts and striated ducts, as mucus does not undergo modification in the duct system.

Sublingual salivary glands

In domestic mammals, the sublingual gland (Figures 10.16 and 10.17) is a compound tubulo-acinar **mixed, predominantly mucous, gland**.

> **Species variation**
>
> **Birds**: Particularly in granivores, the salivary glands play an important part in moistening food. The **maxil-**

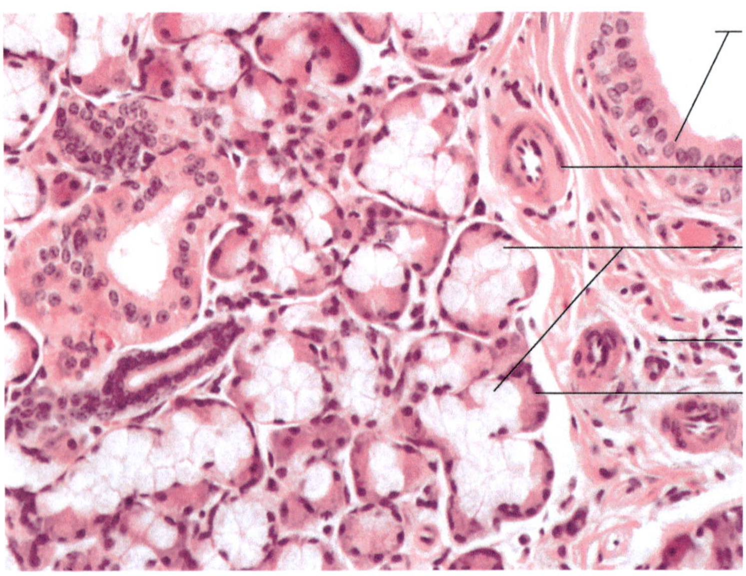

10.16 Branched tubulo-acinar mixed sublingual gland (ox). Haematoxylin and eosin stain (x300).

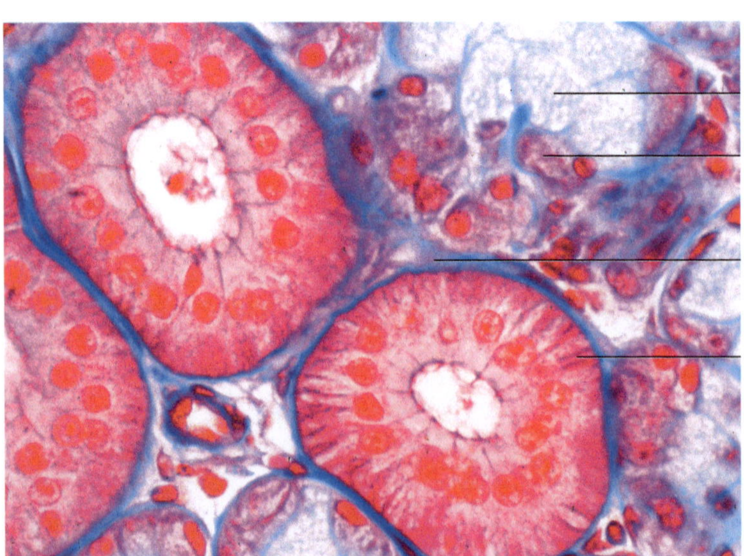

10.17 Striated duct in a mixed sublingual gland (ox). Azan stain (x480).

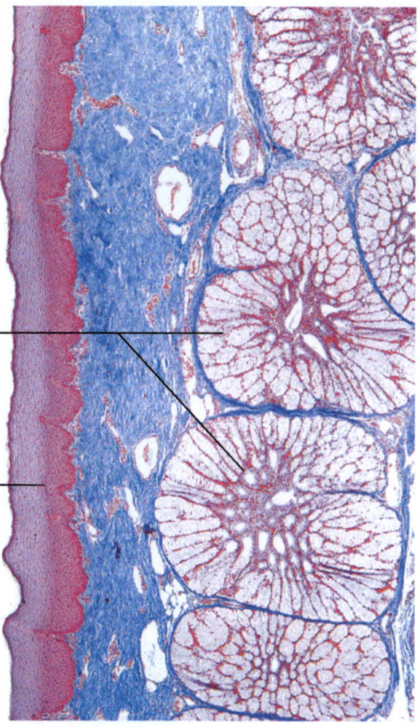

10.18 Floor of the mouth with mucous glands (chicken). Azan stain (x40).

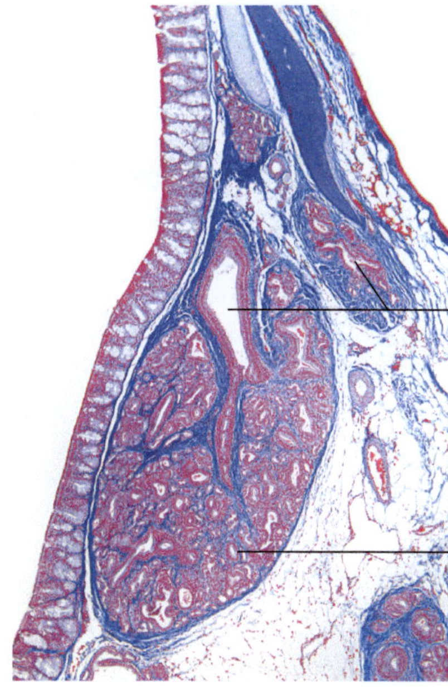

10.19 Pharyngeal glands (chicken). Azan stain (x40).

lary gland (**glandula maxillaris**) is located rostrally in the roof of the mouth. It empties via a duct caudal to the bill tip organ of the upper beak. An abundance of taste buds surrounds the duct orifice. At the angle of the mouth, the glandula angularis oris is similarly drained by a single duct. The palate contains the openings of multiple ducts of the lateral and medial palatine glands (glandulae palatinae). Numerous taste buds surround these orifices. The secretions of the mandibular glands (glandulae mandibulares) (Figure 10.18) and lingual glands (glandulae linguales) pass through many ducts to the floor of the mouth. Additional glands, located more caudally, empty into the oropharynx via several ducts (Figure 10.19).

Pharynx

Due to its relationship to the nasal and oral cavities, the epithelium of the pharynx varies with region. In the nasopharynx, the **pharyngeal mucosa** is lined by pseudostratified ciliated epithelium containing goblet cells. Serous and mixed glands are present in the propria-submucosa.

The epithelium of the **oropharyngeal mucosa** is stratified squamous. The lamina propria encloses lymphoid tissue that varies with species in its degree of organisation (lymphoid follicles, tonsils) (see *Veterinary Anatomy of Domestic Mammals: Textbook and Colour Atlas*). The connective tissue layer is underlaid by elastic fibres and merges indistinctly with a tela submucosa containing mucous glands.

External to the pharyngeal submucosa is an inner fascial layer, a layer of striated muscle, an outer fascial layer and a tunica adventitia.

Tubular digestive organs

The tubular digestive organs can be divided into cranial (oesophagus and stomach), middle (duodenum, jejunum, ileum) and caudal (caecum, colon, rectum) portions and the **anal canal** (Figure 10.1).

Structure of tubular digestive organs

Except for regional, functionally determined specialisations, the wall of tubular digestive organs is consistent in its basic structure (Figure 10.20). From interior to exterior, it is composed of the following layers:

- **tunica mucosa:**
  - epithelium (epithelium mucosae),
  - lamina propria (lamina propria mucosae),
  - muscular lamina (lamina muscularis mucosae),
- **tela submucosa,**
- **tunica muscularis:**
  - circular layer (stratum circulare),
  - longitudinal layer (stratum longitudinale) and
- **tunica adventitia.**

Within body cavities, the following layers are present in place of a tunica adventitia:

- **tela subserosa,**
- **tunica serosa:**
  - lamina propria serosae and
  - epithelium (mesothelium serosae).

These layers form a **musculomembranous** tube that also occurs in similar form elsewhere in the body (e.g. urinary tract).

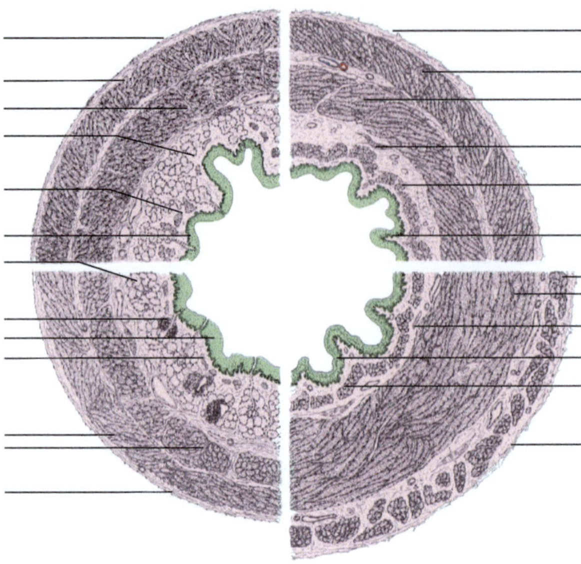

10.20 Comparative structure of the oesophagus (schematic) (refer to text).

Tunica mucosa

The tunica mucosa lines the internal surface of the tubular digestive organs. As well as providing protection, the mucosal epithelium contributes to the synthesis of digestive enzymes and absorption of nutrients. The underlying mucosal layers participate in these functions (see below). A continuous basal lamina separates the epithelium from the lamina propria mucosae. A distinction is made between:

- **glandular mucosa (tunica mucosa glandularis):**
  - simple columnar epithelium,
  - lamina propria mucosae with glands,
  - lamina muscularis mucosae and
- **non-glandular mucosa (tunica mucosa non-glandularis):**
  - papillated stratified squamous epithelium,
  - lamina propria mucosae lacking glands (when glands are present, they are located in the tela submucosa) and, in some cases,
  - lamina muscularis mucosae.

Glandular mucosa is lined by a **simple columnar epithelium** with microvilli. It forms the internal layer of the wall of the monogastric stomach (non-glandular regions are also present in the horse and pig) and of the intestine, where it performs secretory and absorptive functions. By secretion of mucus, for example, the epithelium protects the epithelial cells in the stomach from gastric acid. In the intestine, the epithelium absorbs various substances including amino acids, glucose, fatty acids, water, vitamins and electrolytes.

The epithelium is supported by the underlying **lamina propria mucosae**, which is composed of loose connective tissue and houses blood and lymph vessels, nerves, immune cells, mast cells and isolated smooth muscle cells. **Tubular glands** protrude into the lamina propria. Their cuboidal to columnar epithelial cells secrete various substances including hormones. The **lamina muscularis mucosae** is the deepest layer of the mucosa, lying adjacent to the tela submucosa. It contains smooth muscle cells.

The **non-glandular mucosa** is characterised by a papillated **stratified squamous epithelium**. Glands are absent in the **lamina propria mucosae**. The lamina muscularis mucosae may be continuous, intermittent or lacking. Occasional glands are located in the tela submucosa, **deep to the non-glandular mucosa**. Non-glandular mucosa is present in the oral cavity, pharynx, oesophagus, forestomachs, non-glandular region of the stomach and in parts of the anus, where it has a protective function.

Tela submucosa

The tela submucosa consists of loose connective tissue containing abundant blood and lymph vessels, and multipolar nerve cells within **autonomic ganglia (Meissner's plexus, plexus nervorum submucosus)**. The plexus nervorum submucosus sends nerve fibres to the lamina propria mucosae, giving rise to a subepithelial neural network. These nerve fibres provide autonomic innervation to the **glandular cells in the mucosa**, and to **smooth muscle cells** located in the muscular layer and in the walls of blood vessels. They also form synapses with nerve processes extending from the plexus nervorum myentericus.

Bundles of collagen fibres in the tela submucosa are arranged predominantly in lattice-like layers. This permits the tissue to adapt to changes in volume and weight within the gastrointestinal tract. The tela submucosa thus serves both to supply the physiological requirements of the adjacent layers, and to enable these layers to move and flex with respect to one another. It also supports the longitudinal progression of ingesta through the digestive tract.

The tela submucosa contains abundant **free immune cells** (macrophages, lymphocytes and plasma cells), diffuse lymphatic tissue and lymphoid follicles, reflecting the continuous immune responses occurring in the tubular digestive organs. Together with the lamina propria, the tela submucosa plays an important role in immune defence because the mucosa is constantly exposed to microorganisms including bacteria and viruses. Foreign animal and vegetable proteins entering the gastrointestinal tract may also elicit innate and adaptive immune responses. Proteins lose their antigenic effect only after they have been enzymatically degraded into amino acids, which are then absorbed across the mucosa.

Tunica muscularis

Except for species-specific modifications in the oesophagus and anus, the tunica muscularis is composed of **smooth muscle** comprising an **inner circular layer** (**stratum circulare**) and an **outer longitudinal layer** (**stratum longitudinale**). In the oesophagus, smooth muscle may be replaced by striated muscle. Blood and lymphatic vessels course between the muscular layers. **Autonomic ganglia** (**Auerbach plexus**, **plexus nervorum myentericus**) are also present.

Chemical and mechanical stimuli activate the **plexus nervorum myentericus**, from which efferent impulses act upon muscle cells of the tunica muscularis and vessel walls, and on glands. This intramural autonomic system is regulated by sympathetic and parasympathetic nerve fibres. Sympathetic fibres have an inhibitory effect on the plexus nervorum myentericus (relaxation of smooth muscle) and result in vasoconstriction. Parasympathetic fibres acting on the plexus nervorum myentericus increase gut motility and promote glandular secretion.

The muscle layers are responsible for aboral transport of ingesta, via waves of contraction that take place along varying lengths of the tract. Peristaltic contractions also promote mixing of the ingesta with digestive enzymes.

Tunica adventitia

The tunica adventitia consists of loose connective tissue and serves to connect the tubular digestive organs with surrounding tissues. It encloses vessels, nerve fibres, nerve plexuses and adipose tissue. In regions outside the pleural and peritoneal cavities (neck, caudal pelvic cavity) it forms the outermost layer of the digestive tract.

Tunica serosa

Within the pleural and peritoneal cavities (including the cranial pelvic cavity) the exterior of the tubular digestive organs is coated with tunica serosa. This is composed of a superficial layer of simple squamous epithelium which, due to its mesodermal origin, is also referred to as **mesothelium**. The primary functions of the mesothelium are pinocytotic absorption and phagocytosis of substances in the body cavities, and secretion of serous fluid. The mesothelium is connected to the underlying layers of the digestive tract by a thin connective tissue **lamina propria serosae**, which also facilitates movement of adjacent layers with respect to one another. A tela subserosa composed of loose connective tissue lies between the tunica serosa and the tunica muscularis.

Oesophagus

The oesophagus transports food from the pharynx to the stomach. This is achieved by peristaltic contraction of the muscles in its wall. Accordingly, the tunica muscularis is

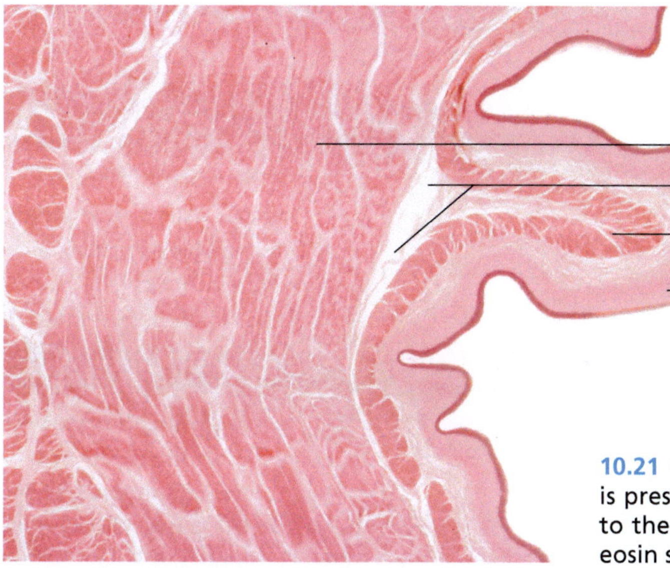

10.21 Oesophagus (horse). A lamina muscularis mucosae is present throughout. The tunica muscularis is striated to the level of the root of the lung. Haematoxylin and eosin stain (x12).

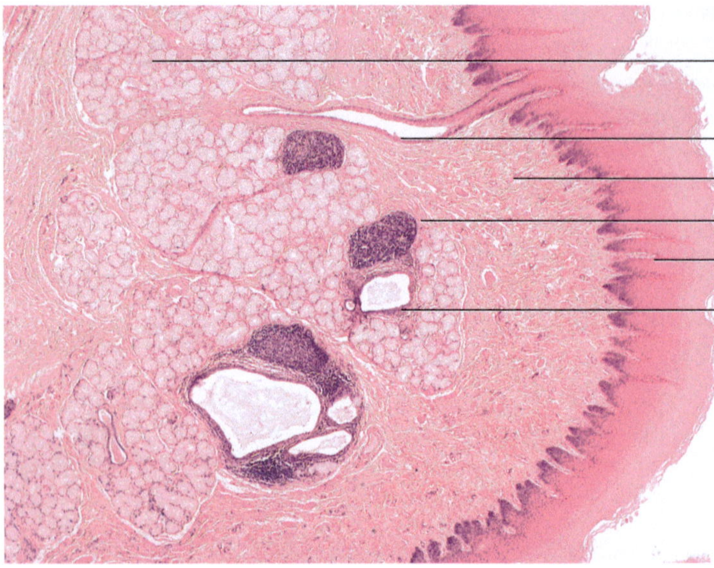

10.22 Proximal oesophagus (pig). In the pig, glands are present mainly in the cranial half of the oesophagus. Haematoxylin and eosin stain (x40).

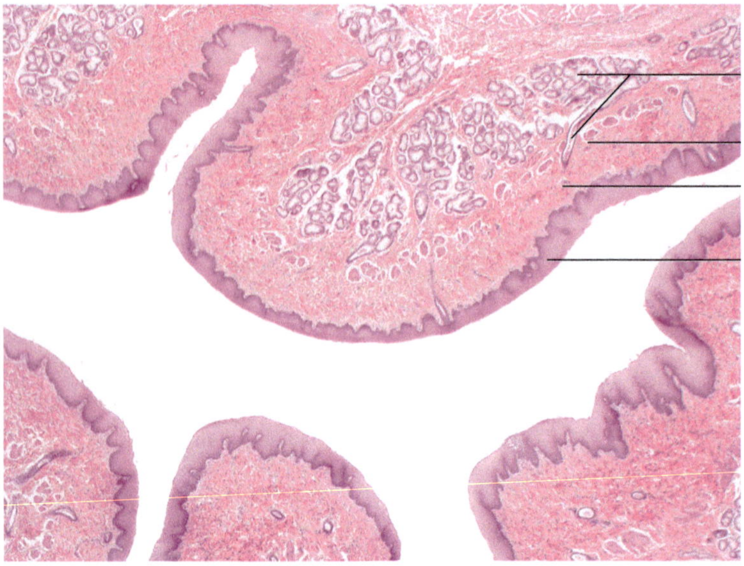

10.23 Distal oesophagus (dog). The lamina muscularis mucosae begins in the distal half of the oesophagus, and submucosal glands are present throughout. Haematoxylin and eosin stain (x20).

well developed. The oesophagus exhibits the typical wall structure of the tubular digestive organs, though considerable species-related differences are evident (Figures 10.21 to 10.23 and Table 10.1).

Connective tissue cushions within the tela submucosa give rise to irregular **longitudinal mucosal folds** that protrude into the lumen of the oesophagus. The height of the folds is increased by contraction of smooth muscle cells in the tunica muscularis. The oesophagus is lined by a papillated, **thick stratified squamous epithelium**. A thin lamina muscularis mucosae is usually present around the lamina propria. The thickness of the mucosa varies with species, depending on the composition of the diet. Keratinisation of the epithelium also exhibits species variation and appears to be influenced by other factors including diet. Least keratinisation is observed in carnivores and birds.

The **submucosa** is a thick connective tissue layer containing abundant collagen and elastic fibres. This layer houses mucous or mixed, tubulo-acinar **oesophageal glands** (**glandulae oesophageae propriae**), the distribution and structure of which varies with region and species. The excretory ducts are lined with cuboidal epithelium. Accumulations of **lymphoid cells** are seen near the glands. Particularly in the pig, lymphoid follicles are evident (Figure 10.22).

Table 10.1 Comparative histological structure of the wall of the oesophagus.

Epithelium	Glands	Musculature	Special features
Domestic mammals			
Stratified squamous epithelium	Tubulo-acinar mucous or mixed glands in the tela submucosa – proximally in most domestic mammals; throughout the length of the oesophagus in the dog	Thin lamina muscularis mucosae (absent cranially in the dog); inner circular and outer longitudinal layers in tunica muscularis, striated muscle cranially, smooth muscle caudally in most species; sphincter at entrance to stomach	In the cat and horse, striated muscle extends for most of length of oesophagus; in dogs and ruminants, muscle is entirely striated; lymphoid follicles abundant in the submucosa in pigs
Birds			
Stratified squamous epithelium	Tubular in the rhea, alveolar in owls, tubulo-acinar in chickens	Tunica muscularis: inner circular layer and outer longitudinal layer (lacking in some species; refer to text)	Oesophageal tonsils at distal end of oesophagus; structure of wall of oesophagus extends into the crop

The **tunica muscularis** is composed of an inner circular and an outer longitudinal layer. Muscle fibre bundles are predominantly arranged in elongated spirals that appear oblique in histological section. The bundles spiral in opposite directions, crossing over in some cases.

Depending on species, the muscle is smooth and/or striated. To accommodate the juxtaposition of different muscle types, collagen networks within the endomysium of the striated muscle cells merge with elastic tendons. These reduce the strong tensile force exerted by this muscle type, and interconnect with other fibro-elastic networks. The outer layer of the oesophagus comprises a **tunica adventitia** in the neck and a **tunica serosa** within the body cavities.

Species variation

Cat: A lamina muscularis mucosae is present throughout the length of the oesophagus; glands are limited to the pharyngo-oesophageal region. Striated muscle extends through to the distal third of the oesophagus before becoming smooth.

Dog: The lamina muscularis mucosae appears in the distal half of the oesophagus. Submucosal glands are present throughout. The tunica muscularis is composed entirely of striated muscle, smooth muscle only appearing at the entrance to the stomach (Figures 10.20 and 10.23).

Pig: The lamina muscularis mucosae appears in the distal half of the oesophagus. Submucosal glands extend to beyond halfway along the oesophagus; throughout much of the oesophagus the tunica muscularis comprises striated muscle, becoming smooth near the pars cardiaca of the stomach. The ducts of the oesophageal glands are commonly surrounded by lymphatic tissue (diffuse tissue or lymphoid follicles) (Figures 10.20 and 10.22).

Ruminants: The lamina muscularis mucosae is present throughout; submucosal glands are limited to the pharyngo-oesophageal region. The tunica muscularis consists entirely of striated muscle (Figure 10.20).

Horse: The lamina muscularis mucosae is present throughout. Submucosal glands are present only in the pharyngo-oesophageal region. To the level of the root of the lung, the tunica muscularis consists of striated muscle, gradually transitioning to smooth muscle thereafter (Figures 10.20 and 10.21).

Birds: The stratified epithelium varies considerably in thickness between avian species (Figures 10.24 to 10.26 and Table 10.1). The **lamina propria mucosae** contains numerous **mucous glands** that exhibit profound species-related structural variation. These may be tubular (e.g. rheas), alveolar (long-eared owls) or tubulo-alveolar (e.g. chickens). Regardless of species, the glandular epithelium is **columnar**. Lymphoid follicles (**tonsillae oesophagealis**) are present at the gastric end of the oesophagus. In chickens, the tunica muscularis consists of an inner circular and outer longitudinal layer of smooth muscle. In some species, the longitudinal layer is lacking; the circular layer and lamina muscularis mucosae are thickened in these birds. Shortly before passing into the body cavity, the oesophagus dilates to form the **crop**. In granivorous birds, the crop can be very large. The wall of the crop is similar in structure to the oesophagus (Figure 10.27). The mucous glands of the crop (**glandulae ingluviales**) resemble oesophageal glands. They are located near the 'crop channel' in chickens, and in the fundic region of the crop in pigeons.

The histological differences in the structure of the oesophagus are summarised in Table 10.1.

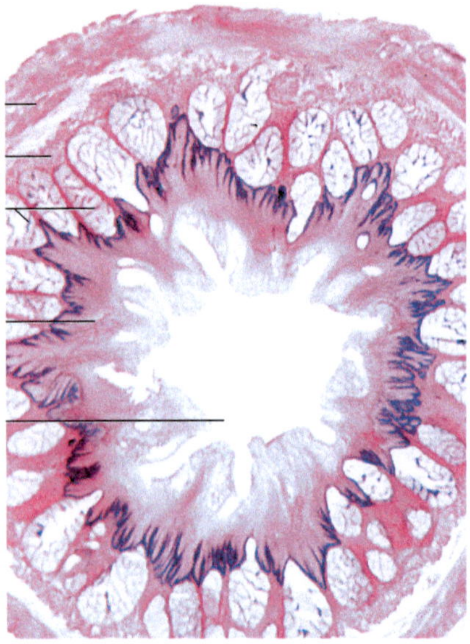

10.24 Oesophagus (chicken). Haematoxylin and eosin stain (x25).

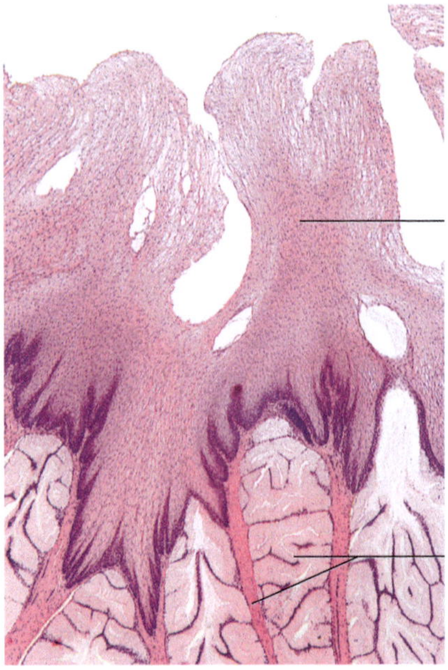

10.25 Oesophageal mucosa (chicken). Haematoxylin and eosin stain (x180).

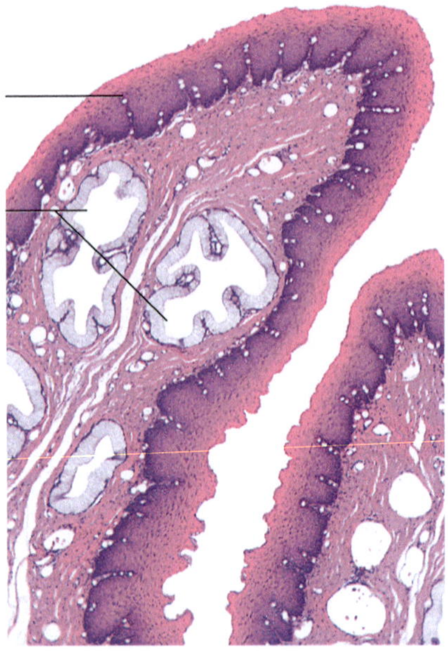

10.26 Oesophageal mucosa (duck). Haematoxylin and eosin stain (x100).

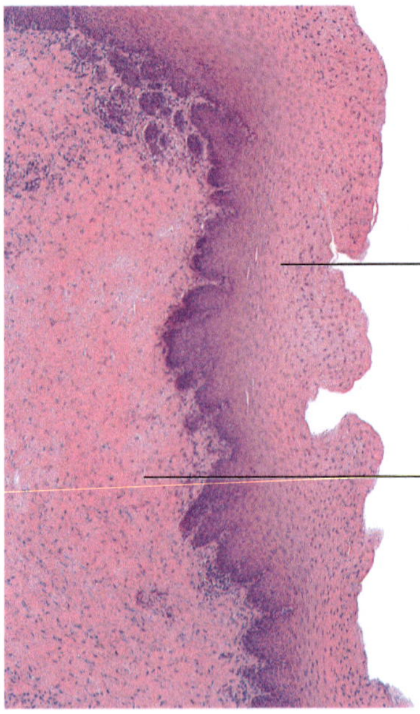

10.27 Crop mucosa (chicken). Haematoxylin and eosin stain (x180).

Stomach (gaster, ventriculus)

The stomach develops as a dilation of the primitive gut tube. Its function is to prepare ingested foodstuffs for delivery to the intestine, thus supporting the digestive function of the intestinal tract. Digestive processes that take place during the temporary storage of food in the stomach include breakdown of proteins and emulsification of fat by gastric secretions. Differences in the structure of the stomach, including the gastric mucosa, reflect the varying dietary strategies of the domestic mammals. Carnivores, omnivores and horses have a single-chambered stomach while the stomach of ruminants has multiple compartments.

The internal surface of the stomach is lined entirely by **glandular mucosa** (carnivores) or a combination of **glandular** and **non-glandular mucosa** (horses, pigs, ruminants) (Figure 10.29). In the horse, non-glandular mucosa is present in the saccus caecus, from which it continues a short distance into the body of the stomach. In the pig, glands are absent in an area surrounding the cardia and in part of the pars proventricularis. In both species, most of the mucosa is glandular.

The mucosa of the **multi-chambered stomach** of ruminants is **non-glandular** throughout the forestomach (reticulum, rumen and omasum) and **glandular** in the abomasum.

Glandular stomach (pars glandularis)

The **gastric mucosa** (**tunica mucosa gastrica**) and underlying tela submucosa are thrown into longitudinal **folds** (**plicae gastricae**). The mucosal surface is divided into areas (**areae gastricae**) onto which **gastric pits** (**foveolae gastricae**) open. At the base of the pits, tubular gastric glands extend into the lamina propria. The distribution of gastric pits and the shape, size and structure of the glands in the individual regions of the stomach are variable, **depending on species** (Figures 10.28 to 10.38 and Table 10.2).

The **tunica mucosa** is lined with **simple columnar epithelium** incorporating numerous mucus-producing cells. The surface of each individual cell (**epitheliocytus superficialis gastricus**) typically bulges towards the lumen and is coated with a layer of highly viscous **mucus** that resists the effects of gastric acids. Mucous neck cells of the gastric glands also contribute to the mucous lining. The epithelial cells contain abundant metabolic organelles and a central nucleus, and are firmly held together by tight junctions (zonulae occludentes) and gap junctions (nexus). The

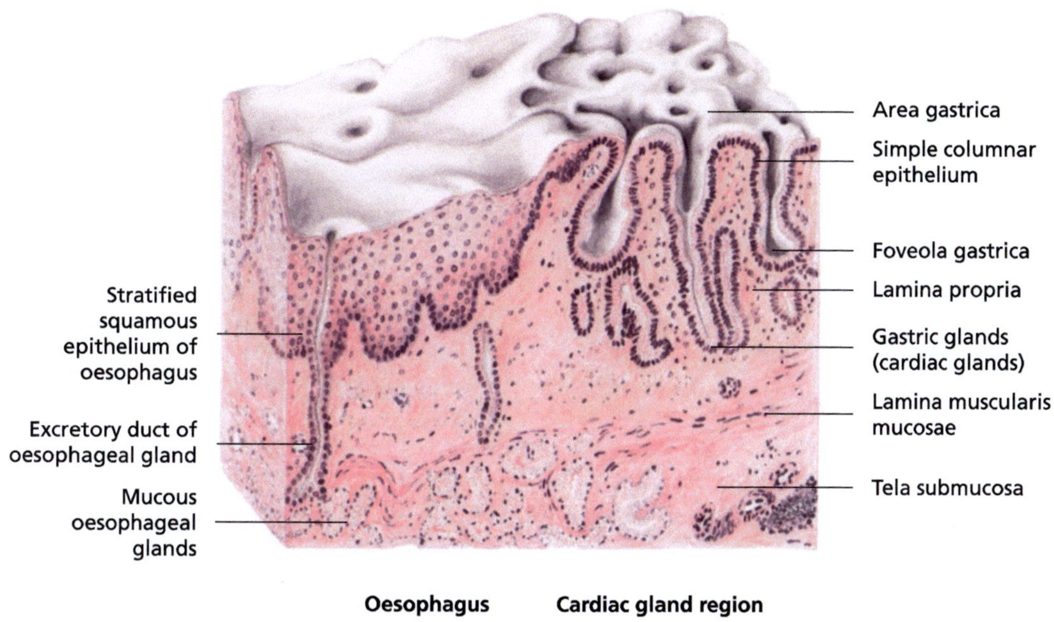

10.28 Junction of the oesophagus with the cardiac gland region (pars cardiaca) of the stomach (dog; schematic).

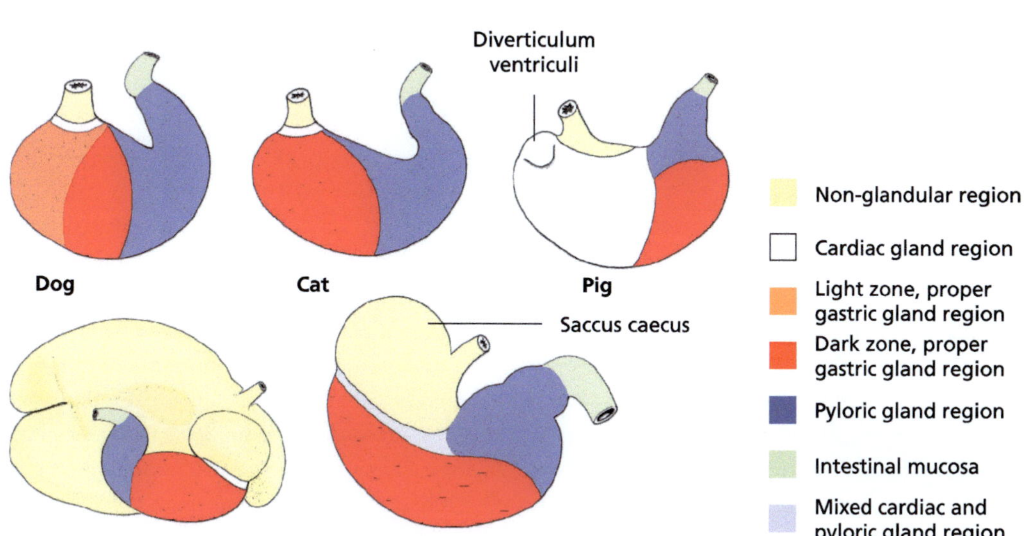

10.29 Comparative representation of the gastric mucosa (schematic; König and Liebich, 2009).

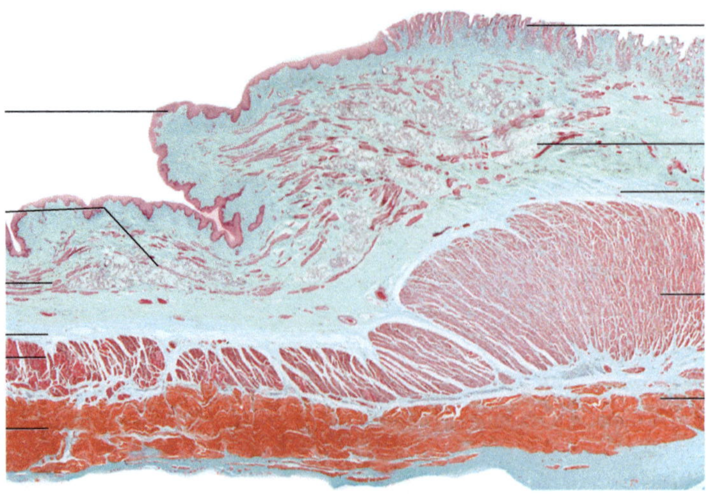

10.30 Zone of transition from non-glandular oesophageal mucosa to the glandular mucosa of the cardiac region of the stomach (dog). Goldner's Masson trichrome stain (x13).

Table 10.2 Comparative structure of the glandular stomach of domestic mammals.

Region	Epithelium	Glands	Muscle	Special features
Cardiac	Simple columnar epithelium, gastric pits	Tubular, branched mucous glands (cardiac glands), endocrine cells	Distinct lamina muscularis, tunica muscularis composed of circular, longitudinal and oblique smooth muscle fibres, cardiac sphincter	Extensive in the pig, smaller in the dog and horse
Body (and fundus in carnivores)	Simple columnar epithelium, gastric pits	Tubular glands with isthmus, mucous neck cells, chief and parietal cells (proper gastric or fundic glands), endocrine cells	Similar to cardiac region	Light and dark zones are observed in the dog
Pyloric	Simple columnar epithelium, gastric pits	Short, branched and unbranched tubular mucous glands (pyloric glands) emptying into deep gastric pits, endocrine cells	Similar to cardiac region, the middle layers of smooth muscle form the pyloric sphincter (sphincter pylori)	Torus pyloricus present in pigs and ruminants

mucous coating serves as an additional barrier by preventing lysis of the epithelial layer by the acid gastric juice. Compromise of this protective function affects the structural and functional integrity of the gastric mucosa.

The **tubular gastric glands** (**glandulae gastricae**) in the **lamina propria** are surrounded by a delicate connective tissue network. Type I and type III collagen fibres and elastic fibres form a meshwork containing large numbers of immunologically active cells (lymphocytes, plasma cells, granulocytes and mast cells). In places, these cells cluster together to form diffuse lymphoid tissue and occasional lymphoid follicles may be observed (pig). Extensive capillary networks surround the glands. Numerous autonomic nerve fibres are also present, originating from ganglia in the tela submucosa (**plexus nervorum submucosus, Meissner's plexus**). The capillary networks and neural networks influence the secretory activity of the glands.

Isolated smooth muscle cells are found throughout the lamina propria, extending to just beneath the mucosal surface. These cells facilitate transport of secretions within the tubular glands and fine-tune the contractility of the tunica mucosa. They represent offshoots of the lamina muscularis mucosae, the continuous layer of muscle that forms the outermost portion of the mucosa.

In carnivores a **subglandular layer** (stratum subglandulare) may be observed. This layer has two components: an inner stratum granulosum, located at the base of tubular glands containing mainly lymphocytes and plasma cells, and an outer stratum compactum, a dense layer rich in collagen fibres located adjacent to the lamina muscularis mucosae (Figure 10.31).

The **lamina muscularis mucosae** is relatively prominent in domestic mammals. Individual muscle fibre bundles follow a criss-crossing spiral path, forming a contractile system that manifests as two to three distinguishable layers. This muscle layer contributes to the folding of the mucosa and supports gastric emptying.

The stomach has a typical **tela submucosa** containing vessels, nerves, adipose tissue and localised accumulations of lymphatic tissue. The tela submucosa permits movement of the layers of the stomach wall with respect to one another. It conforms to the shape of the gastric wall, as determined by its degree of contraction, thus contributing to the topography of the mucosal surface.

The **tunica muscularis** consists of an inner circular and an outer longitudinal layer of smooth muscle. The passage of muscle fibres within these layers varies with region and species, due to the presence of **obliquely oriented fibre bundles** (**fibrae obliquae**). Towards the pylorus, the **inner circular muscle layer** thickens to form the **m. sphincter pylori**. In the pig and ox, the thickened muscle protrudes into the lumen as the torus pyloricus. The oblique muscle fibres form a loop (ansa cardiaca) at the cardia of the stomach, contributing to the **m. sphincter cardiae** (particularly well developed in the horse). The oblique fibres also form the muscular foundation of the **lips of the gastric groove** (prominent in pigs and, particularly so, in ruminants; refer to *Veterinary Anatomy of Domestic Mammals: Textbook and Colour Atlas*). The outermost layer of the stomach comprises a **tunica serosa**.

The **tubular gastric glands** in the **tunica mucosa** vary in structure and exhibit species-related differences in their regional distribution. Three types of glands are recognised:

- cardiac glands (glandulae cardiacae),
- proper gastric (fundic) glands (glandulae gastricae propriae) and
- pyloric glands (glandulae pyloricae).

CARDIAC GLANDS

The zone containing the cardiac glands is referred to as the **cardiac gland region** (**pars cardiaca**) of the stomach (Figure 10.29). In carnivores and ruminants, the cardiac glands are restricted to an annular zone at the entrance to the stomach (abomasum in ruminants). In the horse, strips of mucosa containing cardiac glands adjoin the saccus caecus. Cardiac glands extend over a larger region of the mucosa in pigs, incorporating the diverticulum ventriculi and half of the body of the stomach (Figure 10.29).

The **cardiac glands** are typically branched and heavily coiled tubular glands that empty via a short 'neck' into the base of the gastric pits. The terminal portion of the glands is expanded. The glandular epithelium is **cuboidal** to **columnar** and produces an **alkaline mucous secretion** that also contains the enzyme lysozyme. Parietal cells (dogs) and chief cells (pigs) are sometimes present within the epithelium. In addition to these exocrine glandular cells, the cardiac gland region of the stomach of domestic mammals contains **endocrine glandular cells** that can be identified using silver staining and immunohistocytochemical techniques. These cells form part of the gastrointestinal endocrine system. Their secretory product, including serotonin, somatostatin and endorphins, passes into the capillary network of the stomach wall.

PROPER GASTRIC (FUNDIC) GLANDS

Proper gastric (fundic) glands occur over approximately two thirds of the gastric mucosa in carnivores, in a small region near the greater curvature in pigs and across most of the body of the stomach in horses. While this portion of the glandular mucosa is referred to as the proper gastric gland (fundic) region, it only includes the fundus in carnivores (Figure 10.29).

The **proper gastric glands** are tightly packed and are longer and less branched than cardiac glands (Figures 10.31 and 10.32). They extend through the lamina propria to the lamina muscularis, surrounded by connective tissue, vessels, nerves, smooth muscle cells and cellular infiltrates. Several glands empty via a common isthmus into the gastric pits.

The **proper gastric glands** are composed of three regions characterised by structurally and functionally distinct cell types:

- **isthmus**: isthmus cells (epitheliocytus nondifferentiatus),
- **neck** (**cervix**): neck cells (mucocytus cervicalis),
- **body** and **fundus** (**pars principalis**):
  - chief cells (exocrinocytus principalis),
  - parietal cells (exocrinocytus parietalis) and
  - endocrine cells (endocrinocytus gastrointestinalis).

Isthmus

The isthmus is the portion of the gland located in the gastric pits from which the gland itself develops. Its typically low cuboidal epithelium is continuous with the epithelial lining of the gastric pits. The cells increase in height throughout this transition. The cells of the isthmus are daughter cells of the mucous neck cells and are usually not fully differentiated (epitheliocyti nondifferentiati).

Like the epithelial cells lining the gastric pits, these cells produce **mucus** and thus contribute to **protection of the epithelium**. In addition, isthmus cells serve to replace cells abraded at the mucosal surface. They may also replace deeper **glandular cells** (neck, parietal and chief cells) (Figures 10.31 and 10.32).

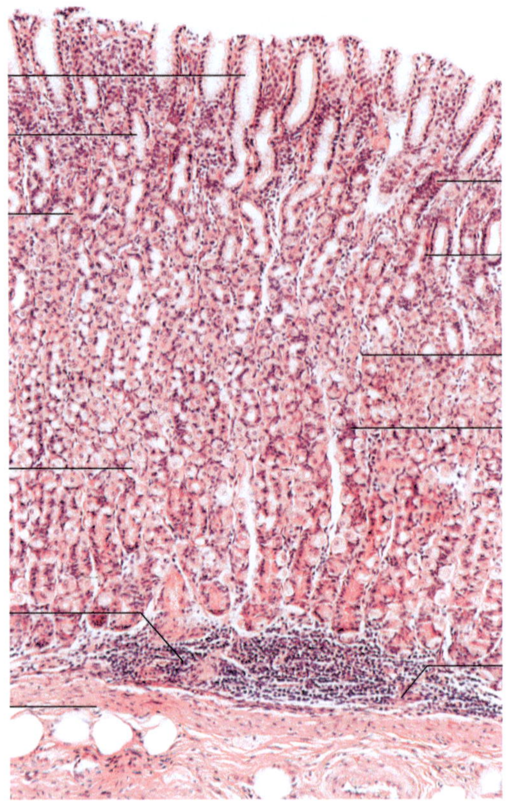

10.31 Proper gastric (fundic) gland region of the stomach (dog). Haematoxylin and eosin stain (x100).

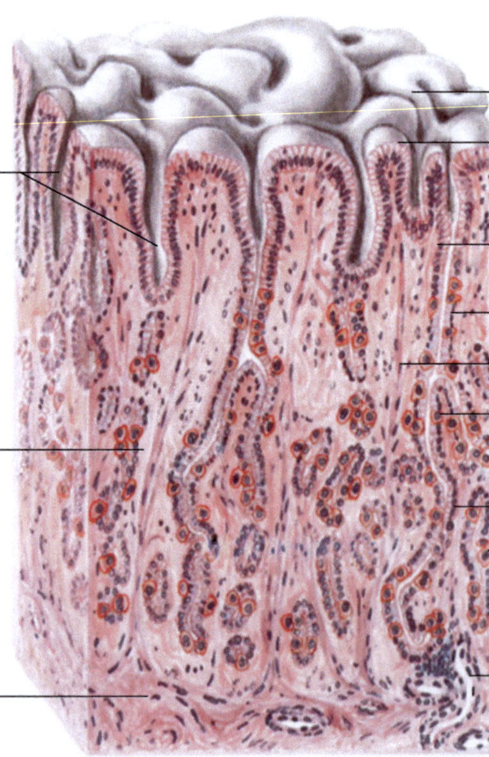

10.32 Proper gastric (fundic) gland region of the stomach (dog; schematic).

Neck

The neck region contains parietal cells (see below) and **mucous neck cells (mucocyti cervicales)**. Occurring individually or in groups, mucous neck cells differ in structure and function to isthmus cells. Neck cells are cuboidal to low columnar and typically stain only weakly. The nucleus occupies a basal position and the accumulation of secretory granules causes the apical surface of the cell to bulge into the lumen.

The mucus produced by neck cells is **acidic**, of **relatively low viscosity** and comparatively high in glycosaminoglycans. The layer formed by the combination of this mucus, and that produced by isthmus and surface cells, protects the epithelium against the proteolytic and hydrolytic activity of the proteases and H^+ ions secreted by parietal cells (see below).

Body and fundus

The epithelial lining of the body and fundus of the proper gastric glands incorporates numerous **exocrine chief cells** and **parietal cells**. Also present are **endocrine cells** of the enteroendocrine system of the gastrointestinal tract.

The **chief cell (exocrinocytus principalis)** is cuboidal or pyramidal with slightly basophilic cytoplasm (Figures 10.32, 10.33 and 10.35). The oval nucleus is usually located in the basal third of the cell. Typical of cells with high secretory activity, chief cells are rich in organelles associated with protein synthesis (ribosomes, rough ER). Chief cells contain **zymogen granules** that, in the active secretory phase, cause apical bulging of the cells. Chief cells secrete **pepsinogen**, the precursor of pepsin.

The **parietal cell (exocrinocytus parietalis)** is a rounded to pear-shaped, strongly acidophilic cell that is interposed between, or lies peripheral to, chief cells (Figures 10.32, 10. 33, 10.35 and 10.37). The nucleus is spherical. **Parietal cells** occur throughout the wall of tubular glands, particularly in the middle section, and are characterised by the presence of abundant mitochondria containing particularly numerous cristae. Tubulovesicular structures accumulate beneath the plasmalemma during the inactive stage of the parietal cell.

In addition, parietal cells contain a system of **intracellular canaliculi (canaliculi intracellulares)** that increases the surface area across which secretion can occur. During the active secretory phase, the number of microvilli lining the canaliculi increases while the tubulovesicular system regresses (Figure 10.35). Dissociated hydrochloric acid (H^+ and Cl^-) is secreted into the canaliculi. Depending on species, parietal (and/or chief cells) also secrete intrinsic factor required for absorption of vitamin B_{12}.

Intra-epithelial endocrine cells (endocrinocyti gastrointestinales) are found particularly in the middle and terminal sections of the gland. Together with endocrine cells of the pylorus and small intestine, and endocrine cells of the pancreas, these cells belong to the **gastroenteropancreatic (GEP) endocrine system**. Endocrine cells found in the region of the proper gastric glands include enterochromaffin (EC) cells (serotonin), D cells (somatostatin) and G cells (gastrin) (Figure 10.38, see also Figure 2.22); their relative number varies with species.

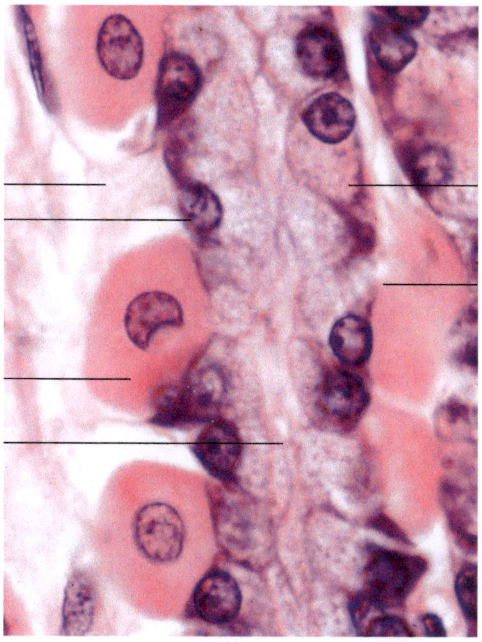

10.33 Proper gastric (fundic) gland with chief cells and peripherally located parietal cells (dog). Haematoxylin and eosin stain (x1200).

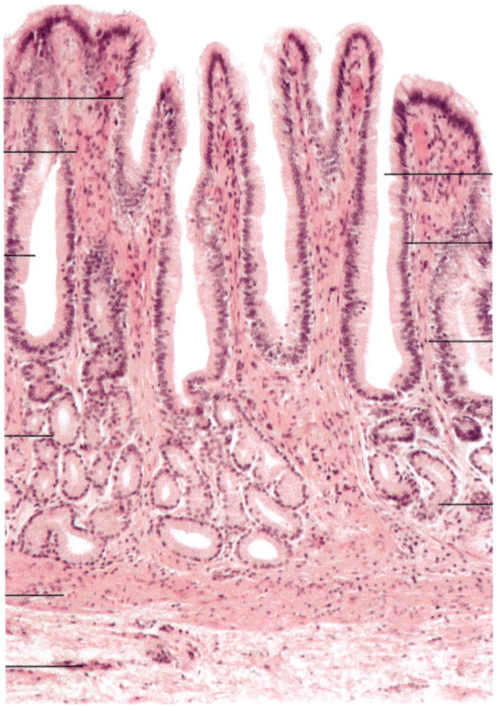

10.34 Pyloric gland region of the stomach with expanded gastric pits and short, coiled pyloric glands (dog). Haematoxylin and eosin stain (x250).

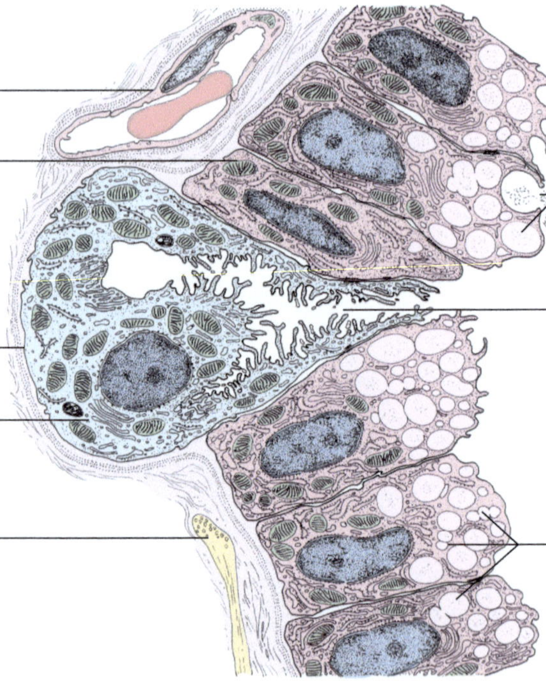

10.35 Chief cells in the proper gastric (fundic) gland region with adjacent parietal cells in different secretory phases (schematic).

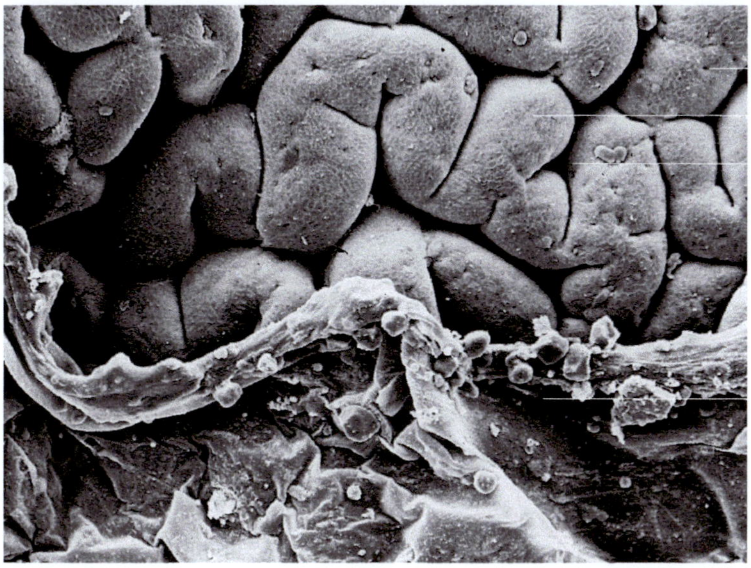

10.36 Scanning electron microscope image of the gastric mucosa (dog; x1500).

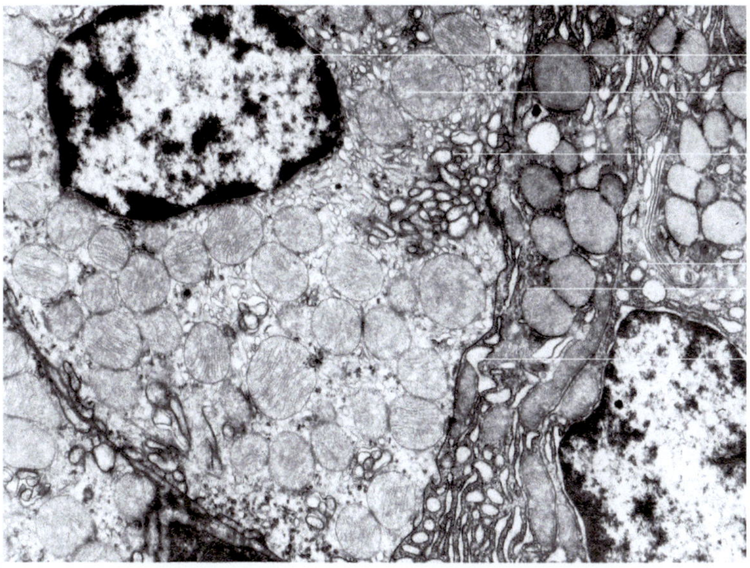

10.37 Fine structure of a parietal cell and adjacent chief cell in the proper gastric (fundic) gland region of the stomach (dog; x11,000).

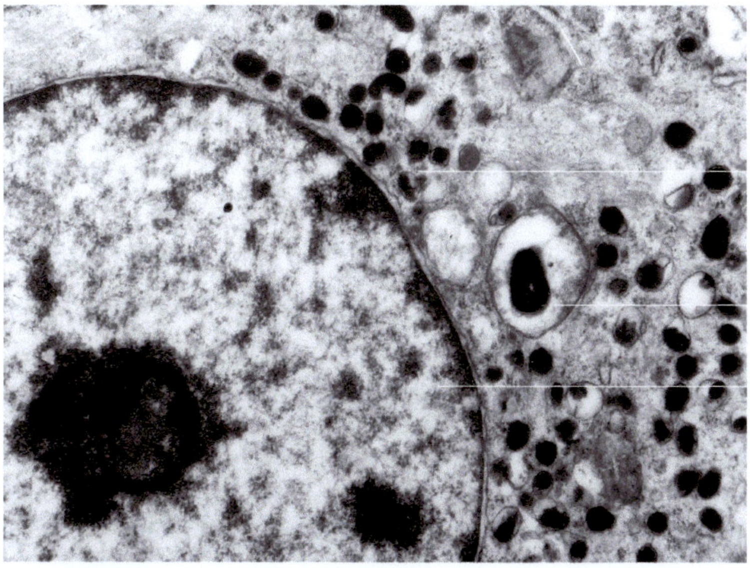

10.38 Fine structure of a gastrin cell (G cell) (dog; x10,000).

PYLORIC GLANDS (GLANDULAE PYLORICAE)

The relatively short **pyloric glands** are located in the pylorus, extending to a varying extent into the body of the stomach (Figure 10.29). They typically open into elongated, dilated gastric pits (Figure 10.34). Pyloric glands are branched and extensively coiled. The deep portion of the lumen is usually expanded. The **glandular cell** (**exocrinocytus pyloricus**) is cuboidal to columnar with an oval nucleus (may be flattened due to accumulation of mucus). These cells primarily secrete a mucous substance that also contains lysozyme. Characteristic of the glandular epithelium is the presence of **endocrine G cells**. Release of **gastrin** from G cells into the bloodstream stimulates the activity of parietal cells.

The histological features of the gastric glands are summarised under Table 10.2.

GASTRIC MUCUS

Gastric mucus comprises the secretory product of surface epithelial cells, mucous neck cells and other gastric gland cells (Figure 10.36). It is composed of neutral long-chain glycoproteins with amino sugar, hexose and sialic acid residues. The highly viscous mucus produced by surface cells forms the layer that lies on the epithelium. This is overlaid by a less viscous layer produced by the gastric glands.

The **protective function of the gastric mucus** includes buffering of free H^+ ions arising from the secretion of carbonic acid by the tunica mucosa. Under normal physiological conditions, the gastric mucus provides an effective barrier against the denaturing effects of gastric acid. Factors favouring acid production can disrupt this relationship, resulting in auto-digestion of the gastric mucosa. Production of gastric mucus is regulated by neural, hormonal and immune mechanisms.

GASTRIC JUICE

The components of gastric juice include organic and inorganic substances. Of greatest significance are H^+, Cl^-, Na^+, K^+, Mg^{2+}, HPO_4^{2-}, SO_4^{2-}, pepsin, lipase, water and, in young animals, rennin. Gastric juice also mixes with gastric mucus. The production of H^+ and Cl^- involves special features at the **internal surface of the plasmalemma** of parietal cells.

Upon stimulation of **parietal cells** (e.g. by gastrin or histamine) the **tubulovesicular system** (see above) transforms into a secretory component of the **intracellular canaliculi**. Evidence indicates that H^+ and Cl^- are actively transported against a concentration gradient into the lumen of the gland. Carbonic acid, H_2CO_3, is formed within the parietal cell from CO_2 and H_2O in a reaction catalysed by the enzyme carbonic anhydrase. Carbonic acid dissociates into H^+ and HCO_3^-. Transport of H^+ ions through the walls of the intracellular canaliculi into the gland lumen occurs via H^+/ K^+-ATPase proton pumps. For each transported H^+ ion, a HCO_3^- ion is exchanged at the basal surface of the cell to be taken up by the bloodstream. Cl^- ions function optimally in the pH range 1.8–3.5; this range is achieved through the buffering effect of gastric mucus and saliva.

REGULATION OF GASTRIC JUICE PRODUCTION

Control of gastric acid secretion can be divided into cephalic, gastric and intestinal phases.

In the **cephalic phase**, the senses of vision, olfaction and gustation influence the motor and secretory activity of the stomach. Activation of the vagus nerve via the nucleus dorsalis induces secretion of gastrin by G cells in the pyloric antrum. Concurrently, H^+ and pepsinogen are secreted by parietal and chief cells.

The **gastric phase** is the period during which ingesta are present in the stomach. During this phase, gastric secretion is influenced by vagal, hormonal (gastrin, histamine), mechanical, chemical (amino acids, protein rich nutrients) and immune factors. Excessively acid conditions in the stomach have an inhibitory effect on gastrin secretion.

Acetylcholine, gastrin and histamine are key transmitters in the control of gastric secretion. The activity of these molecules is controlled in turn by mediators such as prostaglandins and leukotrienes. In addition to regulating gastrin secretion by G cells, the vagus nerve influences blood supply to the stomach. Direct contact of dietary peptides with the gastric mucosa has a stimulatory effect. Acting as antigens, these induce local **immune responses** that are mediated by products of lymphatic cells within the tunica mucosa (e.g. leukotrienes, gamma-interferon, lymphokines) and via paracrine signalling by mast cell secretions (histamine, prostaglandins and leukotrienes). Together, these responses give rise to increased **acid** and **pepsinogen** secretion. Protection of the gastric mucosa against decreasing pH (cytoprotection) is facilitated by concurrent stimulation of gastric mucus production and increased mucosal perfusion. The combination of these various regulatory mechanisms preserves the functional integrity of the mucosa.

In the **intestinal phase**, the stomach contents induce secretion of gastrin by the small intestinal mucosa. The enterogastric reflex results in a gradual decrease in gastric motility. Gastric acid secretion is reduced by inhibitory substances such as cholecystokinin and gastric inhibitory peptide (GIP).

Ruminant forestomach

The primary function of the ruminant forestomach is the enzymatic cleavage of vegetable matter by microbial flora to form predominantly short-chain fatty acids. These are taken up, together with other products of microbial metabolism, by the mucosa of the forestomach, particularly the rumen, and transferred to the bloodstream. In the omasum, the gruel-like ingesta are mechanically compressed and water is absorbed. The **forestomach** constitutes the **non-glandular portion** of the multi-chambered ruminant stomach. Enzymatic digestion of the liquid portion of the ingesta occurs in the glandular **abomasum**. The mucosa of the abomasum represents the **glandular** portion of the ruminant stomach. The forestomach consists of three compartments:

- reticulum,
- rumen and
- omasum.

The internal surface of the forestomach is lined by **non-glandular mucosa** (**pars non-glandularis**) (Figures 10.39 to 10.42 and Table 10.3). The papillated **stratified squamous epithelium** is keratinised depending on the functional demands on the mucosa. In the **tela submucosa**, branching blood vessels give off arterioles that lead to subepithelial capillary networks, which drain into post-capillary venules. Veins merge in the tela submucosa and course through the muscle layer towards the exterior. As is typical for the musculomembranous gastrointestinal tract, lymphatic vessels and autonomic intramural ganglia are present in the tela submucosa. External to the tela submucosa is a **tunica muscularis** and a **tunica serosa**.

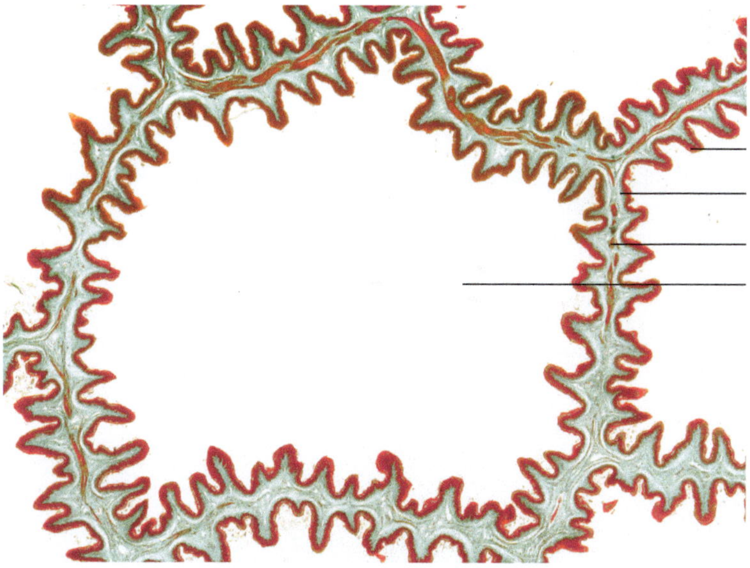

10.39 Horizontal section of reticular crests (goat). Numerous small papillae are present on the crests that form the pentagonal reticular cell. A continuous lamina muscularis envelops each cell and combines with smooth muscle surrounding adjacent cells to form a network. Goldner's Masson trichrome stain (x20).

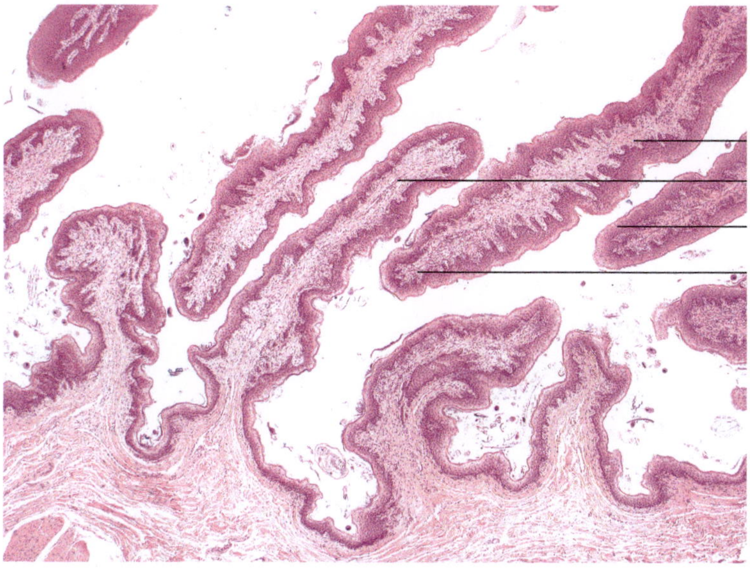

10.40 Wall of ventral sac of the rumen (sheep). Characteristic ruminal papillae are evident. These are frequently sectioned in such a way that they appear to have no contact with the mucosa. Haematoxylin and eosin stain (x20).

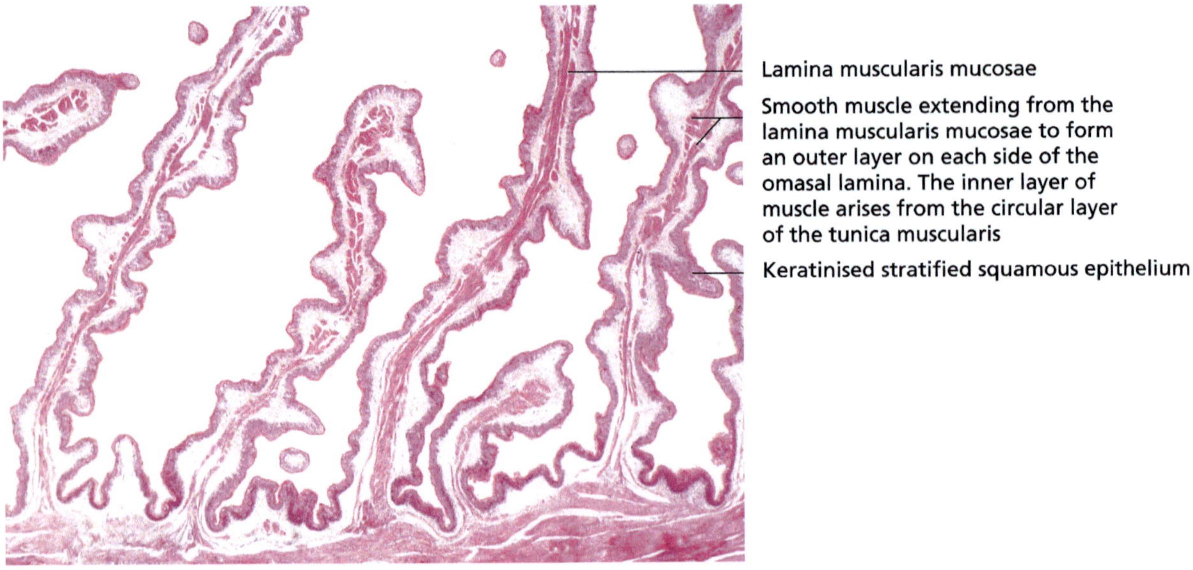

10.41 Wall of omasum (ox). The largest of the omasal laminae contain smooth muscle (lamina muscularis mucosae and fibres extending from the circular layer of the tunica muscularis). Muscle is absent in the smaller laminae. Haematoxylin and eosin stain (x32).

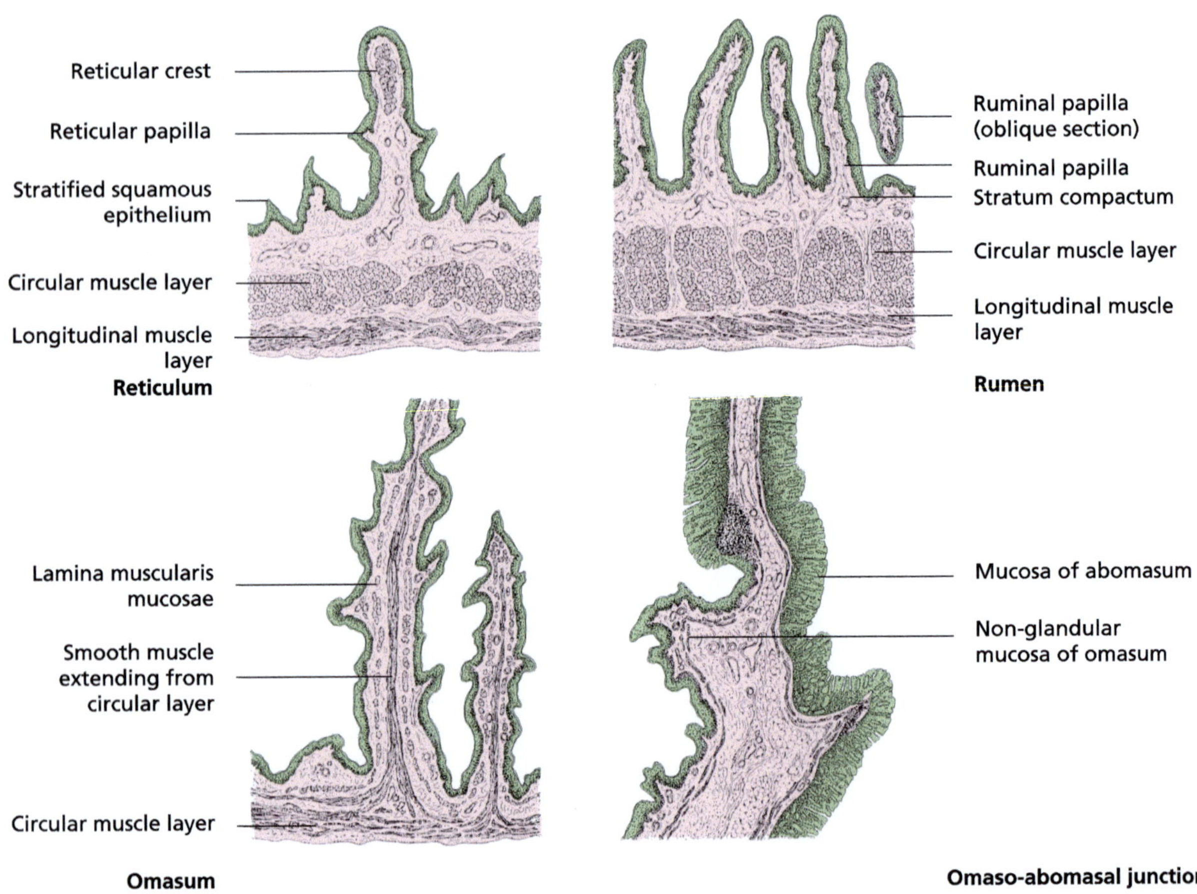

10.42 Structure of the compartments of the forestomach of the ox (schematic).

Table 10.3 Comparative structure of the compartments of the ruminant forestomach and abomasum.

Compartment	Epithelium	Glands	Muscles	Special features
Rumen	Keratinised stratified squamous	No glands	Lamina muscularis mucosae absent, circular and longitudinal layers of smooth muscle in tunica muscularis	Conical or elongated finger-like papillae, varying in length and morphology
Reticulum	Keratinised stratified squamous	No glands	Lamina muscularis mucosae present in upper portion of the primary reticular crests, tunica muscularis is weaker than in the rumen	Presence of papillae on surface of crests
Omasum	Keratinised stratified squamous	No glands	Lamina muscularis extends to varying degree into the higher order (I–III) omasal laminae	Prominent tunica muscularis, fibres of circular layer extend into higher-order omasal laminae
Abomasum	Simple columnar epithelium, gastric pits	Cardiac, proper gastric and pyloric glands	Inner circular layer, outer longitudinal layer	

RETICULUM

The reticulum is characterised morphologically by **reticular crests** (**cristae reticuli**) that form the four- to six-sided boundaries of **reticular cells** (**cellulae reticuli**) (Figures 10.39 and 10.42). Secondary and tertiary crests further divide the reticular cell into smaller chambers. Stratified squamous epithelium lines the reticular crests. The sides of the crests are studded with small **conical papillae**.

Originating from the oesophagus, a lamina muscularis is present in the upper portion of the primary crests. The muscle bundles surround each reticular cell and form networks with those of adjacent cells. The lamina propria blends without clear distinction with the tela submucosa. The tunica muscularis is composed of an inner circular and outer longitudinal layer. Additional striated muscle fibres, remnants of the oesophageal musculature, radiate into the reticulum. The outer layer of the reticulum comprises a **tunica serosa**.

RUMEN

The rumen is distinguished by the presence of **papillae** (**papillae ruminis**). These tongue-shaped structures (Figures 10.40, 10.42 and 10.43) vary considerably in form, length, distribution and density. The surface of the rumen is lined by **non-glandular mucosa**. The connective tissue of the lamina propria incorporates condensed layers of collagen fibres and smooth muscle cells; a delicate subepithelial capillary network is present. The **tunica muscularis** consists of **smooth muscle**, with some oesophageal skeletal fibres extending into the ruminal atrium.

The smooth muscle comprises an inner circular and outer longitudinal layer. A tunica serosa forms the outermost layer in the region facing the peritoneal cavity. Between the rumen and the spleen, a **tunica adventitia** is present.

The mucosa of the rumen has important functions and is responsive to dietary factors. Within 4–5 weeks, a high-energy, low-cellulose diet induces growth of the papillae, proliferation of a thickened, non-keratinised epithelium and elaboration of the subepithelial capillary network. In response to an energy-poor, high-fibre feed, the papillae become shorter and plump keratinised cells appear in the epithelium. These changes reflect the adaptability of the structural elements of the papillae and represent normal processes occurring in wild ruminants due to seasonal changes in diet. Comparable cycles of proliferation and regression are also observed in high-performance animals during the dry and subsequent lactation period.

The key determinant of functionally induced morphological adaptations of the ruminal papillae is the concentration of **short-chain fatty acids**, particularly β-hydroxybutyric acid, in the forestomach. Fatty acids are formed in the rumen and in the ruminal epithelium by microbial (bacterial and protozoal) digestion of feedstuffs containing carbohydrate. Numerous other substances are also produced by anaerobic fermentation in the rumen and reticulum, most of which are absorbed across the tunica mucosa. These include water, methane, carbon dioxide, lactic acid, non-protein nitrogen compounds (ammonium

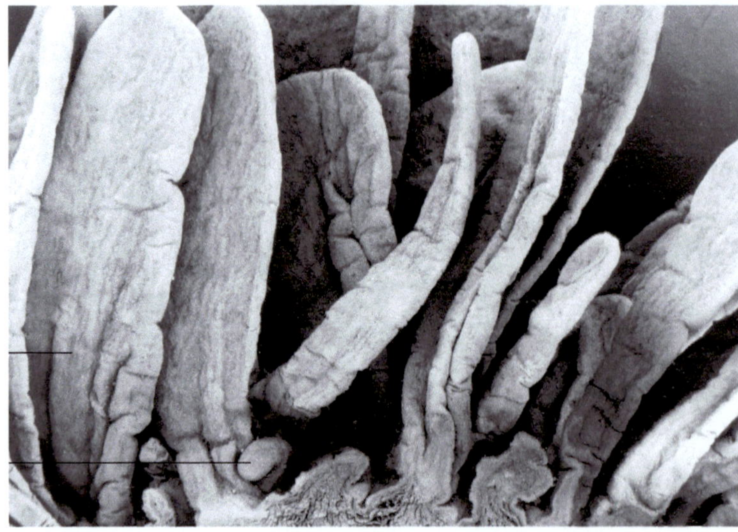

10.43 Scanning electron microscope image of ruminal papillae (ox; x10).

salts, urea, biuret) and vitamins B and K. The three main fatty acids produced in the rumen and reticulum are:

- acetic acid (ca. 60% intraruminal fatty acids), utilised for synthesis of acetyl CoA for lipid metabolism,
- propionic acid (ca. 25% of intraruminal fatty acids), used in the liver for synthesis of glucose (gluconeogenesis) and
- butyric acid, converted by the ruminal epithelium into β-hydroxybutyrate (ketone).

A particularly important characteristic of the **ruminal microorganisms** is the capacity to convert non-digestible vegetable carbohydrates into ammonia and microbial protein that can be utilised by the animal. In this process, the tunica mucosa acts as a **semipermeable epithelial absorption barrier**. Absorption occurs primarily in the rumen, to a lesser extent in the reticulum and omasum and minimally in the abomasum. The degree of development of the ruminal papillae has a considerable influence on the **capacity for absorption** of fatty acids by the rumen, and thus upon the **regulation** and **stability** of ruminal pH. As the fatty acid concentration rises, the papillae proliferate to prevent the accumulation of acid in the ruminal contents.

Through the processes of **proliferation** and **regression**, the ruminal papillae contribute to regulation of the **energy balance**. As absorption by proliferating papillae increases, fatty acids become the **primary energy source**. Control of feed intake serves as an additional regulatory mechanism: ruminants stop feeding when ruminal pH is too low.

OMASUM

The interior of the omasum is divided by **omasal leaves** (**laminae omasi**) into narrow chambers. There are several orders of laminae (one to four or five), each subsequent order decreasing in size.

The surface of the folds is lined with **stratified squamous epithelium** and is covered with small keratinised papillae. The connective tissue core of the laminae forms a lamina propria.

Smooth muscle cells accompany the robust connective tissue layer to the free edge of the laminae. These fibres are continuations of the **lamina muscularis mucosae** and the inner **circular layer of the tunica muscularis**.

All but the smallest laminae are thus reinforced by three layers of muscle. The tunica muscularis consists of a relatively thick inner circular muscle layer and a thinner outer longitudinal muscle layer. A tunica serosa forms the outermost layer. The omasal laminae serve to press the fluid from the pulpy ingesta. In addition, short-chain fatty acids and electrolytes are absorbed across their surface.

The structural features of the wall of the forestomach are summarised in Table 10.3.

OMASO-ABOMASAL JUNCTION

The omasum is separated from the **abomasum** by two mucosal folds. In the ox, the mucosa on the omasal side of the omaso-abomasal orifice is **non-glandular mucosa** while that on the abomasal side is **glandular**. In small ruminants, the glandular mucosa extends beyond the free edge of the mucosal folds. Lymphatic tissue accumulates at the junction between the two mucosal epithelia. The connective tissue within the mucosal folds contains barrier arteries that contribute to the rigidity of the tissue.

Avian stomach

In granivorous and herbivorous species such as chickens, pigeons, geese and ducks, the stomach has two distinct divisions, the **glandular stomach** and the **muscular stomach**.

GLANDULAR STOMACH (PROVENTRICULUS, PARS GLANDULARIS)

The proventriculus continues from the oesophagus without a clear anatomical boundary. In most species, the mucosa is arranged in folds (Figures 10.44 and 10.45 and Table 10.4). The mucosal surface is lined by mucus-secreting **simple columnar epithelium** with microvilli. **Tubular glands** situated in the lamina propria deliver their mucous secretory product onto the mucosal surface (Figures 10.44 and 10.45). These comprise:

- superficial proventricular glands (glandulae proventriculares superficiales) and
- deep proventricular glands (glandulae proventriculares profundae).

The superficial proventricular glands are simple tubular mucus-producing glands that open into folds in the mucosa. The prominent layer of deep proventricular glands, or 'deep proprial glands', is bounded by a lamina muscularis mucosae. Portions of this muscle layer cleave off and extend towards the surface, largely surrounding the deep glands and protruding between the deep and more superficially located glands. While proventricular glands are usually not lobed, distinct lobulation occurs in chickens and geese. The openings of these glands are located on mucosal elevations (papillae proventriculares).

The cuboidal epithelium of the proventricular glands secretes pepsinogen and HCl (oxynticopeptic cells). These cells contain numerous mitochondria and rough ER. Additional cell types produce gastric hormones (e.g. somatostatin, bombesin and vasoactive intestinal peptide).

The loose connective tissue of the tela submucosa contains the submucosal nerve plexus (plexus nervorum submucosus; Meissner plexus) and numerous vessels. In the tunica muscularis, a well-developed inner circular layer (stratum circulare) is surrounded by a thinner outer longitudinal layer (stratum longitudinale). The myenteric nerve plexus (plexus nervorum myentericus; Auerbach plexus) lies between the two muscular layers. Externally, the proventriculus is lined by a single-layered tunica serosa that is continuous with the intestinal peritoneal sac.

The proventriculus is typically separated from the ventriculus by a narrow gastric isthmus (isthmus gastris). This transitional zone (zona intermedia) is usually free of mucosal elevations and folds and is devoid of glands. In the chicken, the narrowing at the isthmus is attributable to a high concentration of elastic fibres and a relatively thin muscular layer.

MUSCULAR STOMACH (VENTRICULUS, PARS MUSCULARIS)

Tunica mucosa: The **gastric mucosa** is irregularly subdivided by folds (**rugae ventriculi**). These are absent near the tendinous centres (see below).

The luminal surface of the ventriculus is covered by a tough, greenish-yellow layer known as the **cuticle** (cuticula gastris) that acts akin to a grinding plate for the breakdown of food (Figures 10.46 and 10.47). The cuticle consists of solidified secretions of clusters of **tubular glands in the lamina propria** (glandulae ventriculares). Secretory product is released onto the mucosal surface as compacted cylinders, or **columnae verticales**, that harden to form rods. This solidified secretion combines with the **matrix**

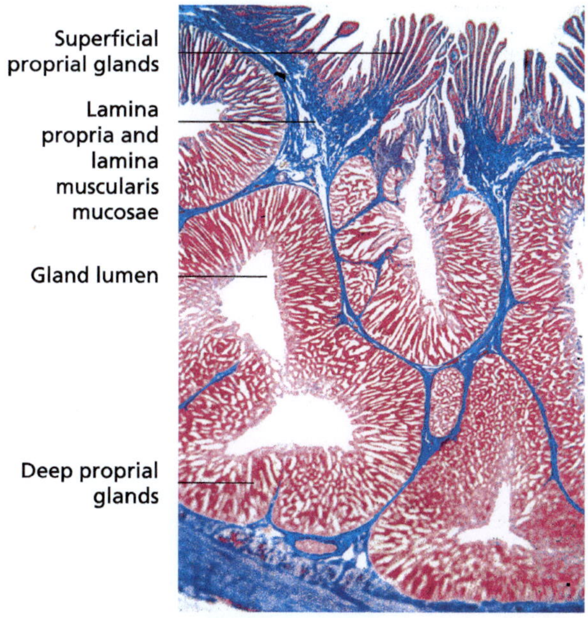

10.44 Mucosa of glandular stomach (chicken). Azan stain (x20).

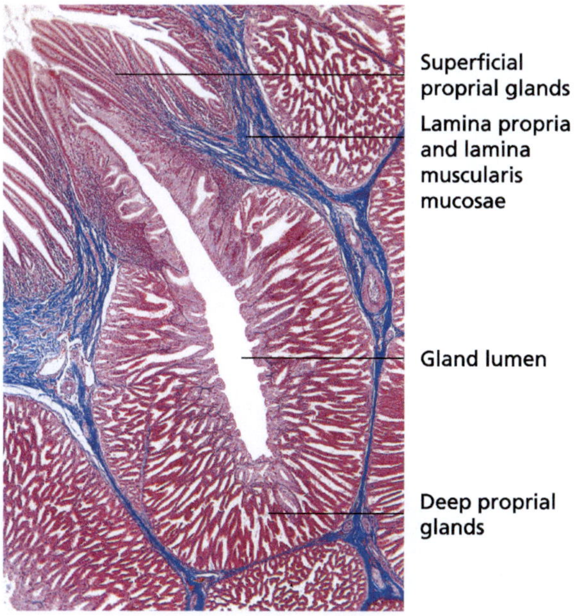

10.45 Mucosa of glandular stomach (chicken). Azan stain (x40).

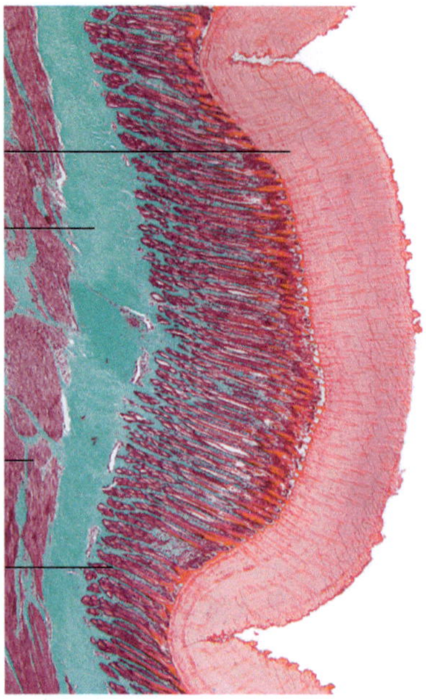

10.46 Muscular stomach (chicken). Goldner's Masson trichrome stain (x20).

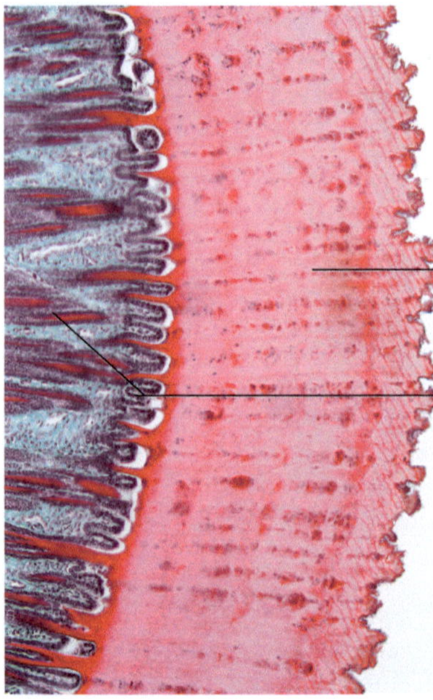

10.47 Cuticle of the muscular stomach (chicken). Goldner's Masson trichrome stain (x40).

Table 10.4 Comparative structure of the avian glandular and muscular stomach.

Compartment	Epithelium	Glands	Muscle	Special features
Glandular stomach	Simple columnar	Superficial and deep tubular glands, deep proprial glands extensively lobulated in the chicken and goose, mucous secretion; endocrine cells	Lamina muscularis mucosae protrudes between clusters of deep glands, dividing these into distinct lobules; inner circular layer of muscle in tunica muscularis is well developed	Cuboidal epithelium, secretes pepsinogen and HCl (oxynticopeptic cells)
Muscular stomach	Simple columnar	Clusters of tubular glands; secretion forms a rigid grinding plate (cuticle) composed of a keratin-like complex (koilin); endocrine cells	Wall subdivided into two major and two minor muscles composed of smooth muscle fibres; the inner muscle layer is particularly well developed; tendinous centres present laterally	Together with ingested stones (grit), the cuticle contributes to mechanical breakdown of stomach contents

horizontalis (softer secretions of the simple columnar gastric mucosal epithelium) to form a continuous layer of varying thickness.

Biochemically, the cuticle is composed of a keratin-like carbohydrate-protein complex (**koilin**). Small stones (**grit**) ingested with the food further assist with mechanical grinding.

Tela submucosa: The tela submucosa forms an immobile connection with the connective tissue components of the lamina propria mucosae (a lamina muscularis mucosae is absent). As a result, the gastric mucosa is tightly anchored to the overlying layer, the tunica muscularis.

Tunica muscularis: The wall of the muscular layer consists predominantly of smooth muscle tissue that can be divided macroscopically into four separate muscles. The inner circular layer is usually more developed than the outer longitudinal layer. The individual muscles are referred to as the:

- m. crassus caudodorsalis,
- m. crassus cranioventralis,
- m. tenuis craniodorsalis and
- m. tenuis caudoventralis.

The strong **m. crassus caudodorsalis** and **m. crassus cranioventralis** extend from one **tendinous centre** (centrum tendineum) to the other, forming the dorsal and ventral borders of the ventriculus. Lying between the thick muscles are the weaker **m. tenuis craniodorsalis** and **m. tenuis caudoventralis**. In grain feeders, the ventriculus is the site of mechanical breakdown of food. Further digestion of protein also occurs in this portion of the stomach. The cuticle terminates at the **ostium pyloricum**. The mucosa of the pylorus contains **pyloric glands** (**glandulae pyloricae**) and numerous endocrine cells responsible for local hormone production (e.g. gastrin cells, somatostatin cells).

The histological features of the wall of the avian glandular and muscular stomachs are listed in Table 10.4.

Small intestine (intestinum tenue)

The small intestine comprises three structurally and functionally distinct segments, the duodenum, the jejunum and the ileum. Considerable species variation exists in the macroscopic appearance of these components (for more detail see anatomy textbooks).

The function of the small intestinal mucosa, supported by the activity of the muscular layers, is digestion of nutrients and absorption of the resulting breakdown products.

For the most part, the digestive processes that commence in the proximal portion of the gastrointestinal tract are completed by reactions occurring in the small intestine. Further digestion takes place in the large intestine (within fermentation chambers in the pig and horse). Ruminants represent a special case, due to the role played in digestion by the forestomach.

Breakdown of nutrients is completed by the combined action of gastric juice (pepsin) and secretions of the intestinal glands (including 1,6-glucosidase, aminopeptidase, dipeptidases and phosphodiesterases) and the pancreas (including lipase, α-amylase, trypsin, chymotrypsin, carboxypeptidase,

Table 10.5 Comparative structure of the intestinal wall in domestic mammals.

Segment	Epithelium	Glands	Muscle	Special features
Small intestine (villi present throughout in domestic mammals)				
Duodenum	Simple columnar with brush border, isolated goblet cells	Tubular, branched or unbranched glands (crypts of Lieberkühn), extend into the lamina propria, tubulo-alveolar glands (Brunner's glands) in submucosa, endocrine cells	Lamina muscularis mucosae present – sends smooth muscle cells into intestinal villi, inner circular and outer longitudinal tunica muscularis with plexus nervorum myentericus	Isolated lymphatic nodules (GALT), submucosal glands (mucous in dog and ruminant, may be mixed in the pig and horse).
Jejunum	Similar to duodenum, microvilli longer and finer	Similar to duodenum but no glands in submucosa	Similar to duodenum	Increasing numbers of lymphatic follicles
Ileum	Similar to jejunum	Similar to jejunum	Similar to duodenum	Well-developed GALT, Peyer's patches (all domestic mammals, particularly horse and calf)
Large intestine (villi absent in all domestic mammals)				
Caecum	Simple columnar with low brush border	Numerous goblet cells, simple tubular intestinal glands	Lamina muscularis mucosae present, inner circular and outer longitudinal smooth muscle layers	GALT near ileocaecal orifice in the dog, pig and ruminant, more developed in the colon in the cat and horse; taeniae (musculoelastic bands) and haustra in pig and horse
Colon	Simple columnar with low brush border	Marked increase in goblet cells, simple tubular intestinal glands	Similar to caecum	Taenia (musculoelastic bands) and haustra in pig and horse
Rectum	Similar to colon	Similar to colon	Muscle more prominent than in caecum and colon	

nucleases and phosphatases). In addition, bile produced by the liver and, in some cases, enzymes present in foodstuffs, contribute to the digestive process.

Food components are hydrolysed to form low-molecular weight substrates. The associated metabolic processes are regulated by neural and hormonal mechanisms.

In animals with simple stomachs, **breakdown of proteins** into **amino acids** is completed in the small intestine. Polypeptides produced by the action of pepsin on proteins in the stomach are hydrolysed in the small intestine by trypsin and chymotrypsin, giving rise to oligopeptides, and by peptidases to produce L-amino acids. **Polysaccharides** are broken down by pancreatic α-amylase and intestinal 1,6-glucosidase into monosaccharides (maltose, isomaltose, glucose). Following emulsification in the stomach, triglycerides are cleaved in the small intestine by pancreatic lipase to form β-monoglycerides and fatty acids. Digestion of fats is further aided by bile salts and cholesterol. Additional pancreatic enzymes (nucleases and phosphatases) catalyse the conversion of **nucleic acids** into **nuclear bases** and **pentoses**.

These processes rely on continuous mixing of chyme with hydrolytic secretions that function optimally in a neutral to slightly alkaline environment. End products available for absorption are taken up at the luminal surface of the mucosal epithelium and pass through the basal portion of the cell to reach the blood or lymph system.

Absorption is an **active process** that utilises **concentration gradients** and/or the **membrane potential** of the plasmalemma.

Short-chain fatty acids formed by the hydrolysis of fats pass through the epithelium into the blood capillaries and then directly to the liver. **Long-chain fatty acids** and **monoglycerides** are taken up into the epithelial cells by pinocytosis and converted into triglycerides in the smooth endoplasmic reticulum. These are furnished with a lipoprotein coat in the Golgi apparatus and transported as **chylomicrons** through the intracellular compartment to the lymphatic capillaries.

As well as **secreting digestive enzymes** and absorbing the products of digestion, the epithelial cells – to an even greater extent than in the stomach – synthesise and secrete mucus for **cytoprotection** of the intestinal surface. In addition, **tissue hormones** are produced by the mucosa, primarily by the epithelial cells of the intestinal glands. The mucosa also absorbs water, electrolytes and vitamins. Furthermore, in terms of surface area, the enteral **mucosa constitutes** the **largest lymphatic organ of the body** and actively participates in immune responses.

The small intestine exhibits the typical layered musculomembranous structure of the tubular digestive organs. Apart from certain segment-specific differences, the morphology of the small intestine is similar, and the following description applies to the duodenum, jejunum and ileum.

A summary of the structural features of the segments of the intestine is provided in Table 10.5.

Tunica mucosa

The various functions of the small intestine depend largely on structural specialisations that greatly **increase its internal surface area.** These include transversely oriented macroscopically visible **folds** (**plicae circulares**) that gradually decrease in height in the caudal segments of the intestine. In ruminants, the folds are permanent. The core of the folds is composed of loose connective tissue in the tela submucosa that protrudes into the intestinal lumen. In addition, the entire small intestinal mucosa is covered with **intestinal villi** (**villi intestinales**), finger-like evagina-

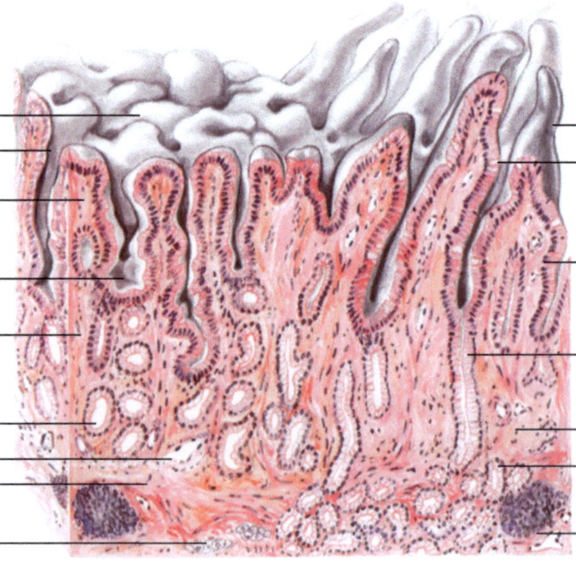

10.48 Opening of the pylorus into the proximal duodenum (dog; schematic).

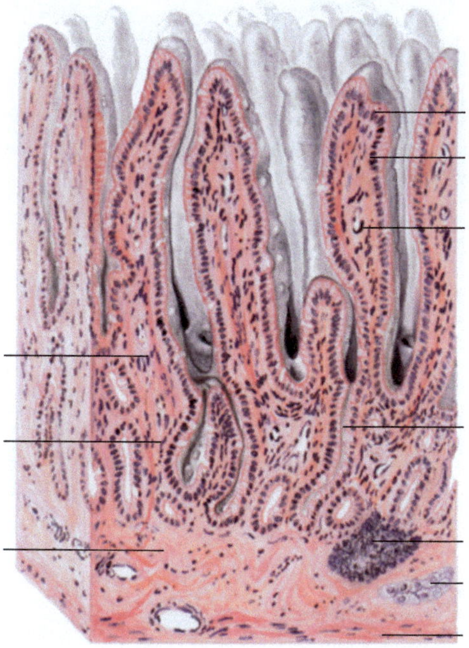

10.49 Jejunal mucosa in a dog (schematic).

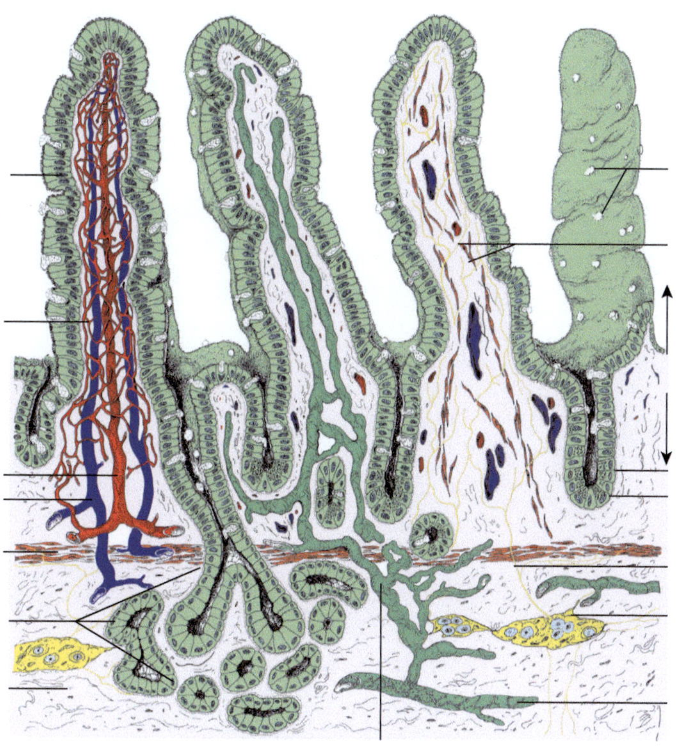

10.50 Structure of intestinal villi with emphasis on intestinal glands, Brunner's glands, vascularisation, lymph vessels, innervation and extension of smooth muscle cells from the lamina muscularis mucosae into the villus (schematic).

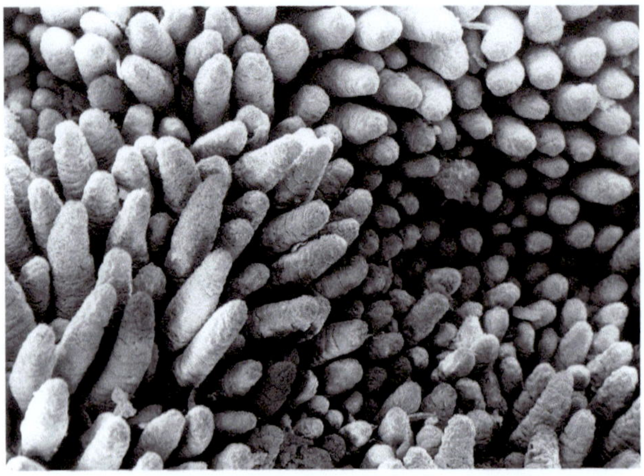

10.51 Scanning electron micrograph of intestinal villi after removal of the intestinal contents (sheep; x14).

tions of the lamina propria lined with simple epithelium (epithelium mucosae) (Figures 10.48 to 10.50).

Intestinal villi (length 0.5–1.5 mm, density 20–40/mm^2) contribute significantly to the total mucosal surface area. In carnivores the villi are long and slender, while those of ruminants are short and wide. In all domestic mammals, the villi are longest in the jejunum, and shorter in the duodenum and ileum (Figures 10.48 to 10.51).

MUCOSAL EPITHELIUM (EPITHELIUM MUCOSAE)

Microvilli projecting from the mucosal **epithelial cells** form a dense border that considerably increases the absorptive intestinal surface area. Thus, the internal lining of the small intestine is enlarged by the combination of plicae circulares, intestinal villi and microvilli lining the epithelial cells of the villi.

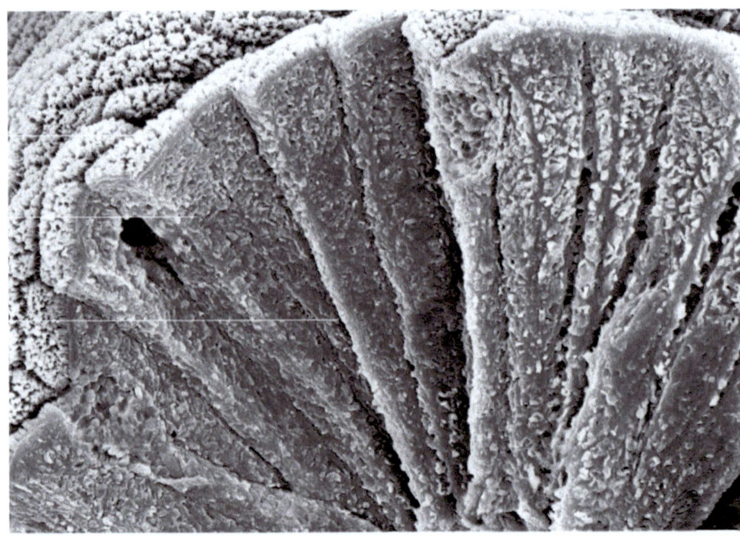

10.52 Scanning electron micrograph of the sides of columnar enterocytes in the intestinal mucosa (sheep; x2500).

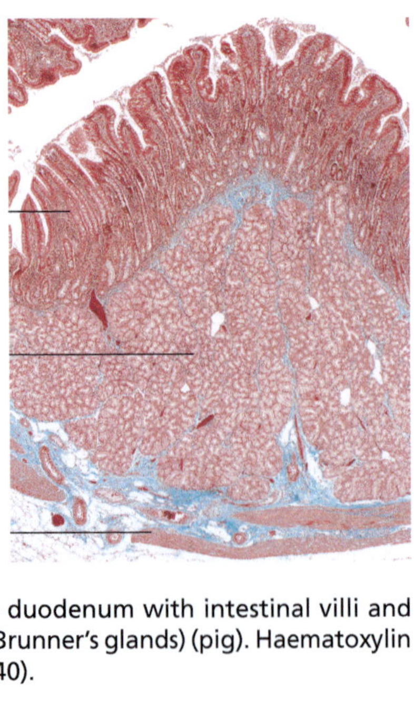

10.53 Wall of the duodenum with intestinal villi and duodenal glands (Brunner's glands) (pig). Haematoxylin and eosin stain (x40).

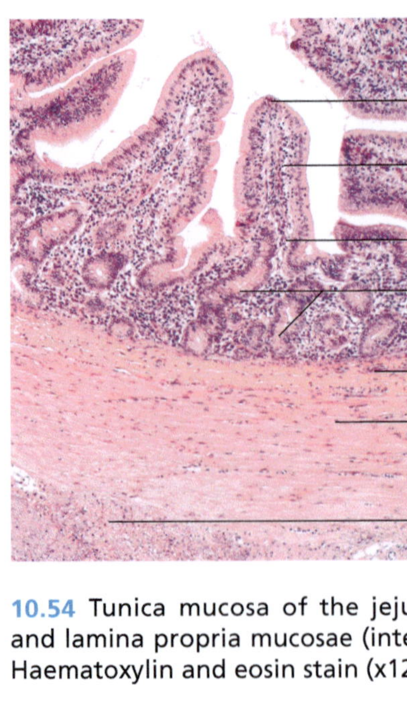

10.54 Tunica mucosa of the jejunum with mucosa and lamina propria mucosae (intestinal villi) (sheep). Haematoxylin and eosin stain (x120).

In addition to the projections from its surface, the mucosa is characterised by invaginations of the lamina propria in the form of straight, **non-branching tubular intestinal glands** (**glandulae intestinales, crypts of Lieberkühn**) (Figures 10.50 and 10.54 to 10.57). **Undifferentiated epithelial cells** (**epitheliocyti nondifferentiati**) at the base of the glands undergo constant mitotic division. Daughter cells migrate towards the lumen to the tip of the intestinal villi where they replace continuously desquamating cells, thus serving to regenerate the **absorptive surface**.

The lifespan of an intestinal epithelial cell is generally 10–14 days in neonates and 2–5 days in adults. The relatively long lifespan in juveniles facilitates intra-epithelial multiplication of microbial pathogens within the mucosa. As protection of the intestinal surface by mucus is typically lacking at this time, the protracted cellular lifespan can increase vulnerability to gastrointestinal infection (e.g. diarrhoea) in newborn animals. As the intestinal glands also undergo postnatal development, the capacity for rapid replacement of shed epithelial cells is not yet fully developed.

The intestinal villi and the walls of the intestinal glands are lined by a simple columnar epithelium incorporating several cell types that vary in structure and function:

- enterocytes (epitheliocyti columnares villi),
- goblet cells (epitheliocyti caliciformes),
- endocrine cells (endocrinocyti gastrointestinales) and
- Paneth cells (exocrinocyti cum granulis acidophilis).

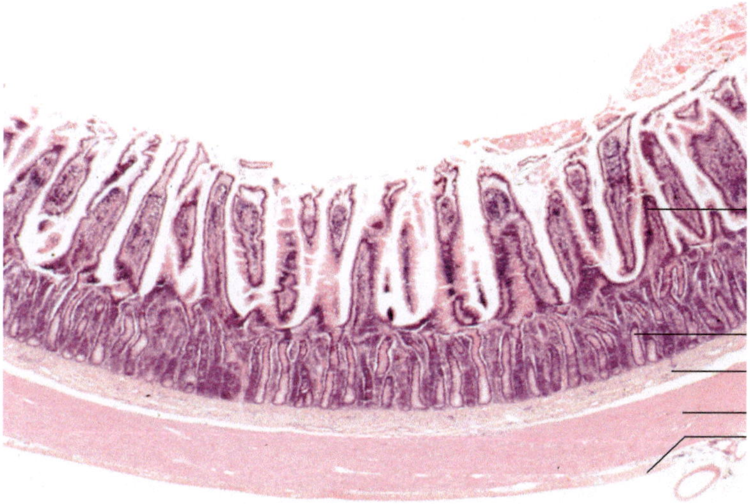

10.55 Transverse section of jejunum (cat). Haematoxylin and eosin stain (x12).

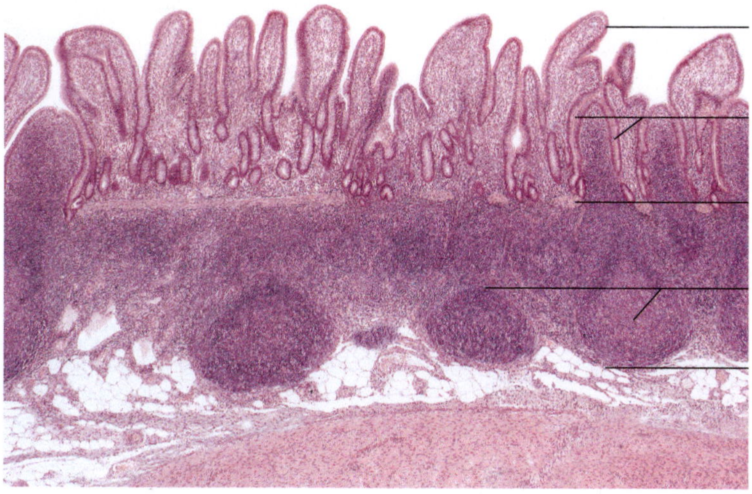

10.56 Transverse section of ileum (pig). Haematoxylin and eosin stain (x42).

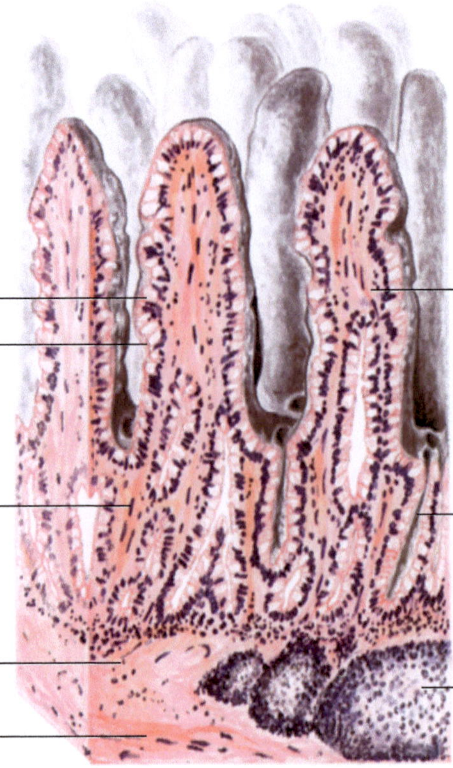

10.57 Mucosa of the ileum in the dog (schematic).

Enterocytes, or intestinal absorptive cells, and secretory goblet cells form the **epithelial lining of the intestinal villi**. They also form substantial components of the walls of the intestinal glands. In addition, the glands contain endocrine cells and, frequently, cells of Paneth.

Enterocytes

Enterocytes are **columnar cells** that form the absorptive lining of the intestinal tract (Figure 10.54). The cells contain an ovoid euchromatic nucleus, abundant mitochondria, rough and smooth endoplasmic reticulum and a well-developed Golgi apparatus. Apically, enterocytes are tightly joined by **zonulae occludentes** and **junctional complexes**, preventing the movement of fluid between the intestinal lumen and the intercellular space. Exchange of low-molecular weight molecules and ions between enterocytes occurs via **gap junctions** (**nexus**). Finger-like lateral cell processes increase the surface area of the cell and facilitate intercellular transport. At their base, enterocytes are in close contact with the basal lamina to which they are mechanically bound by hemidesmosomes.

Regularly spaced and densely arranged **microvilli** are present on the apical surface of the cell (see Figure 2.29). Microvilli are approximately 1–1.5 μm long and 0.1 μm in diameter. Each cell bears around 2000–3000 microvilli, resulting in a density of up to 200 million per mm^2 of the epithelial surface. This **brush border** can be observed with the light microscope.

Microvilli contain **longitudinally oriented** bundles of **actin filaments** that insert into the plasmalemma at the tip of each microvillus. At the base of the microvilli, the actin filaments are connected to myosin filaments of the cytoskeleton via the **terminal web**. These contractile elements of the microvilli bring about movement of the cytoplasm and promote cellular uptake of the end products of digestion.

The **plasmalemma of the microvilli** is associated with enzymes including disaccharidases, phosphatases, aminopeptidases and lipases. These play a major role in the **hydrolysis** (**digestion**) of food components and absorption of the products of nutrient breakdown. The external surface of the plasmalemma is coated with a prominent **glycocalyx** that is resistant to proteolytic and mucolytic enzymes and thus has a **protective function**.

Goblet cells

Goblet cells are interposed between enterocytes in the epithelial lining of the intestinal villi and crypts (Figure 10.50). The number of goblet cells increases from the duodenum towards the ileum. In the large intestine these form almost the entire population of cells lining the walls of the intestinal glands. Goblet cells are **monocellular glands** that produce mucus rich in glycoproteins and glycolipids. The mucus is secreted by the merocrine mode onto the surface of the intestinal mucosa, where it protects the epithelium against enzymatic autodigestion and colonisation of epithelial cells by pathogens. The mucus occupies receptors used by microorganisms or binds toxins, thus preventing their adhesion to the epithelial surface. Through its **lysozyme** content, mucus also has **bactericidal properties**. In addition, mucus binds to microorganisms and transports them aborally, assisted by peristaltic movements of the intestine.

Endocrine cells

Endocrine cells are present in the lining of the intestinal glands of the proximal small intestine. These cells synthesise **peptide hormones** and **serotonin** (**5-hydroxytryptamine**), which regulate secretion of digestive enzymes and peristaltic activity. Together with similar cells in the stomach and pancreas, the endocrine cells of the intestine (enteroendocrine cells) form the **gastroentero-pancreatic** (**GEP**) **endocrine system**.

The **intra-epithelial** endocrine cells deliver their secretory granules to the immediately adjacent **subepithelial capillary network**. Based on immunohistochemical techniques and, in some cases, on affinity for chromium and silver salts, the contents of the cytoplasmic secretory granules have been identified as particular peptide hormones and biogenic amines (e.g. serotonin) or their precursors.

A feature common to these cells is the presence of usually basally located **granules** containing amino acid decarboxylases. These enzymes are involved in the synthesis of biogenic amines. Endocrine cells that contain amino acid decarboxylases are referred to as **APUD cells** (amine precursor uptake and decarboxylation). These hormone-producing cells are characterised by the presence of surface receptors and the capacity to secrete polypeptides in response to an appropriate stimulus.

Several specific hormone-producing cell types have been identified, particularly in the deeper portions of the intestinal glands of the duodenum. In addition to basal granules (150–450 nm), features common to these cells include a usually spherical nucleus and close contact with the basal lamina. Endocrine cells vary between species in their distribution in the gastric and intestinal glands, their size and shape, their electron density and in the contents of their granules.

D cells synthesise **somatostatin**, which inhibits the synthesis of gastric secretions (e.g. gastrin). D cells also occur in the pancreas and gastric mucosa.

G cells secrete **gastrin**; in addition to the pars pylorica of the stomach, these are found in the duodenum and jejunum. Gastrin stimulates the secretory activity of parietal cells and mucous cells of the gastric mucosa, as well as cells of the intestinal mucosa and pancreas.

I cells produce **cholecystokinin** (**CCK**), which promotes production of bile by the liver, contraction of the gall bladder and secretion of digestive enzymes by the pancreas.

Secretin, produced by S cells, stimulates production and secretion of pancreatic juice, $NaHCO_3$ and bile.

Enterochromaffin cells (**EC cells**) stain with silver and chromium salts. Their granules contain serotonin, which increases gut motility (refer to Chapter 9, 'Endocrine system' and biochemistry texts.)

Paneth cells

Paneth cells, or acidophilic granular cells, are located at the base of the intestinal glands. They are characterised by the presence of numerous acidophilic granules that accumulate towards the apex of the cell. Paneth cells produce a serous, glycoprotein-rich exocrine secretion that also contains lysozyme. This enzyme exerts bactericidal effects by dissolving the bacterial cell wall and thus influences the microbial flora of the intestine. Paneth cells are present in the horse. They have not been demonstrated definitively in ruminants and pigs and are absent in carnivores.

LAMINA PROPRIA MUCOSAE

The lamina propria mucosae consists of loose connective tissue. It forms the core of the intestinal villi (Figures 10.49 and 10.50). Much of the lamina propria is occupied by the **intestinal glands**. Between the glands, the loose connective tissue is condensed and houses blood and lymph vessels, nerve fibres, myofibroblasts and smooth muscle cells. This layer also contains numerous immune cells, in aggregates of varying density, and reticular fibres.

The **microvasculature** serves primarily to support the secretory activity of epithelial cells and to transport products of digestion, water, electrolytes and vitamins. Accordingly, each villus contains a dense and substantial **capillary network**. An arteriole passes centrally to the tip of each villus where it arborises into capillaries. The capillaries anastomose to form a subepithelial network that extends along the sides of the villus to its base, where blood drains via postcapillary venules into one or more venules. These combine to form veins of the submucosal vascular plexus. Arteriovenous anastomoses regulate the flow of blood.

Also passing through the centre of each villus is a lymphatic capillary or **lacteal**. The lacteal begins at the tip of the villus as a blind-ended vessel and opens at the base of the villus into a plexus that joins collecting lymphatic vessels in the tela submucosa (Figure 10.50). The lacteal is lined with simple squamous epithelium that is specialised for the uptake of chylomicrons.

The loose tissue of the lamina propria is pervaded by networks of fine **autonomic nerve fibres** that have their perikarya in the **plexus nervorum submucosus** (**Meissner's plexus**) (Figure 10.50). These nerve fibres supply exocrine and endocrine gland cells and regulate the function of smooth muscle, including the muscular component of blood vessel walls.

Smooth muscle cells (**myocyti villi**) originating from the lamina muscularis mucosae pass through the lamina propria along the longitudinal axis of the villus. These cells undergo rhythmic contraction, resulting in shortening and lengthening of the villus. Through these contractions, the cells act as a pumping station that aids in transport of blood and lymph into deeper vessels (Figure 10.50). **Myofibroblasts** lying perpendicular to the smooth muscle cells extend to the sides of the villus. These may also play a role in contraction of the villus.

The lamina propria contains dense aggregates of **lymphatic tissue** rich in T and B lymphocytes, plasma cells, monocytes, macrophages, mast cells, neutrophils and eosinophils. This is a manifestation of the **immune responses** that occur continuously within the gastrointestinal mucosa. The lymphatic tissue of the intestinal mucosa is collectively termed **GALT** (gut-associated lymphoid tissue) and resembles the **BALT** (bronchus-associated lymphoid tissue) of the respiratory tract (see Chapter 8, 'Immune system and lymphatic organs').

In carnivores, and to a limited extent in horses, a **stratum compactum** is present at the base of the **lamina propria** near the lamina muscularis. This is an extension of the stratum compactum of the gastric mucosa, which it resembles morphologically.

> **Species variation**
>
> **Birds**: Particularly in the chicken, numerous mucosa-associated lymphatic follicles may be present near Meckel's diverticulum, in the distal jejunum and at the entry to the caecum. These tonsil-like lymphatic organs (Peyer's patches) are part of the immune system of the avian gastrointestinal tract, in which discrete lymph nodes are absent in most species.

LAMINA MUSCULARIS MUCOSAE

The layers of the lamina muscularis mucosae resemble those of the gastric mucosa. Species variation in muscle layer thickness is observed.

INNATE AND ADAPTIVE PROTECTIVE MECHANISMS OF THE INTESTINAL MUCOSA

Throughout the life of the organism, the intestinal mucosa is exposed to a multitude of foreign materials and microorganisms (antigens within foodstuffs, viruses, bacteria, fungi, parasites). To prevent these from entering the body, the tunica mucosa incorporates innate and adaptive mechanisms that form a **mucosal barrier**. The bactericidal effect of mucus and the acid pH of the gastric juice have been described above. Other innate phenomena include inactivation of enteropathogenic viruses by **bile** and the bacteriostatic properties of **lactoferrin** secreted by the intestinal mucosa. **Interferon** also contributes to local immune defence. In addition, competition from normal gut flora frequently prevents colonisation of the mucosa by pathogens.

In its entirety, the mucosal barrier protects **against absorption** of antigens, modifies antigens (antigen handling) and hinders trans-epithelial uptake of antigens via the formation of complexes with **secretory immunoglobulin A** (**IgA**) (see below).

Adaptive mechanisms comprise cellular responses that result in localised production of **immunoglobulins**. These antibodies, predominantly IgA, are synthesised by plasma cells in the lamina propria. IgA is taken up by epithelial cells, coupled with transport peptides and delivered by exocytosis from the intestinal glands to the intestinal lumen.

Secretory IgA is resistant to proteolytic secretions and thus has a long duration of action. It prevents bacteria from binding to the mucosa, agglutinates bacteria and neutralises viruses and toxins. IgA forms the first line of immune defence in protecting the surface epithelium against agents of disease. Other immunoglobulins (IgM, occasionally IgG) are of lesser importance in the local immune response. As the immune system of neonates is not fully developed, early development of localised immunity in the gastrointestinal tract is particularly important.

Tela submucosa

The structure of the collagen fibre-rich connective tissue of the tela submucosa is typical for the tubular digestive tract. In addition to adipose tissue, **vessels** and **neural networks** (plexus nervorum submucosus), the submucosa contains solitary **lymphatic nodules** (noduli lymphatici solitarii) and **aggregated lymphatic nodules** (noduli lymphatici aggregati, Peyer's patches). These are described in more detail below (see 'Ileum'). Mucous glands are present in the tela submucosa of the duodenum (glandulae submucosae) (see below).

Tunica muscularis and tunica serosa

The structure of the tunica muscularis and tunica serosa corresponds to the earlier description applying generally to the gastrointestinal tract. Macroscopically, the thickness of the layers varies with species, in some cases to a considerable degree (see anatomy textbooks).

Distinguishing features of segments of the small intestine

DUODENUM

The duodenal mucosa is extensively folded with marked plicae circulares. The intestinal villi are uniform, dense and relatively broad. Abundant intestinal glands are present, and the epithelium contains isolated goblet cells.

A defining **histological feature** of the duodenum is the presence of **glandulae submucosae** (**Brunner's glands**) (Figures 10.48 and 10.53). Brunner's glands lie in the **tela**

submucosa and may sometimes protrude through the lamina muscularis into the lamina propria. They are limited to the first 1.5–2 cm of the duodenum in the dog and are more widely distributed in other species, extending over 20–25cm in the goat, 60–70 cm in the sheep, 4–5 m in the ox, 3–5 m in the pig and 5–6 m in the horse.

Brunner's glands are usually densely packed, gradually thinning out to individual glands more distally. In most domestic species, they are branched tubulo-acinar glands. In carnivores the tubular form is dominant, while in ruminants the glands tend to be acinar. Brunner's glands are mucous in dogs and ruminants. In pigs and horses the secretion may be mixed. The glands produce a viscous, slippery secretion rich in neutral glycoproteins (carnivores). The alkaline mucus (pH 8–9) buffers the acidic gastric juice, protects the intestinal mucosa and creates an optimal environment for the action of pancreatic enzymes. In contrast, the mucus produced by the Brunner's glands of ruminants is typically acidic.

JEJUNUM

The basic structure of the jejunum is generally typical for the musculomembranous tubular digestive tract (Figures 10.49 and 10.54). The finger-like intestinal villi are longer and finer than in the duodenum. Isolated small lymphatic follicles occur deep in the mucosa and in the submucosa, particularly in the pig. Goblet cells are more numerous than in the duodenum.

ILEUM

Mucosal folding is notably reduced in the ileum. The intestinal villi are shorter, less dense and broader than in the jejunum and goblet cells are more plentiful (Figures 10.56 and 10.57). The ileum is characterised by the presence in the tela submucosa of **aggregated lymphatic nodules** (Peyer's patches) that usually protrude far into the tunica mucosa to reach the surface of the intestine. They frequently bulge into the intestinal lumen, displacing the intestinal villi. In these regions, the tunica mucosa (particularly the epithelium) is extensively infiltrated with lymphoid cells. Peyer's patches are tonsil-like structures that provide localised immune surveillance and defence (see Chapter 8, 'Immune system and lymphatic organs').

Large intestine (intestinum crassum)

The large intestine comprises the caecum, colon and rectum. Macroscopically, the structure of certain segments varies dramatically with species (e.g. the caecum in the pig and horse; refer to anatomy textbooks). These differences are reflected only to a certain extent in the histological structure of the intestinal wall, particularly in the tunica muscularis. The layers of the wall of the large intestine essentially conform to the basic structure of a musculomembranous tube (Table 10.5).

The activity of intestinal and pancreatic secretions gradually reduces in the large intestine. Ongoing digestion of residual foodstuffs, particularly hydrolysis of cellulose, is taken over by carbohydrate- and protein-cleaving intestinal bacteria and protozoa. In the caecum and colon of the horse and pig, short-chain fatty acids are formed anaerobically by microbial digestive processes similar to those occurring in the forestomach of ruminants. These are subsequently absorbed; vitamins B and K are also formed by bacteria in the large intestine.

Other important functions of the large intestinal mucosa include **absorption** of **water** and **electrolytes**, in exchange for calcium and bicarbonate, associated thickening of the intestinal contents and **secretion** of **mucus** from goblet cells for lubrication of the faeces. Absorption of nutrients and vitamins also takes place.

Tunica mucosa

A feature common to all segments of the large intestine of domestic mammals – in contrast to birds – is the **absence of intestinal villi** (Figures 10.58 to 10.60). The internal surface of the intestine is thus **predominantly smooth**, with some longitudinal folds formed by protrusions of the tela submucosa. Throughout the large intestine, elongated, relatively straight and unbranched **intestinal glands** extend into the lamina propria. The glands are tightly packed, filling the lamina propria to a large extent. The mucosal surface is lined by **simple columnar epithelium**. Uniformly arranged microvilli form a brush border on the apical surface of the absorptive epithelial cells. This significantly increases the surface area of the cells and the total surface area available for absorption of water and electrolytes from the intestinal lumen.

The surface enterocytes continue into the **intestinal glands** as a **simple columnar glandular epithelium** (**exocrinocyti columnares**). Distally these epithelial cells become less frequent and are replaced by an increasing number of goblet cells.

Goblet cells (**exocrinocyti caliciformes**) are the dominant cell type in the intestinal glands of the middle and distal segments of the large intestine (Figures 10.60 and 10.61). The epithelial cells are constantly replaced from a population of undifferentiated cells at the base of the gland. The structure of the lamina propria is typical of musculomembranous tubular organs. A continuous lamina muscularis mucosae is present.

Tela submucosa

Isolated lymphatic nodules (noduli lymphatici solitarii) and aggregated nodules (noduli lymphatici aggregati) are scattered throughout the tela submucosa.

Tunica muscularis

In the pig and horse, the inner circular layer of the tunica muscularis of the caecum and colon forms a continuous

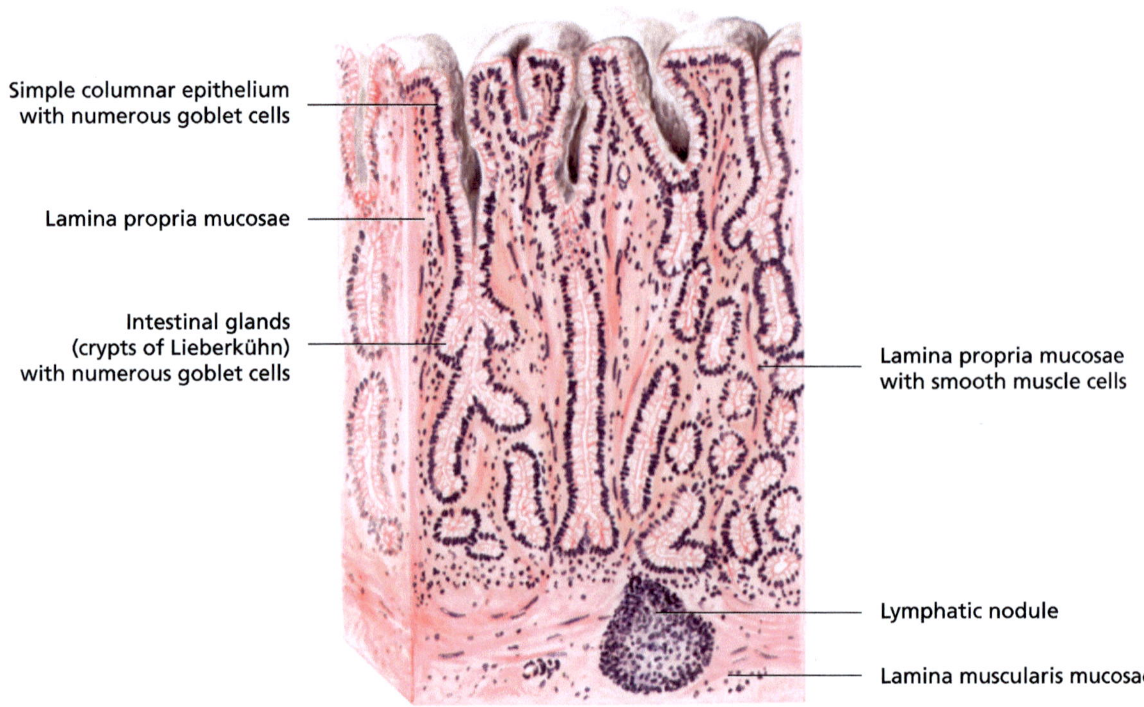

10.58 Mucosa of the colon in a dog (schematic).

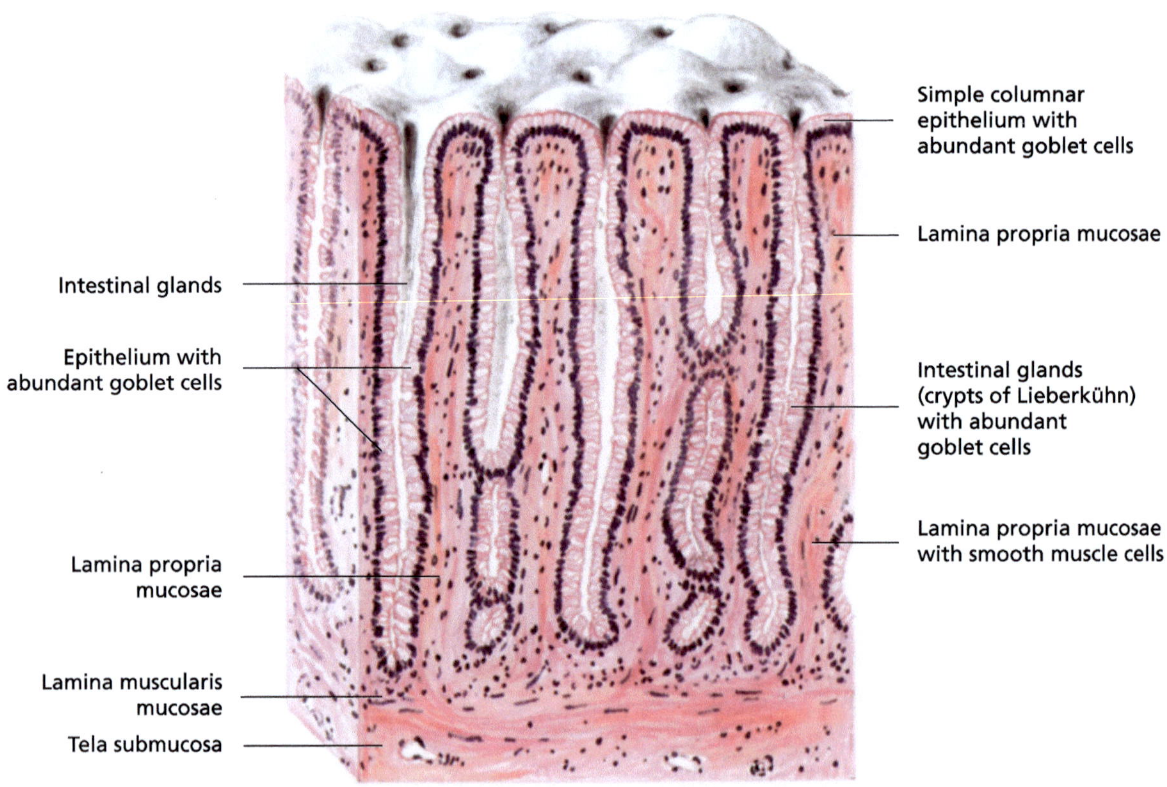

10.59 Mucosa of the rectum in the dog (schematic).

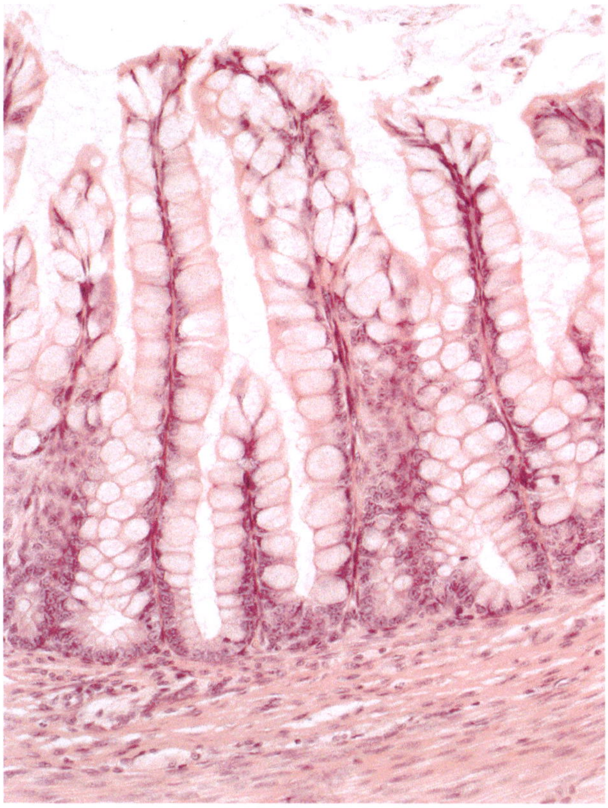

10.60 Colon (cat). Throughout the large intestine, intestinal villi are absent and goblet cells are considerably more numerous than in the small intestine. Haematoxylin and eosin stain (x200).

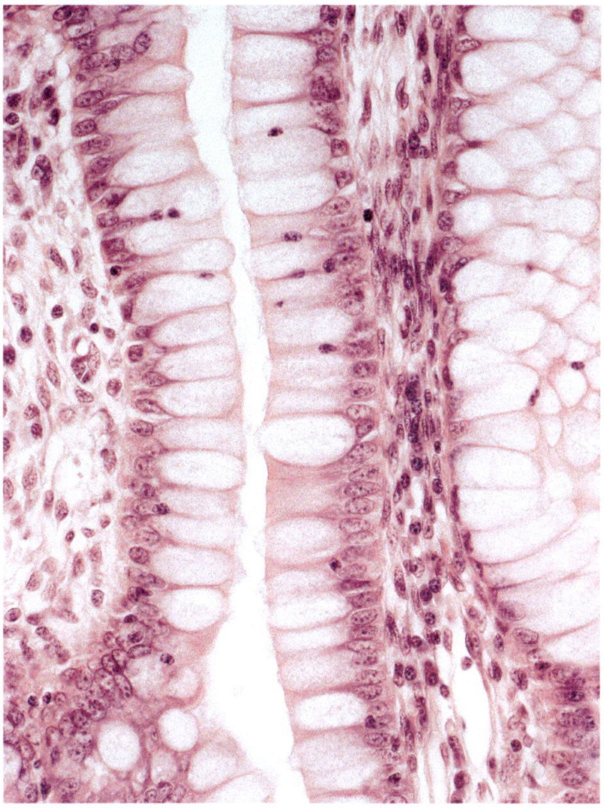

10.61 Elongated intestinal glands (crypts of Lieberkühn) in the large intestine with abundant goblet cells (dog). Haematoxylin and eosin stain (x300).

sheet while the outer longitudinal layer is differentiated into thick **bands** (**taeniae**) of smooth muscle. The caecum and colon of the pig have three and two bands respectively. In the horse, the caecum and ventral ascending colon have four bands. At the pelvic flexure and left dorsal colon there is only one band, while two bands are present at the diaphragmatic flexure. The **taeniae** are reinforced by abundant elastic fibres that often replace the muscle fibre bundles.

Distinguishing features of segments of the large intestine

CAECUM

The caecum is relatively large in the pig and markedly enlarged in the horse. This macroscopic phenomenon is accompanied by adaptations of the tunica muscularis (see above). Lymphatic nodules are scattered evenly throughout the proximal caecum of carnivores, pigs and ruminants and the distal end of the caecum in the horse and cat.

COLON

As with the caecum, the tunica muscularis of the colon of the horse and pig is modified to form longitudinal bands of smooth muscle strengthened by elastic fibres. The intestinal glands contain numerous goblet cells (Figure 10.60).

RECTUM

The tunica muscularis of the rectum is relatively thick and lacks taeniae. A characteristic feature of the rectum is the considerable density of goblet cells, both in the surface epithelium and the walls of the intestinal glands (Figure 10.59). Outside the peritoneal cavity (retroperitoneal portion of the rectum), the outer tunica serosa is replaced by a tunica adventitia. The loose connective tissue surrounding the rectum is usually interspersed with multilocular adipose tissue that extends into the connective tissue associated with the anus.

A summary of the histological features of the wall of the intestine is provided in Table 10.5.

Anal canal (canalis analis)

The epithelium of the mucosa lining the anal canal varies between its proximal and distal boundaries, forming **three distinguishable zones**:

- zona columnaris,
- zona intermedia and
- zona cutanea.

Within these zones, the mucosa of the large intestine transitions into the epidermis of the external skin. The most proximal segment of the canal (zona columnaris) commences at the **anorectal line**. Here the glandular mucosa of the rectum (lined with simple columnar epithelium) abruptly changes into the non-glandular mucosa of the anal canal (lined with stratified squamous epithelium). The zona columnaris is followed by the narrow zona intermedia. From its distal boundary (the **anocutaneous line**), the zona intermedia is continued by the **zona cutanea** which has keratinised stratified squamous epithelium.

The **zona columnaris** contains numerous **longitudinal folds** (**anal columns**) underlaid by bundles of smooth muscle and a submucosal vascular (or venous) plexus. Grooves located between the folds are termed **anal sinuses**. The tela submucosa of the columnar zone contains reticular tissue and isolated lymphatic nodules. The **zona intermedia** is lined with papillated non-keratinised stratified squamous epithelium. Diffuse lymphatic tissue and lymphatic nodules are present in the deeper connective tissue layers of this middle zone of the anal canal. Tonsil-like structures are present in the pig and dog. In both species, the submucosa contains **tubulo-acinar anal glands** (**glandulae anales**). The secretion of these glands is mucous in the pig and lipid in the dog. The intermediate zone is separated from the cutis of the external skin by the anocutaneous line.

The beginning of the **zona cutanea** is characterised by the appearance of structures associated with hairy skin (hairs, sweat and sebaceous glands). In the dog, and to a lesser extent in the cat, the wall of the cutaneous zone of the anal canal also contains hepatoid modified sebaceous glands, the **circumanal glands** (**glandulae circumanales**). These glands lack excretory ducts. Their secretory products appear to be hormones that participate in the modification of steroids. In carnivores, paired **anal sacs** (**sinus paranales**) lined with stratified squamous epithelium are present ventrolateral to the anal canal.

Located in the wall of the anal sacs are the **glands of the anal sacs** (**glandulae sinus paranales**) These apocrine modified sweat glands function as scent glands. In cats, the anal sacs also contain **sebaceous glands**.

Avian intestine

The avian intestine is relatively short compared to that of domestic mammalian species. Its length is influenced by diet, being relatively long in granivores and grass-feeders and shorter in carnivores. A peculiarity of the intestine of birds is the presence of **intestinal villi throughout the length of the small and large intestine**. Central lacteals are absent in birds. The **epithelium** is simple columnar and, in addition to chief and goblet cells, contains a sparse population of endocrine cells. **Intestinal glands**, smooth muscle cells and lymphatic tissue are present in the **lamina propria mucosae** throughout the intestine.

A thin lamina muscularis mucosae separates the mucosa from the **tela submucosa**. In addition to vessels and nerve plexuses (Meissner's plexus), the submucosa of most avian species houses **duodenal glands** (**glandulae duodenales**). Exceptions include chickens, ducks and geese (Figures 10.62 to 10.66).

In the typically thin **tunica muscularis**, the circular layer is thicker than the longitudinal layer. This layer also contains autonomic intramural neural networks (Auerbach plexus) and vessels.

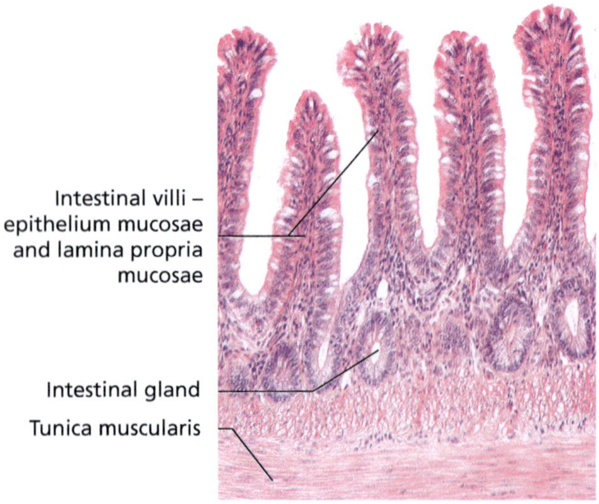

10.62 Duodenum (chicken). Haematoxylin and eosin stain (x40).

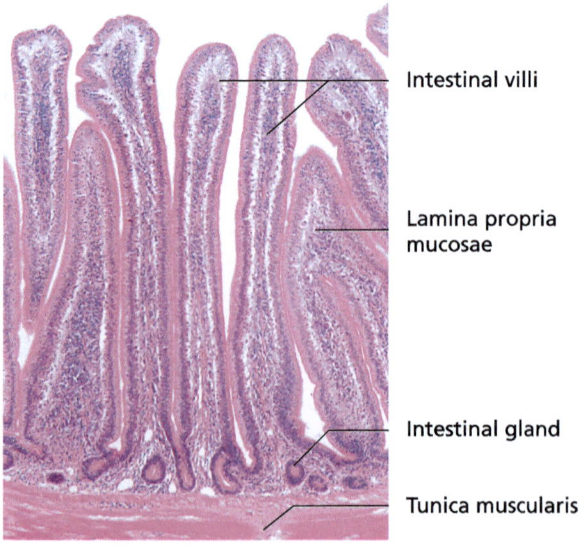

10.63 Jejunum (chicken). Haematoxylin and eosin stain (x25).

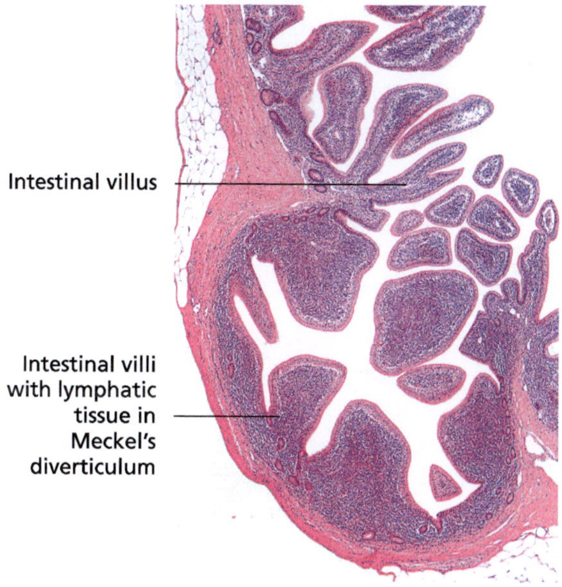

10.64 Jejunum at the level of Meckel's diverticulum. Haematoxylin and eosin stain (x10).

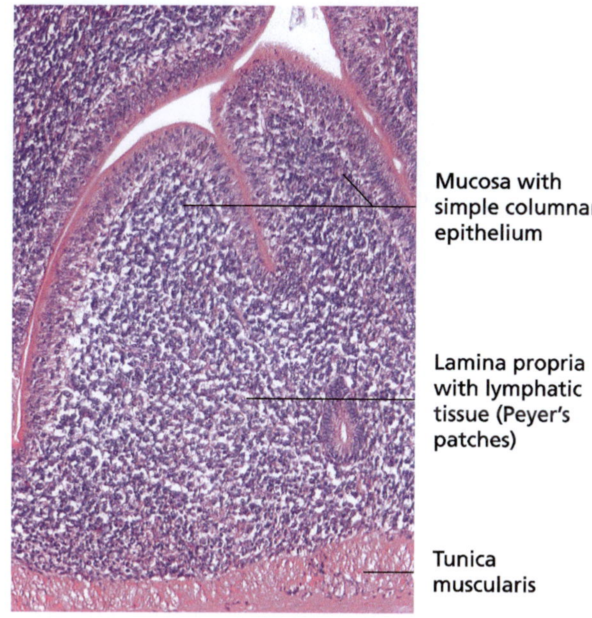

10.65 Ileum with villi (chicken). Haematoxylin and eosin stain (x40).

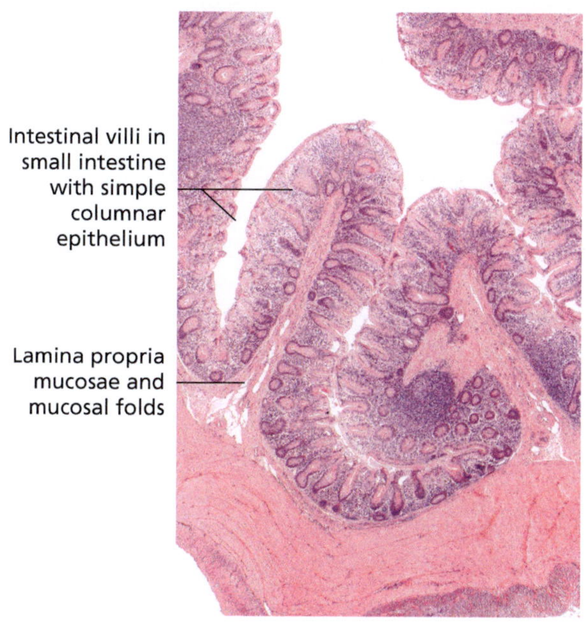

10.66 Caecum with intestinal villi (chicken). Haematoxylin and eosin stain (x25).

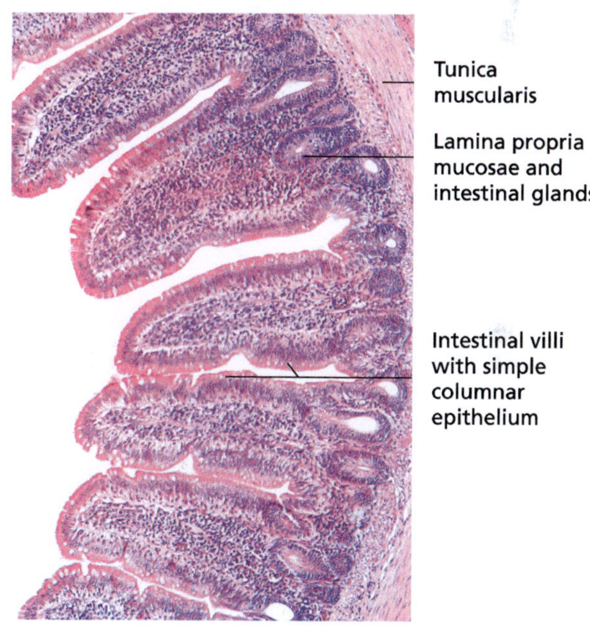

10.67 Cloaca (coprodeum) with intestinal villi (chicken). Haematoxylin and eosin stain (x42).

Cloaca

The common excretory passage for the avian digestive and urogenital systems, the cloaca, is divided by two mucosal folds into three sections:

- coprodeum,
- urodeum and
- proctodeum.

In the chicken, the rectum merges with the first segment of the cloaca, the **coprodeum** (Figure 10.67) with no visible boundary. The intestinal villi are particularly broad in this region. Distally the villi become shorter. The dorsal wall of the subsequent segment, the **urodeum**, contains the ostia of the paired ureters. Adjacent to these openings, the deferent ducts of male birds open on conical papillae. In females, the left side of the urodeum receives the **left oviduct**. In the final section, the **proctodeum**, the rectal lining transitions to a non-glandular mucosa that is continuous with the external skin. The opening of the **cloacal bursa** (**bursa cloacalis, bursa of Fabricius**) is in the dorsal wall of the proctodeum (see Chapter 8, 'Immune system and lymphatic organs'). Glands (**glandulae proctodaeales**) are present in the dorsolateral wall.

At the **external opening of the cloaca**, there is a dorsal and ventral **lip** (**labium venti dorsale** and **ventrale**) each of which contains **glands** (**glandulae venti**). In the chicken, the lips contain numerous sensory Herbst corpuscles.

Glands associated with the intestine

Liver (hepar)

The liver of domestic mammals and birds is one of the few glands of the body that performs a diverse range of functions. Most of these relate to one cell type, the **liver cell** or **hepatocyte** (**hepatocytus**). In greatly simplified terms, the liver performs three central functions that have a significant influence on metabolic processes throughout the body:

- synthesis and immediate secretion (e.g. proteins),
- synthesis, storage and secretion (e.g. glycogen) and
- metabolism and detoxification (e.g. steroids, drugs).

From nutrients absorbed in the intestine, the liver synthesises various endogenous substances: glycogen is produced from the monosaccharide glucose and amino acids are coupled to form complex proteins. Some of these proteins pass into the circulation as plasma proteins (albumin, fibrinogen, prothrombin, enzymes and glycoproteins). Lipoproteins and ketone bodies are metabolised within the hepatocytes.

An important function of liver cells is the synthesis and secretion of bile via a specialised system of capillaries and collecting channels. Hepatocytes secrete bile acids, bilirubin and water, as well as cholesterol and steroid hormones. After synthesising glycogen and triglycerides, liver cells may periodically – often in a diurnal pattern – store these substances in the cytoplasm before releasing them into the blood. Liver cells also act as reservoirs of fat-soluble vitamins (A, D and K). A further key function of liver cells is deamination of amino acids. Additional processes occurring within liver cells include hydroxylation, acetylation, methylation and oxidation-reduction, thus resulting in detoxification of numerous metabolic products that are then eliminated from the body in the bile or through the kidneys.

Embryologically, the liver is a compound organ that develops from **endodermal** and **mesodermal components**. Hepatocytes originate from the endoderm from buds of the **hepatopancreatic ring** of the embryonic foregut. The developing liver cells and pancreatic cells separate from the gut but remain attached by ducts (**ductus choledochus, ductus pancreaticus**). Both the liver and pancreas exert a continuous influence on metabolism.

Early in embryonic development, the endodermal liver cell anlage is divided into sheets of liver cells by the ingrowth of mesodermal umbilical vessels (vv. omphalomesentericae). Endothelial cells lining the capillaries that enter the liver tissue retain their **mesodermal** character, becoming sinusoidal capillaries (liver sinusoids).

Through its mesodermal components, the functions of the liver are expanded to include:

- phagocytosis and
- embryonic haematopoiesis.

Cells migrate from the bone marrow to the liver and, as components of the **mononuclear phagocyte system** (**MPS**), perform non-specific functions such as uptake of molecules, particles and cell fragments from circulating blood (**Kupffer cells**). Haematopoiesis occurs in the liver from early in the middle phase to the end of embryonic development.

The distribution of the embryonic vascular network gives rise to the characteristic lobulation of the liver. This manifests to a varying extent in different species, depending on the degree of connective tissue development. The capacity of the liver to perform its many different functions relies upon a close association between the intra-hepatic vascular network and the spatial arrangement of liver cells.

Structure of the liver

The liver is enclosed in a **capsule** (**tunica fibrosa**) containing collagen fibres and some elastic fibres. The outside of the capsule is lined by a **tunica subserosa** and a simple tunica **serosa**. Bundles of **type 1 collagen fibres** extend from the connective tissue capsule into the parenchyma as interstitial tissue. Afferent and efferent vessels, bile passages and nerve fibres pass through the connective tissue. The arrangement of connective tissue fibres and passages divides the liver into distinct **lobules** (**lobuli hepatici**, see below). The interlobular septa are particularly well developed in the pig (Figure 10.70). In this species, lobulation can be appreciated macroscopically on the surface of the liver. In other mammalian species, lobulation is less distinct (Figure 10.71) but is nevertheless evident in terms of structure and function.

VESSELS OF THE LIVER

The liver receives venous and arterial blood through the hepatic porta (hilus of the liver). These vessels divide and extend widely throughout the parenchyma. Blood entering through both the venous and arterial systems drains into a common outflow.

Within the liver, the nutrient-rich functional blood supply from the intestine and associated unpaired abdominal organs (**portal system**) combines with the oxygen-rich nutritional supply originating from the **hepatic artery**.

Upon entering the liver at the porta, the **portal vein** divides within the interstitial tissue into **interlobular veins**.

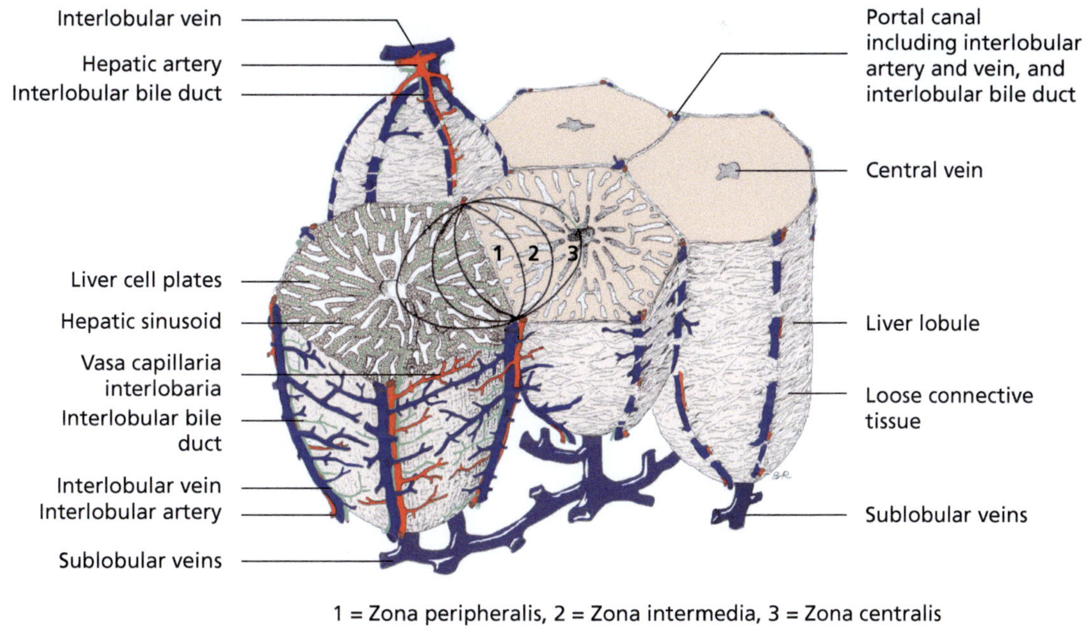

10.68 Three-dimensional reconstruction of liver lobules illustrating the three metabolically active zones (zona peripheralis, zona intermedia and zona centralis) and vascular supply.

The **hepatic artery** passes into the liver together with the portal vein. Its branches, the **interlobular arteries**, accompany the interlobular veins. Both vascular systems lie at the external boundary of the liver lobules and, together with an **interlobular bile duct** (**ductus interlobularis bilifer**) occupy the **portal canal** (Figure 10.68). Within the interlobular connective tissue, the interlobular arteries and veins undergo terminal division into arterioles and venules, then **capillaries** (**vasa capillaria interlobularia**) that enter the liver lobules at right angles to the portal canal.

Immediately after entering the lobule, the arterial and venous systems unite with the **sinus capillaries** (**hepatic sinusoids**, **vasa sinusoidea**) (Figure 10.68), which contain mixed arterio-venous blood.

The sinusoids are thin-walled vessels with a relatively large lumen. They are radially arranged, passing inwards from the outer edge of each liver lobule. At the middle of the lobule the sinusoids converge to form the **central vein** (**v. centralis**) (Figures 10.68, 10.70, 10.71 and 10.73). Within the lobules, the sinusoids pass between hepatic cell plates, or **laminae** (**laminae hepatis**), permitting extensive exchange between the blood and hepatocytes. The central veins merge to form the contractile **sublobular veins** (Figure 10.68) and then **hepatic veins** that drain collectively into the **caudal vena cava**.

The liver contains an extensive network of **lymph vessels**. Lymph drains into deep lymph vessels in the interstitial connective tissue, which pass to the superficial zones of the liver. Lymph vessels leave the liver at the hepatic porta. Superficial lymph capillary networks associated with the tunica subserosa also converge at the hilus of the liver. Together with the deep lymph vessels, they drain into the **hepatic lymph nodes** (**lnn. hepatici**).

LIVER LOBULE (LOBULUS HEPATICUS)

The liver is composed of lobules. Lobule formation is influenced by the distribution of hepatic vessels during embryonic development. Hepatic lobules are structural and functional units comprising hepatocytes of ectodermal origin and mesodermally derived sinusoids. They are defined in different ways (Figure 10.69), according to the vascular structure, or structures, that form(s) the central axis (**portal canal**, **branches of the interlobular arteries and veins** or the **central vein**). The resulting units are the:

- **portal lobule** (= functional unit, emphasises the glandular, exocrine nature of the liver),
- **hepatic acinus** (vascular focus, reflects the metabolic function of the liver) and
- **classic polyhedral liver lobule with central vein** (morphological unit of the liver).

In the **portal lobule** (represented by lines connecting the central veins of three adjacent liver lobules), the **portal canal is at the centre** and the drainage area of its component bile canaliculi is circumscribed. In this view of the liver lobule, emphasis is placed on the **glandular** (secretory) function of the liver (Figure 10.69, A).

The definition of the lobule as a **hepatic acinus** views the lobule as a vascular unit supplied by the interlobular arteries and veins (Figure 10.69, B). An acinus comprises an **interlobular artery and vein**, their terminal branches (as its central axis) and portions of the **two immediately**

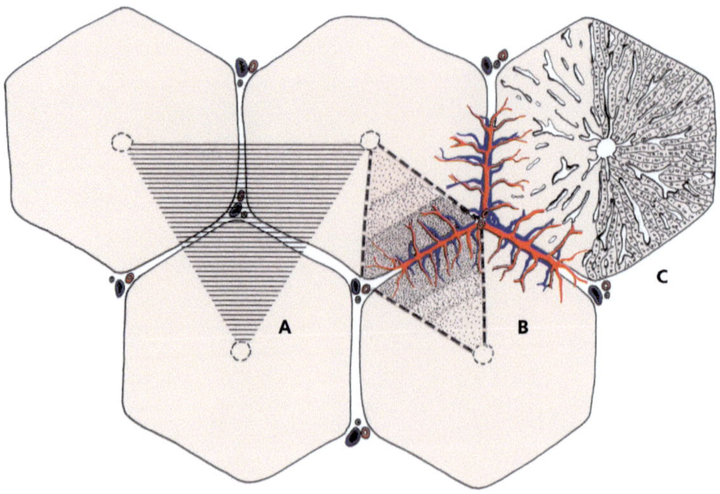

10.69 Subdivision of the liver (schematic). A: portal lobules with portal canal, B: terminal vessels with hepatic acini and C: polygonal lobules with central veins. The portal lobule (A) is centred around the portal canal containing the interlobular bile duct, highlighting the secretory/glandular function of the liver. When the lobule is viewed in the context of the hepatic acini and associated terminal vessels (interlobular arteries and veins) (B), attention is drawn to the metabolic role of the liver. The division of the liver into polygonal lobules (C) is oriented around the central vein and represents a structurally descriptive categorisation of the liver (see text for further detail).

adjacent classic lobules. This incorporation of two neighbouring lobules into a common vascular zone defines a region of the liver based on its **metabolic activity**. Based on changes in the composition of blood from the periphery to the centre of the lobule, the acinus is divided into **three continuous zones** (zona peripheralis, zona intermedia and zona centralis).

Functional distinction of liver lobules on a vascular basis is particularly significant with respect to normal processes and pathological changes occurring within the liver. Processes occurring at the periphery of the lobule include oxidation, components of gluconeogenesis and acetylation of fatty acids.

Anaerobic stages of metabolic processes, including detoxification and lipogenesis, dominate towards the centre of the lobule. The level of metabolic activity exhibits diurnal variation. Certain pathological processes preferentially affect particular zones.

The division of the liver into **classic lobules**, with a central vein and a peripheral boundary comprising interstitial connective tissue, is **morphological** and purely **descriptive** (Figure 10.69, C). From a three-dimensional perspective, the classic liver lobule is a polyhedral arrangement of liver cells measuring approximately 1.5 to 2 mm in length and 0.8 to 1.5 mm at its widest point.

In histological cross-section, classic lobules appear **polygonal** and are generally densely packed. In the pig, the lobules are separated by extensive interstitial connective tissue. **Portal canals** (**portal areas**), containing an **interlobular artery and vein**, **bile duct**, lymph vessels, nerve

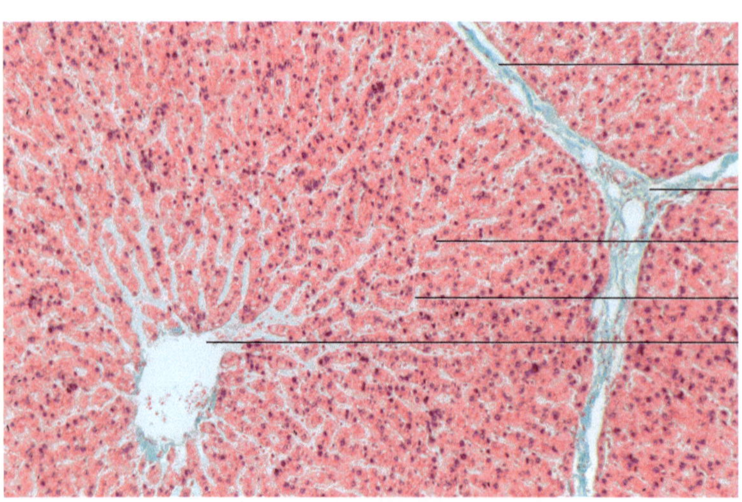

10.70 Liver lobule (pig). Goldner's Masson trichrome stain (x120).

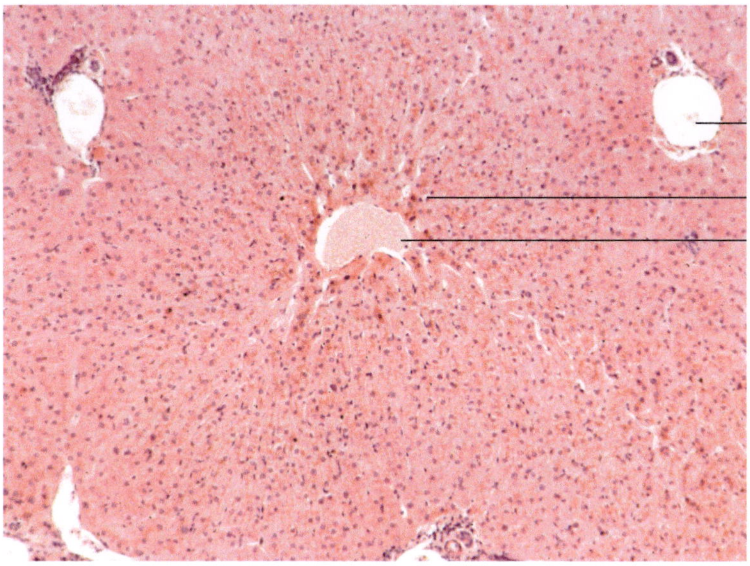

10.71 Liver lobule (dog). The lobular structure is indistinct, marked only by the central vein and portal canals. Haematoxylin and eosin stain (x100).

fibres and associated connective tissue, are present at some of the corners of the polygon (Figure 10.72).

Within the classic lobule, the hepatocytes are arranged in plates (lamina) surrounded by sinusoids. Blood flows from the periphery of the lobule towards the central vein (Figure 10.68).

LIVER SINUSOID (VAS SINUSOIDEUM)

The blood capillaries of the liver have several special characteristics. They are extensively interconnected, up to 0.5 mm long and, depending on the functional status of the liver, 5–15 µm wide with irregular outpouchings. Increases in lumen diameter greatly slow the flow of blood, considerably facilitating exchange of substances with the hepatocyte. At least one surface of each hepatocyte faces a sinusoid. Morphologically, sinusoids are characterised by the following features:

- endothelial cells with pores, endothelial vesicles and intercellular openings,
- discontinuous basal lamina and
- the presence of Kupffer cells.

WALL OF SINUSOID

Hepatic sinusoids are lined with flattened **endothelial cells** that frequently contain non-fenestrated micropinocytic vesicles (coated vesicles). Numerous irregularly spaced pores (diameter up to 0.5 µm) are usually present. **Intercellular spaces** occur sporadically throughout the endothelial lining. **As the basal lamina is discontinuous**, pores and intercellular spaces permit the free passage of substances between the lumen of the sinusoid and the perisinusoidal space of Dissé (see below).

KUPFFER CELLS (MACROPHAGOCYTI STELLATI)

A distinctive **feature of the endothelium** is the presence of **Kupffer cells**. As components of the **MPS system**, these cells have a **phagocytic function** (Figure 10.78). Kupffer cells develop from bone marrow-derived cells and from mesodermal stem cells of the liver.

Based on their three-dimensional morphology, Kupffer cells are also referred to as stellate macrophages. They may become partly detached from the endothelium or bulge into the sinusoid. Kupffer cells **phagocytose** circulating cell fragments, damaged blood cells, bacteria, immune complexes, fibrin and dissolved substances. They store and release iron. In contrast to endothelial cells, Kupffer cells contain abundant organelles, particularly phagosomes, lysosomes and peroxisomes. They are characterised by high peroxidase activity.

As cells of the MPS system, **Kupffer cells** also participate in breakdown of haemoglobin originating from erythrocytes. This results in the formation of bilirubin, which is released by the Kupffer cells and passes into hepatocytes. In the smooth ER of the hepatocyte, bilirubin (insoluble in water) is enzymatically converted into soluble bilirubin glucuronide and transported through the bile ducts to the intestine, from whence it is excreted as urobilinogen.

In addition, Kupffer cells synthesise PGD_2, PGE_2 and other prostaglandins, interleukin-1 and -2, leukotriene D_4 and C_4 as well as interferon and tumour necrosis factor.

PERISINUSOIDAL SPACE (SPATIUM PERISINUSOIDEUM)

Between the wall of the sinusoids and the surface of the hepatocytes is a narrow space (0.5–1 µm), the **perisinusoidal space** (**space of Dissé**; **spatium perisinusoideum**) (Figure 10.78).

The perisinusoidal space plays an important part in regulating interactions between the sinusoid endothelium and

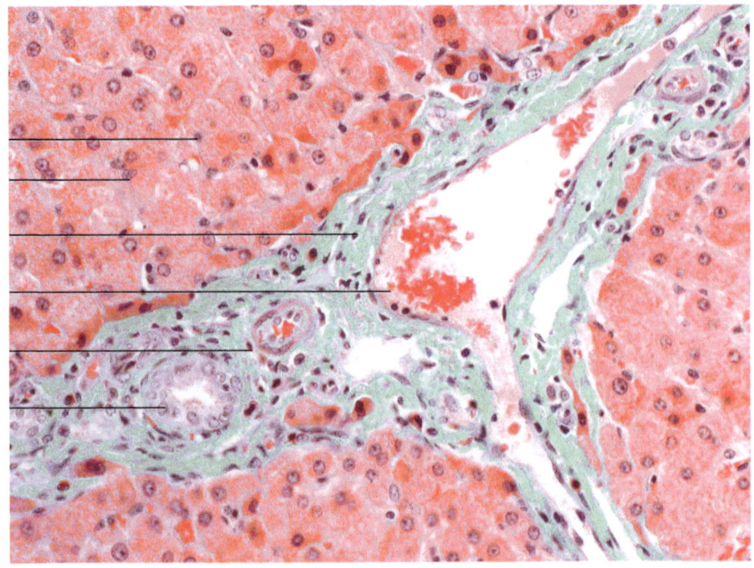

10.72 Portal canal (pig). The bile duct is characterised by simple cuboidal epithelium. Goldner's Masson trichrome stain (x250).

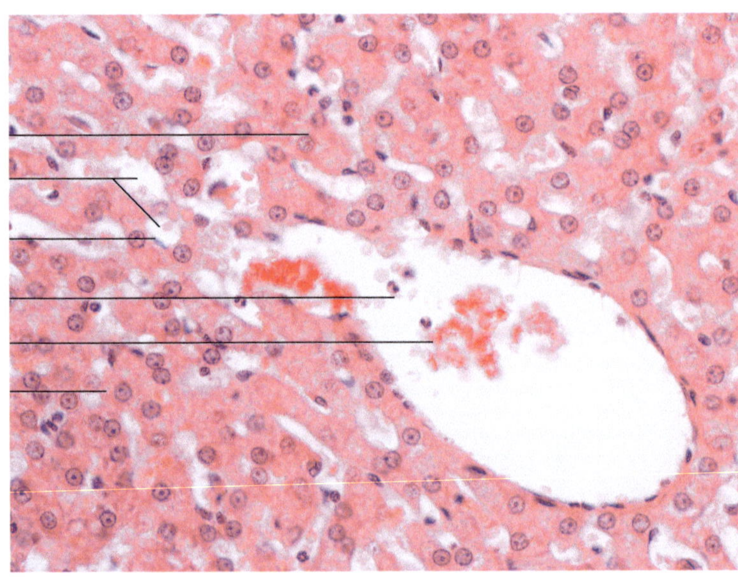

10.73 Middle of a hepatic lobule with hepatic sinusoid opening into central vein (dog). Haematoxylin and eosin stain (x400).

the hepatocyte by facilitating phagocytosis and substance transport and influencing the microcirculation.

The space encloses collagen fibres (type III), fibrocytes, adipocytes (Ito cells) and adrenergic nerve fibres. It is constantly bathed in protein-rich fluid (plasma). Hepatocyte microvilli project into the space, promoting metabolic exchange with the sinusoids. Pathological processes may result in an increase in the collagen fibre content of the perisinusoidal space, leading to a reduction or interruption of the metabolic function of the affected parenchyma.

Ito cells

Adipocytes within the perisinusoidal space (Ito cells) serve as a reservoir of fat and vitamins A, D and K (in cytoplasmic vacuoles). In certain pathological processes, these cells can differentiate into myofibroblast-like cells that appear to contribute to hepatic fibrosis.

Hepatocyte (hepatocytus)

Liver cells, or hepatocytes, are arranged in **plates** or **laminae** (**laminae hepatis**). The laminae form a spongiform three-dimensional system that encloses the network of hepatic sinusoids. The plates radiate outwards from the **central vein**. Hepatocytes have a long lifespan. Degenerating or dead cells can, to some extent, be replaced slowly by mitosis.

Individual **hepatocytes** (Figures 10.74, 10.75 and 10.79) are 15–30 μm, polyhedral and have a typically spherical nucleus rich in euchromatin. One distinct nucleolus is usually present. Through amitosis, hepatocytes may contain two or more nuclei, depending on the functional status of the cell. Hepatocytes contain abundant metabolically active organelles, reflecting the diversity of functions they perform.

The dense network of **rough endoplasmic reticulum** within hepatocytes is indicative of their role in protein synthesis. The rough ER participates in formation and transport of α- and β-globulins, ceruloplasmin, fibrinogen, coagulation factors and cellular enzymes (e.g. glutamate dehydrogenase). These cellular products are continuously processed by the Golgi apparatus and released into the perisinusoidal space, from whence they reach the blood.

Smooth endoplasmic reticulum is diffusely distributed in the cytoplasm (Figure 10.79). This is the site of **lipoprotein** synthesis and **detoxification of noxious substances**. Individual substances produced by the smooth ER include phospholipids, triglycerides, cholesterol, cholesterol esters and free fatty acids. The smooth ER also contributes to synthesis of steroid hormones and transformation and breakdown of sterols. The lipoproteins are assembled in the Golgi apparatus, enclosed in a membrane and exocytosed into the perisinusoidal space.

The membranes of the smooth ER also serve in the modification, breakdown, detoxification and expulsion of metabolic products and foreign substances (e.g. steroids, drugs). Enzymatic detoxification involves processes such as acetylation, methylation, demethylation, reduction and/or oxidation.

A major function of the smooth ER is **formation of bile**. In this process, cholesterol is converted to bile acids and bile salts, which are actively transported into the bile canaliculi together with water and bilirubin.

With respect to metabolic exchange, the key organelle within hepatocytes is the well-developed **Golgi apparatus**

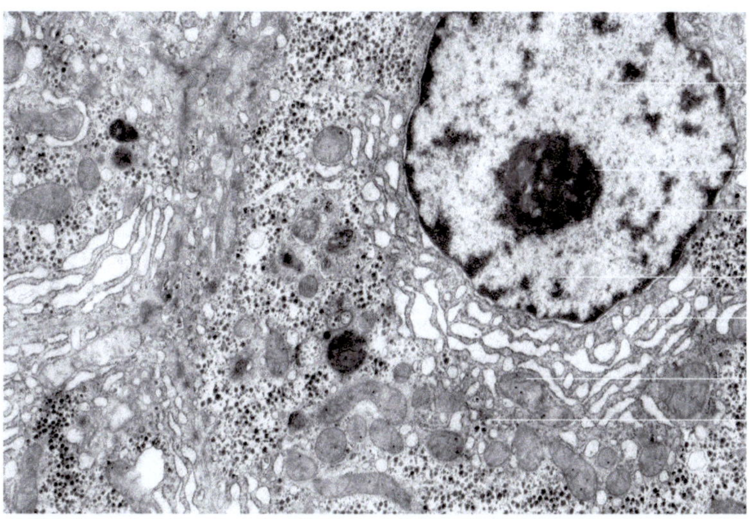

10.74 Fine structure of a hepatocyte (horse; x6000).

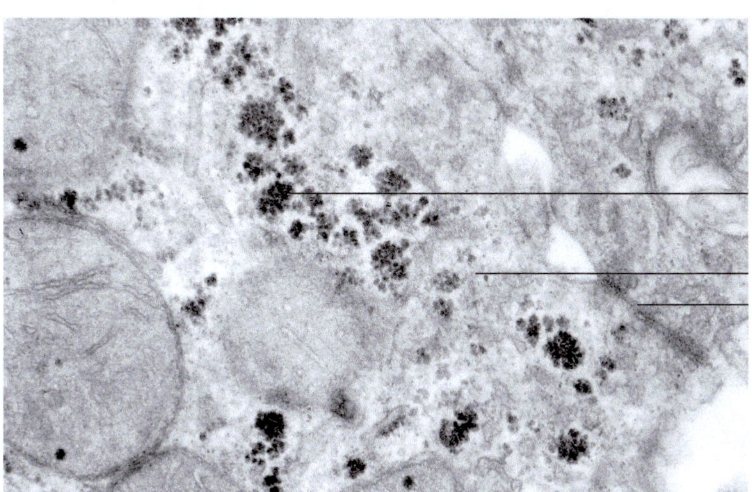

10.75 Fine structure of the cytoplasm of a hepatocyte (horse; x14,000).

(Figures 10.74, 10.78 and 10.79). The Golgi apparatus is responsible for turnover and storage of substances undergoing intracellular transport. The membrane systems of the Golgi apparatus participate in the formation of proteoglycans and the manufacture of lipoproteins and bile acids. In addition, they are the site of production of intracellular membranes and numerous enzymes (e.g. acid phosphatases, thiaminopyrophosphatases).

Hepatocytes contain abundant, usually oval **mitochondria**. Their number and structure vary according to the level of cellular activity (up to 3000 mitochondria per cell). Hepatocyte mitochondria are replaced approximately every 10 days. These organelles contribute to metabolism by providing energy. Enzymes associated with the mitochondrial membranes and matrix are involved in the cellular respiratory chain, the citric acid cycle and β-oxidation.

Lysosomes are plentiful near the bile canaliculi (see below). These serve in intracellular digestion of exogenous or endogenous substances. The breakdown of proteins, glycoproteins, glycolipids, nucleic acids and lipids takes place within lysosomes. In addition, lysosomes form residual bodies, or lipofuscin. Organelles referred to as microbodies contain metabolic enzymes including oxidases, uricase and catalase.

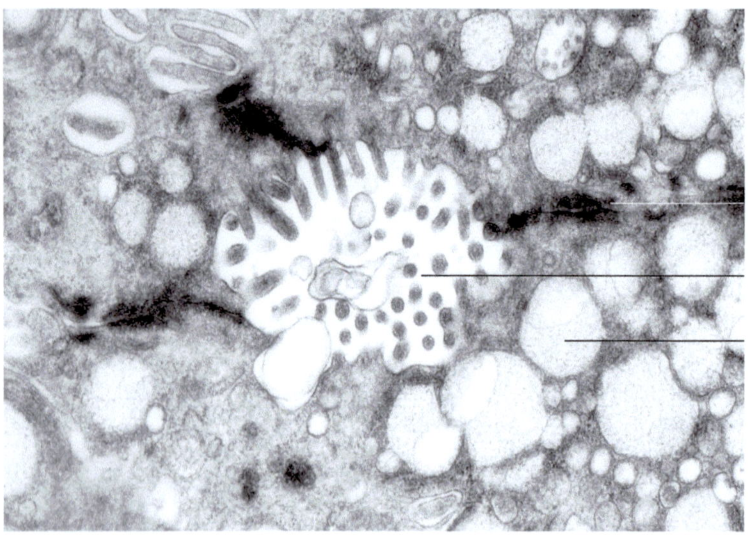

10.76 Fine structure of a bile canaliculus (horse; x15,000).

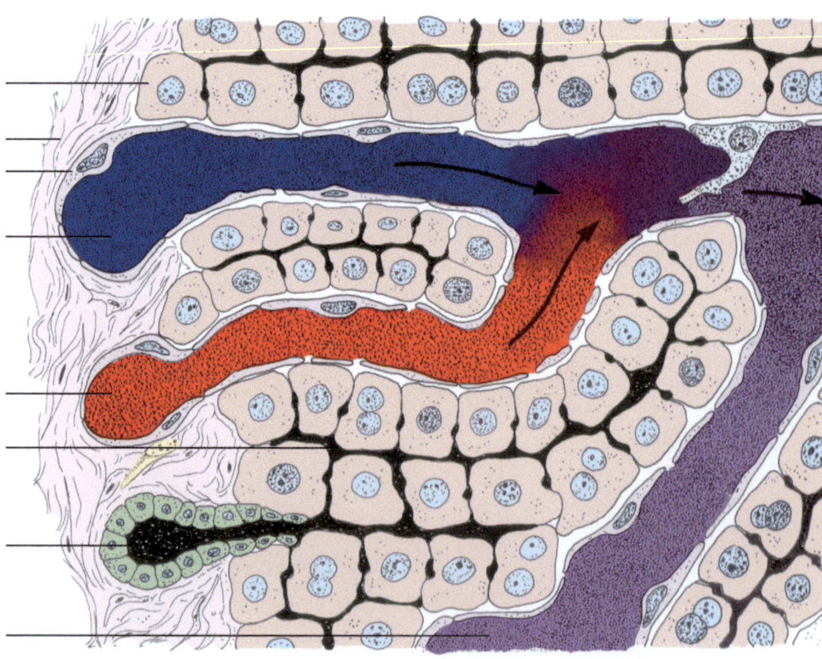

10.77 Interlobular artery and vein supplying a liver lobule, and bile canaliculi passing between hepatocytes and opening into bile ductules (schematic).

The **cytoplasm of hepatocytes** is rich in paraplasmic inclusions (see Chapter 1, 'The cell') such as **lipid vacuoles** and **glycogen**. Glycogen (Figures 10.75 and 10.79) takes the form of small granules (20–30 nm) that are typically arranged in rosettes. Glycogen content exhibits diurnal variation.

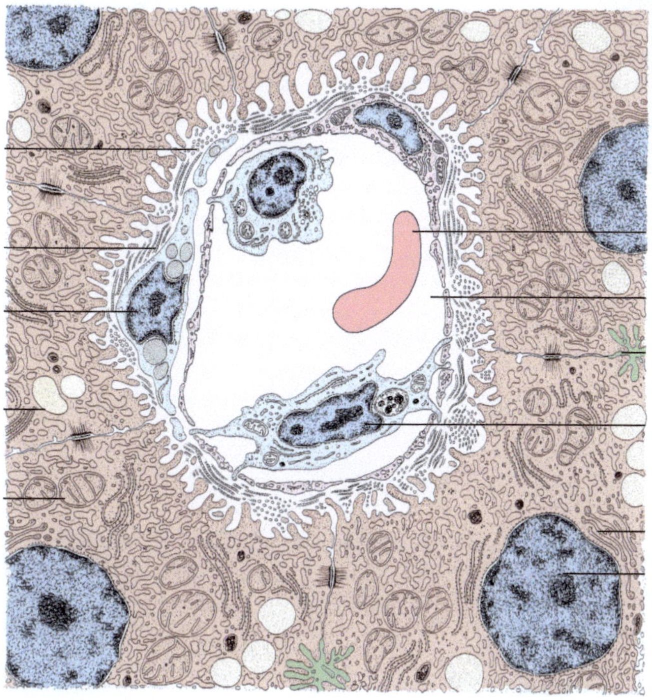

10.78 Hepatic sinusoid with perisinusoidal space and surrounding hepatocytes (schematic).

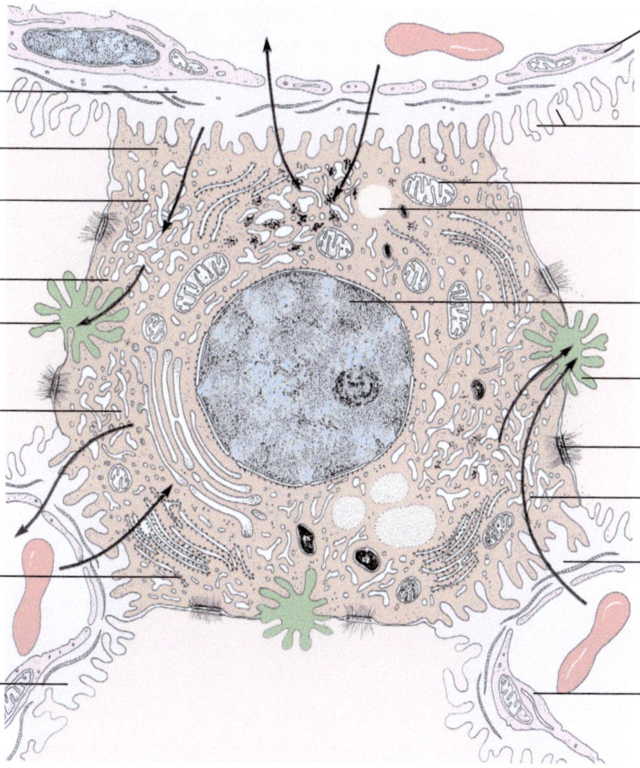

10.79 Structure of a hepatocyte and adjacent sinusoid (schematic).

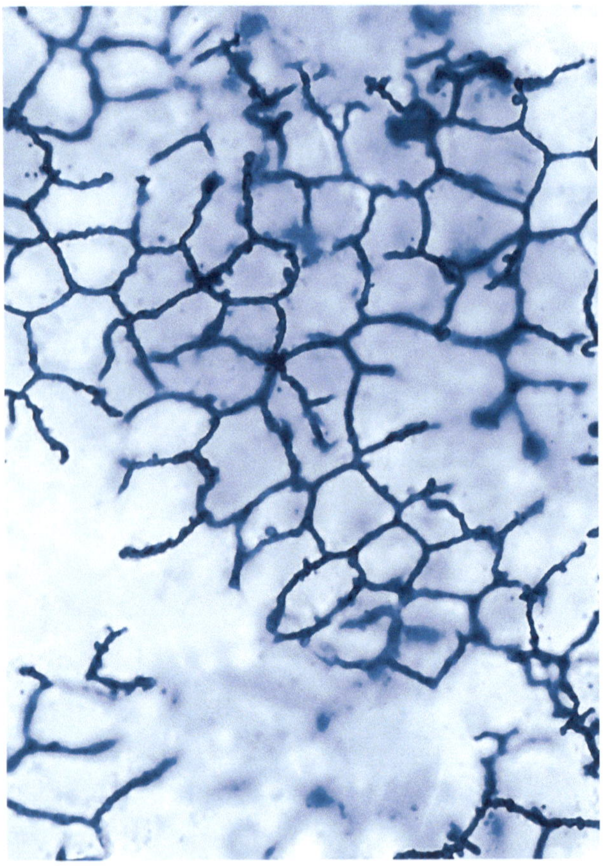

10.80 Reticular arrangement of bile canaliculi in the liver (pig). Injected specimen (x560).

The **plasmalemma** of the hepatocyte has three structurally and functionally distinct zones. At least one, sometimes two to three, **surfaces** of the hepatocyte face the **perisinusoidal space** (Figure 10.79). Microvilli on these surfaces serve in the absorption of substances, in the exchange of ions, or as hormone receptors (insulin, glucagon, secretin).

Uptake of substances across these surfaces occurs by pinocytosis or transmembrane transport. Depending on the level of metabolic activity, vesicles and irregular cell processes may be present. Cellular products are constantly delivered to the blood across this structurally dynamic interface.

The **remaining surfaces** are divided into **areas of contact** between adjacent cells (contact surfaces) and areas that secrete bile (canalicular surfaces). Intercellular contacts include **tight junctions** (**zonulae occludentes**), **zonulae adherentes** and **nexus** (**gap junctions**) (Figures 10.75 and 10.76).

At the canalicular surface, bile is excreted into a specialised drainage system. The walls of this system comprise modified hepatocyte plasmalemma while the **tubular lumen** is formed by expansion of the intercellular space. The resulting channel is referred to as a **bile canaliculus** (**canaliculus bilifer**) (Figures 10.76 and 10.79). Microvilli project into the canaliculi, increasing the capacity for bile excretion. The membrane lining the canaliculi is rich in membrane-active enzymes (ATP) and resistant to the effects of bile acids. Intercellular junctions prevent leakage of bile into the intercellular space adjacent to the bile canaliculi.

Bile ducts

The following structures and processes are responsible for the formation, excretion and transport of bile:

- intracellular production of bile acids in the smooth ER and Golgi apparatus of the hepatocyte,
- vesicular intracellular transport to the bile canaliculi (canaliculi biliferi) lined by modified plasmalemma,
- luminal intrahepatic transport of bile through small bile ductules (ductuli biliferi) lined by cuboidal epithelium, followed by larger ductules (ductuli interlobulares; one of the components of the portal canal),
- passage of bile into the hepatic duct (ductus hepaticus),
- luminal extra-hepatic transport of bile acids in the cystic duct (from the gall bladder) and bile duct and
- delivery of bile into the duodenum (duodenal papilla).

Within liver lobules, bile flows through a network of tubular **bile canaliculi** (see above) (Figures 10.76, 10.79 and 10.80). Near the surface of the lobules, these channels drain into small **bile ductules** (**ductuli biliferi**). Bile moves against the direction of blood flow, driven by the pressure created by production of new bile. The bile canaliculi are not bounded by endothelium. Their walls are formed by the modified surface membrane of hepatocytes. The bile ductules are lined by simple cuboidal to columnar epithelium.

Bile ductules pass from the liver lobules into the interstitial connective tissue and combine to form larger **interlobular ducts** (**ductus interlobularis bilifer**). Each interlobular duct lies within a portal canal, accompanied by an interlobular artery and vein. Several **interlobular ducts** combine to form the **hepatic ducts** (**ductus hepaticus**), that exit the liver at the **porta**.

Together, the bile canaliculi, bile ductules, interlobular ducts and hepatic ducts form the **excretory system** of the liver. Obstruction of any of these passages results in back pressure that is damaging to liver cells and may cause bile to enter the blood (icterus).

Outside the liver, the hepatic ducts are joined by the **cystic duct** (**ductus cysticus**) (from the gall bladder) to form the **bile duct** (**ductus choledochus**). These extra-hepatic passages are lined with simple columnar epithelium. The bile duct mucosa is surrounded by loose connective tissue with elastic fibres and thin layers of smooth muscle. Occasional goblet cells and mucoid glands are present.

Species variation

Birds: The structure of the liver and bile passages of birds is similar to that of mammals. The main distinction is the limited amount of interlobular connective tissue, and thus poor differentiation of hepatic lobules, in birds. The plates of hepatocytes may be composed of a single layer (sparrows) or a double layer (chicken) (Figures 10.81 and 10.82). The surface of the avian liver is covered by a **tunica serosa**, resting upon a thin **stratum fibrosum**. The liver is enclosed by the hepatic peritoneal sac. Double layers of serous lamellae anchor the liver within the coelomic cavity.

Gall bladder (vesica biliaris, vesica fellea)

The gall bladder stores bile. In addition, bile is concentrated in the gall bladder by the reabsorption of water. The **gall bladder is absent in the horse**. In the empty gall bladder, the mucosa is thrown into folds (**plicae tunicae mucosae**). Invaginations and crypts (**cryptae tunicae mucosae**) allow the mucosa to expand without excessive stretching of the gall bladder wall.

The layers of the gall bladder wall are as follows:

- **tunica mucosa**: simple columnar epithelium with microvilli and goblet cells,
- **lamina propria mucosae**: contains mucoid glands (particularly in ruminants),
- **tunica muscularis**: musculo-elastic tissue, smooth muscle arranged in spiral lattices,
- **tunica adventitia**: where gall bladder adjoins the liver and
- **tunica serosa**: on the free surface of the gall bladder.

The **tunica mucosa** (Figure 10.83) is lined by a simple columnar epithelium that typically has a distinct brush border. This reflects the intense absorptive activity of the epithelial cells. The prominent intercellular spaces are hyperosmolar (via

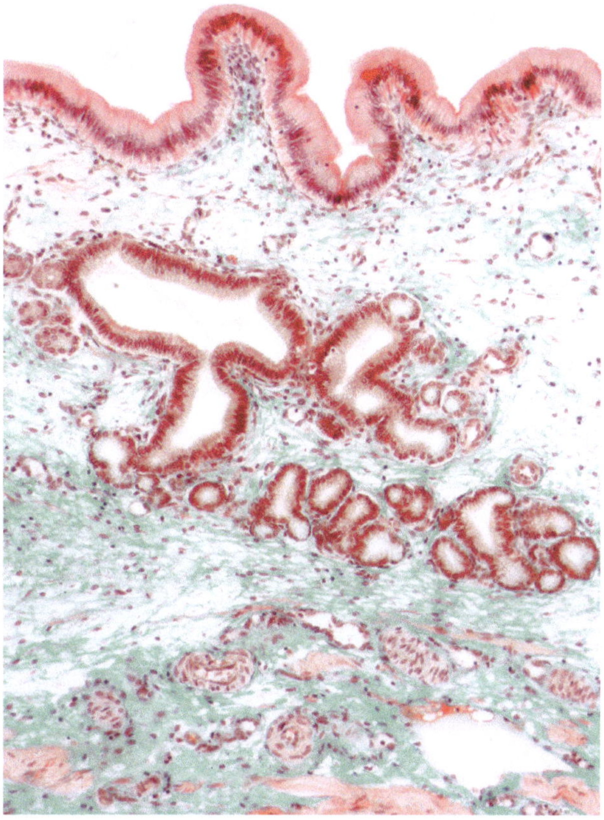

10.81 Wall of gallbladder with simple columnar epithelium and mucous glands (ox). Goldner's Masson trichrome stain (x120).

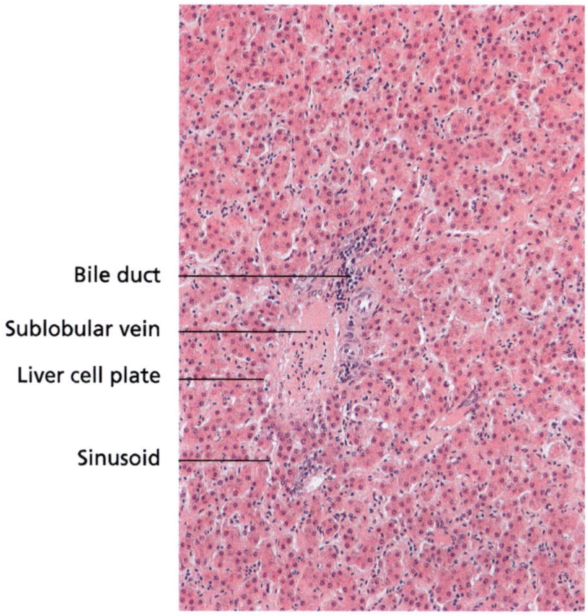

10.82 Liver with sparse connective tissue between hepatic lobules (chicken). Haematoxylin and eosin stain (x120).

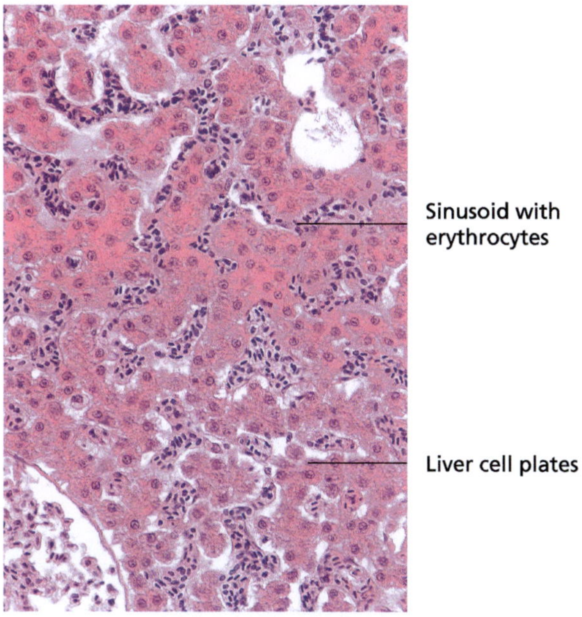

10.83 Section of liver taken from the centre of a lobule (chicken). Haematoxylin and eosin stain (x200).

Na^+ ion pump in lateral plasma membrane), drawing water from the cells. The nuclei lie in the basal third of the cell. In addition to absorptive **epithelial cells**, the lining of the gall bladder contains isolated **secretory mucous cells** (**goblet cells**). Mucus produced by these cells, and by mucoid glands in the lamina propria, protects the surface of the epithelial cells against the effects of bile acids.

The mucous glands in the lamina propria are scant in carnivores and pigs, and numerous in ruminants. The subepithelial tissue is richly supplied with blood vessels and autonomic nerve fibres that regulate the secretory activity of the glands and the absorptive function of the epithelial cells.

External to the lamina propria is a layer of **smooth muscle**. Due to the spiral arrangement of these fibres, this layer usually appears irregular in histological section. The contractile capacity of the smooth muscle layer is supported by a delicate network of elastic fibres. The connective tissue layer external to the muscle layer contains extensive fat deposits. In the regions that are in contact with the liver, the outermost layer of the gall bladder comprises a **tunica adventitia**. A **tunica serosa** covers the surfaces of the gall bladder that face the peritoneal cavity.

Pancreas

The pancreas is a gland that, together with the liver, develops from the hepatopancreatic ring of the embryonic foregut. In contrast to the liver, in which hepatocytes perform several different functions, the cells of the pancreas are divided into those that have an exocrine (secretory) or an endocrine (incretory) role. These groups of cells are referred to as the **exocrine pancreas** (**pars exocrina pancreatis**) and the **endocrine pancreas** (**pars endocrina pancreatis**). The endocrine component of the pancreas is described in Chapter 9, 'Endocrine system'. The exocrine portion consists of a:

- compound tubulo-acinar gland with:
  - serous end-pieces with basally located rough ER and zymogen granules,
- a system of ducts:
  - intercalated duct (ductus intercalatus) with characteristic centro-acinar cells,
  - numerous non-striated intralobular ducts,
  - several interlobular ducts and
  - an excretory duct (ductus pancreaticus).

The compound tubulo-acinar glandular parenchyma is similar in structure to that of the parotid gland (Figures 10.84 to 10.87, 10.89). The cells of the acinar end pieces have characteristics typical of protein-synthesising serous cells (Figure 10.84). The basal third of the cell contains the rough endoplasmic reticulum and most of the ribosomes, and hence this region is basophilic. The rough ER is the site of production of the components of pancreatic juice (e.g. trypsinogen, chymotrypsinogen, ribonucleases or desoxynucleases). These are coated with a membrane in the Golgi apparatus for transport to the apical cytoplasm.

These inactive secretory granules, termed **zymogen granules**, render the cytoplasm acidophilic (Figure 10.86). After being transported to the cell surface, zymogen granules are released into the intercalated ducts by exocytosis. The quantity of zymogen granules in the cytoplasm varies with feed intake; their numbers rapidly decrease after feeding and build up during periods of starvation. Also added

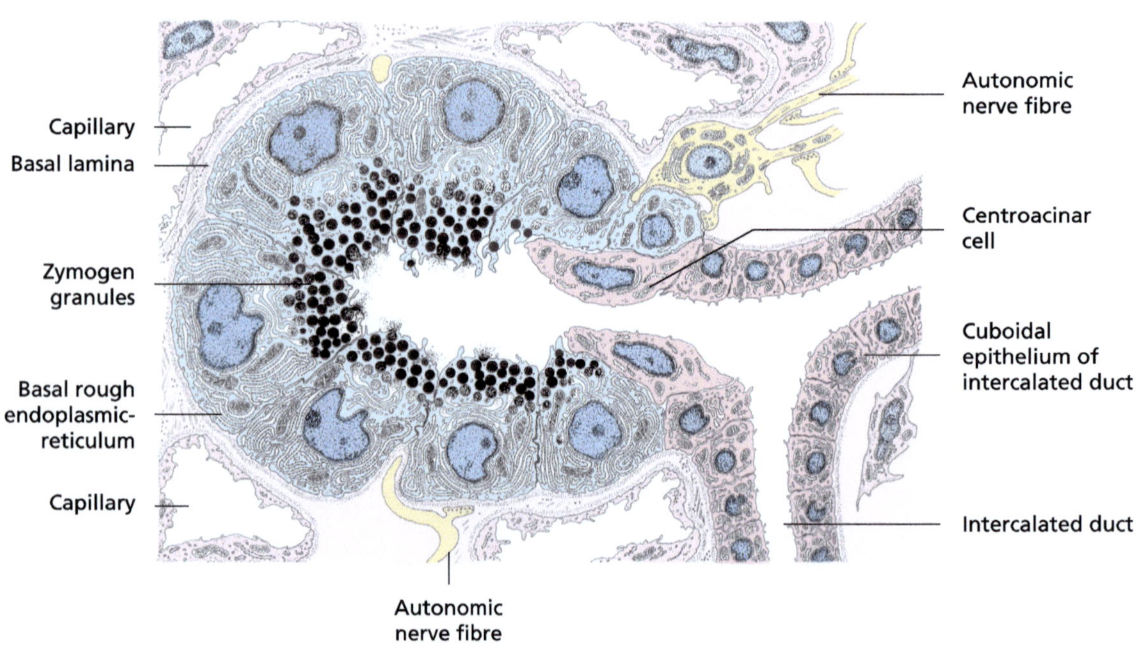

10.84 Exocrine pancreas with associated vessels and nerve fibres (schematic).

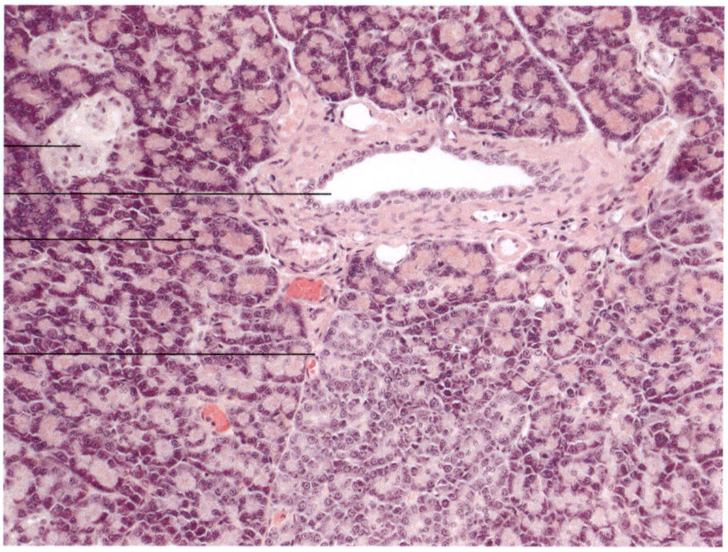

10.85 Pancreas (cat). The exocrine pancreas has a tubulo-acinar gland structure. The end-pieces produce a serous secretion. Haematoxylin and eosin stain (x18).

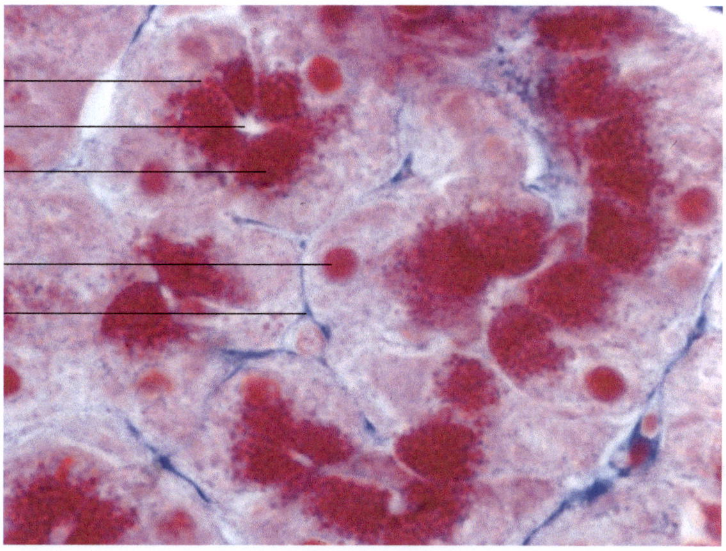

10.86 Serous end-pieces in the exocrine pancreas (calf). The basal cytoplasm contains abundant rough ER, the apical cytoplasm contains acidophilic zymogen granules. Azan stain (x1200).

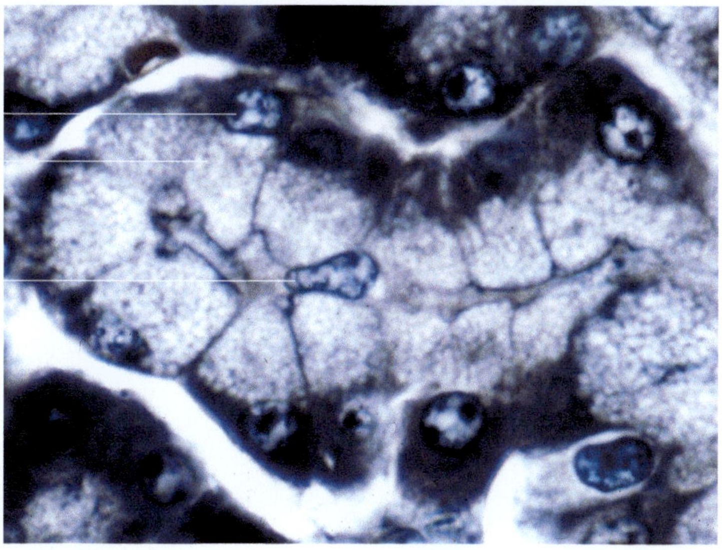

10.87 Pancreatic acinus (dog). Iron haematoxylin stain (x1200).

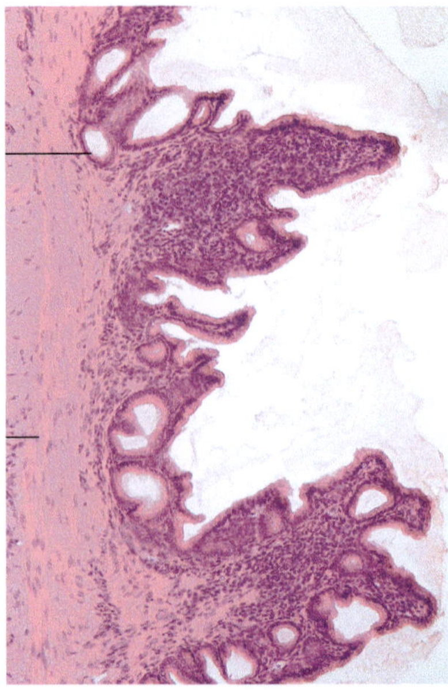

10.88 Gall bladder (chicken). Haematoxylin and eosin stain (x42).

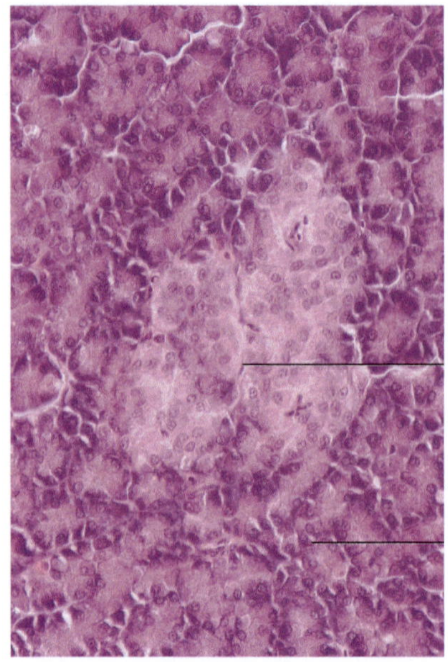

10.89 Pancreas (chicken). Haematoxylin and eosin stain (x300).

to the pancreatic juice are carboxypeptidases, phospholipases, amylases, collagenases and esterases (from the Golgi apparatus and endoplasmic reticulum), as well as water and electrolytes. Within the pancreas, enzymes are present in their inactive form, becoming activated by secretions of the intestinal mucosa. The synthesis and secretion of pancreatic juice components is stimulated by the vagus nerve, and by gastrin, secretin and cholecystokinin.

Centro-acinar cells, considered components of the intercalated ducts, frequently extend into the acinar end pieces (Figures 10.84 and 10.87). The epithelium of the **intercalated duct** (**ductus intercalatus**) is simple cuboidal. Intercalated ducts are continued by **intralobular ducts**. There are no striated ducts. The epithelium of the larger **interlobular ducts** is columnar and often contains goblet cells. The ducts are surrounded by loose networks of collagen fibres containing blood vessels and nerve fibre bundles.

Species variation

Birds: The gall bladder lies on the facies visceralis of the right lobe of the liver. **Many varieties of pigeons and parrots lack a gall bladder**. Where present, the gall bladder exhibits a structure similar to that of mammals (Figure 10.88).

The secretions of the **exocrine portion** of the avian pancreas pass via three ducts (ductus pancreaticus dorsalis, ventralis and accessorius) into the ascending duodenum. As in mammals, the **endocrine portion** (Figure 10.89), the islets of Langerhans, produce insulin, glucagon and somatostatin. The islets are largest and most numerous in the splenic lobe of the pancreas.

Respiratory system (apparatus respiratorius)

11

The principal function of the respiratory organs is the uptake of oxygen from the atmosphere to sustain aerobic cellular metabolism, and the expulsion of carbon dioxide produced during cellular respiration. The vascular system serves as a **vehicle for transport** of gases between the **respiratory system** and the cells of the body. Respiratory activity influences the concentration of oxygen and carbon dioxide in the blood, thus regulating blood pH.

The respiratory system is divided into two structurally and functionally distinct components:

- conducting airways for transport of inspired and expired gases and
- an interface for passive exchange of gases between the air and the blood (blood–air barrier).

The **conducting airways** begin at the nasal cavity and continue through the pharynx, larynx and the trachea to the bronchi within the lungs. Throughout its course, inspired air is filtered, humidified, warmed or cooled and subjected to sensory sampling by the olfactory region (fundus nasi). The respiratory mucosa performs innate and acquired immune functions.

Organs lying adjacent to the upper respiratory tract, including the paranasal sinuses, auditory tube, vomeronasal organ, nasolacrimal ducts and the guttural pouches (in the horse), perform ancillary functions that complement the role of the conducting airways. The larynx is specialised for vocalisation.

The conducting airways end in a series of increasingly narrow tubes that open into blind sacs referred to as **alveoli**. These terminal segments constitute the **respiratory system** in the strictest sense, as this is where gas exchange occurs. The alveoli are thin-walled chambers surrounded by a dense network of capillaries. The blood-air barrier is formed by the epithelium of the alveoli and the endothelium of the adjacent blood vessels with its underlying basal lamina.

The pulmonary capillaries also play a role in regulation of the circulatory system. The endothelium synthesises serotonin, histamine and bradykinin, and converts angiotensin I into angiotensin II.

Conducting airways

Structure of the conducting airways

Most of the internal surface of the conducting airways is lined by **respiratory mucosa**. A small portion, restricted to the olfactory region of the nasal cavity, is classified as **olfactory mucosa**.

The structure of the respiratory mucosa is consistent throughout the conducting airways (Figure 11.1 and Table 11.1), comprising:

- ciliated pseudostratified columnar epithelium (respiratory epithelium) underlaid by
- a fibro-elastic network, mixed glands, smooth muscle cells, and numerous aggregates of lymphatic tissue and
- occasional capacitance vessels (veins), particularly in the nasal cavity.

Except for the nasal vestibule, pharynx and larynx, the conducting airways are lined from the nasal cavity to the distal bronchi by **respiratory epithelium** (Figure 11.2). This typically **pseudostratified columnar** epithelium contains various cell types:

- ciliated epithelial cells,
- secretory cells (mainly goblet cells),
- brush cells with microvilli,
- basal cells (acting as reserve cells) and
- APUD cells.

The free surface of most **epithelial cells** bears **cilia** that beat in a coordinated fashion to transport inhaled foreign matter, or particles originating from within the body, towards the pharynx. To facilitate this function, particles are bound to cilia by mucus produced by numerous **secretory cells** within the epithelium. Secretory cells (predominantly goblet cells) are found mainly in the upper airways, preventing build-up of mucus in the lungs. Together with subepithelial mixed glands, the mucus produced by goblet cells also serves to humidify inspired air.

Brush cells, featuring prominent microvilli, are specialised chemosensory cells. **Basal cells** serve as reserve cells, capable

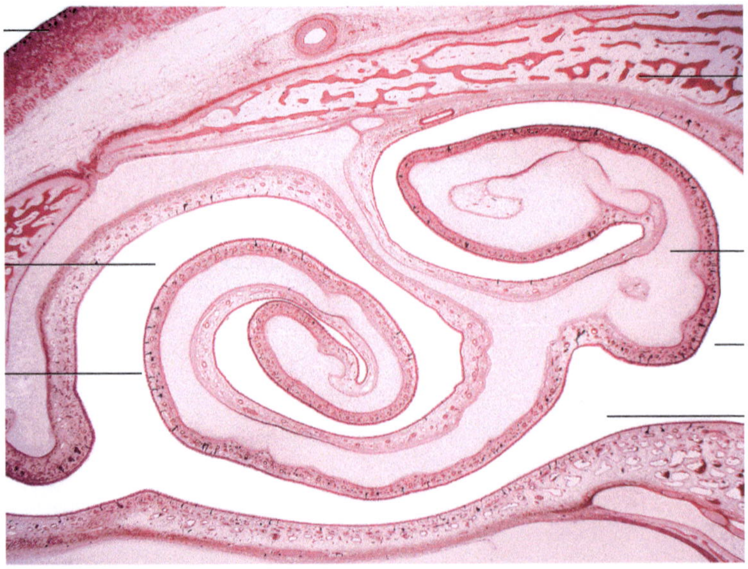

11.1 Low-magnification view of the nasal concha (calf). Haematoxylin and eosin stain (x10).

Table 11.1 Histological features of the conducting airways of domestic mammals.

Segment	Epithelium	Glands	Connective and supportive tissue	Special features
Nasal cavity: nasal vestibule	Keratinised, pigmented, stratified squamous epithelium	Sweat glands and sebaceous glands	Hyaline cartilage, dense connective tissue	Vibrissae
respiratory region	Respiratory mucosa with cilia, microvilli, secretory (mainly goblet) cells	Serous, mucous or mixed tubulo-acinar glands	Tightly adherent to underlying cartilage or periosteum	Cavernous stratum with capacitance veins
olfactory region	Olfactory mucosa with sensory cilia	Tubulo-acinar, predominantly serous glands	Similar to respiratory region	Bipolar neurons (neurosensory cells) with club-like dendritic bulbs, basal cells and sustentacular cells
Nasopharynx	Respiratory mucosa with cilia, microvilli and secretory cells	Branched mucous, serous and mixed glands	Underlaid by skeletal muscle and dense connective tissue	Lymphatic tissue in the form of tonsils (varies with species)
Larynx	Stratified squamous epithelium and respiratory epithelium with secretory cells	Predominantly mucous glands	Hyaline and elastic cartilage, dense connective tissue	Diffuse lymphoid tissue and lymphoid follicles
Trachea	Respiratory mucosa with cilia, microvilli and secretory cells (mainly goblet cells)	Tubulo-acinar mucous and seromucous glands	Hyaline cartilage, dense connective tissue and smooth muscle spanning the free edges of the cartilaginous rings (m. trachealis)	Number and shape of tracheal rings varies with species

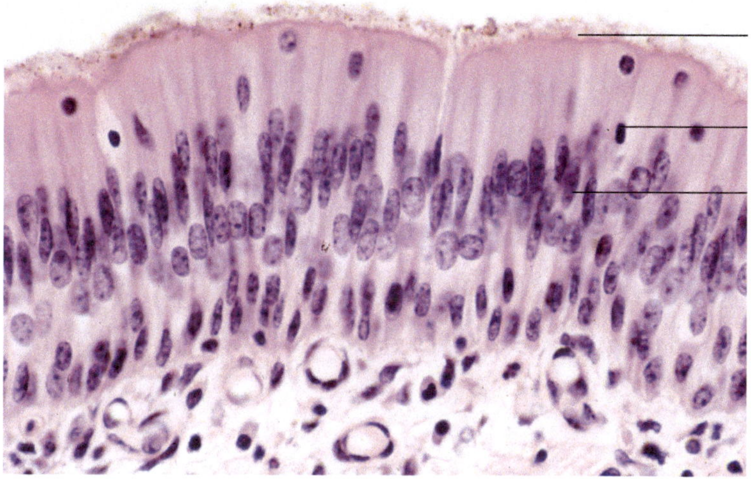

11.2 Nasal septum (calf). Respiratory epithelium (pseudostratified columnar) is ciliated and usually coated with a thin layer of mucus. Subepithelial capillaries are abundant. Haematoxylin and eosin stain (x480).

of dividing and differentiating into other cell types. **APUD cells** (amine and precursor uptake and decarboxylation cells) containing amino acid decarboxylases are also present.

A subepithelial fibro-elastic network anchors the epithelium firmly to underlying periosteum or cartilage. This layer contains glands, mostly of the **seromucous** type, as well as a prominent vascular network incorporating capacitance veins. Isolated smooth muscle cells are also found in this tissue. Depending on location, the outermost layer of the conducting airways is comprised of cartilage.

This basic structure is modified, according to function, in individual segments of the conducting system.

Segments of the conducting airways

The conducting airways are composed of the:

- nasal cavity (cavum nasi),
- paranasal sinuses (sinus paranasales),
- vomeronasal organ (organa vomeronasalia),
- pharynx,
- larynx,
- trachea and
- bronchi and bronchioles.

Nasal cavity (cavum nasi)

Nasal vestibule

The rostral portion of the nasal cavity, the nasal vestibule (**vestibulum nasi**), is lined by stratified squamous epithelium. Initially, this is keratinised (cutaneous zone), becoming non-keratinised deeper in the vestibule. The epithelium is usually pigmented and distinctly papillated. Caudally, the vestibular epithelium gradually reduces in height and transitions into respiratory epithelium of the nasal cavity proper.

The taut, elastic lamina propria contains abundant blood vessels and nerve fibres as well as isolated serous glands. This layer is firmly connected to underlying muscle or cartilage.

The **lateral nasal gland** (**glandula nasalis lateralis**) empties into the nasal vestibule. Its secretory product serves to moisten the nasal openings.

> **Species variation**
>
> **Birds**: Pigeons lack a nasal gland. In most birds the nasal gland consists of a **lateral** and **medial lobe**, each with a single duct.
>
> **Dog**: The **lateral nasal gland** is particularly well developed in the dog. Its serous secretion passes into the nasal vestibule and moistens the nasal planum.
>
> **Horse**: The rostral portion of the nasal cavity and the **nasal diverticulum** (**diverticulum nasi**) are lined with hairy skin incorporating sebaceous glands and sweat glands.

Respiratory region

The respiratory region constitutes the major portion of the nasal cavity proper. In this region, the lumen of the nasal cavity is subdivided by the ectoturbinates and endoturbinates. The surfaces of the nasal conchae, nasal meatuses and nasal septum are lined by **respiratory epithelium**.

The loose subepithelial connective tissue contains tubulo-acinar serous, mucous or mixed **glands** (**nasal glands**). These may occur individually or as groups, separated by **lymphoid tissue** (Figure 11.3). The respiratory mucosa is tightly bound to the underlying perichondrium or periosteum.

The vascular system of the respiratory mucosa, particularly well developed in the dog and horse, incorporates

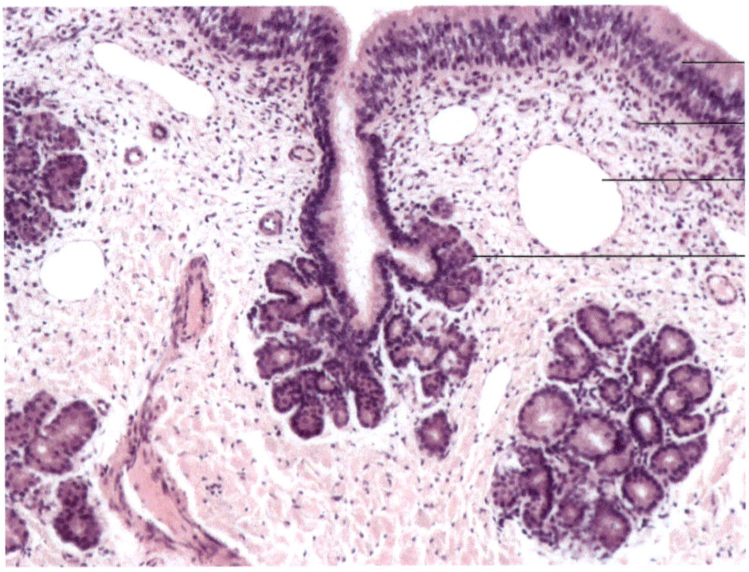

11.3 Nasal mucosa (calf). The mucosa of the conducting airways is characterised by respiratory epithelium, branched tubulo-acinar seromucous glands and a well-developed vascular network. Haematoxylin and eosin stain (x120).

structural and functional specialisations (Figures 11.3 and 11.7). Small muscular arteries passing rostro-caudally through the loose connective tissue give rise to a delicate subepithelial capillary network with a fenestrated epithelium. The capillaries drain into a plexus of expanded, sinus-like veins. Temporary contraction of **longitudinally oriented muscle cushions** in the walls of the veins ('**capacitance veins**') slows the flow of blood in the venous plexus, resulting in swelling of the mucosa. This reflex mechanism, together with the mucous layer on the epithelial surface, serves to warm and humidify air entering the nasal cavity. Arteriovenous anastomoses facilitate this process.

Olfactory region

The olfactory region is responsible for the sense of smell. The mucosa lining the olfactory region (tunica mucosa olfactoria) is composed of:

- pseudostratified columnar epithelium (olfactory epithelium) incorporating neurosensory olfactory cells (bipolar nerve cells), sustentacular cells and basal cells,
- tubulo-acinar serous glands (olfactory glands, glandulae olfactoriae) in the propria-submucosa and
- axon fascicles (fila olfactoria) in the submucosa.

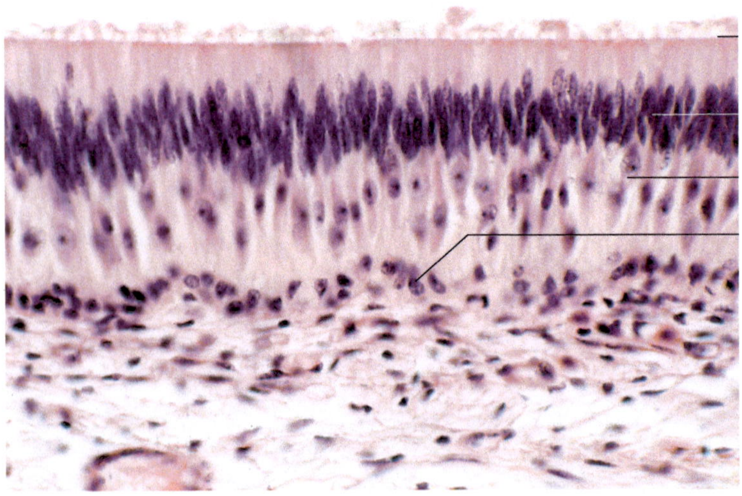

11.4 Olfactory mucosa (dog). The epithelium contains sustentacular cells, bipolar neurons and basal cells (considered to serve as reserve cells for replacement of other cell types, including neurons). Haematoxylin and eosin stain (x275).

The olfactory mucosa covers the ethmoturbinates, dorsal endoturbinates and part of the caudal segment of the nasal septum. Modified **bipolar neurons** serve as neurosensory cells that detect odours (Figure 11.4). Axons leave the basal portion of the cell forming bundles that pass through the submucosa (see description of olfactory epithelium in Chapter 16, 'Receptors and sense organs').

The lamina propria houses branched tubulo-acinar **olfactory glands** (**glandulae olfactoriae**). The thin, watery glandular secretion contains enzymes (proteases) that are important for breaking down odoriferous substances and binding them to neurosensory cells. In addition, the secretory product of these cells has a cleansing function, facilitating the detection of subsequent olfactory stimuli.

Species variation

Birds: The **cranial portion** of the nasal cavity (**nasal vestibule**) is lined with non-glandular mucosa. Caudally, in the **respiratory region**, this transitions to a ciliated pseudostratified epithelium with secretory cells (Figures 11.8 and 11.9). This is continued in the olfactory region by olfactory epithelium. The histological structure of the epithelium differs little from that of mammals. Typically yellowish in colour, the **olfactory**

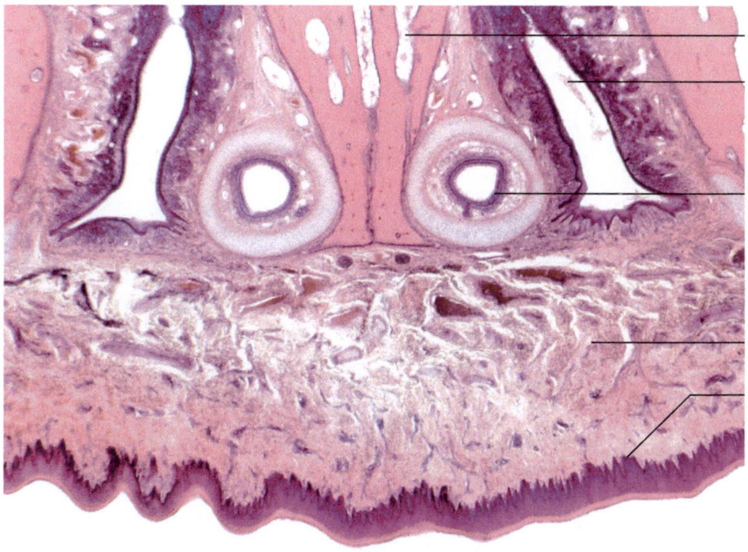

11.5 Vomeronasal organ (cat). The paired vomeronasal organ lies at the base of the osseous nasal septum. Haematoxylin and eosin stain (x15).

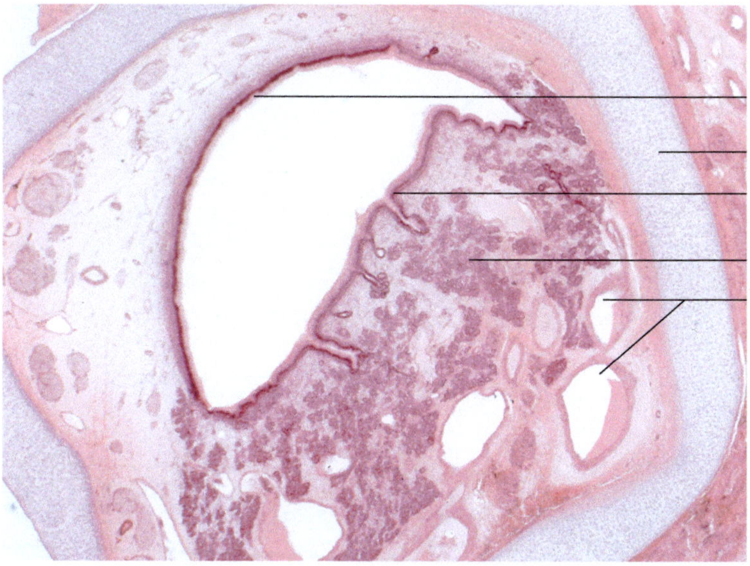

11.6 Vomeronasal organ (calf). The interior of the vomeronasal organ is lined medially by olfactory mucosa and laterally by respiratory mucosa. Glandular aggregates and expanded veins lie between the respiratory mucosa and the external cartilage. The respiratory mucosa contains poorly myelinated subepithelial nerve fibre bundles. Haematoxylin and eosin stain (x40).

region of chickens and water birds comprises a small circumscribed area on the caudal nasal concha and the caudal portion of the nasal septum. Both the olfactory region and the olfactory bulb of birds are relatively small and limited in function. In comparative terms, the olfactory system is more developed in carnivores (including fish eaters) than in granivorous species.

Paranasal sinuses (sinus paranasales)

The paranasal sinuses are lined with a low respiratory epithelium. Glands are rarely present. The lamina propria is closely associated with the periosteum. In carnivores this layer contains tubulo-acinar serous glands (in the maxillary sinus). Their secretions pass from the sinus into the nasal cavity.

Vomeronasal organ (organum vomeronasale)

The vomeronasal organ aids in identification of **scents and odours**. It bears receptors for specific pheromones and is believed to play a role in detecting oestrus, particularly in lower order vertebrates. In domestic mammals, the vomeronasal organ is relatively poorly developed.

The vomeronasal organ is a paired tubular structure, lying parallel to the base of the nasal septum (Figure 11.5). Its rostral opening empties into the nasal and oral cavities via the incisive duct. In the horse, the connection to the oral cavity is lacking. The caudal end of the vomeronasal organ is blind.

The lumen of the vomeronasal organ is lined with respiratory mucosa on its lateral aspect and with olfactory mucosa on its medial internal surface (Figure 11.6).

In the **respiratory mucosa**, prominent clusters of glands lie between the epithelium and a dense network of capacitance vessels. Secretions produced by these glands serve to moisten the mucosa and solubilise odoriferous chemicals.

The structure of the neurosensory **olfactory mucosa** is similar to that of the olfactory region of the nasal cavity. Poorly myelinated fibres of the terminal nerve (n. terminalis) traverse the connective tissue of the lamina propria. These sensory fibres pass to the area cribrosa and then to the olfactory bulb. The exterior of the vomeronasal organ is surrounded by a cuff of hyaline cartilage (vomeronasal cartilage).

Pharynx

The dorsal compartment of the pharynx, the **nasopharynx** (**pars nasalis pharyngis**) is lined with respiratory mucosa. The lamina propria and tela submucosa contain abundant lymphoid nodules. Nodular aggregates form the pharyngeal tonsils. The lymphoid tissue is immediately surrounded by tubulo-acinar, predominantly mixed glands. The tunica muscularis is composed of skeletal muscle. On the outer surface of its muscular wall, the nasopharynx is lined by a dense tunica adventitia. At the level of the soft palate (structure described in Chapter 10, 'Digestive system'), the **nasopharynx** is continued by the **oropharynx**, in which the respiratory and digestive tracts intersect. In this portion of the pharynx, the epithelium is stratified squamous. Mixed glands and lymphoid tissue are located in the submucosa. The submucosa is permeated by a dense meshwork of elastic fibres that strengthens the pharyngeal wall. Lying external to the submucosa are the striated bundles of the pharyngeal muscles, followed by a layer of fibro-elastic tissue.

Larynx

The larynx is a bilaterally symmetrical tubular organ that is continuous rostrally with the pharynx and caudally with the trachea. The structural framework of the larynx consists of the laryngeal cartilages. Ligaments interconnect

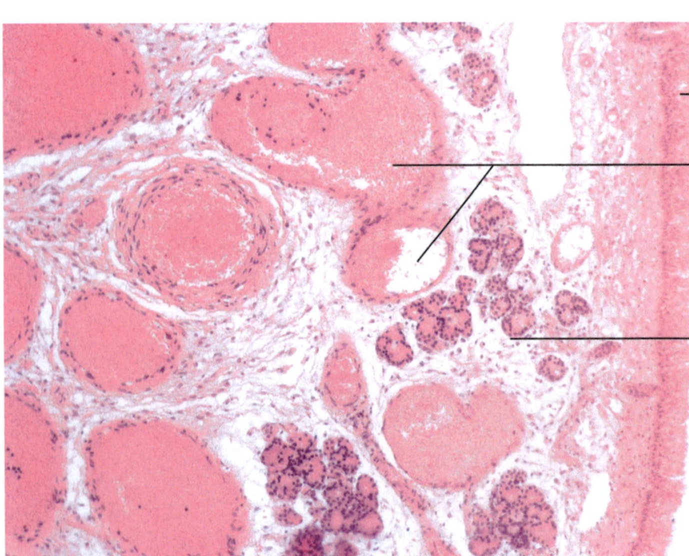

11.7 Nasal mucosa (calf). Beneath the mucosa of the nasal septum is a prominent venous plexus. Contraction of smooth muscle in capacitance veins slows blood flow resulting in congestion of the nasal mucosa. Haematoxylin and eosin stain (x80).

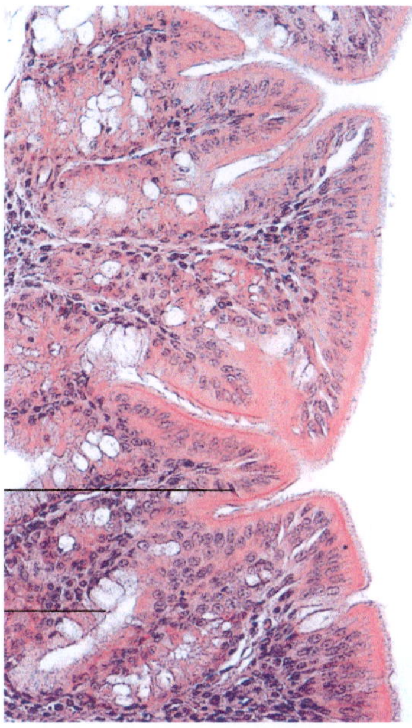

11.8 Nasal cavity (chicken). Haematoxylin and eosin stain (x120).

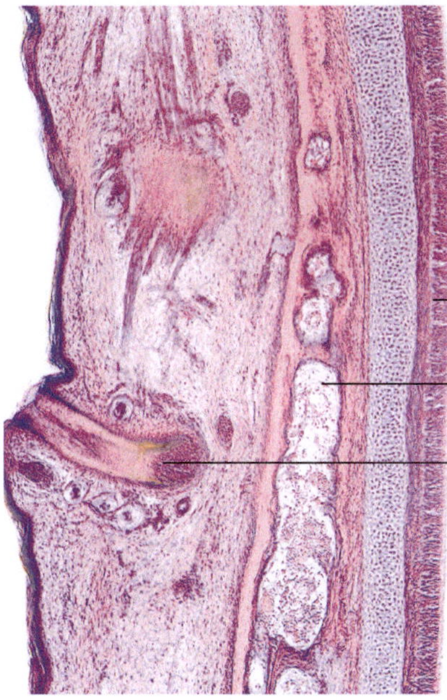

11.9 Nasal cavity (chicken). Haematoxylin and eosin stain (x80).

the laryngeal cartilages and join the larynx to the bones of the hyoid apparatus, rostrally, and the tracheal cartilage, caudally. Paired skeletal intrinsic laryngeal muscles pass between the laryngeal cartilages. The outer connective tissue layer of the laryngeal muscles is continuous with a loose tunica adventitia.

The **epithelium** lining the individual segments of the larynx exhibits functional modifications. Species variation is also observed. In all species, the epiglottis, laryngeal vestibule and the edges of the vocal folds are lined with **non-glandular mucosa** with non-keratinised stratified squamous epithelium. On the aborally directed surfaces of the larynx (those facing the trachea), the lining consists of **respiratory epithelium**. This type of epithelium continues to the bronchioles.

While the histological structure of the walls of the larynx is essentially consistent among domestic mammals, differentiation of the connective tissue underlying the epithelium contributes to species variation in the shape of the laryngeal lumen.

Species variation

Pig and carnivores: The laryngeal ventricles are lined with stratified squamous epithelium.

Horse: The laryngeal ventricles are lined with respiratory epithelium.

Birds: The larynx manifests as a prominent mound caudal to the tongue in the ventral oropharynx. Two rows of caudally directed, usually conical papillae (papillae pharyngeales) are located on the caudal half of the mucosal elevation.

Epiglottis

The base of the epiglottis is joined to other segments of the larynx by connective tissue. On its orally directed surface, the epiglottis is lined with non-glandular mucosa with a well-developed **stratified squamous epithelium**. This is consistent, in functional terms, with its exposed position within the pharynx. On the laryngeal surface, the epithelium becomes flatter (Figure 11.10). In all species except the horse, the laryngeal surface contains isolated taste buds. The lamina propria houses numerous mainly mucous and mixed glands that frequently protrude into indentations in the cartilage. The connective tissue is layered and is permeated by **elastic fibres**. Diffuse lymphoid tissue and isolated nodules are common. Tonsils are also observed in pigs and small ruminants. The epiglottis is supported by elastic cartilage. In carnivores, a cartilaginous outer casing encloses multilocular adipose tissue.

The larger **laryngeal cartilages** (thyroid cartilage, cricoid cartilage and substantial portions of the arytenoid cartilage) are composed of **hyaline cartilage** (Figure 11.11). Like the epiglottis, the cuneiform, corniculate and vocal processes of the arytenoid cartilage are supported by **elastic cartilage**. The individual cartilages are connected by fibro-elastic ligaments. The **vocal folds** and **vestibular folds** are composed of **elastic fibres**. Solitary or clumped tubulo-acinar mixed glands occur in the loose connective tissue and between the cartilage and the laryngeal musculature. These are absent in the vocal folds. In contrast to the musculature of the more distal respiratory tract (trachea, bronchi), the laryngeal muscles are striated (see *Veterinary Anatomy of Domestic Mammals: Textbook and Colour Atlas*).

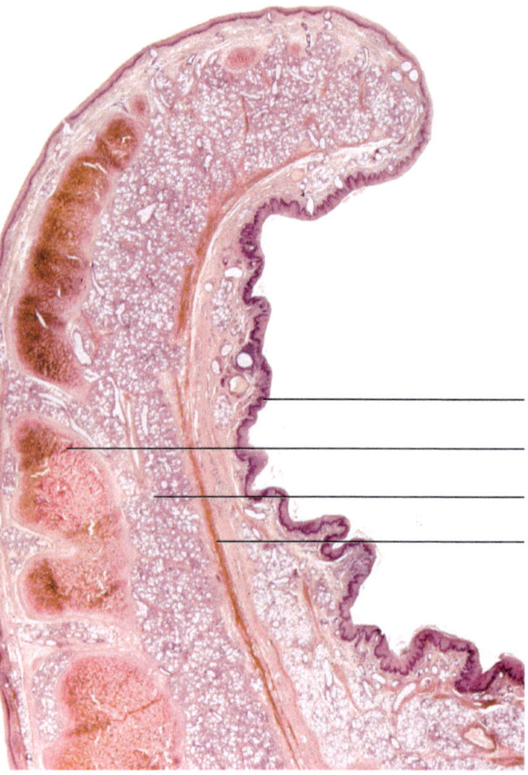

11.10 Epiglottis (calf). The oral surface of the epiglottis is lined with stratified squamous epithelium underlaid by mucous glands. Elastic cartilage forms the structural core. Striated muscle fibres radiate into the base of the epiglottis from the root of the tongue. Orcein-haemalum stain (x8).

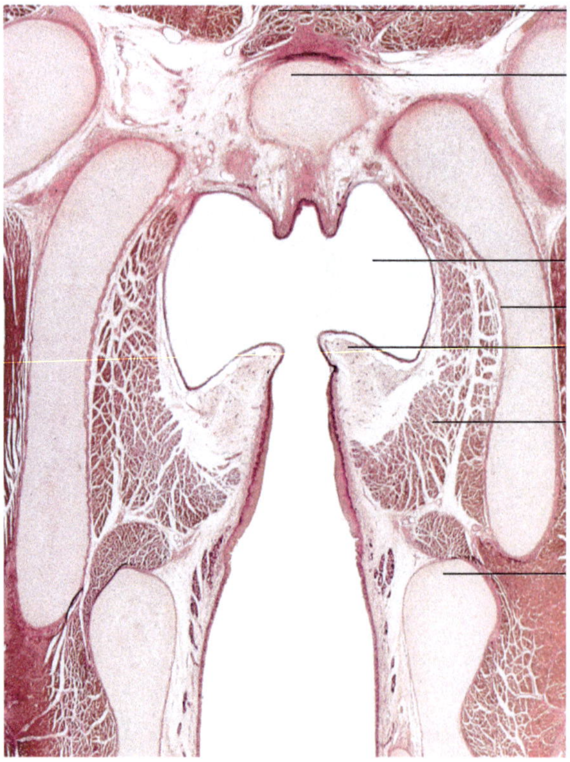

11.11 Larynx, dorsal section (young dog). Haematoxylin and eosin stain (x22).

Trachea

The trachea is a semiflexible tube that commences at the caudal end of the larynx and ends at the tracheal bifurcation. Structurally, the trachea is composed of concentric layers of tissue (Figures 11.12 and 11.13).

The trachea is lined with **ciliated pseudostratified epithelium** containing numerous **goblet cells** (**respiratory epithelium**). Basal cells and columnar cells with microvilli are also present. Neuroendocrine cells, including **enterochromaffin** and **APUD cells** (amine and precursor uptake and decarboxylation cells) are more numerous in young animals. These cells are in contact with nerve endings and produce biogenic amines. The **lamina propria** is composed of an irregular meshwork of fine collagen fibres

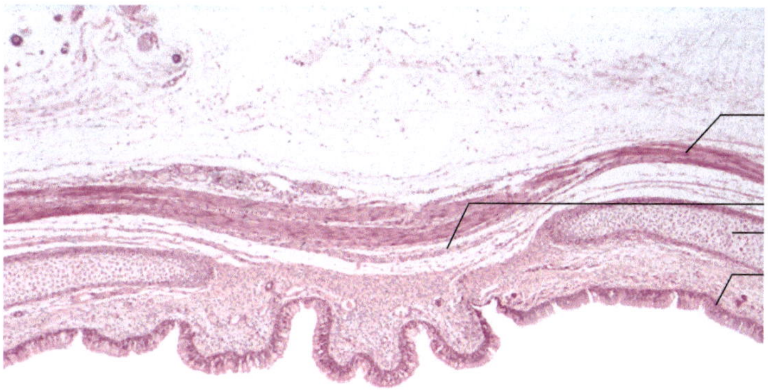

11.12 Trachea (young dog). Rings of hyaline cartilage form the structural framework of the trachea. The free edges of the rings are open dorsally. The gap between these is bridged by connective tissue (paries membranaceus) and the m. trachealis. In this section, the respiratory mucosa is folded. Haematoxylin and eosin stain (x50).

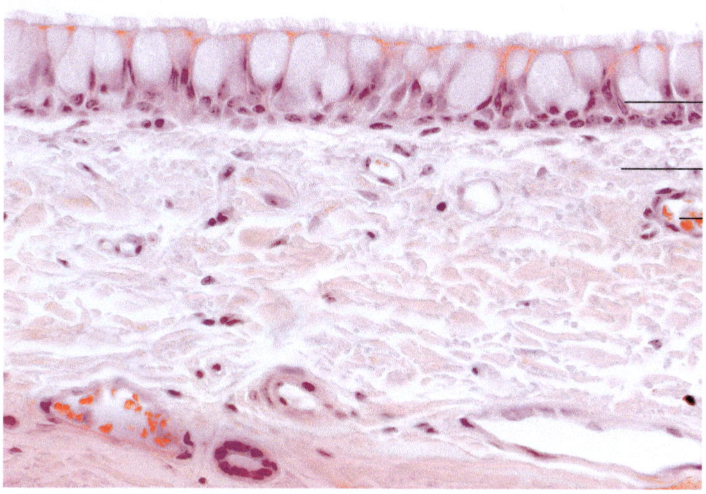

11.13 Trachea (dog). The wall is lined by respiratory epithelium with goblet cells, resting on a layer of loose connective tissue containing glands. These layers are surrounded by the cartilage of the tracheal rings. Haematoxylin and eosin (x240).

housing small vessels and nerves. Between this meshwork and the epithelium is a layer of densely woven longitudinally oriented elastic fibres.

Solitary tubulo-acinar **tracheal glands** (**glandulae tracheales**) are located within the lamina propria and submucosa. The epithelial cells of the tubular portion mainly produce a mucous secretion rich in acid glycoproteins, whereas the glycoproteinaceous secretions of the acinar end-pieces are neutral and serous. The glands frequently protrude between the cartilaginous tracheal rings, sometimes reaching the tunica adventitia. The cuboidal epithelium of the excretory ducts is surrounded by smooth muscle cells. In domestic mammals, tracheal glands are found particularly in the proximal portion of the trachea.

The semi-flexible status of the trachea results from **rings of hyaline cartilage** that encircle the tracheal mucosa. These are developed to a varying degree, depending on species. The surface of the tracheal cartilages is lined with perichondrium. In the spaces between the rings, the perichondrium continues as the fibro-elastic **annular ligaments** (**ligamenta anularia**). Dorsally, the tracheal rings are usually incomplete. The free ends of the cartilage are joined by a tough elastic connective tissue membrane (**paries membranaceus**), lined on its internal surface by smooth muscle (**m. trachealis**). In carnivores the muscle is external to the paries membranaceus (Figure 11.12). The tunica adventitia surrounding the tracheal cartilages is fibro-elastic, facilitating movement of the trachea with respect to adjacent tissues.

Species variation

Birds: The **tracheal mucosa** is lined with ciliated pseudostratified epithelium with columnar cells, narrow basal cells and mucus-producing goblet cells (Figure 11.14). Serving as small endo-epithelial glands, the goblet cells form small, crypt-like depressions (mucous crypts). The lamina propria underlying the epithelium contains mucous glands, lymphoid follicles and diffuse lymphoid tissue. Bands of **muscle** (**mm. tracheales**) pass along the exterior of the trachea. The tracheal rings are complete.

The syrinx is located at the level of the bifurcation of the trachea into the primary bronchi. In the chicken, the last four tracheal rings are considered to be part of the syrinx. The subsequent rings are no longer complete. Instead, they are joined at one or both ends to a median **bridge** known as the **pessulus**. Extending cranially from the pessulus is a mucosal fold, the **membrana**

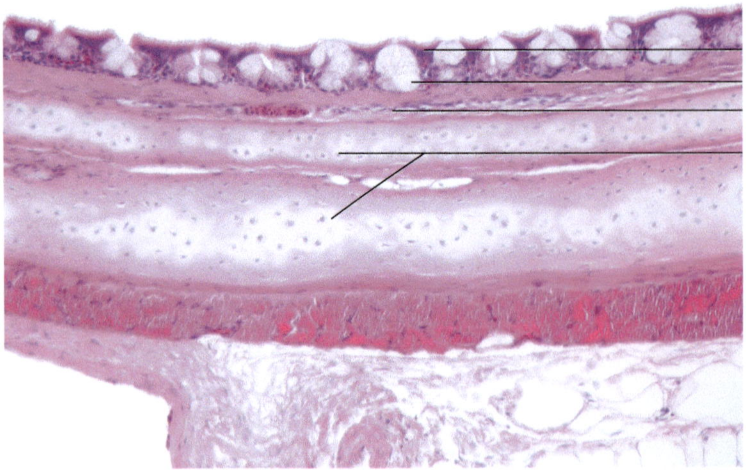

11.14 Trachea (chicken). Haematoxylin and eosin stain (x70).

semilunaris. Together, the cartilaginous components of the syrinx form the **tympanum**. Left and right **lateral tympaniform membranes** (membrana tympaniformis lateralis) extend from the tympanum to the lateral side of the bronchial cartilages. Paired **medial tympaniform membranes** (membrana tympaniformis medialis) pass from the pessulus to the (incomplete) medial aspect of the bronchial cartilages. Elastic connective tissue pads termed **labia** project from the membranes into the lumen of the syrinx. During phonation, the membranes and labia function in a similar manner to the **vocal folds** of the mammalian larynx. **Syringeal muscles** are present in song birds and **absent** in domestic poultry.

Lung (pulmo)

At the tracheal bifurcation, the trachea divides into **two primary bronchi** (**bronchi principales**). The primary bronchi branch to form the intra-pulmonary **lobar bronchi** (**bronchi lobares**).

The lobar bronchi typically divide into two further branches, each of which divides again (into bronchi segmentale and subsegmentales). This dichotomous process of division continues, accompanied by a decrease in the diameter of the airway, until the small bronchioles (**bronchioli veri**) are formed. The small bronchioles divide extensively, giving rise to the terminal bronchioles (**bronchioli terminales**). These represent the final portion of the conducting component of the respiratory system, which is continued by the respiratory portion (region of gas exchange) (Figure 11.15).

The respiratory portion commences with the appearance of the first sac-like evaginations (**alveoli**) in the wall of the respiratory bronchioles (**bronchioli respiratorii** or **alveolares**). Further divisions result in the formation of narrow tubular airways termed alveolar ducts (**ductus alveolares**). The walls of the alveolar ducts consist of adjacent alveolar openings. The alveolar ducts open into alveolar sacs (**sacculi alveolares**) (Figure 11.16).

The intra-pulmonary segments of the conducting airways, the bronchi and bronchioles, represent approximately 6% of the volume of the lung. Over 85% of lung volume is formed by the **respiratory parenchyma** – the respiratory bronchioles, alveolar ducts, alveolar sacs and alveoli.

The lung is enclosed by the visceral pleura (**pleura visceralis**), composed of a single layer of squamous to cuboidal mesothelial cells and a variably thick layer of collagen and elastic fibres. Connective tissue septa extend from the pleura into the lung. This **interstitial connective tissue** (**interstitium**) **divides** the lobes of the lung into lobules. Intra-pulmonary vessels and nerves accompanying the connective tissue septa account for around 10% of lung volume.

Species variation

Ruminants and pig: The pulmonary interstitial tissue is prominent.

Horse and carnivores: The pulmonary interstitium is relatively sparse.

Bronchi

The main differences in the structure of the bronchi (bronchi principales, lobares, segmentales and subsegmentales), compared with the trachea, are the shape of the cartilaginous elements and the arrangement of the smooth muscle fibres (Figures 11.16 to 11.19). From innermost to outermost, the bronchi consist of the following components:

- respiratory epithelium,
- lamina propria with mixed glands (bronchial glands),
- elastic fibre network and smooth muscle layer and
- rings of hyaline cartilage with associated elastic fibres.

Distally, the height of the **respiratory epithelium** lining the bronchial lumen gradually decreases (Figure 11.18).

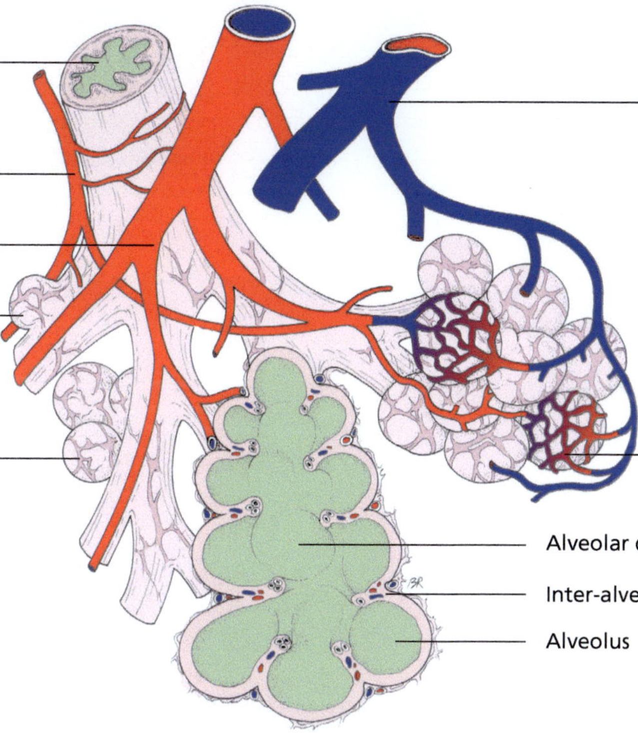

11.15 Peripheral bronchial tree with alveoli and vascular supply (schematic).

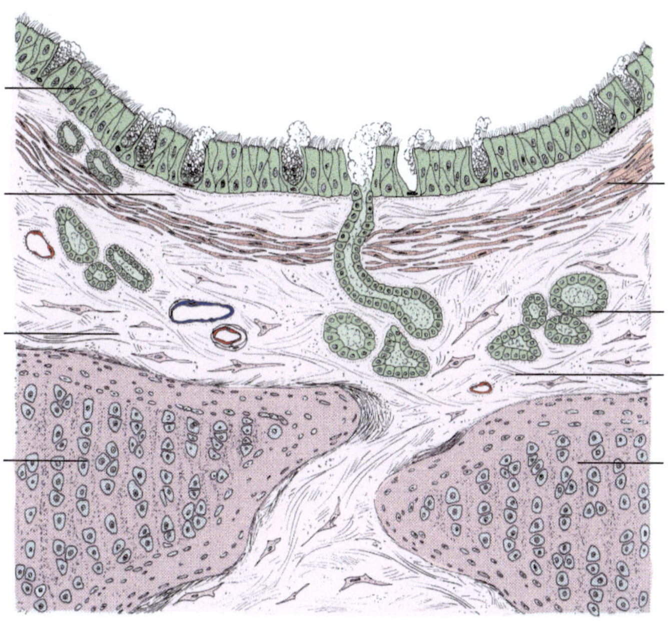

11.16 Wall of bronchus (schematic).

Mixed bronchial glands (**glandulae bronchiales**) are present in the lamina propria and in the submucosa. These produce a watery, serous secretion rich in protein- and glycoprotein-containing mucus. Within the lumen of the bronchi, proteinaceous serum components, immunoglobulin A, lactoferrin and glycoproteins are added. These substances aid in **protecting the epithelial cells** by preventing attachment of viruses and bacteria to the epithelium or by a direct bacteriostatic effect.

The **lamina propria** contains abundant connective tissue composed mainly of collagen, but also **elastic fibres**. Blood vessels, lymph vessels, nerves and solitary lymphoid follicles are also present. Externally adjacent to the lamina propria is a layer of **smooth muscle** (Figure 11.16). Proximally, the orientation of the muscle is circular, transitioning into a spiral lattice in the smaller bronchi. The muscle fibres conform to the alignment of the elastic fibres. The mucosa often appears folded due to contraction of the bronchial muscles (Figures 11.17 and 11.18).

Incomplete rings of hyaline cartilage form the structural core of the bronchi. Near the trachea, they are almost complete. With increased branching of the bronchial tree, the rings become smaller and less substantial (cartilage 'plates'), eventually becoming **fragmented**. The cartilage fragments are connected by predominantly **elastic fibres** that project into the perichondrium, contributing to the flexibility of the bronchi. The smallest, most peripheral cartilage fragments are composed of elastic cartilage. The tunica adventitia contains connective tissue, vessels and nerves (Figures 11.16 to 11.19).

Bronchioles (bronchioli veri, bronchioli terminales)

In the bronchioles, the lumen of the conducting airways is reduced to a diameter of less than 1 mm. The wall of the small bronchioles (bronchioli veri) and terminal bronchioles (bronchioli terminales) comprises:

- ciliated epithelium with Clara cells,
- lamina propria with elastic fibres and smooth muscle cells surrounded by loose connective tissue and
- no glands or cartilaginous elements.

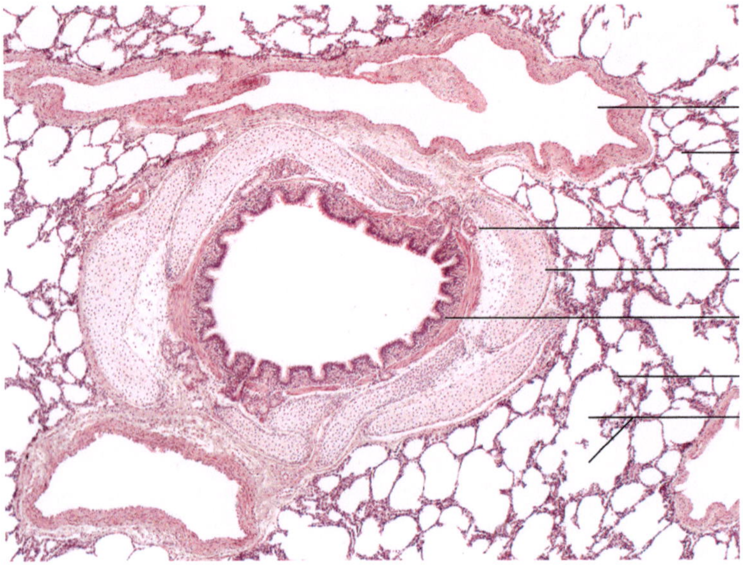

11.17 Lung (ox). Bronchi are characterised by the presence of mixed glands and hyaline cartilage rings or fragments. Haematoxylin and eosin stain (x30).

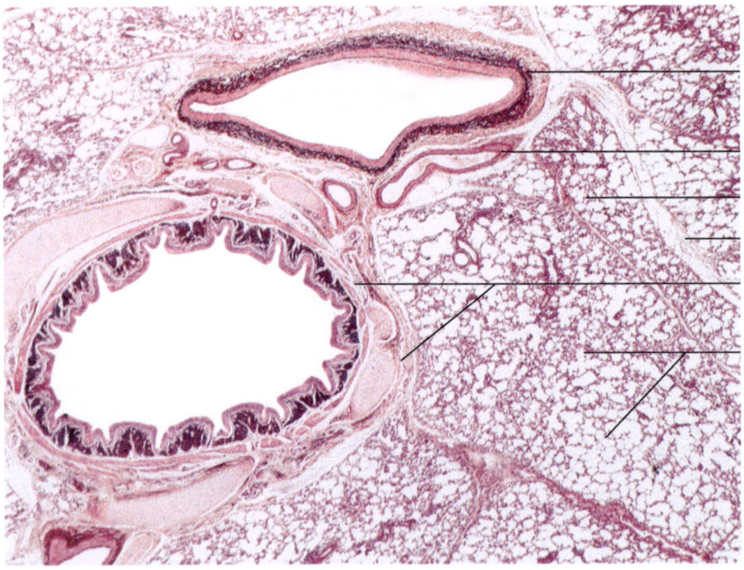

11.18 Lung (calf). The staining technique used in this section highlights the elastic fibres, which are particularly prominent in the larger bronchial branches. Resorcin–fuchsin–nuclear-fast red (Weigert's elastic) stain (x30).

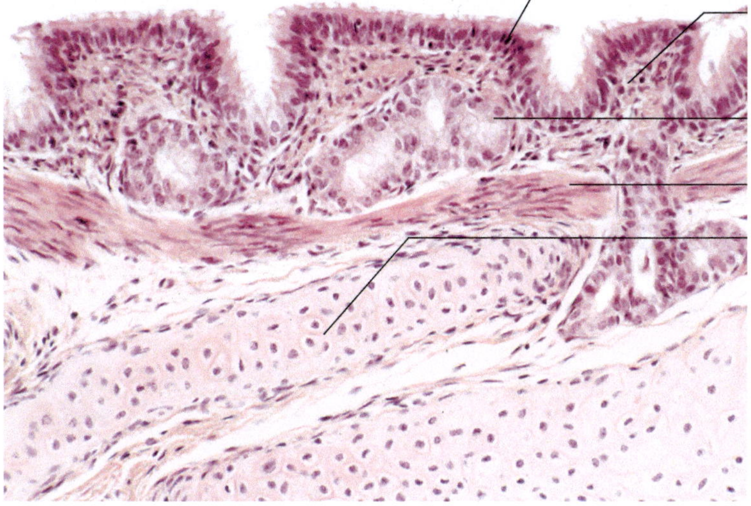

11.19 Wall of a bronchus (pig). The respiratory epithelium rests upon a lamina propria of loose connective tissue with coiled, tubular mucous glands that occasionally protrude through to the hyaline cartilage fragments. Smooth muscle encircles the bronchus forming a contractile ring. Haematoxylin and eosin stain (x80).

With continued branching of the bronchioles, the pseudostratified columnar epithelium becomes flatter, eventually transforming into simple columnar or cuboidal epithelium (Figures 11.20 and 11.21). In addition to ciliated epithelial cells, the bronchiolar epithelium contains non-ciliated columnar cells (**Clara cells**) (Figure 11.25). These are most numerous in the smaller bronchioles. Released by the apocrine mode, the secretory product of Clara cells contains proteolytic and mucolytic enzymes that reduce the viscosity of the bronchial mucus. In contrast to the bronchi, **glands** and **cartilage** are **absent** from the walls of the bronchioles. The loss of goblet cells is followed by the disappearance of cilia. Bronchioles have a distinct muscle layer comprising several sheets of mainly circularly oriented **smooth muscle cells**. This muscle layer is important for regulating ventilation of the conducting airways. Contraction of the circular muscle rapidly constricts the bronchioles, increasing resistance to air flow (Figures 11.20 and 11.21) (excessive constriction results in bronchial asthma in humans).

In the final segments of the conducting airways, the **terminal bronchi**, the epithelium is reduced to a **single layer** of **cuboidal cells** and the number of elastic fibres in the lamina propria increases. In conjunction with the well-developed bronchiolar muscle, the constrictive effect of the elastic fibres contributes to folding of the mucosa.

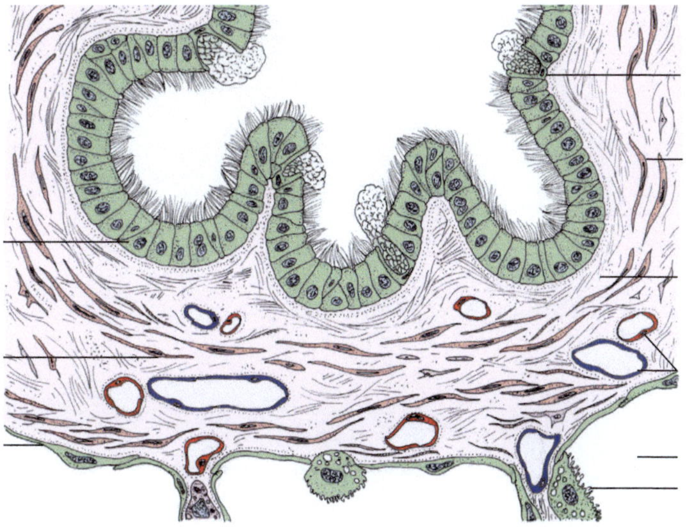

11.20 Wall of a terminal bronchiole (schematic). Occasional goblet cells may be observed in the proximal portions. In contrast to the bronchi, subepithelial glands and cartilage are absent.

Gas exchange interface

Having passed through the conducting airways, inspired air reaches the region in which gas exchange takes place. The components of this interface (Figures 11.22 to 11.27 and Table 11.2) comprise:

- respiratory bronchioles with:
  - simple epithelium,
  - elastic fibres and smooth muscle cells,
  - the first alveoli with alveolar epithelium,
- alveolar ducts and alveolar sacs with:
  - simple squamous epithelium (alveolar epithelium) and
  - elastic fibres and smooth muscle cells.

Respiratory bronchioles

The terminal bronchioles divide dichotomously into two or more respiratory bronchioles, each of which subsequently divides into two (generations I–III). The respiratory bronchioles are largely similar in structure to the terminal bronchioles. They are distinguished by deep outpouchings (alveoli) lined by a flattened **alveolar epithelium**. With each subsequent generation (I–III) the number of alveoli increases. The respiratory bronchioles thus serve both as **conducting airways** and as sites of **gas exchange** (Figure 11.22).

Species variation

Carnivores: Respiratory bronchioles are extensively developed.

Horse: Occasional respiratory bronchioles are seen.

Ruminants and pig: Respiratory bronchioles are rare.

Alveolar ducts and alveolar sacs

The final respiratory bronchioles branch to form up to ten alveolar ducts (ductus alveolares) (Figure 11.22). The walls of the alveolar ducts consist of closely spaced openings, each leading into an alveolus lined with **simple squamous epithelium** (**alveolar epithelium**). Externally, the alveolar ducts are surrounded by a network of collagen fibres with some elastic fibres. Together with smooth muscle cells, this network acts as a sphincter. Terminal branching (3- to 5-fold) of the alveolar ducts gives rise to **alveolar sacs** (**sacculi alveolares**), the terminal segments of the respiratory system (Figures 11.22 to 11.24).

Alveoli (alveoli pulmonis)

Alveoli are the site of **gas exchange** within the respiratory system. These are sac-like evaginations located in the final segments of the bronchial tree – the respiratory bronchioles, alveolar ducts and alveolar sacs. Alveolar components include:

- Type I alveolar epithelial cells (Type I pneumocytes),
- Type II alveolar epithelial cells (Type II pneumocytes),
- a surface film of phospholipid (surfactant),
- alveolar macrophages and
- an inter-alveolar septum with macrophages, capillary networks and pores.

The walls of alveoli (Figures 11.24, 11.26 and 11.27) are lined by two cell types.

Type I (**squamous**) **alveolar epithelial cells** (**pneumocytes**) (**cellulae respiratoriae** or **squamosae**) are extremely thin, flattened cells. The nucleus bulges slightly into the lumen (Figure 11.27). Type I cells form a continuous layer that lines approximately 95% of the internal

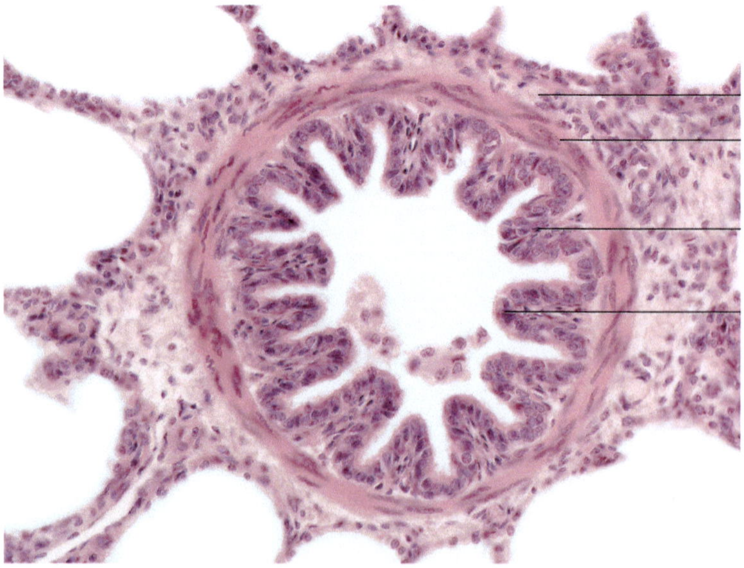

11.21 Bronchiole (lung, ox). The respiratory mucosa is deeply folded, due to the constrictive effect of elastic fibre bundles and smooth muscle. In contrast to bronchi, glands and cartilage are lacking. Haematoxylin and eosin stain (x275).

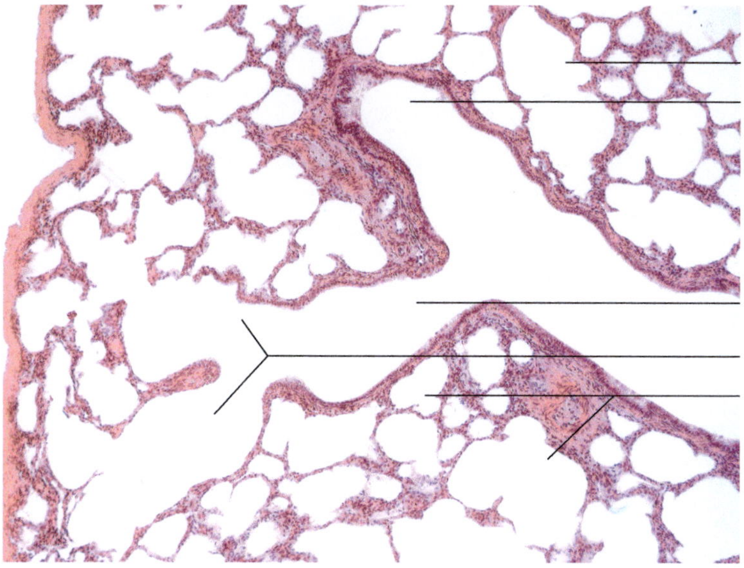

11.22 Transition from a terminal bronchiole to alveolar ducts with clusters of alveolar sacs (lung, ox). Haematoxylin and eosin stain (x80).

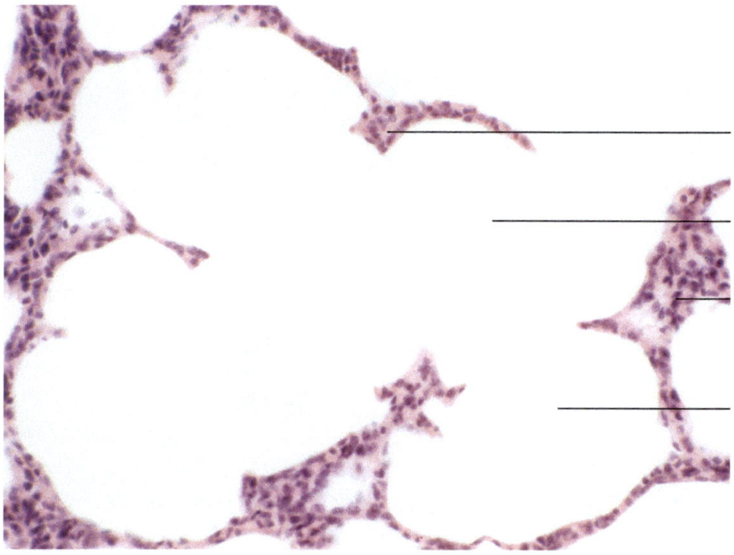

11.23 Pulmonary alveolae with inter-alveolar septa (lung, pig). Haematoxylin and eosin stain (x320).

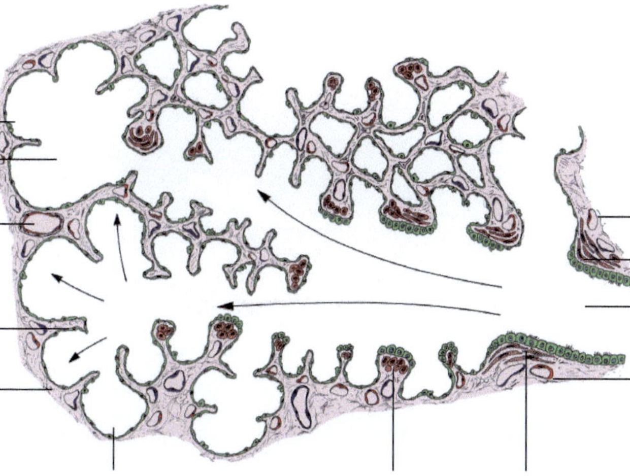

11.24 Terminal branching of a respiratory bronchiole to form alveolar ducts (tips of long arrows), alveolar sacs and numerous alveoli.

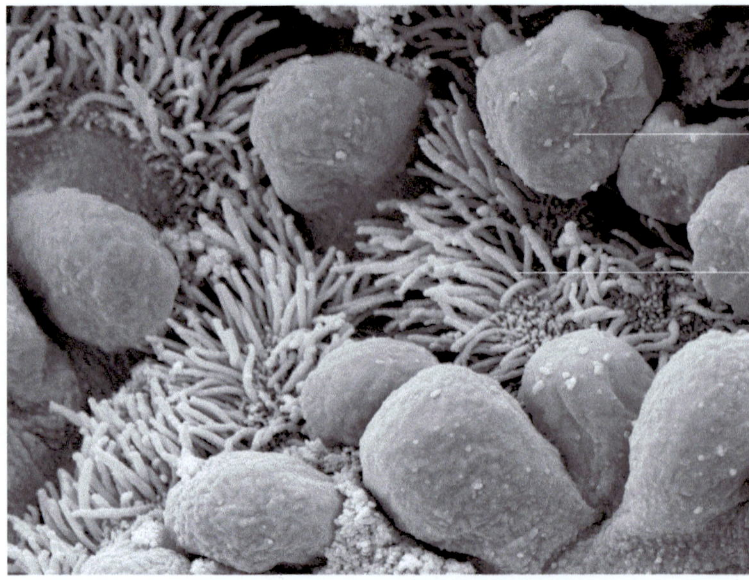

11.25 Scanning electron micrograph of the wall of a bronchiole (x2000). (Courtesy of S. Reese, Munich).

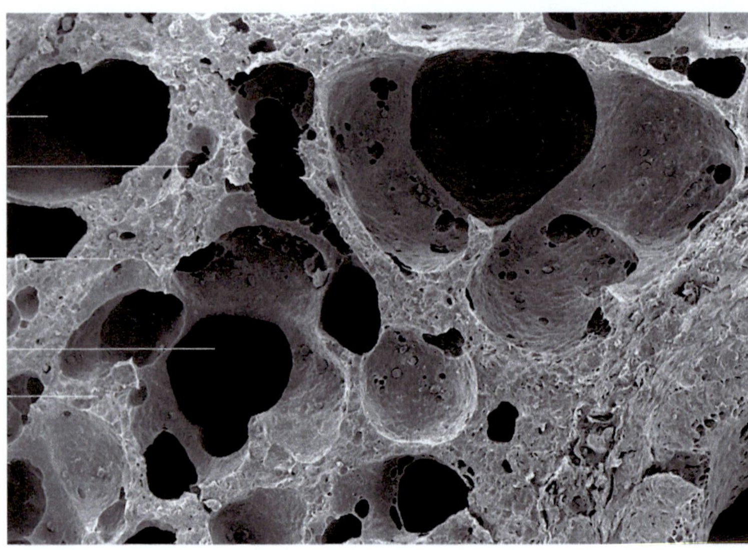

11.26 Scanning electron micrograph of the interior of pulmonary alveoli (lung, pig) (x1000).

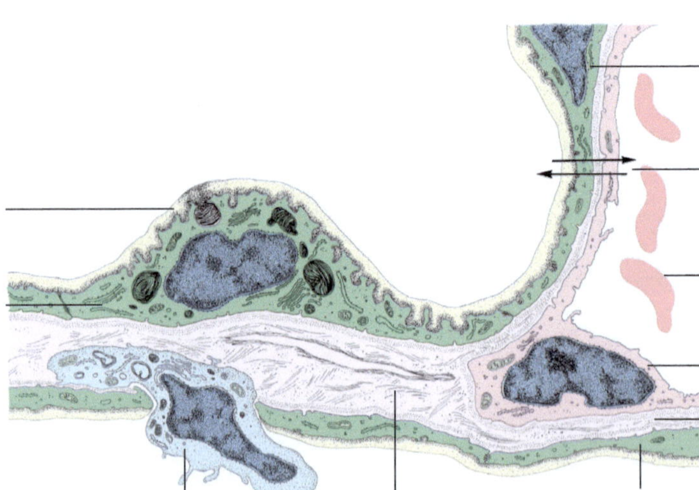

11.27 Blood–air barrier with Type I and II alveolar epithelial cells and capillary wall (schematic).

alveolar surface. Aside from numerous micropinocytotic vesicles, signifying their role in trans-epithelial transport, these cells have few organelles. Type I alveolar epithelial cells are closely associated with the thin underlying basal lamina. They form part of the blood–air barrier.

Type II alveolar epithelial cells (**cellulae magnae** or **granulares**) are relatively large, wedge-shaped or spheroid cells (10–12 µm) that occur in small clusters (Figure 11.27). They are rich in organelles, including abundant characteristic, apically located multivesicular and lamellar bodies (cytosomes, 0.2–1.0 µm). The content of these osmiophilic secretory granules is high in phospholipids (saturated lecithins), glycosaminoglycans and acid phosphatases. The secretory product is exocytosed to the free alveolar surface, where it disperses widely forming a surface-active phospholipid film (**pulmonary surfactant**). Surfactant has a detergent effect, reducing the surface tension of the alveolar wall by a factor of 5–10. Type II alveolar cells can divide and transform into Type I cells.

Impurities, such as aspirated particles and fluids, are removed from the alveolar surface by pulmonary **alveolar macrophages** (components of the mononuclear phagocyte system). These cells migrate from the interstitial connective tissue and attach to the internal alveolar wall (Figure 11.27). Alveolar macrophages are expelled via the conducting airways, together with mucus and desquamated epithelial cells.

> **Species variation**
>
> **Calf, sheep, goat, cat and pig**: In the lungs of these species, clusters of lymphocytes and lymphoid nodules are found in the walls of the airways and in association with blood vessels. This tissue is referred to as **BALT** (bronchus-associated lymphoid tissue).

The **alveolar septum** (**septum inter-alveolare**) constitutes the common wall of two adjacent alveoli (Figures 11.24 and 11.27). A distinction is made between septa in the alveolar ducts and septa between neighbouring alveoli. The inter-alveolar septa increase the surface area of the gas exchange interface.

Both alveolar surfaces of inter-alveolar septa are lined with **Type I** and **Type II alveolar epithelial cells** resting on a thin basal lamina. A connective tissue **interstitium** is formed by a delicate network of collagen (types I and III), reticular and elastic fibres and fibrils. The spaces in this meshwork are occupied by fibroblasts, fibrocytes, granulocytes, lymphocytes and mast cells. Phagocytic macrophages, originating from migrating blood monocytes, are frequently observed. Inter-alveolar septa house **dense capillary networks** that are closely apposed to the alveolar epithelium (Figure 11.27). Also present are contractile cells that support the function of basket-like networks of elastic fibres in compressing the lumen of the alveoli during exhalation. These cells are innervated by non-myelinated nerve fibres. Pores in the inter-alveolar septa facilitate air circulation and pressure equilibration between adjacent alveoli. At their free ends, the septa become expanded; smooth muscle cells occurring at these locations act as sphincters.

Blood–air barrier

Gas exchange occurs across the blood–air barrier. The process is facilitated by the close apposition of the alveolar epithelium, and its thin basal lamina, with the wall of the alveolar capillaries.

The **exchange of gases** between the alveoli and erythrocytes occurs across the following interfaces (Figure 11.27):

- surfactant coating the surface of the alveolar epithelium,
- cytoplasm of the flattened alveolar epithelial cells,
- basal lamina of the alveolar epithelium,
- basal lamina of the capillary wall,
- cytoplasm of the capillary endothelium,
- blood plasma and the
- plasmalemma of erythrocytes.

The adjacent basal laminae are often fused. Interstitial connective tissue is sometimes found between these.

The rate of gas exchange is determined by:
Any change in the diameter of the blood vessels, cellular surface area or membrane permeability has the potential to impact on respiratory function.

Bronchial system and gas exchange in birds

The **pulmonary bronchi** of birds consist of:

- the diameter of the capillary lumen,
- the rate of blood flow in the capillaries,
- partial pressures and
- the thickness of the cell membranes and interstitial connective tissue.

The **primary bronchi** are also referred to as **first-order bronchi**. They penetrate the **horizontal septum** and pass through the lung to its caudal margin, where they open into the abdominal air sacs.

The walls of the primary bronchi contain **incomplete rings of cartilage** that are absent from all subsequent bronchial divisions. In the primary bronchi, the lumen is surrounded by **respiratory epithelium**, underlaid by elastic and collagen fibres, seromucous glands and lymphoid tissue. The **smooth muscle** of the primary bronchi is mostly circular. An adventitia of loose connective tissue is present.

Secondary bronchi, or **second-order bronchi**, extend from the primary bronchi. According to the direction in which they pass, they are grouped into:

- two primary bronchi (bronchi primarii),
- secondary bronchi (bronchi secundarii),
- parabronchi (parabronchi) and
- air capillaries (pneumocapillares).

- numerous laterodorsal secondary bronchi,
- 7–10 mediodorsal secondary bronchi,
- 4–7 lateroventral secondary bronchi and
- 4 medioventral secondary bronchi.

Third-order bronchi, or **parabronchi**, are also referred to as 'air pipes'. Parabronchi arising from mediodorsal secondary bronchi within the dorsal palaeopulmo meet and anastomose with their ventral counterparts in the interior of the lung (refer to anatomy texts). The parabronchi are arranged in a parallel hexagonal array of **elongated tubules**. In most species their diameter is around 0.5 mm (1–1.5 mm in the chicken).

Parabronchi have several distinctive features (Figures 11.28 and 11.29):

- they anastomose with one another,
- chambers called atria open from their walls into infundibula and air capillaries,
- they contain gas exchange units,
- their diameter is uniform within species and
- they manifest as hexagonal tubes.

Table 11.2 Histological features of the bronchial tree and gas exchange system of domestic mammals.

Segment	Epithelium	Glands	Connective tissue and muscle	Special features
Bronchi	Respiratory epithelium with cilia, microvilli, goblet cells, neuro-endocrine cells	Tubulo-acinar seromucous glands	Hyaline cartilage plates and fragments, with helically and circularly oriented smooth muscle bundles underlain by dense interstitial connective tissue	Cartilage supported by elastic fibre network
Bronchioles	Transforms from pseudostratified into simple columnar or cuboidal partly ciliated epithelium, Clara cells, neuro-endocrine cells	Absent	No cartilage, helically and circularly oriented smooth muscle fibres, loose interstitial connective tissue	Connective tissue supported by elastic fibre network
Terminal bronchioles	Simple cuboidal epithelium, Clara cells, neuro-endocrine cells	Absent	Smooth muscle cells and connective tissue, elastic fibre network	Particularly well developed in ruminants, pigs and horses
Respiratory bronchioles	Simple cuboidal epithelium, Clara cells, Types I and II alveolar epithelial cells	Absent	Smooth muscle cells and connective tissue, reinforced by elastic fibre network	Number of alveoli increases with each generation (I–III), abundant in carnivores, occasionally seen in the horse, rare in the pig and in ruminants
Alveolar ducts	Simple squamous epithelium (alveolar epithelium), Types I and II alveolar epithelial cells, macrophages	Absent	Elastic fibre network, muscle cells in inter-alveolar septa (acts as sphincter)	Up to 10 alveolar ducts are formed from the branching of each respiratory bronchiole, branching of alveolar ducts gives rise to alveolar sacs
Alveoli	Simple squamous epithelium (alveolar epithelium), Types I and II alveolar epithelial cells, macrophages	Absent	Loose connective tissue with prominent elastic fibre network	Blood–air barrier

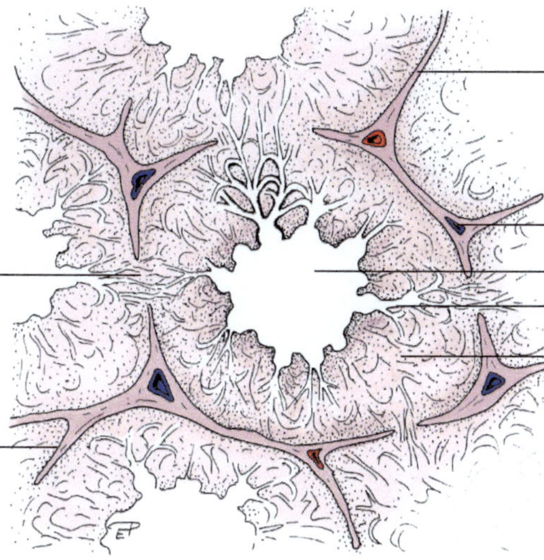

11.28 Parabronchi of the chicken (schematic).

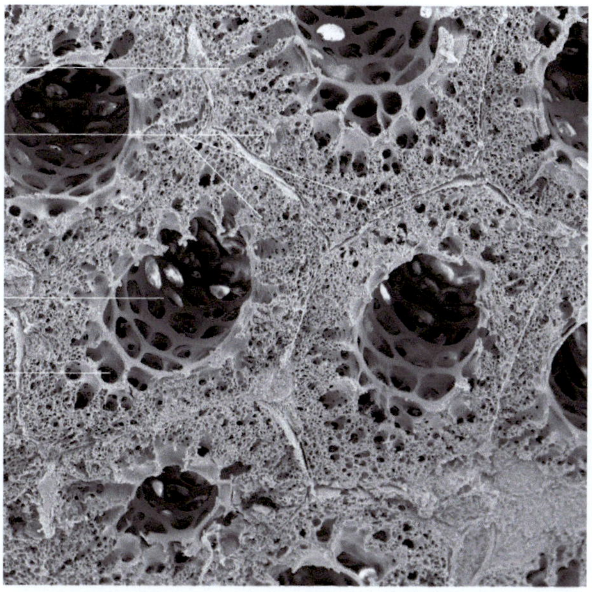

11.29 Scanning electron micrograph of the parabronchi of the lung of a chicken (x50). (Courtesy of S. Reese, Munich).

The epithelial lining of the parabronchi is **simple squamous**. Numerous small air chambers (**atria**) bulge outwardly from the atrial lumen. The atria are lined with squamous to cuboidal epithelium containing **lamellated osmiophilic bodies** (**surfactant**) for reduction of surface tension. The epithelium is surrounded by muscle cells and elastic fibres.

Several funnel-shaped **infundibulae** open from the atria and radiate into the periphery of the parabronchi. These give rise to an anastomosing three-dimensional network of tubular **air capillaries** (**pneumo-capillaries**).

The diameter of the air capillaries, characteristic for each species, ranges from 3 to 10 µm. Due to the high surface tension within these small-calibre tubes, their diameter remains relatively constant. The air capillaries are intimately intermeshed with a dense network of **blood capillaries**, permitting **gas exchange** to take place. The avian **blood–air barrier** is considerably thinner than that of mammals and consists of three elements:

- endothelial cells of the blood capillaries,
- the fused basal membranes of the blood and air capillaries and
- the epithelial lining of the air capillaries.

Relative to body weight, the surface area for gas exchange in birds is around ten times greater than in mammals. In the chicken, it constitutes 18 cm^2/g of body weight.

Air sacs (sacci pneumatici, sacci aerophori)

The air sacs are **thin-walled deformable** cavities. They are joined by connective tissue with adjacent organs or muscles but can also be partially covered with a tunica serosa. By penetrating the bones, the air sacs also serve to **pneumatise the skeleton**. The **walls of the air sacs** contain collagen and elastic fibres, as well as smooth muscle cells.

Urinary system (organa urinaria)

12

The urinary system comprises the organs that produce and modify urine (**kidneys**) and the passages through which the urine is conveyed and excreted (**renal pelvises**, **ureters**, **bladder** and **urethra**).

Kidney (ren)

The kidneys have several functions. They perform a central role in the **excretion of waste products** and contribute to **homeostasis** by maintaining the normal composition of body fluids. Production of urine by the kidneys involves processes of **filtration**, **secretion**, **reabsorption** and **concentration**.

Specific functions of the kidney include:

- excretion of organic products of metabolism (e.g. bilirubin, urea), inorganic compounds (e.g. trace elements, alkaline earth metals [e.g. Mg^{2+}, Ca^{2+}], alkali metals [e.g. Na^{+}, K^{+}]) and non-metabolisable exogenous substances (e.g. pharmacological agents),
- maintenance of osmotic pressure and H^{+} concentration of body fluids by selective reabsorption and/or excretion of ions and water,
- regulation of acid–base balance,
- synthesis of hormones for regulation of blood pressure (renin–angiotensin system) and control of erythropoiesis (erythropoietin) and
- production of 1,25-dihydroxycholecalciferol for regulation of blood calcium.

Macroscopic structure of the kidney

The kidneys are paired, roughly bean-shaped organs (exception: right kidney of the horse). They lie in the retroperitoneal space and are typically surrounded by a layer of fat (**capsula adiposa**). In addition to acting as a reservoir, this peri-renal adipose tissue supports and protects the kidneys. The surface of the kidney is surrounded by a tough connective tissue capsule (**capsula fibrosa**) composed of collagen fibres and occasional elastic fibres. Subjacent to the fibrous capsule is a thin layer of loose connective tissue containing smooth muscle cells. The connection between this layer and the parenchyma is limited to delicate fibre bundles, allowing the capsule to be easily separated from the kidney, particularly in species with **kidneys lacking external fissures** (horse, small ruminants, pig, carnivores) (Figures 12.1 and 12.2). Pathological processes may cause the capsule to adhere more firmly to the parenchyma.

Extension of the loose connective tissue into the parenchyma gives rise to a loose meshwork of collagen fibres that surrounds the renal corpuscles and tubules, and forms the adventitia of blood vessels and nerves (**renal interstitium**). In the ox, sheep and dog, there are also bundles of smooth muscle fibres around collecting tubules.

On the medial aspect of the kidney, the indented renal hilus (**hilus renalis**) is continuous with the deep **renal sinus** (**sinus renalis**). The sinus is occupied by the **renal pelvis** (**pelvis renalis**) and/or the renal calyces (**calices renales**). The hilus is traversed by the **ureter**, blood vessels, lymph vessels and nerve fibres. These are usually surrounded by fat (Figures 12.1 and 12.3).

The basic structural units of the kidney of domestic mammals are the **renal lobes** (**lobi renales**). These consist of an outer **cortex** and a pyramidal inner **medulla**. A **papilla** (**papilla renalis**) at the tip of the medulla protrudes into the calyces (or pelvis, depending on species). The boundaries of adjacent lobes are marked by interlobar arteries and veins.

Species variation

During development, the renal lobes undergo fusion to produce a single, discrete organ. The degree of fusion varies with species. In most domestic species, the cortices are completely fused and the surface of the kidney is smooth and uninterrupted. In the ox, partial fusion results in deep, externally visible fissures.

Horse, goat, sheep, cat and dog: The tips of the medullary pyramids are fused to form the renal crest (**unilobar kidney**).

Pig and ox: The apices of the medullary pyramids remain separate and project into renal calyces (**multilobar kidneys**).

Birds: **Renal lobules** may be visible on the surface of the kidney as small dome-shaped bulges (diameter 1–2 mm). However, not all renal lobules reach the surface of the kidney. In functional terms, the avian kidney

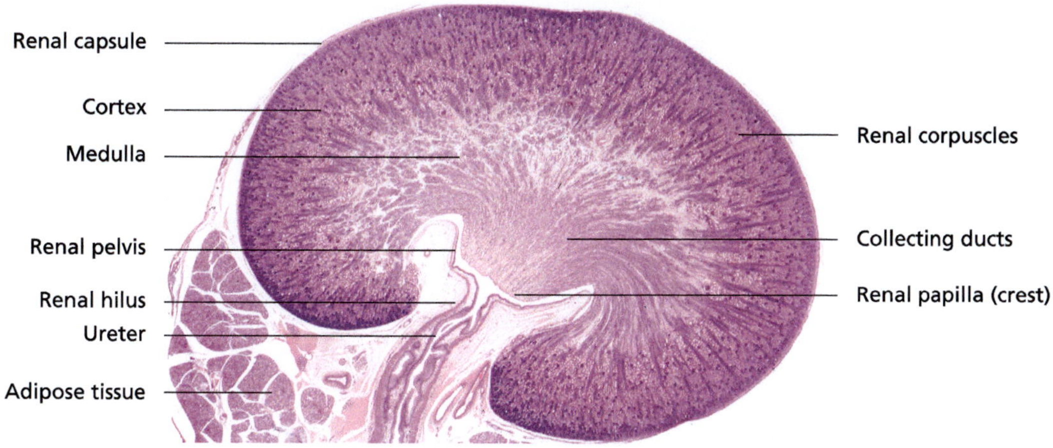

12.1 Low power view of the kidney, pelvis and proximal ureter (juvenile dog). Haematoxylin and eosin stain (x3).

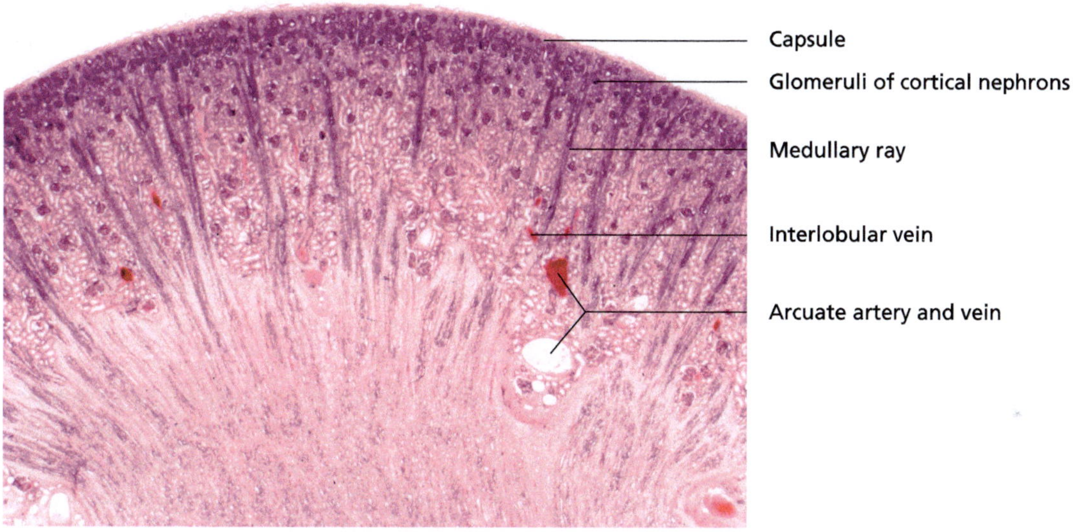

12.2 Renal cortex and medulla (dog). Haematoxylin and eosin stain (x32).

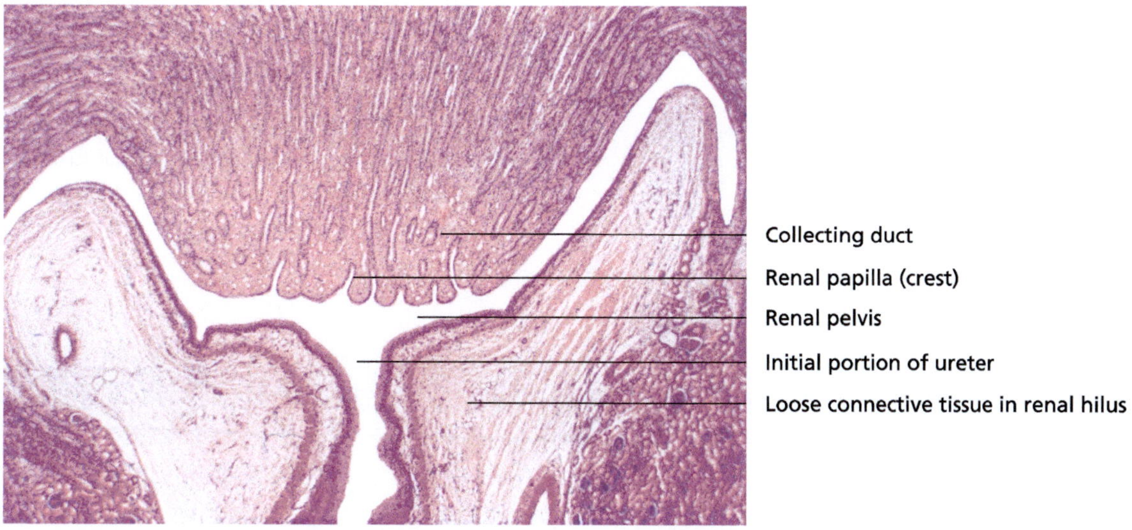

12.3 Renal papilla (crest), pelvis and proximal ureter (juvenile dog). Haematoxylin and eosin stain (x40).

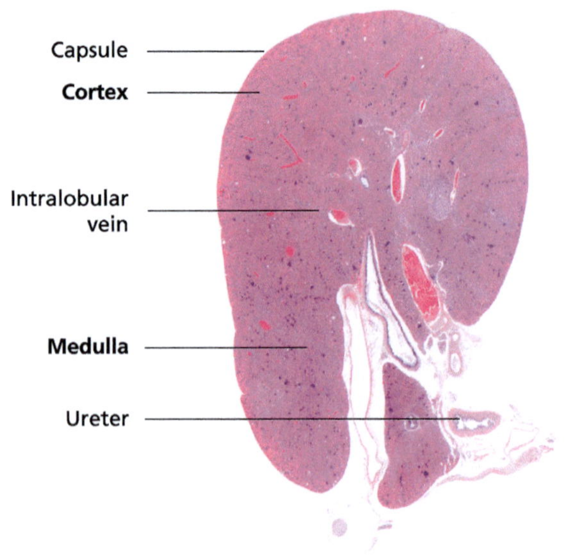

12.4 Kidney (chicken). Haematoxylin and eosin stain (x8).

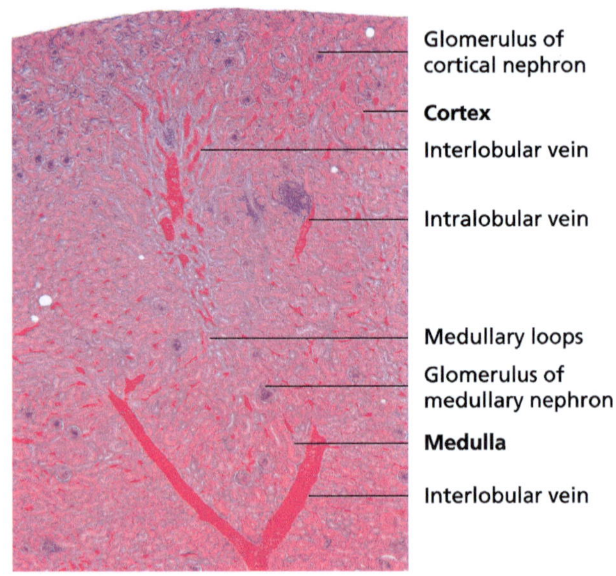

12.5 Kidney (chicken). Haematoxylin and eosin stain (x15).

can be divided into **renal lobes** (lobi renales) and **renal lobules** (lobuli renales) based on the branching pattern of the ureter. **Renal lobes** are defined as a portion of medulla that drains into secondary branches of the ureter, plus the region of the cortex that is drained by that medullary tissue. Each lobe is composed of several **renal lobules** that include both medullary tissue and the cortical tissue that it drains. Individual lobules drain into tertiary branches of the ureter, which then combine to form the aforementioned secondary ureteral branches. The medullary component of each renal lobule consists of cone-shaped bundles of **medullary collecting tubules** (tubuli colligentes medullares) enclosing blood vessels and loops of Henle of juxtamedullary nephrons. Passing through the centre of each lobule are an efferent vein of the renal portal system (intralobular vein) and an afferent artery that supplies the lobule (intralobular artery). In histological section (Figures 12.4 and 12.5), renal lobes and lobules are seen at different levels. Consequently, the cortical and medullary regions appear to be **intermingled**. In birds that have a high capacity for water conservation, the medullary regions (and thus the loops of Henle) are particularly well developed, with each medullary region draining only a relatively small area of cortex. This arrangement presumably allows for production of more concentrated urine.

Vascular supply and innervation

Blood vessels

Blood enters the kidney at the hilus through the **renal artery**, which then divides into the **interlobar arteries** (Figure 12.6). At the boundary between the cortical and medullary regions, the interlobar arteries branch to form the **arcuate arteries**. The arcuate arteries give off **interlobular arteries** that pass between the medullary rays towards the surface of the kidney. Numerous **afferent arterioles** arise from the interlobular arteries and pass towards the **vascular pole** of the glomeruli. Within the glomeruli these vessels give rise to the **glomerular capillaries**. The **efferent arterioles** arborise to form a capillary network that surrounds the renal tubules in the cortex and medulla.

Upon reaching the renal capsule, the **interlobular arteries** form a plexus (**ramus capsularis**). In the cat, the venous component of the plexus is particularly well developed. In some species, particularly the horse, there is a stellate subcapsular venous network (**vv. stellatae**) that opens into the **interlobular veins**. The **renal medulla** is supplied by straight vessels (arteriolae rectae) that arise from the efferent arterioles. These provide blood to the peri-tubular capillary networks of the medulla. The capillaries drain into venulae rectae (Figure 12.6). The arteriolae rectae and venulae rectae are collectively referred to as the **vasa recta**.

Venous vessels generally accompany the arterial supply. Drainage occurs via **intralobular, arcuate** and **interlobar veins** and ultimately the **renal vein** (see *Veterinary Anatomy of Domestic Mammals: Textbook and Colour Atlas*).

While the arteries of the kidney do not interconnect, the venous system contains numerous anastomoses as well as 'padded' barrier veins. Receiving approximately 20% of the cardiac output, the kidneys are among the most highly perfused organs of the body.

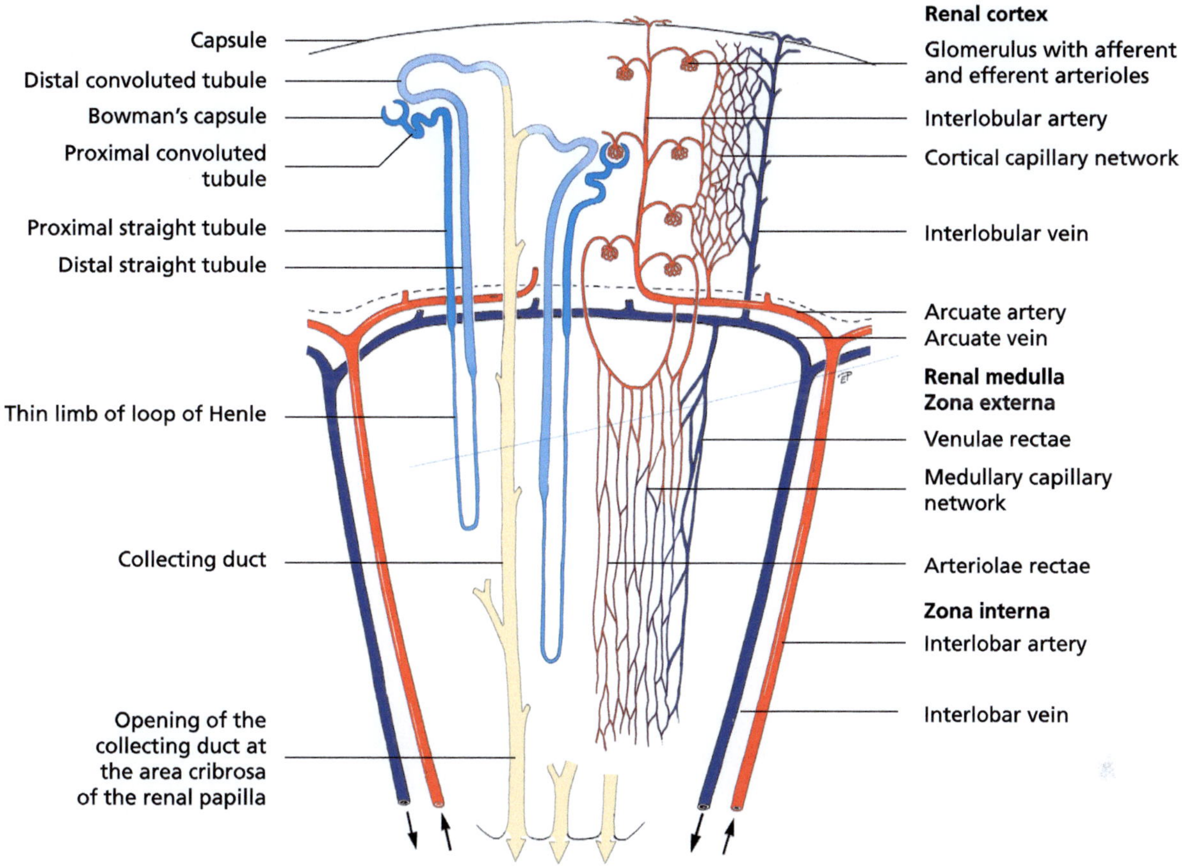

12.6 Blood supply of the kidney (schematic) (König and Liebich, 2009).

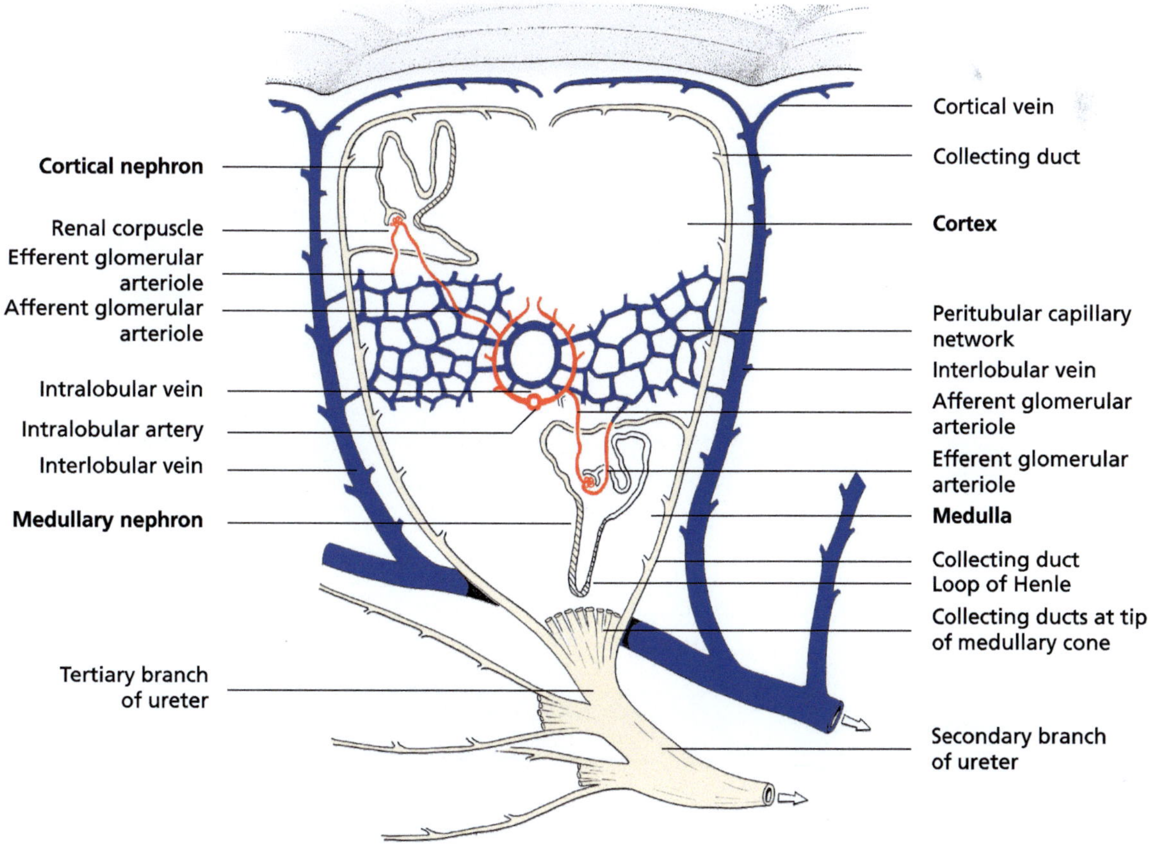

12.7 Renal lobule of a chicken (schematic). (Adapted from King and McLelland, 1978).

Species variation

Birds: Branching of the intralobular vessels resembles that of mammals. The intralobular artery gives off afferent arterioles (arteriolae glomerulares afferentes). Post-glomerular efferent arterioles (arteriolae glomerulares efferentes) give rise to capillaries that anastomose with the capillaries of the renal portal system, together forming the peri-tubular capillary network that surrounds the tubules of the nephron (Figure 12.7).

Lymph vessels

The lymph vessels travel together with the arteries and veins. In the capsule, they form a superficial drainage system.

Nerves

The kidney, particularly the blood vasculature, is innervated by numerous unmyelinated sympathetic nerve fibres originating from the coeliac plexus. Some branches extend through the interstitium to the juxtaglomerular apparatuses. Occasionally, smaller nerve fibre bundles are closely apposed to the walls of renal tubules. Visceral afferent fibres are found in the capsule and the renal pelvis. Parasympathetic fibres appear to be lacking. It has been demonstrated through kidney transplantation that transection of nerve fibres does not impact on kidney function.

Microscopic structure of the nephron and collecting duct system

The functional unit of the kidney, consisting of the **nephron** and **collecting duct system**, is structurally similar in all domestic mammals. The nephron and collecting system are connected in series. Together with the renal interstitium and the peri-tubular capillary network, they serve to produce and modify the urine. The number of functional units per kidney varies with species (approximate number of nephrons per kidney: horse – 2.7 million, ox – 4 million, small ruminants – 0.5 million, pig – 1 million, dog – 180,000 to 400,000).

Embryologically, the **nephron** develops from the **metanephrogenic blastema**. Under the influence of the ureteric bud and its derivatives, the metanephrogenic blastema transforms into a **tube**. The blind end of each developing nephron undergoes balloon-like expansion, later differentiating into the bi-layered **Bowman's capsule**. This component of the nephron is invaginated by a **capillary bundle** (**glomerulus**). The inner (visceral) layer of the nephron-anlage becomes closely associated with these capillaries. The inner and outer (parietal) layers of Bowman's capsule, together with the capillaries, later form the **renal**

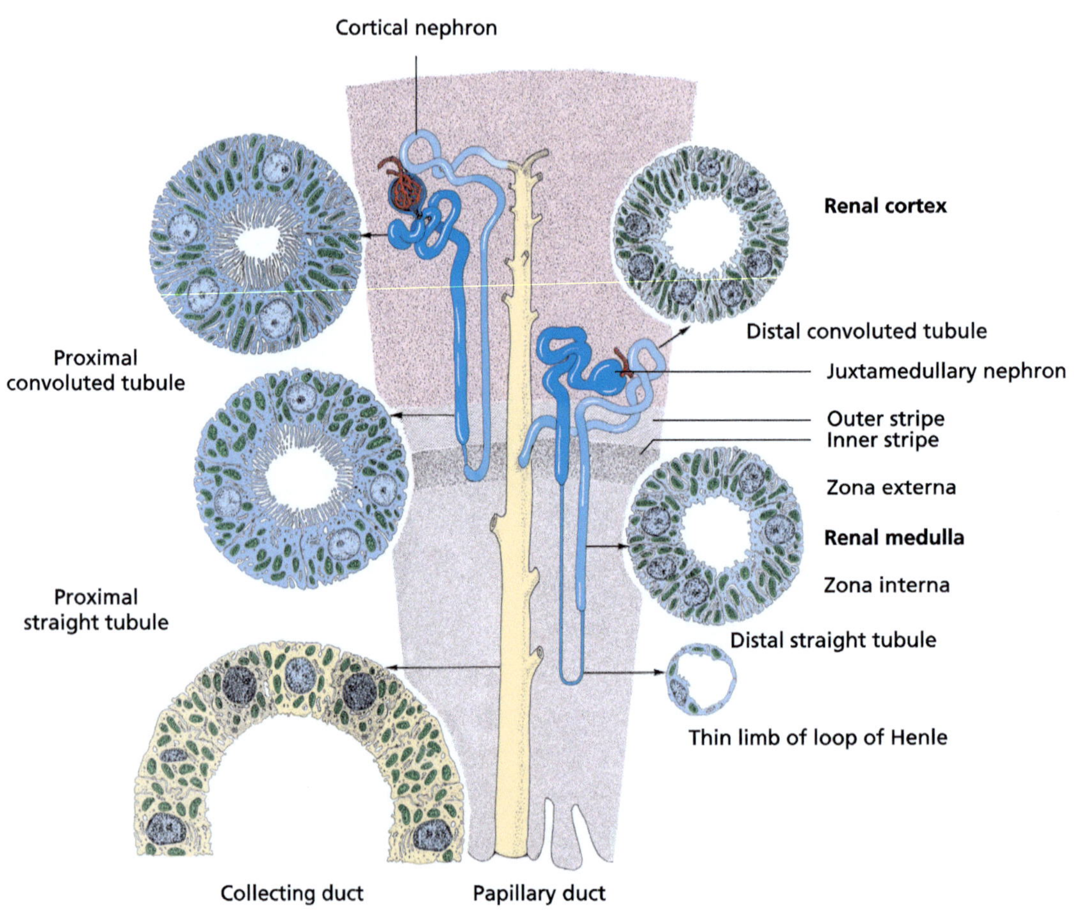

12.8 Structure of the kidney and distribution of the components of the nephron and collecting duct system in the renal cortex and medulla (schematic).

corpuscle (**corpusculum renale**) (Figures 12.9 to 12.12). The nephron becomes elongated and convoluted, developing a descending and ascending limb, and joins the tubuli of the extensively branched derivatives of the ureteric bud. The latter differentiate to form the collecting duct system that drains into the renal pelvis (and/or calyces) (refer to embryology textbooks for further detail). Nephrons can be divided into two types:

- cortical nephrons with short loops of Henle and
- juxtamedullary nephrons with long loops of Henle.

Cortical nephrons are relatively short and extend only a short distance into the renal medulla, generally as far as the boundary between the internal and external medullary zones (see below).

Juxtamedullary nephrons are particularly numerous in carnivores. Their long, thin loops extend deep into the medulla. The straight portion of the proximal tubule (see below) is continuous with the descending, thin limb of the loop of Henle.

Based on the size and number of renal corpuscles, the arrangement of proximal and distal tubules, the length of the loop of Henle and the distribution of vessels, the **renal parenchyma** can be divided (Figure 12.8) into the:

- **renal cortex (cortex renalis):**
  - medullary rays (= pars radiata),
  - cortical labyrinth (= pars convoluta),
- **renal medulla (medulla renalis):**
  - zona interna and
  - zona externa; outer and inner stripe.

The **cortex** is composed of the pars radiata (medullary rays), comprising straight segments of the proximal and distal tubules as well as collecting ducts, and the pars convoluta (cortical labyrinth), containing renal corpuscles, convoluted portions of the proximal and distal tubules and initial segments of the collecting duct system.

The **renal medulla** contains ascending and descending limbs of the loops of Henle, collecting ducts and papillary ducts. The **zona interna** contains loops of Henle of long-looped nephrons, collecting ducts and the papillary ducts. The **zona externa** is composed largely of loops of Henle of short-looped nephrons and collecting ducts.

Species variation

Variation is observed in the relative number of long- and short-looped nephrons.

Horse and small ruminants: Short-looped nephrons predominate, with renal corpuscles located mainly in the outer cortex.

Ox, pig, dog and cat: Most nephrons are long-looped, with the renal corpuscles located closer to the medulla (**juxtamedullary glomeruli**).

Renal corpuscle (corpusculum renale) and ultrafiltration

Renal corpuscles (Figures 12.9 to 12.13) – also referred to as Malpighian corpuscles – measure approximately 110–150 μm in diameter. They are composed of:

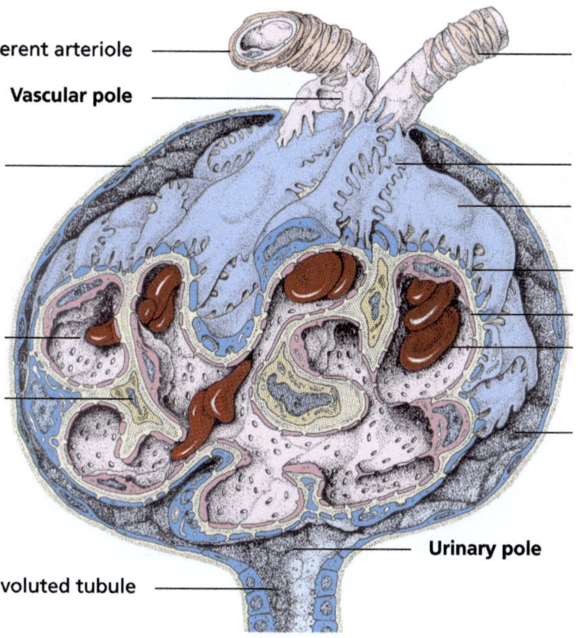

12.9 Structure of a renal corpuscle (schematic).

- a **capillary tuft** (**glomerulus**) between the afferent and efferent arteriole,
- a **double-walled capsule** (**Bowman's capsule, capsula glomeruli**) comprising:
  - an outer parietal layer of simple squamous epithelium,
  - an inner visceral layer composed of podocytes,
  - a urinary space between the two capsular layers,
- intraglomerular mesangial cells and connective tissue and
- a vascular and a urinary pole.

Species variation

Birds: The **renal corpuscles** are smaller, but considerably more numerous, than in mammals.

Capillary tuft (glomerulus)

The **afferent** and **efferent arterioles** enter and exit the renal corpuscle at the vascular pole (located opposite the urinary pole). Thus, the capillary network of the renal corpuscle begins and ends at the vascular pole. The efferent arterioles are continued by the **peri-tubular capillary network** in the cortex and medulla.

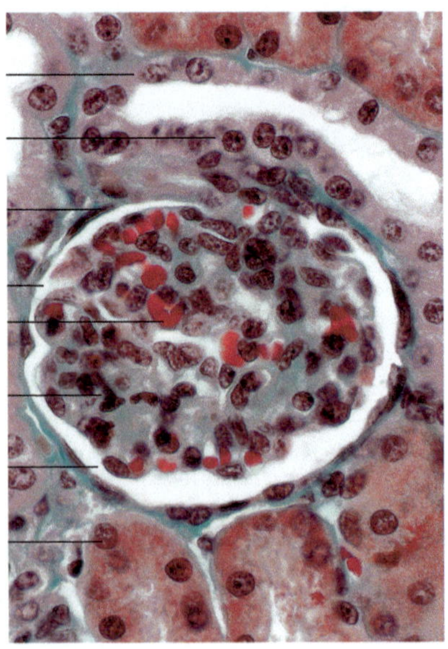

12.10 Glomerulus and Bowman's capsule with macula densa (dog). Goldner's Masson trichrome stain (x800).

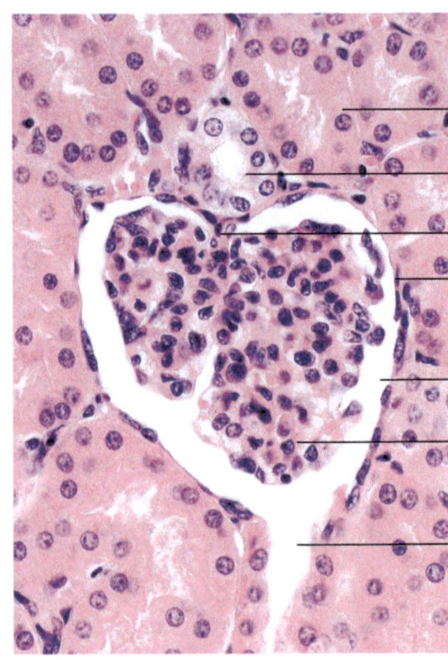

12.11 Renal corpuscle with vascular and urinary poles (dog). Haematoxylin and eosin stain (x800).

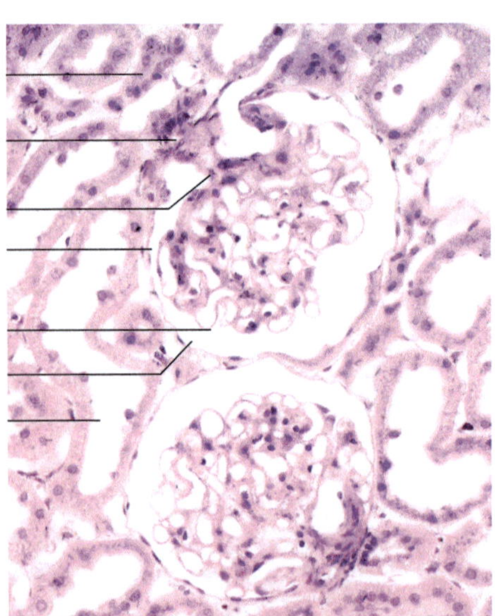

12.12 Renal corpuscle with juxtaglomerular apparatus (dog). PAS stain (x450).

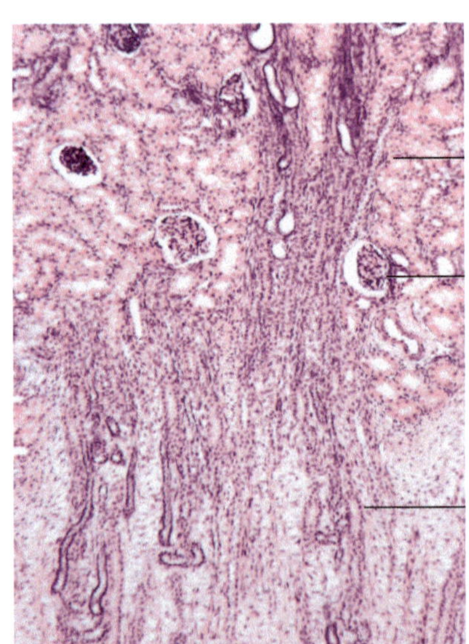

12.13 Transition from renal cortex (with juxtaglomerular renal corpuscles) to medulla (dog). Haematoxylin and eosin stain (x70).

The capillary tuft of the glomerulus (**rete capillare glomerulare**) develops from the division of the afferent arteriole into four to eight branches. These branches form up to 50 anastomosing capillary loops. The structural components of the glomerulus (Figure 12.9) comprise:

- endothelial cells of the capillary wall,
- glomerular basement membrane,
- podocytes (= inner visceral layer of Bowman's capsule) and
- intraglomerular mesangial cells with loose connective tissue.

ENDOTHELIAL CELLS

The wall of the glomerular capillaries is composed of an extremely thin endothelium with numerous round pores. These openings are generally evenly spaced and lack a diaphragm. Substances that can pass through the endothelium include water, sodium, urea and small proteins. The endothelial surface contains negatively charged proteoglycans that limit the filtration of large anionic proteins. The endothelium also synthesises endothelin. Release of endothelin results in vasoconstriction of the afferent and efferent arterioles of the glomerulus.

BASEMENT MEMBRANE (MEMBRANA BASALIS)

The basement membrane (thickness 0.1–0.2 µm) lies against the exterior of the capillary wall, where it acts as a physical boundary and filter (Figure 12.14). The membrane consists of three layers:

- inner lamina rara interna (adjacent to endothelium),
- middle lamina densa and
- outer lamina rara externa (adjacent to podocytes).

The **basement membrane** is composed of fine fibrillar non-aggregated type IV collagen macromolecules as well as collagenous and non-collagenous glycoprotein subunits (laminin and fibronectin). These are embedded in a proteoglycan-rich matrix of sialic acids.

The basement membrane is produced mainly by the capillary endothelium and partly by the podocytes. Mesangial cells serve to remove and phagocytose substances filtered by the membrane.

The lamina densa acts as a mechanical filter. The less electron-dense lamina interna and externa are rich in polyanionic molecules. Thus, the basement membrane serves as a further barrier to proteins based on their negative charge. Neutral or positively charged molecules transit more readily than, for example, negatively charged albumin.

Renal disease, with associated loss of electric charge of the basement membrane, can result in significant albuminuria.

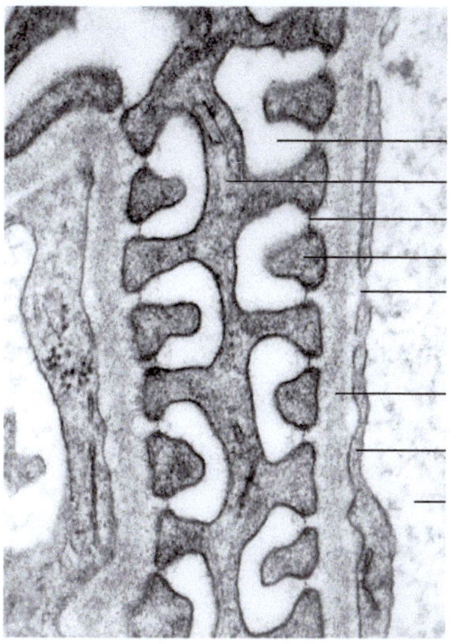

12.14 Fine structure of a glomerular capillary, basement membrane and adjacent podocyte processes with slit diaphragms ('blood–urine barrier') (dog; x18,000).

Bowman's capsule

VISCERAL LAYER (PODOCYTES, PODOCYTI)

The flattened cells of the **visceral layer of Bowman's capsule** (podocytes) cover the external surface of the glomerular capillaries (Figures 12.15 to 12.17). Their nuclei and cell bodies bulge into the urinary space. Extending from the cell bodies are long, actin-rich processes (**primary processes**) that divide to form secondary and tertiary processes (Figures 12.14 to 12.16). At the points of contact with the basement membrane, the tertiary processes expand to form foot processes (the origin of the term '**podocyte**'). Their surfaces bear negatively charged membrane proteoglycans.

The finger-like processes are tightly interdigitated leaving narrow spaces (25 nm) between them. These spaces are spanned by a thin **slit diaphragm** (6 nm thick) that is similar in structure to the diaphragm of fenestrated capillaries (Figure 12.14). The slit diaphragm, containing P-cadherin and nephrin, forms a further filtration barrier. Disruption of this barrier leads to substantial proteinuria and oedema. Podocytes have several functions, including:

- contribution to the glomerular filtration barrier,
- uptake of high-molecular weight molecules,
- regulation of pressure within the renal corpuscle through contractile elements of the cytoskeleton and
- production of fibrillar components of the glomerular basement membrane.

PARIETAL LAYER AND URINARY SPACE (LUMEN CAPSULAE)

At the vascular pole (**polus vascularis**), the visceral layer of Bowman's capsule reflects upon itself to continue as the

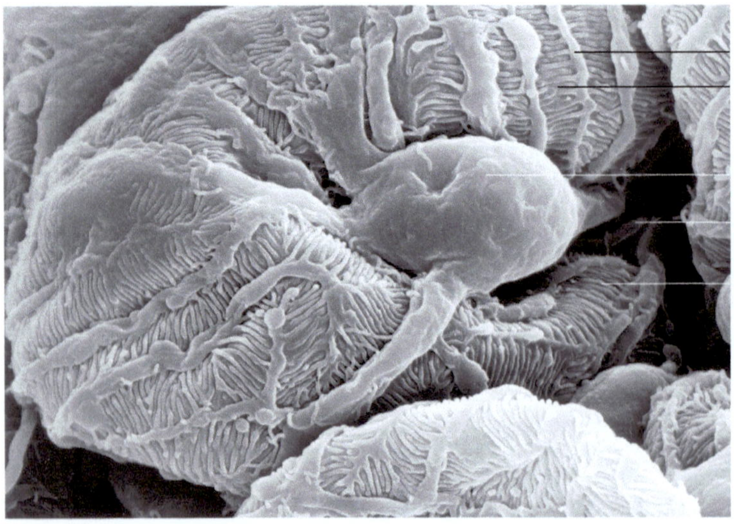

12.15 Scanning electron microscope image of a podocyte covering the wall of a capillary (dog). Podocytes form the inner, visceral layer of Bowman's capsule (x4000).

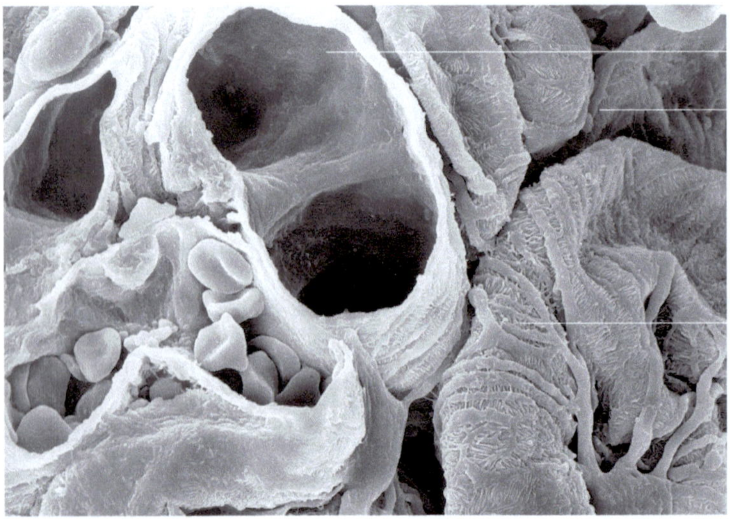

12.16 Scanning electron microscope image of a glomerular capillary tuft (partly opened) with overlying podocytes (dog; x2500).

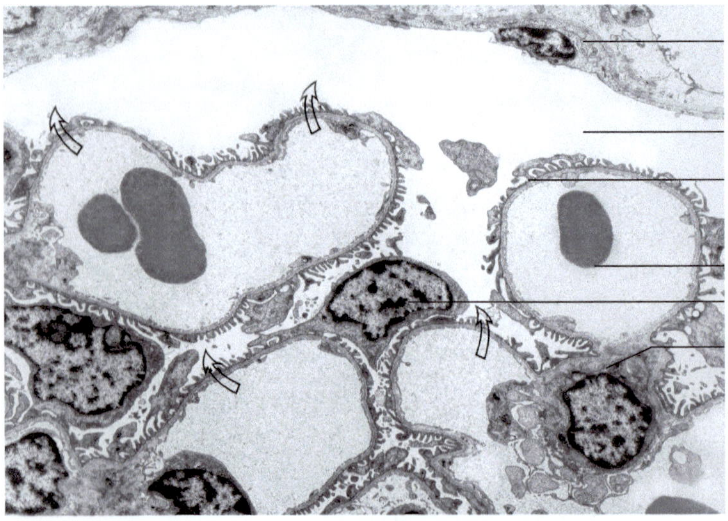

12.17 Fine structure of a renal corpuscle with capillaries, podocytes and mesangium (dog; x3000).

parietal layer. The parietal layer consists of flattened, simple squamous epithelium with an underlying basal lamina and loose connective tissue. The **urinary space** (**capsular lumen**) between the two layers of the capsule serves to collect the ultra-filtrate (= primary urine), which leaves the renal corpuscle at the urinary pole (**polus tubularis**) and passes into the proximal tubule (Figure 12.9).

Mesangium

The term mesangium refers to the **intraglomerular** portion of the renal corpuscle that extends from the vascular pole into the glomerulus, binding the capillary loops together (Figures 12.9 and 12.10). It is derived from mesenchymal connective tissue that migrates into the corpuscle together with the capillaries. The mesangium consists of **mesangial cells** (**mesangiocytes**) and the **mesangial matrix** (**lamella hyalina**). Long processes extending from mesangial cells may in some instances penetrate the endothelium to reach the capillary lumen.

Mesangial cells typically have a bizarre, spindle-like appearance with indented heterochromatic nuclei. The cytoplasm contains a sparse complement of fibrils that permits a limited degree of cellular contraction. Numerous matrix-filled invaginations are present on the cell surface.

The mesangial matrix is in contact with the lamina rara of the glomerular basement membrane, and the mesangium is continuous with the extraglomerular mesangial cells (Goormaghtigh cells, lacis cells). **Functions of the mesangium** include:

- structural support for the glomerular capillaries,
- phagocytosis of substances originating from the capillaries,
- uptake of filtered substances from the glomerular basement membrane (removal of debris),
- production of substances that contribute to immune defence and repair of the glomerulus,
- production of glomerular basement membrane components and
- regulation of capillary resistance/distension.

Binding of angiotensin II with mesangial receptors regulates contraction of blood vessels, thus influencing renal blood flow. Cytokines released in local inflammatory responses result in constriction of the capillary lumen.

Glomerular filtration apparatus (blood–urine barrier)

The glomerular filtration apparatus has three main components:

- capillary endothelium,
- glomerular basement membrane and
- podocytes and filtration slits (Figures 12.9 and 12.14).

The relatively large pores (70–100 nm) of the **capillary endothelium** prevent the movement of cells and large molecules out of the capillary lumen.

The continuous **basement membrane** limits the passage of substances with a molecular weight of greater than 400,000 Da and/or a diameter of more than 10 nm. The main barrier is the lamina densa, which functions primarily as a physical filter. In contrast, the laminae rarae act electrostatically, repelling negatively charged molecules.

The **filtration slit diaphragm** between adjacent foot processes of podocytes permits the transit of substances with a molecular weight below 70,000 Da or a diameter of less than 7.5 nm.

Consequently, the **glomerular filtrate** (**primary urine**) is an ultra-filtrate of plasma. It differs from plasma in that it is largely free of proteins. Molecules such as inulin, free haemoglobin and serum albumin may be detectable in trace amounts. **Primary urine** is isotonic and iso-osmotic with blood. In addition to water and electrolytes, it contains amino acids, glucose and smaller protein molecules.

The volume of **glomerular filtrate** is determined by the filtration surface, the permeability of the filtration unit to water and the effective glomerular filtration pressure. The last of these is influenced by blood pressure, colloid osmotic pressure and pressure exerted by interstitial tissues.

Tubules of the nephron

The tubules of the nephron (Figure 12.8) are comprised of the:

- proximal convoluted tubule,
- proximal straight tubule (thick descending limb of loop of Henle),
- thin limb of loop of Henle (descending and ascending portions),
- distal straight tubule (thick ascending limb of loop of Henle) and
- distal convoluted tubule.

The main function of the **proximal tubule** (**tubulus proximalis**) is to **reabsorb** electrolytes and water, amino acids, peptides, proteins and glucose for **transport** into the interstitium and uptake by the **peri-tubular capillary network**. The proximal tubule also **secretes** various substances, such as NH_4^+ ions, water and salts, as well as heavy metals (e.g. mercury, lead), toxins and foreign matter into the **tubular lumen**. The proximal tubule is divided into segments with different structural characteristics.

The initial portion of the proximal tubule (tubulus contortus proximalis) is tightly convoluted and has a relatively narrow lumen. The loops of the proximal convoluted

Table 12.1 Distinguishing structural features of the tubules of the nephron and collecting duct system in domestic mammals.

Segment	Epithelium	Function
Proximal tubule (diameter 40–60 μm; relatively narrow lumen)	Cuboidal, round nucleus, acidophilic cytoplasm, extensive basal labyrinth comprising infoldings of basal membrane, abundant apically located lysosomes and peroxisomes, prominent apical brush border	Extensive reabsorption of glucose, amino acids, bicarbonate, calcium, water, salts and phosphate, and secretion of organic acids, anions and cations, and pharmacological agents
Thin limbs of loop of Henle (diameter 12–15 μm)	Flattened epithelium (resembling that of endothelium, though somewhat thicker), nuclei protrude slightly into the lumen	Reabsorption of water and salts
Distal tubule (diameter 30–45 μm, relatively wide lumen)	Cuboidal, round nucleus, notably light cytoplasm, prominent basal labyrinth	Ion transport, impermeable to water
Collecting duct (diameter 50 μm in outer regions to 300 μm in inner medulla)	Cuboidal (may be bi-layered distally), round nucleus, contains lipid droplets in older animals, goblet cells present in the horse, bi-layered at the papilla (three layers in pigs)	ADH-dependent transport of water (via increased permeability), aldosterone-dependent reabsorption of sodium and secretion of potassium

tubule meander around the glomerulus and may extend into the subcapsular region of the cortex (where renal corpuscles are lacking). In this tubular segment, around two-thirds of the glomerular filtrate is reabsorbed through the tubular wall and taken up by the surrounding capillary network. The remainder continues distally into the **loop of Henle** (**ansa nephroni**).

The loop of Henle is shaped like a hairpin, with its descending and ascending segments in close proximity. Together with the surrounding capillary network, this arrangement establishes the counter-current exchange mechanism through which urine becomes increasingly concentrated as it passes towards the renal papilla (for more detail, refer to physiology textbooks).

The straight portion of the distal tubule (= thick ascending limb of the loop of Henle) returns to the renal cortex, where it passes close to its associated renal corpuscle. At the point of contact with the corpuscle, specialised tubular epithelial cells (**macula densa**) monitor the sodium concentration of the tubular fluid.

The next segment, the **distal convoluted tubule** (**tubulus contortus distalis**) is the final portion of the nephron. There, the urinary components are either reabsorbed or conveyed into the collecting duct system (Table 12.1).

Species variation

Birds: A morphological distinction is made between **cortical** and **medullary** (or **juxtamedullary**) **nephrons** (Figure 12.7). Cortical nephrons are more numerous (up to 90%) and have smaller renal corpuscles (Figures 12.22 and 12.23). The loops of Henle are short or absent. Medullary nephrons have larger renal corpuscles and the loops of Henle penetrate deep into the medullary tissue. The **cortical nephrons** consist of a proximal convoluted tubule, a short and variable **intermediate segment** and a distal convoluted tubule. The **absence of a loop of Henle** distinguishes them from mammalian cortical nephrons. Also lacking are the basal striations typically seen in the cuboidal epithelial cells of the mammalian proximal convoluted tubule (see below). In **medullary nephrons**, a loop of Henle (also referred to as a medullary loop) is present between the proximal and distal tubules (Figures 12.25 and 12.26). These nephrons resemble those of mammals. The medullary loop consists of a relatively thin portion that descends into the medullary cone and a markedly thicker ascending segment. The latter is continued by the distal convoluted tubule, which opens into peripherally located collecting tubules. At the tip of the medullary cone, the **medullary collecting tubules** (**tubuli colligentes medullares**) from several renal lobules unite to form a **secondary branch** of the ureter (Figure 12.7). The lobules that contribute to each secondary branch are united to form a **renal lobe** (**lobus renalis**). In this sense, according to some authors, there is a degree of organisational similarity with the bovine kidney. The secondary ureteral branches drain into **primary branches** that ultimately open into the **ureter**.

Proximal convoluted tubule

The proximal convoluted tubule (diameter 40–60 μm) is arranged in several loops around its associated renal corpuscle (Figures 12.8 and 12.10 to 12.13). The epithelium consists of relatively large cuboidal to columnar cells. At the apical cell surface there is a brush border (microvilli, up to 1 μm in length) that can be seen with the light microscope. The cytoplasm is acidophilic, and the cell borders are indistinct. Basally, prominent striations are formed by invaginations of the plasmalemma enclosing stacks of elongated mitochondria. The **brush border** is coated by a glycocalyx containing membrane enzymes (e.g. alkaline phosphatase, peptidases). The glycocalyx is visible by electron microscopy.

At the base of the microvilli, the cytoplasm contains numerous **vesicles** and **tubular infoldings of the cell membrane**. In addition, the apical portion of the cell contains large numbers of **lysosomes**, **peroxisomes** and **resorption vacuoles** (Figures 12.20 and 12.21). These organelles are required for the **extensive trans-epithelial uptake** of substances from the tubular lumen. The absorptive capacity of the cell is increased considerably by the density of microvilli in the brush border (up to 7000 per cell). The cells of the proximal tubule are responsible for:

- reabsorption of proteins and amino acids by pinocytosis (transcellular pathway) and
- active transport of sodium into the intercellular space (paracellular pathway).

Proteins passing through the apical cell membrane are taken up and enzymatically degraded by lysosomes. Peptides are cleaved by membrane enzymes (e.g. aminopeptidases, transferases) to form amino acids. Under normal conditions, the urine that is finally excreted is free of proteins.

At the base of the epithelium, extensive interdigitation of branching processes of neighbouring cells gives rise to a **basal labyrinth**. In histological section, this appears as infoldings of the plasma membrane in which mitochondria are localised. The basal labyrinth plays an important role in the **reabsorption of electrolytes and water**. Sodium ions are transported by **ion pumps** (Mg^{2+}-dependent Na^+-/K^+-activated ATPase) into the **expanded extracellular space**. Energy is supplied by ATP produced by the abundant local mitochondria. Chloride ions and water passively follow the actively transported Na^+. The removal of Na^+ and **Cl^- ions** from the base of the cell maintains a gradient between the tubular lumen and the surrounding capillaries, driving absorption of Na^+ from the glomerular filtrate.

By the end of the proximal tubule, over two-thirds of the water filtered by the glomerulus has been reabsorbed from the tubular lumen. This passes through the epithelium into the peri-tubular capillary system. Trans-epithelial fluid transport is facilitated by the oncotic pressure of the highly viscous blood in the postglomerular vessels. Other processes occurring in the wall of the proximal convoluted tubule include:

- reabsorption of bicarbonate and glucose via membrane transport proteins and
- gluconeogenesis in the peroxisomes, via energy supplied by fatty acids.

The epithelium of the proximal tubule also **secretes** various substances. Products of metabolism and foreign substances (e.g. drugs) are **actively secreted**. **Electrolytes**, **NH_4^+ ions** and **H^+ ions** pass passively from the cell into the tubular lumen.

Species variation

Dog: In the **Dalmatian**, the liver enzyme uricase appears to be biologically unavailable, limiting the capacity for

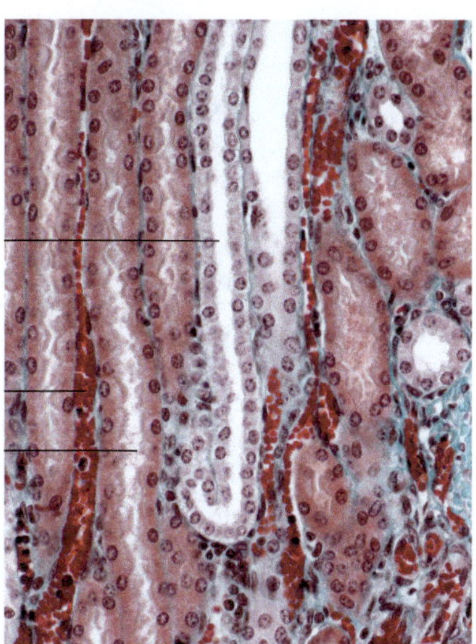

12.18 Section of renal medulla (dog). Goldner's Masson trichrome stain (x480).

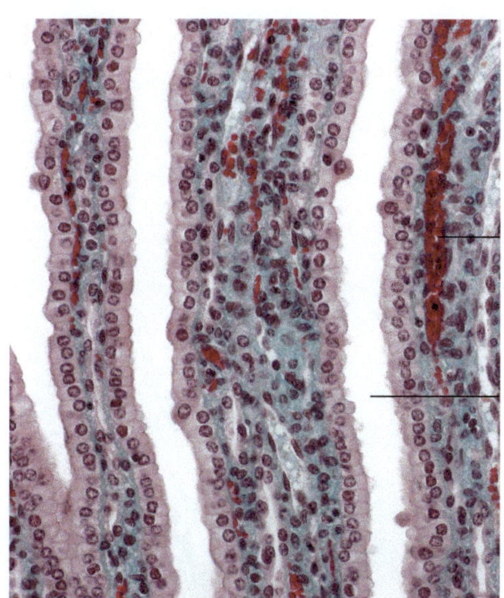

12.19 Straight portion of collecting duct (ductus colligens rectus) in the renal crest (dog). Goldner's Masson trichrome stain (x480).

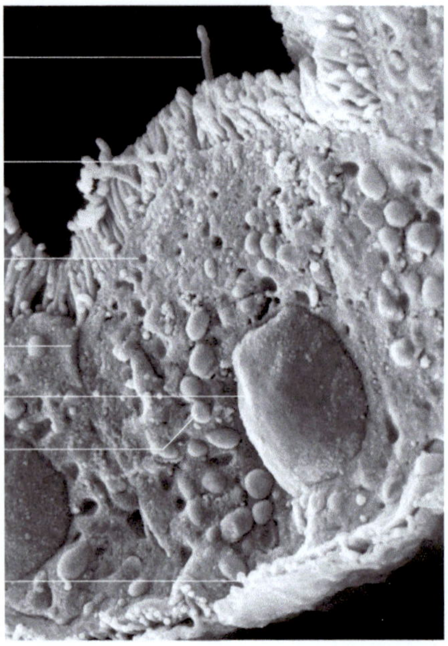

12.20 Scanning electron microscope image of an epithelial cell in the wall of a proximal tubule (dog; freeze fracture, x9000).

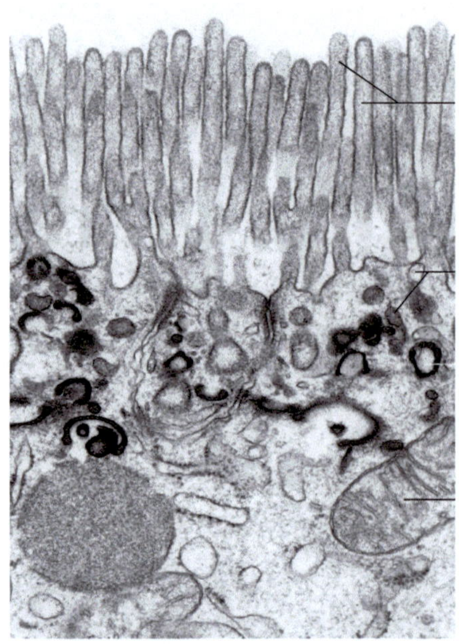

12.21 Fine structure of the apical surface of adjacent epithelial cells of a proximal convoluted tubule with dense brush border and abundant lysosomes and peroxisomes (dog; x16,000).

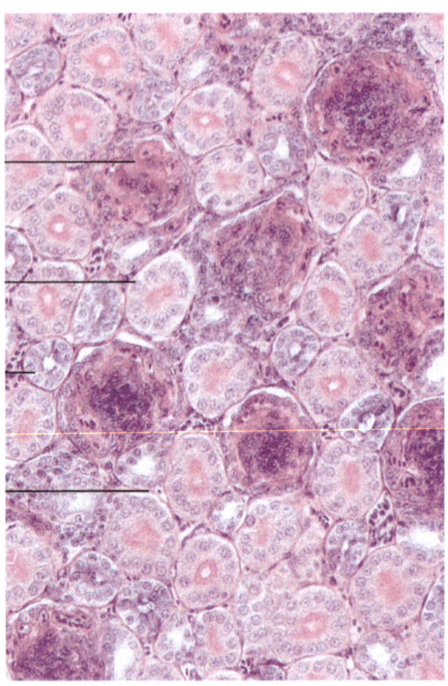

12.22 Kidney (chicken). Haematoxylin and eosin stain (x360).

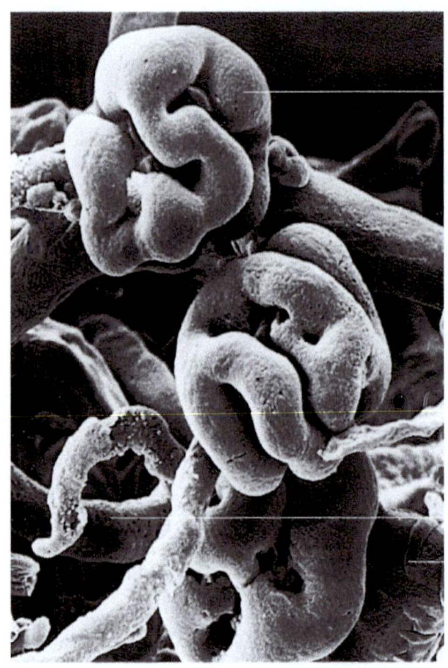

12.23 Scanning electron microscope image of a capillary tuft in the kidney (chicken).

conversion of uric acid to allantoin. Thus, uric acid is excreted in the urine. Reabsorption of uric acid in the proximal convoluted tubule does not occur, due to a lack of the required transport mechanism in this breed. This prevents the accumulation of uric acid in the blood.

Proximal straight tubule

The epithelium of the proximal straight tubule is largely similar to that of the proximal convoluted tubule (Figure 12.8). The height of the epithelium and the extent of the basal invaginations are reduced, compared with the convoluted portion, and there are fewer lysosomes.

Species variation

Carnivores: Numerous lipid droplets are present in the proximal straight tubule (dogs) and proximal convoluted tubule (cats).

Horse and ruminants: The proximal tubule contains only occasional lipid droplets.

Pig: The occurrence of lipid droplets is variable.

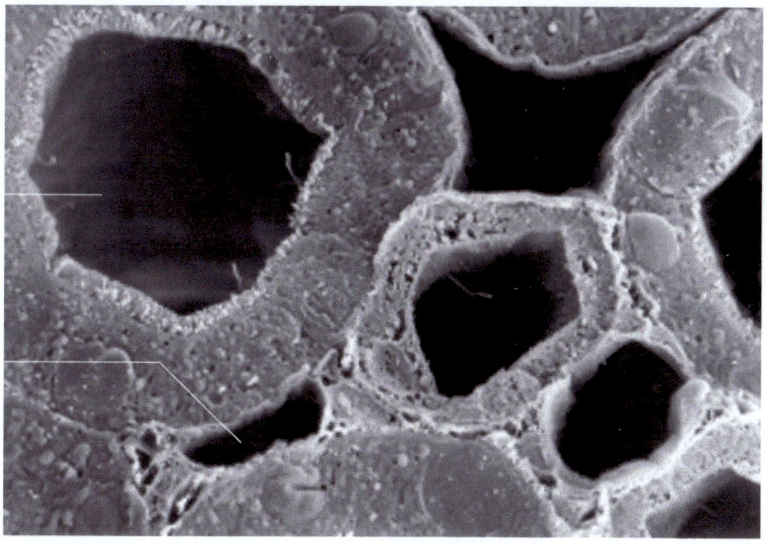

12.24 Scanning electron microscope image of a transverse section of the renal medulla (dog; freeze fracture, x3000).

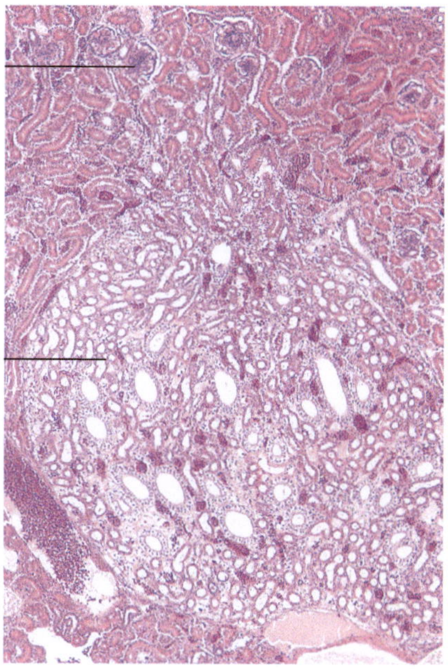

12.25 Medulla (chicken). Haematoxylin and eosin stain (x40).

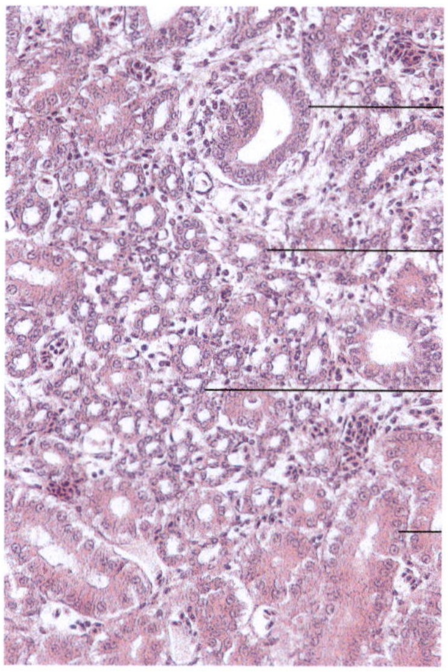

12.26 Medulla (chicken). Haematoxylin and eosin stain (x70).

Thin limb of loop of Henle

The thin limb of the loop of Henle consists of simple squamous epithelium. The width of the lumen is similar to that of the proximal tubule (Figures 12.8 and 12.18) but the external diameter is reduced to around 12–15 μm. The cells lack a brush border, have relatively few organelles and lie immediately adjacent to surrounding capillaries.

The **thin limb of the loop of Henle** serves primarily to **reabsorb water** and **concentrate the primary urine**. The extent to which this occurs is determined by the length of the loop. Desert rodents have particularly long-looped nephrons and extensively developed medullary zones, to minimise excretion of water in the urine.

The **descending** and **ascending thin limbs** are closely apposed. This physical proximity facilitates the concentration of urine by establishing a **counter-current system**, in conjunction with the surrounding capillaries and the collecting duct system. In addition, the epithelial cells of the distal straight tubule (thick ascending limb of the loop of Henle; see below) incorporate a basal labyrinth containing **ion pumps** that actively transport **Na^+ and Cl^-** out of the cell into the interstitium. The distal straight tubule is relatively impermeable to water. Consequently, the osmolarity of the interstitium gradually increases towards the renal papilla. Driven by this mechanism, **water passes through the epithelium of the thin portion of the loop of Henle** into the peri-tubular tissue where it is taken up by medullary vessels (refer to physiology textbooks for more detail).

> **Species variation**
>
> **Birds**: The loops of Henle and associated counter-current mechanism are less extensively developed in birds, thus the **capacity to concentrate urine is lower** than in mammals.

Distal straight tubule and distal convoluted tubule

The ascending thin limb continues as the distal straight tubule, also referred to as the thick ascending limb of the loop of Henle (Figures 12.8 and 12.18). The convoluted portion is located near its associated glomerulus. Both the straight and convoluted portions have a wide lumen (30–45 µm). The epithelium is somewhat lower than that of the proximal tubule. Instead of a brush border, the apical surface bears a few irregularly spaced, small microvilli. The basal labyrinth is particularly prominent, with numerous mitochondria occupying the infoldings of the plasmalemma.

Na^+ ions (via basally located ion pumps) are transported into the interstitium in exchange for K^+, H^+ or NH_4^+. The distal tubule thus plays an important role in **maintaining water and electrolyte balance**. These mechanisms are hormonally regulated. **Aldosterone** influences epithelial Na^+ and K^+ transport (see also below). **Antidiuretic hormone** increases the permeability of the epithelium to water. **Calcitonin** raises, and **parathyroid hormone** lowers, excretion of $Ca2^+$.

Collecting duct system

The collecting duct system (Figure 12.19) comprises the:

- arched collecting tubule,
- straight collecting tubule (collecting duct) and
- papillary duct.

The collecting duct system begins with the short, arched collecting tubule, which opens into the straight collecting tubule or collecting duct (Figure 12.6). Up to ten nephrons drain into each collecting duct. In the cortex, the collecting ducts are grouped together in the medullary rays. They continue to run parallel to one another within the medulla. In the inner zone of the medulla, the collecting ducts merge to form the **papillary ducts**, which empty by a series of openings at the tip of the renal papilla / crest (**area cribrosa**) into the renal calyces / pelvis (Figure 12.3).

In contrast to the **nephron**, the collecting duct apparatus constitutes a branched system of tubules in which the epithelial lining changes gradually from the cortex to the papilla. The epithelial cells are predominantly cuboidal in the cortex and increase in height towards the papilla. The cells have a centrally located nucleus, pale cytoplasm and clear cell boundaries. The simple cuboidal to columnar epithelium of the collecting duct transforms into a double layer of columnar epithelium in the papillary duct (diameter 200–300 µm). Fat droplets may be seen in the collecting ducts of older animals and goblet cells may be present in horses. At the papilla, the epithelium consists of two layers (three in the pig).

The **final stages of urine concentration** take place in the **collecting duct system**. The collecting ducts are surrounded by the hypertonic environment of the renal medulla. Water follows the osmotic gradient into the interstitium. Only small quantities of urea and electrolytes pass into the tubular cells. Recent research has shown that the collecting ducts are the main target of aldosterone in regulating transport of Na^+ and water.

Antidiuretic hormone (**ADH**), secreted by the posterior pituitary gland, increases permeability to water. Lack of ADH or epithelial ADH receptors results in excretion of large volumes of relatively dilute urine (diabetes insipidus).

Juxtaglomerular apparatus (complexus juxtaglomerularis)

The juxtaglomerular apparatus (Figure 12.12) consists of:

- the macula densa,
- juxtaglomerular cells and
- extraglomerular mesangial cells (Goormaghtigh cells, lacis cells).

Located at the vascular pole of the renal corpuscle, the juxtaglomerular apparatus regulates blood pressure and urinary sodium concentration by modifying glomerular filtration rate and sodium reabsorption (**renin–angiotensin system**).

Macula densa

The macula densa is a region of up to 40 **modified epithelial cells** located in the portion of the distal straight tubule that lies adjacent to the vascular pole of the glomerulus, between the afferent and efferent arterioles and the extraglomerular mesangial cells (Figure 12.10). Beyond this point, the distal tubule becomes convoluted.

The epithelial cells are columnar with dense cytoplasm. Short microvilli are present on the cell surface. Basally there is a relatively poorly developed basal labyrinth and a continuous basal lamina. The macula densa acts as a **chemoreceptor**, detecting the **Na^+ ion concentration in the tubular fluid**. A fall in tubular Na^+ triggers release of renin by the juxtaglomerular cells. This activates the angiotensin system which brings about increased Na^+ reabsorption, with water following by osmosis.

Juxtaglomerular cells

Juxtaglomerular cells are modified smooth muscle cells found in the afferent arteriole, near its entry into the glomerulus. These cells are in contact with the vascular endothelium and the macula densa. Juxtaglomerular cells are characterised by **myosin filaments** and **dense granules** containing **renin**. Release of the contents of these granules initiates the **renin–angiotensin system**.

Extraglomerular mesangial cells

Extraglomerular mesangial cells (Goormaghtigh cells, lacis cells) lie between the macula densa and the afferent and efferent arterioles. They are continuous with the intraglomerular mesangium. The function of the extraglomerular mesangial cells is unclear. It has been proposed that they act as reserve cells for juxtaglomerular cells.

Interstitium

The renal interstitium fills the spaces between the renal tubules and collecting ducts. It is composed of **modified** fibrocytes, relatively few collagen fibrils and an extensive matrix containing proteoglycans. There is evidence that interstitial fibroblasts produce erythropoietin, though the significance of this phenomenon under normal physiological conditions has been questioned. **Prostaglandins** and **bradykinin** are also released by cells of the interstitium. These substances regulate renal perfusion and thereby exert an influence on the systemic circulation.

Interstitial cells also product **thrombopoietin** and **renin**.

Urinary passages

Renal pelvis (pelvis renalis)

The renal pelvis can be considered as a proximal expansion of the ureter that forms a funnel around the renal papilla (crest). The visceral, inner layer forms the epithelial lining of the renal papilla. It consists of a variable number of cell layers.

> **Species variation**
>
> **Carnivores and small ruminants**: Narrow recesses (**recessus pelvis**) extend from the main portion of the pelvis. The epithelium of these recesses, and that of the pseudopapillae, is simple cuboidal.
>
> **Equids**: The terminal recesses (**recessus terminales**) of the pelvis are lined with stratified epithelium.

Peripherally, the epithelium of the medullary tissue transforms into the **transitional epithelium** (**epithelium transitionale**) of the outer layer of the pelvis. Transitional epithelium lines the urinary passages as far as the external urethral orifice. Due to its specialised structure, this type of epithelium (see Chapter 2, 'Epithelial tissue') serves as a protective barrier against the hypertonic urine within the urinary passages. The underlying lamina propria consists of loose connective tissue. In the horse, the lamina propria contains **mucous tubulo-acinar glands** (**glandulae pelvis renalis**).

The tunica muscularis comprises smooth muscle. Some degree of layering is evident. A sparse inner longitudinal layer is surrounded by a thin layer of circular fibres. Externally, occasional longitudinal fibres are seen.

The muscle of the renal pelvis is continuous with that of the ureter. Specialised smooth muscle cells act as a pacemaker, resulting in peristaltic transport of urine in the pelvis and ureter. Deep in the renal sinus, the tunica adventitia is thin and contains nerves, adipose tissue and blood vessels. Towards the hilus it becomes considerably more substantial.

> **Species variation**
>
> **Carnivores and ruminants**: The tunica adventitia contains smooth muscle fibres.

Ureter

Aided by a well-developed layer of smooth muscle, the ureter conveys urine that has accumulated in the pelvis to the bladder. The tunica mucosa is lined with **transitional epithelium**. In the non-distended ureter, longitudinal folds are visible in the mucosa (Figure 12.27). The lumen thus appears stellate in histological sections. The lamina propria is loose and typically devoid of glands.

> **Species variation**
>
> **Equids**: The mucosa contains elongated mucous glands (glandulae uretericae) that extend up to 10 cm distal to the renal pelvis (Figure 12.28). These are responsible for the characteristic viscous, stringy consistency of equine urine.

As in the renal pelvis, the tunica muscularis has inner and outer longitudinal layers separated by a circular layer. These are joined by obliquely oriented fibres to form a single functional unit.

> **Species variation**
>
> **Cat**: The inner muscle layer is absent.

Near the ureteric orifices, the longitudinal muscle fibres fan out into the bladder forming the muscular core of the trigone. The ureters open into the bladder obliquely. This arrangement results in compression of the ureteric lumen as the bladder fills. The ureters are considered to contain an autonomous impulse generation system.

The external surface of the ureter is covered with a **tunica adventitia** or a **tunica serosa**, depending on its topographic anatomical relationships.

> **Species variation**
>
> **Birds**: The **ureter** emerges from the ventral aspect of the kidney in the region of the middle renal division. The ureter of the chicken is formed from the union of approximately 17 primary branches, each of which drains

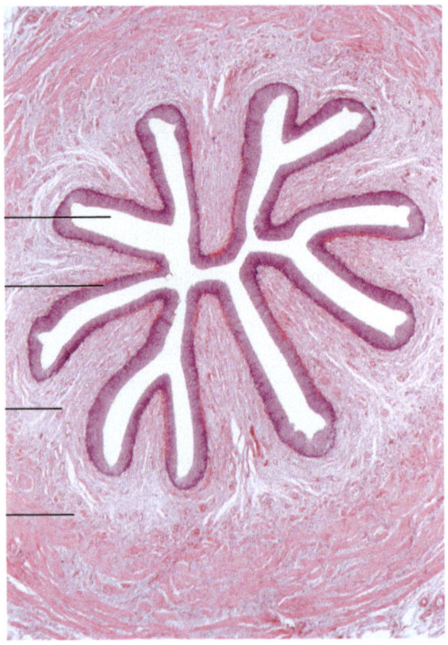

12.27 Cross-section of ureter with transitional epithelium, deeply folded mucosa and layered tunica muscularis (pig). Haematoxylin and eosin stain (x36).

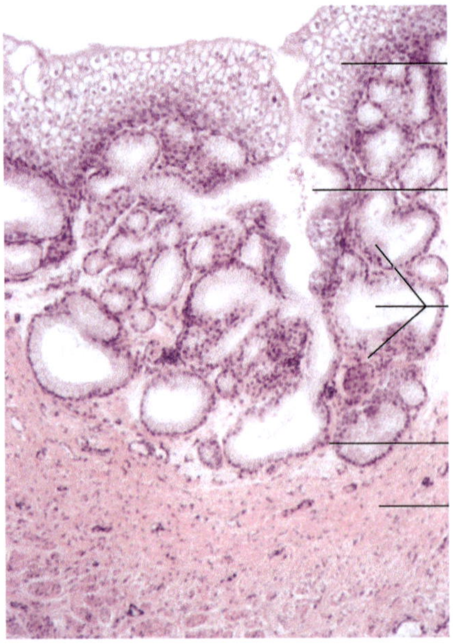

12.28 Wall of ureter with mucous glands (horse). Haematoxylin and eosin stain (x100).

5–6 secondary branches. In the extrarenal portion of the ureter, the lamina propria underlying the **transitional epithelium** is particularly substantial. The loose connective tissue is supported by bundles of elastic fibres and may contain lymphocytic infiltrates. The **tunica muscularis** is thickened along the extra-renal portion by circular and longitudinal smooth muscle bundles. Reinforcement is provided near the cloaca by an additional layer of longitudinal muscle. The ureter enters the dorsolateral wall of the cloaca, opening into the **urodeum**.

Bladder (vesica urinaria)

The bladder is lined internally by **transitional epithelium**. Depending on the degree of filling, the number of cell layers visible in the epithelium ranges from 2–3 in the distended bladder to 10–14 in the contracted state (Figure 12.29). Specialisations of the epithelium serve to protect the underlying tissues against the hypertonic urine. The outer layer of the trilaminar plasmalemma (unit membrane) is thickened. The cellular barrier is reinforced by bundles of subplasmalemmal filaments and membrane

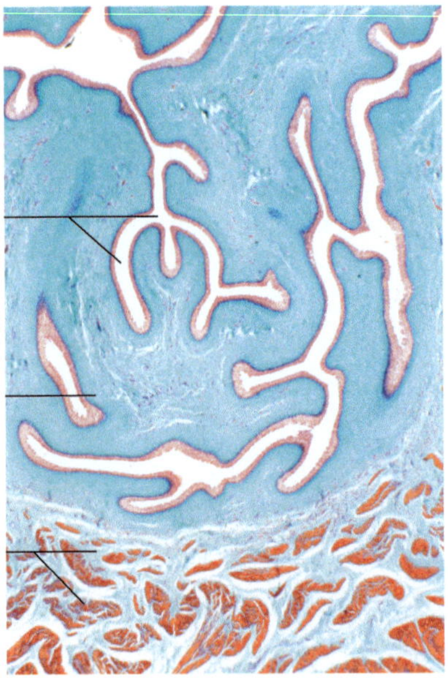

12.29 Contracted bladder with deep mucosal folds resulting in apparent segmentation of the lumen (goat). Goldner's Masson trichrome stain (x30).

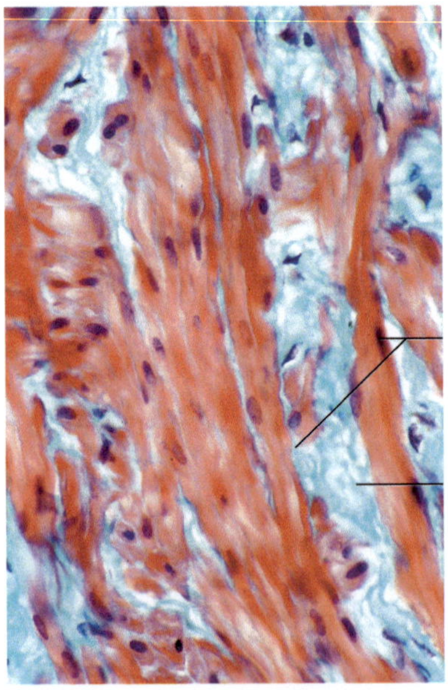

12.30 Smooth muscle of bladder wall with spiral fibre orientation (goat). Goldner's Masson trichrome stain (x250).

vesicles (**crusta**). The **lamina propria** consists of a connective tissue lattice containing delicate elastic fibres. Together with the submucosa, the lamina propria forms a mobile, displaceable layer that facilitates the alternate folding and stretching of the bladder wall. The lamina propria and submucosa are typically separated by a **lamina muscularis mucosae**. Bundles of elastic fibres provide mechanical reinforcement at the neck of the bladder. Lymphoid follicles may be present in the lamina propria. A dense network of capillaries, concentrated in the subepithelial region, is particularly extensive in ruminants.

The **tunica muscularis** consists of relatively thick layers of smooth muscle (longitudinal – circular – longitudinal) comprising interwoven spirally oriented fibres (Figure 12.30).

> **Species variation**
>
> **Horse and pig**: The outer longitudinal layer may be lacking.

The boundary between the muscle layers is sometimes indicated by a vascular plexus. The spiral arrangement of muscle fibres facilitates sustained, uniform contraction of the bladder wall. Near the vertex and neck of the bladder, the muscle fibres from tight loops, though a functional sphincter is not formed.

The bladder wall is **innervated** by an autonomic plexus with ganglion cells located between muscle layers (intramural ganglia). Sympathetic and parasympathetic nerve fibres regulate bladder motility and contraction of vessel walls. The mucosa also contains sensory fibres.

Urethra

Female urethra

The female urethra extends from the neck of the bladder to the external urethral orifice. It consists of a tunica mucosa, submucosa, tunica muscularis and a tunica adventitia.

The **mucosa** is lined by **transitional epithelium**, becoming pseudostratified towards the external urethral orifice. Isolated areas of cuboidal or columnar cells may be observed. The epithelial cells may contain mucus.

> **Species variation**
>
> **Pig and horse**: The epithelium contains goblet cells.
>
> **Sheep and horse**: Near the external urethral orifice, the epithelium changes to **stratified squamous**.

The epithelium rests upon a dense **connective tissue layer**. This is extensively vascularised, particularly in the ox. The lamina propria contains **cavernous spaces**, the extent of which varies with species.

> **Species variation**
>
> **Cat and sheep**: Cavernous spaces are lacking in the initial portion of the urethra. In other species, cavernous tissue is present throughout the urethra, becoming more prominent near the opening into the vestibule.

Occasional smooth muscle cells are present in the subepithelial connective tissue. The **tunica muscularis** consists of inner circular and outer longitudinal layers. In the horse, the oblique orientation of muscle fibres may give the appearance of a third layer. At the opening into the genital tract, the smooth muscle cells intermingle with skeletal muscle fibres (m. sphincter urethrae).

Male urethra

The male urethra is closely connected, both structurally and functionally, with the genital organs and is discussed in Chapter 13, 'Male reproductive system'.

13 Male reproductive system (organa genitalia masculina)

The male reproductive system consists of the:

- **testes** (sperm production),
- **epididymides** (sperm maturation and transport),
- **deferent ducts** (sperm transport),
- **accessory sex glands**:
  - terminal portion of the deferent ducts,
  - prostate gland,
  - vesicular glands,
  - bulbourethral glands and
- **penis**.

Not all accessory glands are present in all species (Figure 13.1). Accessory glands are absent in birds.

Testis

The paired testes are responsible for **production of spermatozoa** and **synthesis of male sex hormones**. Based on structural and functional characteristics, the tissues of the testes are classified as:

- **stroma:**
  - tunica vaginalis,
  - tunica albuginea,
  - tunica vasculosa,
  - septula testis,
  - mediastinum testis,
  - lobuli testis,
  - interstitial connective tissue (intestinum testis) with Leydig cells (endocrinocyti interstitiales),
- **parenchyma:**
  - convoluted seminiferous tubules (tubuli seminiferi convoluti),
  - straight testicular tubules (tubuli seminiferi recti),
  - rete testis and
  - ductuli efferentes testis.

Stroma

The testis is surrounded by a collagen-rich connective tissue capsule, the **tunica albuginea** (ca. 1–2 mm thick). The tunica albuginea lies immediately internal to the visceral layer of the **tunica vaginalis**.

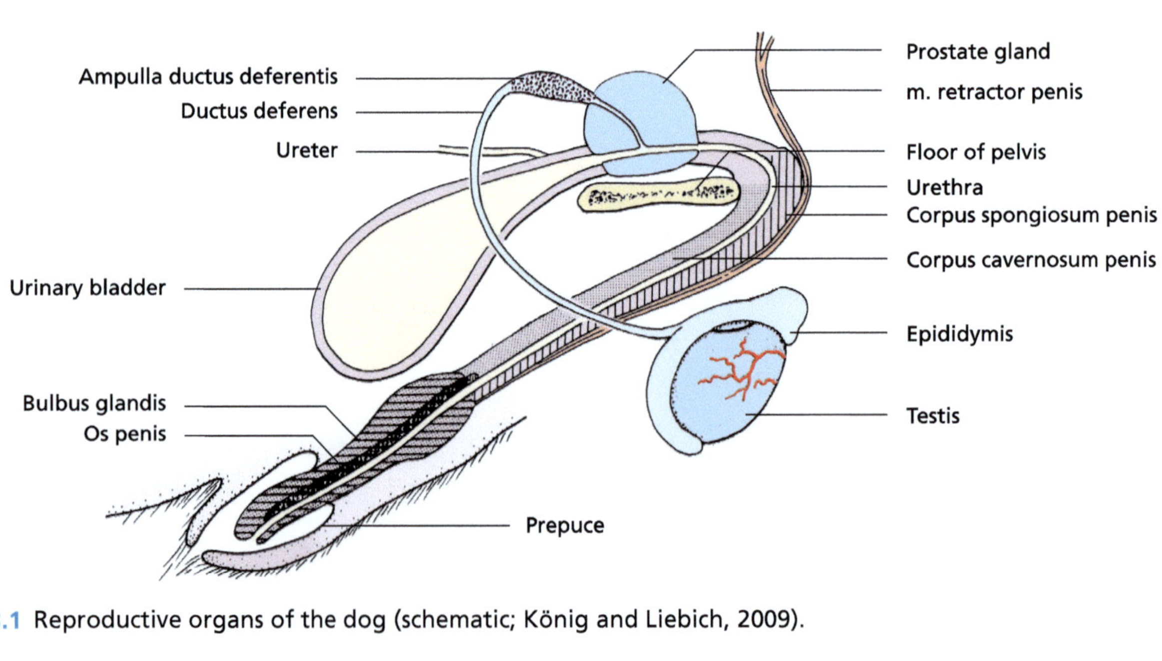

13.1 Reproductive organs of the dog (schematic; König and Liebich, 2009).

Arteries and veins ramify within the tunica albuginea to form a vascular layer (**tunica vasculosa**). This is located superficially in the dog and ram, and more deeply in the stallion and boar. Smooth muscle fibres are also present in the stallion, boar and ram.

Connective tissue septa (**septula testis**) radiate from the tunica albuginea into the interior of the organ where they form the **mediastinum testis**. In ruminants, pigs and dogs, the mediastinum testis begins near the extremitas caudata, extends axially through the testis and recombines with the tunica albuginea at the head of the epididymis. The septula testis divide the testicular parenchyma into numerous pyramidal lobules (**lobuli testis**), each containing between two and five convoluted seminiferous tubules (**tubuli seminiferi convoluti**). These tortuous tubules are surrounded by loose connective tissue, containing vascular and nerve plexuses and interstitial cells (hormone-producing Leydig cells).

Interstitial cells (Leydig cells)

Leydig cells are found in clusters or cords (Figures 13.4 and 13.5). Their number varies with age and species. The proportion of total testis volume represented by Leydig cells is 20–30% in the stallion and boar, and 5% in the bull. Individual cells are connected by gap junctions. Most individual cells lie adjacent to a capillary.

The **interstitial cells** are acidophilic and irregularly polyhedral. The nucleus is spherical and euchromatic with a prominent nucleolus. Numerous lipid vacuoles, lysosomes and peroxisomes are present in the pale cytoplasm. Interstitial cells are characterised by large amounts of **smooth ER** and abundant, typically elongated **mitochondria with tubular projections of the inner membrane**. This tubular mitochondrial morphology is related to the **endocrine function** of the cell. The smooth ER contains 17-β-hydroxysteroid dehydrogenase, which catalyses the transformation of androstenedione into **testosterone**. In the mitochondria, cholesterol is converted into pregnenolone.

Production of androgens (testosterone) by interstitial cells is stimulated by luteinising hormone (LH) produced by the hypophysis. Over 90% of the testosterone in the body is produced by these interstitial testicular cells.

Testosterone regulates spermatogenesis (together with follicle-stimulating hormone, FSH), sexual behaviour, accessory gland function, development of secondary sexual characteristics and anabolism. Secretion of testosterone is subject to negative feedback mechanisms involving the hypothalamus and hypophysis. Interstitial cells also synthesise peptides that act through **paracrine** or **autocrine** (regulation of protein metabolism) mechanisms.

Species variation

Horse and cat: Interstitial cells contain glycogen.

Ox: Interstitial cells have mitochondria with folded cristae, as well as those with a tubular cristal morphology. **Rough ER** is also present. Light intercalated cells have been observed in the loose connective tissue. These are presumed to regulate androgen production by adjacent Leydig cells through paracrine pathways.

Parenchyma

The tightly wound convoluted seminiferous tubules (**tubuli seminiferi convoluti**) lie between the septula testis. Before entering the mediastinum testis, the convoluted tubules straighten to form the **straight testicular tubules** which are joined to the **rete testis** within the mediastinum. The rete testis empties via the **ductuli efferentes testis** into the **epididymis** (Figures 13.2 and 13.3).

Convoluted seminiferous tubules (tubuli seminiferi convoluti)

The convoluted seminiferous tubules are surrounded by a **lamina propria**. The innermost layer of the lamina propria is in contact with the basal lamina of the seminiferous tubules. Fine collagen and elastic fibres are condensed into a thin layer that encloses the so-called **peritubular contractile cells**. These cells contain actin bundles and act as **myofibroblasts**, bringing about contraction of the seminiferous tubules. This facilitates spermiation (release of spermatozoa into the tubular lumen) and transport of spermatozoa through the tubules.

The tubules are around 50–80 cm long and have a diameter of 150–300 μm. **Formation of male gametes (spermatogenesis)** takes place in the spermatogenic epithelium lining the tubular wall. The epithelium is composed of:

- spermatogenic cells and
- sustentacular cells (Sertoli cells, epitheliocyti sustentantes).

SPERMATOGENIC CELLS (CELLULAE SPERMATOGENICAE)

The spermatogenic cells of the tubular (spermatogenic) epithelium differentiate from primordial germ cells that have migrated into the gonads during embryonic development. The spermatogenic cells are located between the sustentacular cells. Spermatogenic cells undergo several phases of division and maturation before being released as male gametes (spermatozoa) into the lumen of the seminiferous tubules. Final maturation occurs during the passage of the cells through the reproductive apparatus. The ability to fertilise an ovum is achieved after capacitation takes place within the female reproductive tract. Multiplication and differentiation of spermatogenic cells

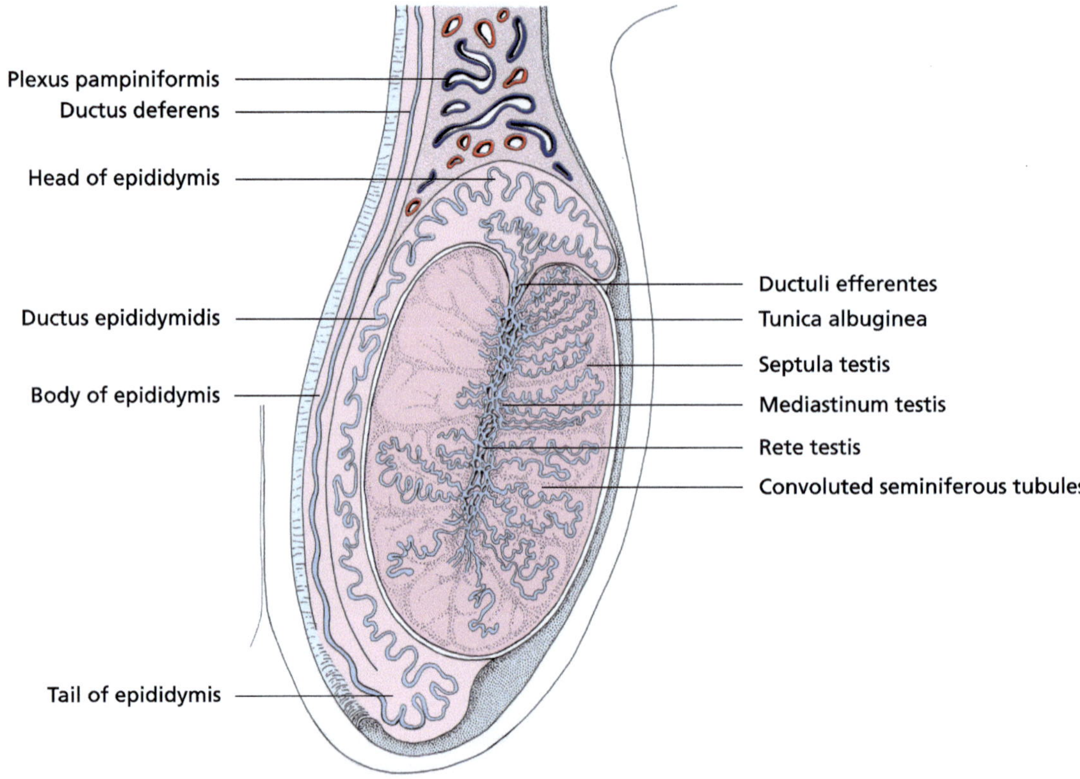

13.2 Schematic representation of the testis, epididymis and ductus deferens of a bull.

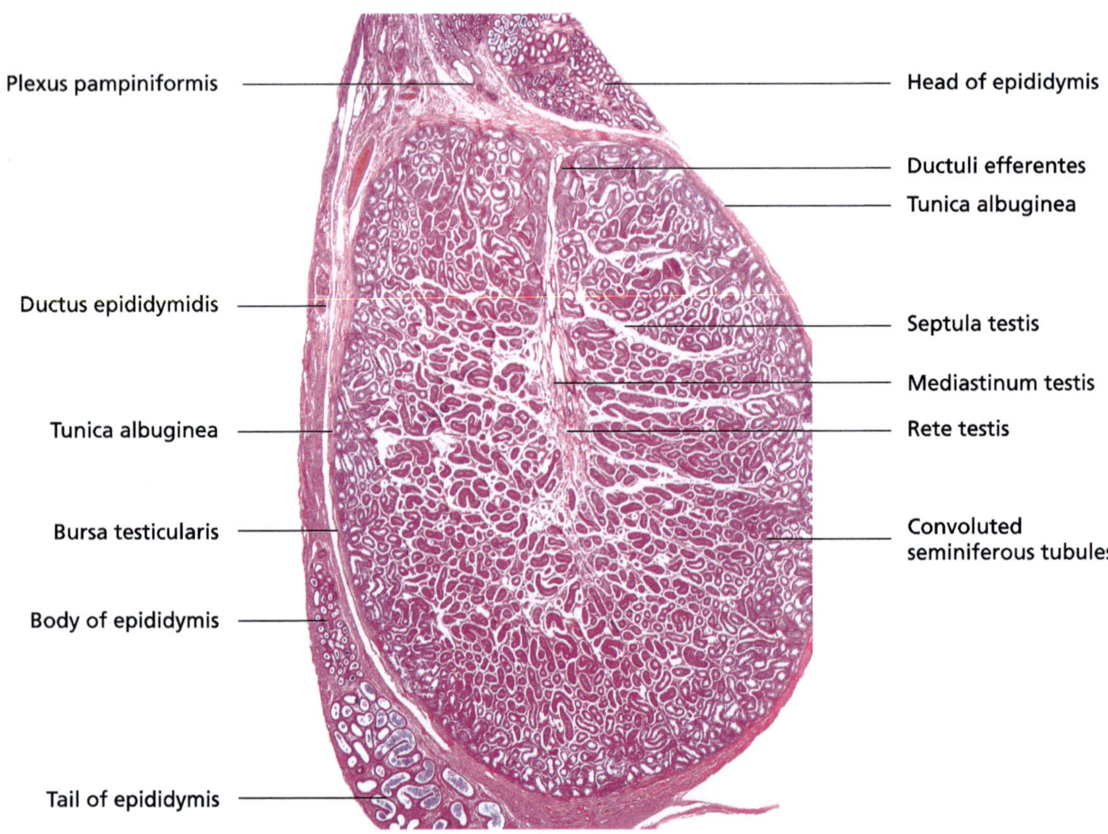

13.3 Testis and epididymis of a bull. Haematoxylin and eosin stain (x8).

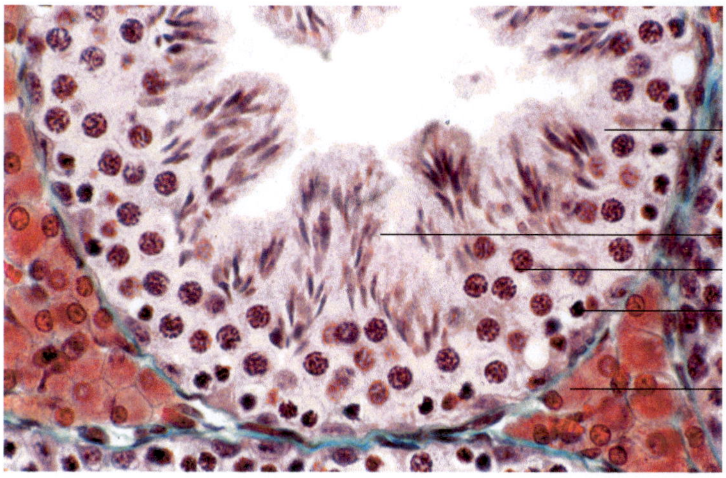

13.4 Seminiferous tubule (boar). The spermatids in the acrosomal phase are arranged in sheaf-like bundles. Goldner's Masson trichrome stain (x440).

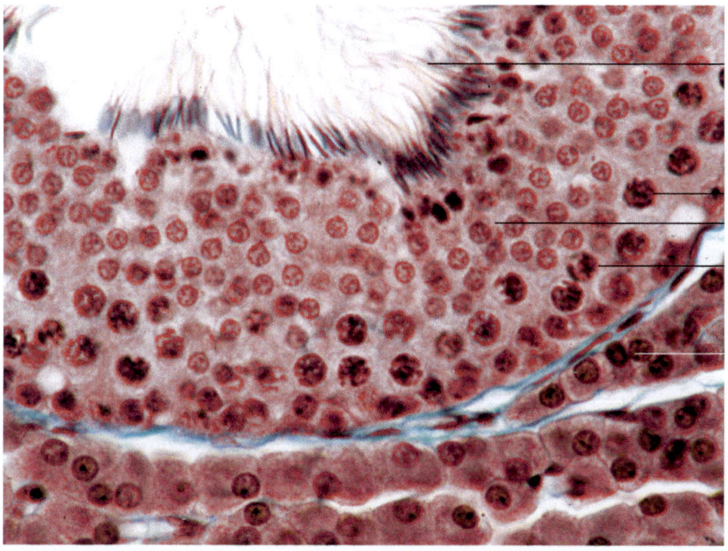

13.5 Seminiferous tubule (boar). Goldner's Masson trichrome stain (x440).

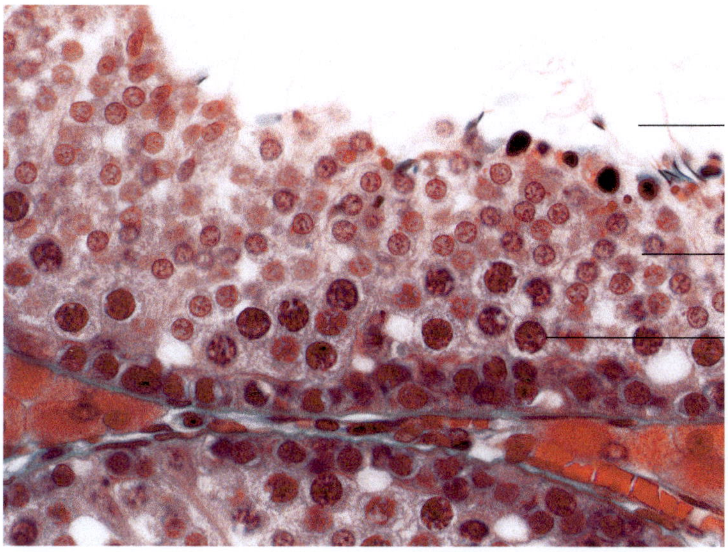

13.6 Seminiferous tubule (boar). Spermatozoa are seen undergoing release into the tubular lumen (spermiation). Goldner's Masson trichrome stain (x440).

is hormonally regulated. The process by which germ cells (spermatogonia) are transformed into spermatozoa is described as spermatogenesis.

SPERMATOGENESIS

The term spermatogenesis describes the processes of multiplication and differentiation that occur in the seminiferous tubules to produce male gametes. These cells then undergo further maturation within the epididymis. Spermatogenesis is divided into two stages:

- spermatocytogenesis and
- spermiogenesis.

Spermatocytogenesis begins with the division of the male spermatogonial stem cells, the **spermatogonia**, into two daughter cells. One of these remains as a new stem cell. The other undergoes further **mitotic divisions**, ultimately giving rise to **primary spermatocytes**. These cells go through a **first maturation** (**meiotic**) **division** to produce **secondary spermatocytes**. Immediately after their formation, secondary spermatocytes undergo a second meiotic division, resulting in the formation of four haploid spermatids (see Chapter 1, 'The cell', 'Meiosis').

During subsequent **spermiogenesis**, spermatids differentiate into **sperm cells** (**spermatozoa**) without further cell division.

Spermatocytogenesis

The number of mitotic divisions of the spermatogonia (and the duration of spermatogenesis) is species-dependent. The following sequence is considered to occur in the bull: one **A_1-spermatogonium** divides into two **A_2-spermatogonia**. One of the A_2-spermatogonia divides to give two further A_1-spermatogonia, that initially remain dormant as new stem cells. The other A_2-spermatogonium divides to form two **A_3-spermatogonia**. One of these degenerates while the other divides mitotically to give rise to **I-, B_1- and B_2-spermatogonia** from which **primary spermatocytes** are formed. At this stage, multiplication of the newly formed A_1-spermatogonia is initiated. **Multiplication of spermatogonia** follows a similar schema in other domestic species, with variations in the number and nomenclature of the individual divisions.

Spermatogonium: Spermatogonia vary in their structure and in their location within the wall of the seminiferous tubule.

A-spermatogonia (diameter 13 μm) are closely associated with the tubular basement membrane and are present at all stages of the seminiferous epithelial cycle (Figures 13.4 and 13.5). These stem cells are spherical and have an ellipsoid, euchromatic nucleus that may contain several nucleoli. The cytoplasm is rich in organelles. **I-spermatogonia** (intermediate spermatogonia) have a smaller, denser nucleus in which the chromatin is more clumped. **B-spermatogonia** are not in contact with the basement membrane. These pear-shaped cells have a heterochromatic nucleus with usually only one nucleolus.

At the end of telophase, spermatogonia undergo incomplete division, leaving cytoplasmic connections between daughter cells. These bridges facilitate exchange of substances between cells and aid in coordinating subsequent steps in the process of cell division. The cytoplasmic connections are only lost towards the end of spermiogenesis, shortly before delivery of spermatozoa into the tubular lumen.

Primary spermatocyte (spermatocytus primarius): Having arisen from the mitotic division of B_2-spermatogonia, primary spermatocytes (Figures 13.4 to 13.6) pass through all stages of meiotic prophase: leptotene, zygotene, pachytene, diplotene and diakinesis. Exchange of paternal and maternal genetic material occurs during this process. This initial phase of meiosis I lasts around 20 days, with the subsequent phases (metaphase, anaphase and telophase) progressing more quickly. Consequently, primary spermatocytes are observed at all stages of the seminiferous epithelial cycle. During meiosis I (first maturation division), the spermatocytes migrate towards the tubular lumen and the volume of the cells gradually increases.

Primary spermatocytes are characterised by nuclei containing chromatin strands of varying density, a large Golgi apparatus, abundant mitochondria and rough ER. They are diploid, the number of chromosomes varying with species (dog 78, cat 38, pig 38, sheep 54, horse, ox and goat 60). The amount of DNA is doubled through the formation of chromatid pairs. Meiosis I (reductional division) gives rise to two secondary spermatocytes, each containing half the original complement of chromosomes (haploid) and half the amount of DNA.

Secondary spermatocyte (spermatocytus secundarius): After a brief interkinetic period, a second maturation division occurs in which secondary spermatocytes are transformed into spermatids. This equatorial division is not preceded by doubling of the DNA, thus the resulting cells are haploid and contain half the amount of DNA of the secondary spermatocyte. As secondary spermatocytes divide almost immediately, they are rarely encountered in histological sections.

Secondary spermatocytes lie near the tubular lumen. They are around 16 μm in diameter and have a spherical, weakly staining nucleus.

Spermiogenesis

During spermiogenesis, **spermatids** undergo conspicuous changes through which they are transformed into **spermatozoa** (Figures 13.4 to 13.7). These modifications occur gradually and mainly involve the nucleus, Golgi apparatus and the centrioles. Spermiogenesis is accompanied by constant exchange of materials between the germ cells and the adjacent sustentacular cells. During this process, the sustentacular cells surround and stabilise the heads of the spermatids while the spermatid tails form a sheaf-like projection beyond the cytoplasm of the sustentacular cells into the tubular lumen.

Spermatid (spermatidium): Spermatids (Figures 13.4 to 13.7) are formed by meiotic division of secondary spermatocytes. They are smaller than spermatocytes. Spermatids are haploid, and the DNA content of the secondary spermatocytes is reduced by half (see also Chapter 1, 'The Cell', 'Meiosis'). Spermatids are initially located near the lumen of the tubule. During spermiogenesis, spermatids undergo a centrifugal–centripetal migration that takes them towards the basement membrane and then back in the direction of the lumen. Maturation processes occurring in the spermatid nucleus and cytoplasm (Figure 13.7) can be divided into the:

- Golgi phase,
- cap phase,
- acrosomal phase and
- maturation phase.

In the **Golgi phase** numerous small vesicles develop in the Golgi apparatus. The vesicles contain dense granules rich in glycoprotein (**pro-acrosomal granules**). Eventually the vesicles merge to form a single **acrosomal vesicle** containing a dense **acrosomal granule**. The acrosomal vesicle translocates to the nucleus and contacts the outer nuclear membrane. This establishes a cellular polarity upon which further differentiation is based. The acrosomal vesicle increases in size and becomes flattened.

During the **cap phase**, the acrosomal vesicle becomes moulded around the nucleus, covering more than half of its proximal aspect. The acrosomal vesicle becomes the **acrosomal (head) cap** with an **inner** and **outer**

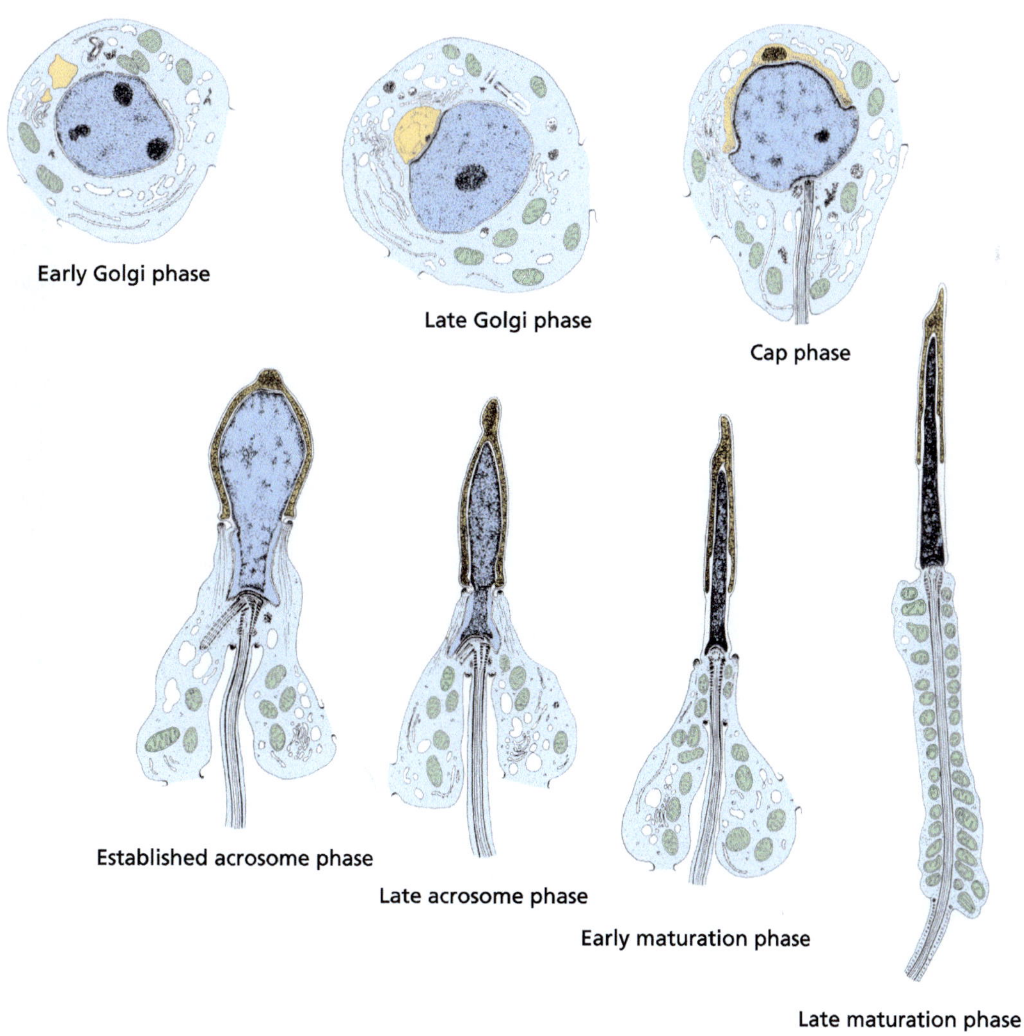

13.7 Developmental phases of spermatids during spermatogenesis in the bull (schematic).

acrosomal membrane. The space between the inner acrosomal membrane and the outer nuclear membrane is the **subacrosomal space**. Beneath the acrosomal cap, the chromatin increases in density. The bulk of the cytoplasm, including the organelles, becomes displaced to the distal aspect of the spermatid nucleus. The diplosome (centriole pair) lies at the distal pole of the nucleus. The **proximal centriole** is in contact with the nuclear membrane at the site of the **implantation fossa**.

During the **acrosomal phase** the nucleus gradually becomes **anterio-posteriorly elongated**, **flattened** and **condensed**. The space between the inner and outer acrosomal membranes is filled completely with glycoprotein-rich material. The acrosomal cap becomes the definitive **acrosome** (see below).

By this stage the spermatid has an elongated appearance. The cytoplasm is in the distal portion of the cell. A transient structure, the **manchette**, forms in the post-acrosomal segment of the nucleus. The manchette arises from a perinuclear ring and ends in the cytoplasm. Composed of microtubules, the manchette influences the final shape of the nucleus and serves as part of the cytoskeleton.

In the neck region of the spermatid, a **flagellum** develops from the distal centriole. The axonemal complex consists of nine outer microtubule doublets and a single central microtubule pair. The future **annulus** (Figure 13.8) begins to form near the proximal centriole.

In the **maturation phase**, **condensation of the nucleus** is completed. The nucleus reaches its final length of 5–10 μm. The **acrosome** (ca. 100 nm thick) is closely associated with the nuclear membrane. The acrosome covers two-thirds of the nucleus and the manchette has receded. The **annulus** is displaced distally, accompanied by mitochondria. The flagellum is fully formed. The **mitochondria**, components of the future **middle piece**, are arranged **helically around the flagellum**. Distal to the mitochondrial covering, the axoneme is surrounded by outer fibres and a fibrous sheath (future **principal piece**). Once the sperm tail has differentiated, the cytoplasm is pinched off and the resulting **residual body** is phagocytosed by sustentacular cells.

Spermatozoon: The spermatozoon (Figures 13.8 to 13.10) is the end-product of spermiogenesis. It is fully differentiated in a morphological sense but is not yet capable of fertilisation. Maturation continues during its passage through the epididymis.

The spermatozoon is composed of the:

- head (caput) and
- tail (flagellum) – neck, middle piece, principal piece and end piece.

The shape and length (60–75 μm) of the spermatozoon varies with species (Figure 13.8).

The **head of the spermatozoon**, the **caput** (Figure 13.8), is composed largely of the **nucleus** and overlying **acrosomal cap**. This portion of the head is continued distally by the **equatorial segment** and the **post-acrosomal region**. The shape of the head varies with species and is determined by the nucleus. Generally, the head is oval when viewed on its flattened surface and pear-shaped in

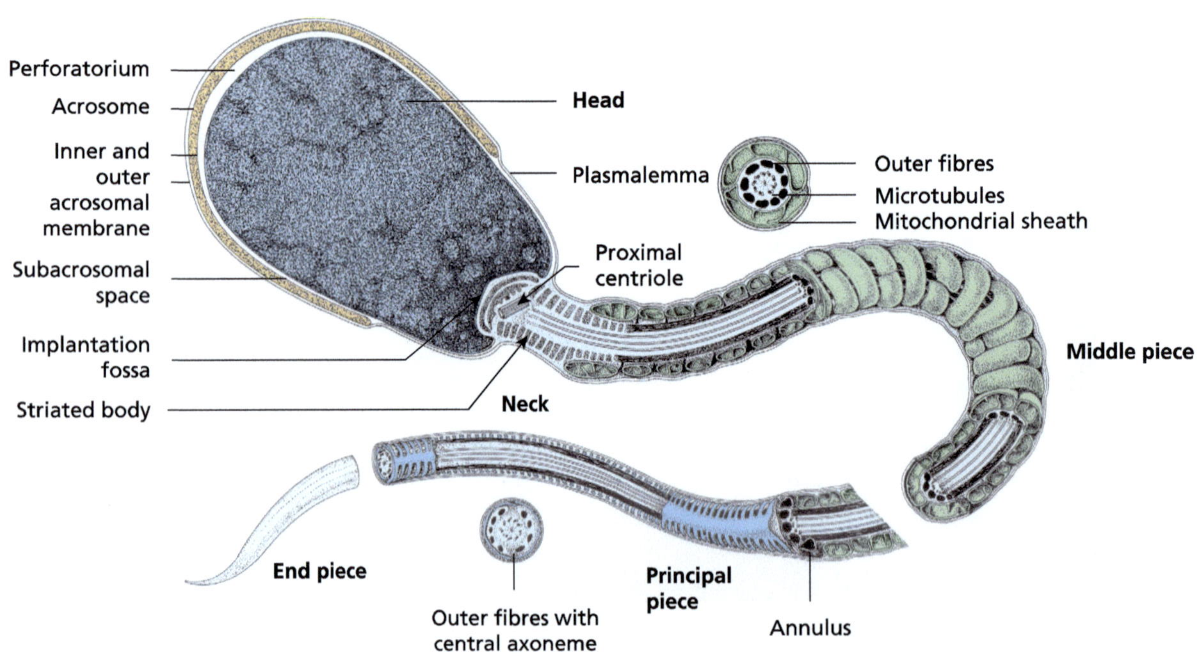

13.8 Schematic representation of the structure of the spermatozoon in the bull.

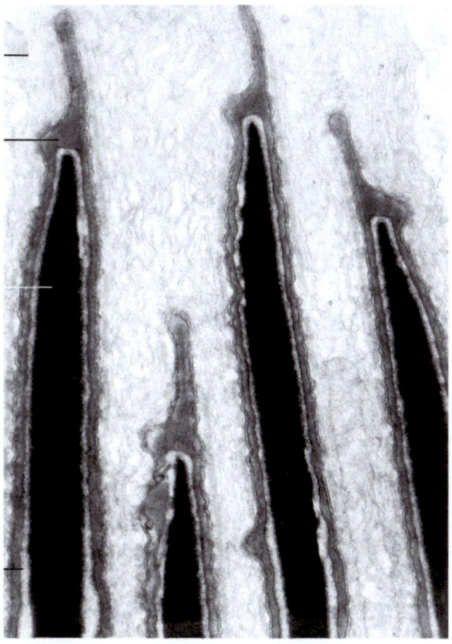

13.9 Heads of spermatozoa in the maturation phase of spermiogenesis (bull; x6000).

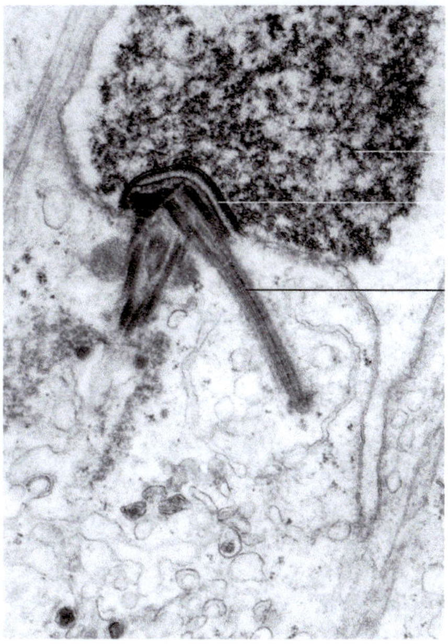

13.10 Anlage of the neck of the tail of a spermatozoon (bull; x11,000).

profile. It is 2–3 μm thick and 5–10 μm long. Most of the nuclear chromatin is strongly **condensed**.

The acrosome covers approximately two-thirds of the nucleus and contains **hydrolytic enzymes**, **hyaluronidase**, **neuraminidase** and **acrosin**. These enzymes are required for penetration by the spermatozoon of the corona radiata and zona pellucida of the oocyte (see Chapter 14, 'Female reproductive system') and are thus essential for fertilisation. In the bull, the proximal portion of the acrosome is elongated (Figure 13.9), forming the **acrosomal process** (0.5 μm in length). This is separated from the tip of the nucleus by the **perforatium**. An invagination at the distal end of the nucleus forms the **implantation fossa** (Figure 13.8).

Non-viable spermatozoon heads stain with eosin, methylene blue and bromophenol blue. Staining properties are used in evaluating the quality of ejaculate.

The **tail** of the spermatozoon consists of a neck, middle piece, principal piece and end piece.

The **neck** (**pars conjungens**) is the articulation between the head and the distal segments of the spermatozoon (Figure 13.8). Forming the proximal portion of the flagellum, the neck is composed of a **capitulum** connected by a **basal plate** to the implantation fossa. The capitulum continues distally as the **striated body** (columna striata) that merges with the **outer dense fibres** (fibrae densae externae) of the middle piece.

The proximal centriole and remnants of the distal centriole are incorporated into these structures. The **axoneme** (filamentum axiale) begins at the centre of the neck.

The axoneme extends through the central axis of the **middle piece** (**pars intermedia**). It has a typical flagellar structure consisting of a central tubule pair surrounded by nine tubule doublets (Figure 13.8). The outer tubules are surrounded by **dense outer fibres** (fibrae densae externae), which are covered by a **mitochondrial sheath** (vagina mitochondrialis). The mitochondria are arranged in spirals. Energy provided by the mitochondria serves to propel the spermatozoa. The mitochondria end at the **annulus**, the distal limit of the middle piece. The middle piece is 5–7 μm in length.

Measuring 50 μm, the **principal piece** (**pars principalis**) is the longest segment of the tail (Figure 13.8). The axoneme continues through the principal piece, the **outer fibres** decreasing towards its distal end. Beneath the plasmalemma, two semicircular elements composed of fibrillar structural proteins form a **peripheral fibrous sheath** (vagina fibrosa). The distal end of the fibrous sheath marks the beginning of the end piece.

The **end piece** (**pars terminalis**) is 5–7 μm long and contains only the microtubule complex. The ordered microtubular structure is lost distally, with plasmalemma surrounding the free ends of the tubules.

Cyclic events of spermatogenesis

Spermatogenesis is characterised by strict regulation and chronological synchronisation of the processes of division and differentiation. Each new generation of cells appears more or less concurrently and undergoes synchronous development. Descendants of a single spermatogonium are referred to as a **phase**. The term **stage** (= **cell association**) describes a particular combination of cell populations, as observed within a histological section of the tubule. Regions of the tubule occupied by a given stage of germ cells are referred to as **segments**. The sum of all segments along the length of the tubule constitutes a **spermatogenic wave**.

Characteristic cell associations arise from generations of cells in different states of differentiation. The **cycle of the seminiferous epithelium** consists of the recurring sequences of cellular associations at a particular point in the tubule.

Based on morphological criteria, the number of stages of the seminiferous epithelial cycle is not necessarily fixed (8–16 in the bull, 8 in the ram, 6–8 in the boar and 8 in the stallion).

Generally, only one stage of the cycle is visible in a histological cross-section of the tubule (Figures 13.4 to 13.6). Except for some irregularities, segments are generally arranged so that they follow the next most developed stage of the cycle.

The **duration of spermatogenesis** is approximately 49 days in the stallion, 52 days in the bull, 52 days in the ram and 34 days in the boar. Final maturation of spermatozoa takes place in the epididymis.

SUSTENTACULAR CELLS (SERTOLI CELLS, EPITHELIOCYTI SUSTENTANTES)

In addition to germ cells, the spermatogenic epithelium contains somatic cells referred to as sustentacular cells or, after their discoverer Enrico Sertoli (1842–1910), as Sertoli cells.

In adult, sexually active mammals, **columnar** sustentacular cells (70–80 µm high) extend from the basement membrane to the tubular lumen. They are pyramidal in shape, tapering towards the lumen from a broad base resting on the basement membrane. Sustentacular cells lie between the differentiating germ cells with which they are in structural and functional contact through specialised intercellular connections (Figures 13.11 to 13.13).

The ovoid to ellipsoid **nucleus** is euchromatic and is typically located basally. Under seasonal influences, or during sexual quiescence, the nucleus may become displaced towards the lumen. Migration of the nucleus also occurs during certain stages of the seminiferous epithelial cycle. The nucleolus is reticulated (net-like). In ruminants, the nucleoli are also characteristically multivesicular.

Numerous thin, branching **cytoplasmic processes** extend from the lateral walls of the sustentacular cells to surround the various stages of spermatogenic cells. These contribute actively to trans-epithelial migration of germ cells and to release of spermatozoa into the tubular lumen (**spermiation**). The cytoplasm contains a well-developed Golgi apparatus, numerous mitochondria and, in pigs and ruminants, abundant rough ER. The **smooth ER** is well developed in all species. Particularly in ruminants, pigs and

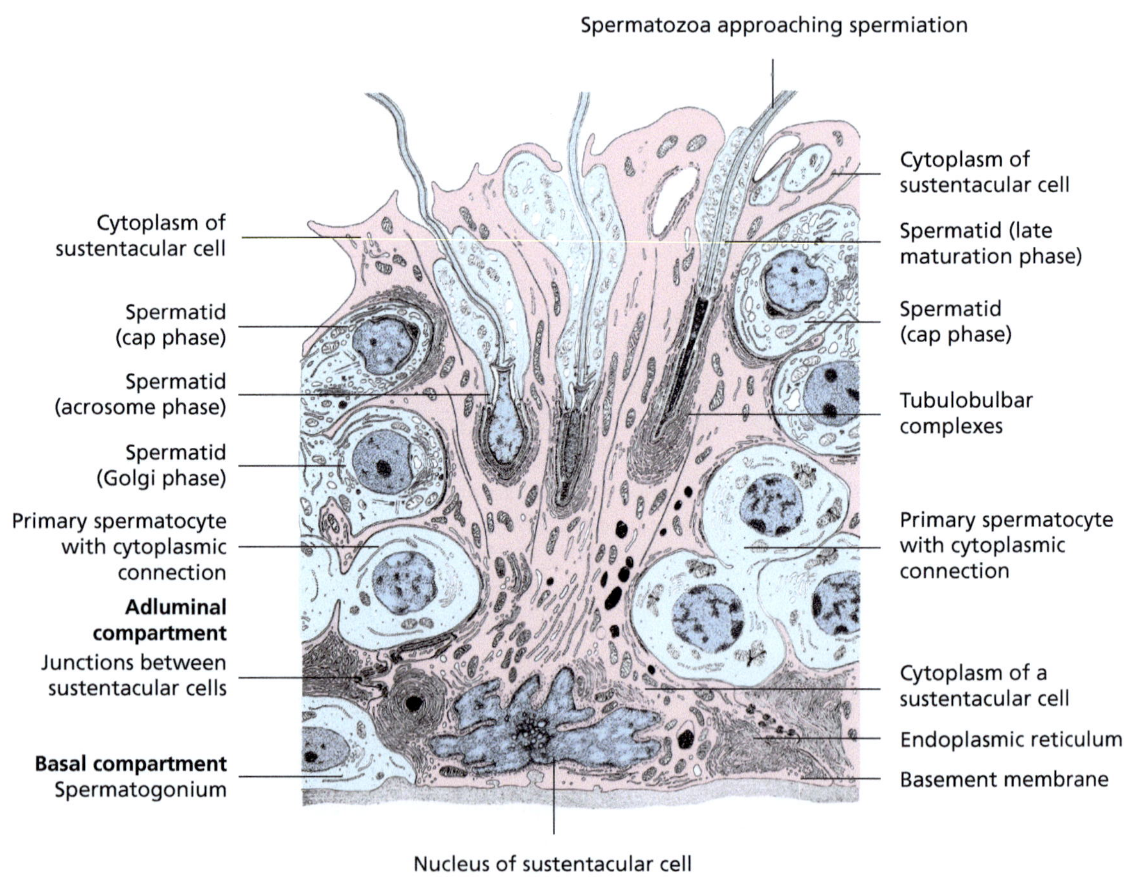

13.11 Sustentacular cell and various stages of spermatogenesis (schematic; based on the bull).

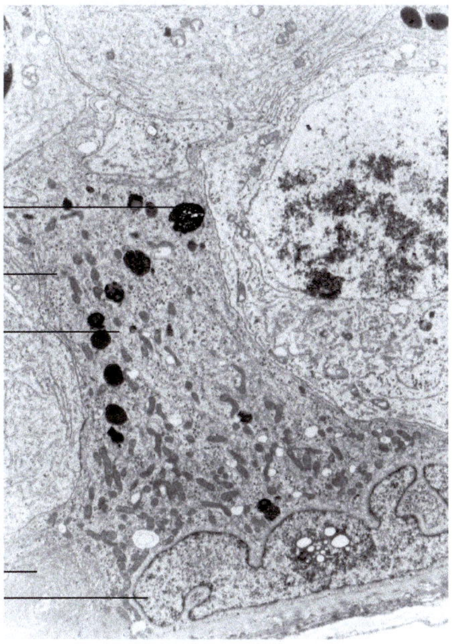

13.12 Fine structure of the basal region of a seminiferous tubule with sustentacular cell and adjacent spermatogonia (bull; x3500).

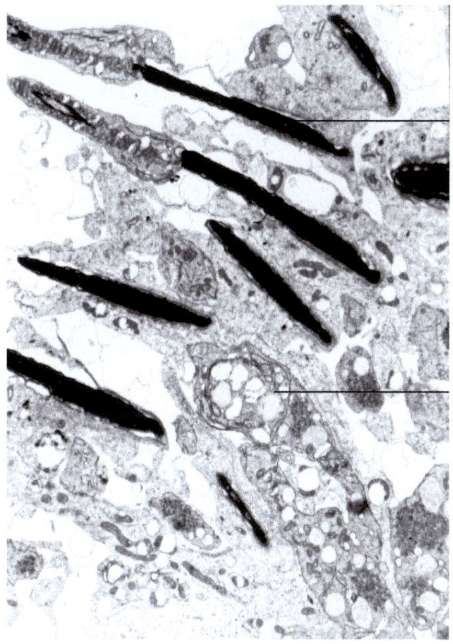

13.13 Fine structure of apical zone of a seminiferous tubule during spermiation (bull; x4000).

dogs, dense stacks of cisternae of smooth ER are observed in close contact with lysosomes and lipid vacuoles. In all domestic species, **stacks of smooth ER** surround the periacrosomal region of spermatids. This phenomenon may play a role in steroid metabolism or enzymatic digestion.

The basal cytoplasmic compartment contains **microbodies**, **membrane aggregates** and **lamellar inclusion bodies**. These organelles are active in resorptive and digestive cell processes. In boars, spindle- or needle-shaped crystals (Charcot–Böttcher crystals) are also present.

Numerous **fat vacuoles** occupy the base of the cell. Their size and number vary considerably with species. **Microtubules** and **microfilaments** contribute to intracellular transport processes and regulate the release of spermatozoa into the tubular lumen (**spermiation**).

Sustentacular cells are brought into close contact with one another by **numerous intercellular junctions**. Basolaterally, tight junctions and desmosomes almost completely divide the space between adjacent sustentacular cells into **basal** and **adluminal compartments** (see below). Also present are gap junctions and, between sustentacular cells and spermatids, tubulobulbar complexes.

FUNCTIONS OF SUSTENTACULAR CELLS

Sustentacular cells contribute in several ways to the multiplication and differentiation of germ cells. These include:

- structural support and nutrition,
- phagocytosis,
- synthesis and secretion of proteins,
- facilitation of intra-epithelial migration of germ cells and release of spermatozoa into the tubular lumen (spermiation),
- secretion of intratubular fluid contents and
- formation of the 'blood–testis barrier'.

Support and nutrition: Aided by an abundance of intercellular connections, sustentacular cells provide mechanical support by acting as a scaffold for the spermatogenic cells in the wall of the seminiferous tubule. Extensive interconnection between sustentacular cells and germ cells facilitates transcellular exchange of substances including nutrients.

Phagocytosis: The testis contains numerous phagocytic cells. Degenerating germ cells are phagocytosed by epithelial cells of the straight testicular tubules and rete testis, and by sustentacular cells. Following spermiation, cytoplasmic remnants of spermatids are broken down by lysosomes within sustentacular cells.

Protein synthesis and secretion: Sustentacular cells synthesise androgen-binding protein with a high binding affinity for testosterone and dihydrotestosterone. This acts as a carrier for delivering androgens to the germ cells and into the epididymis. Sustentacular cells also produce a 'transferrin-like protein', a plasminogen activator (for increasing the motility of germ cells) and inhibin (negative feedback mechanism for regulation of FSH secretion) (for further information refer to endocrinology texts).

Facilitation of germ cell migration and release of spermatozoa: As spermatogenic cells are not capable of independent movement, they rely on sustentacular cells to manipulate them. This is initiated by the establishment of firm connections between sustentacular cells and germ cells. Cytoplasmic streaming results in the direction of spermatocytes towards the tubular lumen. Release of spermatozoa into the tubular lumen (**spermiation**) is a complex process that commences with dissolution of the **tubulobulbar complexes** between the sustentacular cell and the head of the spermatozoon (Figure 13.13).

Secretion of tubular fluid components: Tubular fluid is produced in large quantities. Like intracellular fluid, it is rich in potassium. The tubular fluid carries spermatozoa through the ductuli efferentes into the ductus epididymidis (epididymal duct), where they complete their maturation.

Formation of the blood–testis barrier: The blood–testis barrier separates the **circulatory system** (**blood and lymph**) and the interior of the **convoluted seminiferous tubules**. While in common usage, the term 'blood–testis barrier' is misleading. It consists of the tight seal formed between the plasmalemma of neighbouring sustentacular cells by basolateral **intercellular junctions**. This gives rise to two compartments **within the tubular epithelium**:

- a basal compartment containing spermatogonia and
- an adluminal compartment containing spermatocytes and spermatids (Figure 13.11).

In the **adluminal compartment**, the sustentacular cells provide protection for the spermatocytes and spermatids. Maintenance of the barrier is important for the secretory functions of the sustentacular cells, through which an osmotic gradient is established in the luminal region, and for maintenance of an optimal environment for spermiogenesis. The vulnerable spermatids are protected from autoimmune reactions, toxins and mutagens.

Straight testicular tubules (tubuli seminiferi recti)

The convoluted seminiferous tubules are continued by short, straight testicular tubules (tubuli seminiferi recti) which open into the rete testis. The straight testicular tubules are usually short, though some are elongated in the boar and stallion. In the dog and bull, groups of sustentacular cells form a club-shaped intraluminal projection at the transition from the convoluted to the straight tubules (terminal segment). These contribute to phagocytosis and prevent retrograde flow of tubular fluid.

The straight testicular tubules are lined with simple cuboidal to columnar resorptive epithelium containing lymphocytes and macrophages.

Rete testis

The rete testis consists of anastomosing straight tubules. These are surrounded by the loose connective tissue and elastic meshwork of the mediastinum testis, and by myofibroblasts (Figures 13.3 and 13.14). The epithelium of the rete testis is simple squamous to columnar. Two epithelial layers are present in the bull. The epithelium is **highly secretory** and increases the volume of the tubular fluid. **Androgens** in the **tubular fluid** are absorbed across the epithelium to a limited extent.

Ductuli efferentes testis

At the extremitas capitata of the testis, the **ductuli efferenties testis** penetrate the tunica albuginea and pass into the head of the epididymis (Figures 13–2 and 13–3 to 13–16). A species-dependent number of ductuli efferentes (stallion 12–23, bull 12–13, boar 14–21, dog 15–16) combines

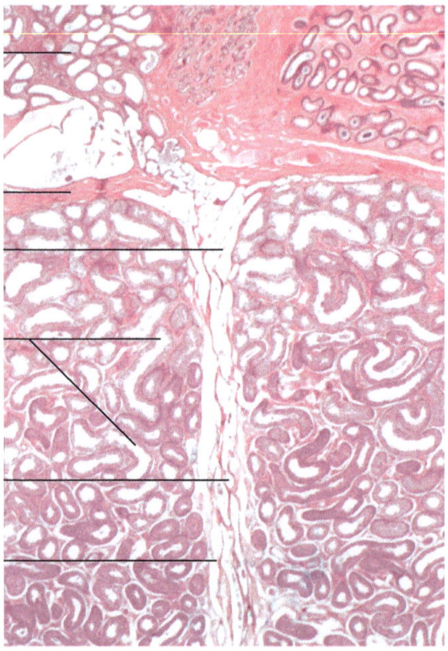

13.14 Testis (bull). Haematoxylin and eosin stain (x30).

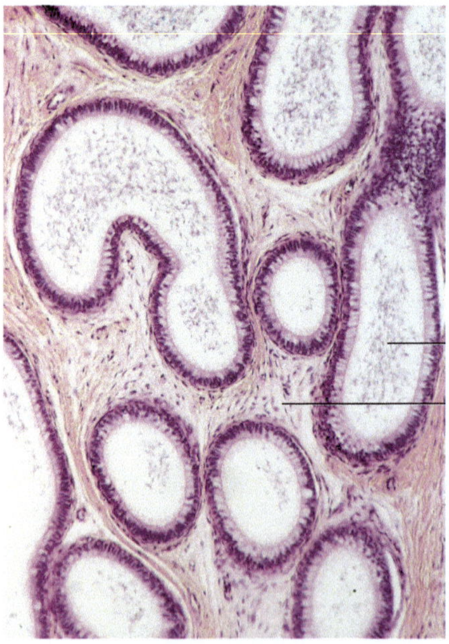

13.15 Ductuli efferentes of the epididymis (stallion). The lumen contains agglutinated spermatozoa. Haematoxylin and eosin stain (x100).

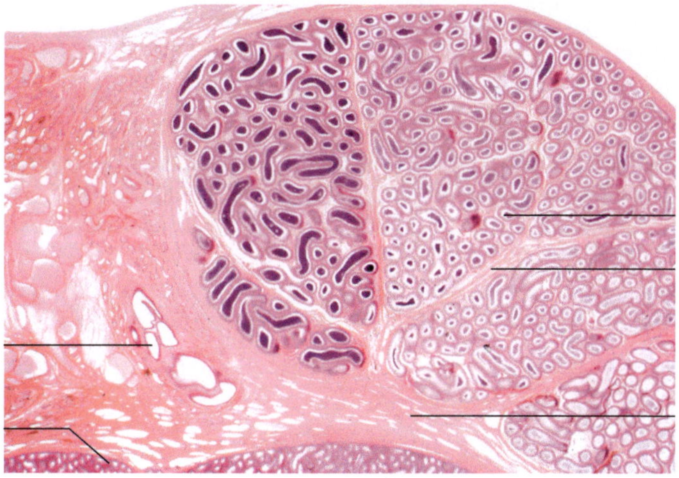

13.16 Low-power view of the head of the epididymis and partial section of the testis (bull). Haematoxylin and eosin stain (x14).

to form the **epididymal duct** (ductus epididymidis; see below). The ductuli efferentes are derived embryologically from the mesonephric tubules. Ductuli efferentes that do not merge into the epididymal duct have blind ends and are referred to as **ductuli aberrantes**.

The ductuli efferentes follow a meandering path within lobules (lobuli epididymidis). They are enclosed within a dense capillary network. In the bull, the ductuli efferentes reach 50–80 cm in length. Three to six thin layers of modified, predominantly circularly oriented, smooth muscle cells (**stratum fibromusculare**) surround the ductular epithelium.

The ductuli efferentes are lined by pseudostratified epithelium. Some of the superficial cells have **cilia** that assist in transporting sperm and tubular fluid towards the epididymal duct. A population of flatter cells (**principal cells**) is characterised by **microvilli**, numerous pinocytotic vesicles and invaginations, endosomes and a well-developed Golgi apparatus. These inclusions and organelles are engaged in the extensive trans-epithelial absorption of tubular fluid. Resorptive activity is indicated morphologically by the appearance of intracellular residual bodies (PAS-positive inclusions). Lymphocytes and macrophages are sometimes seen in the epithelium.

The **ductuli efferentes** have several functions. As well as absorbing ductular fluid, they synthesise nutrients for the spermatozoa. Transport of spermatozoa is promoted by cilia. Spermatozoa taken up from the lumen are phagocytosed.

Testis of birds

The surface of the internally located testis is covered by a layer of serosa (**peritoneum**). The underlying **tunica albuginea** is relatively thin. In the chicken, it contains muscle cells that confer a limited degree of contractility. At the beginning of the breeding season, the tunica albuginea undergoes marked fibrogenesis. Consequently, the tunica appears temporarily to consist of two layers. The tunica albuginea gives off delicate bundles of connective tissue. Clear septa are not formed and there is no **mediastinum testis**.

The **convoluted seminiferous tubules** follow a tortuous course within the loose interstitial connective tissue. They anastomose extensively. During the breeding season the tubules increase in length, in proportion with the increase in size of the testes, up to a total of 250 m in chickens. The intertubular connective tissue contains androstenone-producing **Leydig cells** and **melanocytes**.

The wall of the seminiferous tubules is composed of a membrana propria and spermatogenic epithelium. The **membrana propria** consists of a basal membrane and loose connective tissue incorporating delicate bundles of elastic fibres and numerous contractile cells. This tissue layer forms a structural component of the **blood–testis barrier**. In juvenile and sexually quiescent adult males, the spermatogenic epithelium consists of a single layer of cells, in which the spermatogenic cells and sustentacular cells are in contact with the basal membrane.

In the chicken, the spermatogenic and sustentacular cells become more numerous from the fifth week post-hatching and the epithelial layer increases in height. With the onset of **sexual maturity**, at about 16–24/26 weeks in the cock, the epithelium becomes stratified. This is associated with the mitotic division of spermatogonia and formation of spermatozoa (similar to mammals) (Figures 13.17 and 13.18). The **duration of spermatogenesis**, up to delivery of spermatozoa into the lumen of the convoluted seminiferous tubule, is usually no more than 12 days in the cock.

The short **tubuli seminiferi recti** are lined by cuboidal epithelium (cock). The straight tubules open into the irregularly dilated **rete testis**. In birds, the rete testis is located on the medial aspect of the testis and is divided into **intra-testicular**, **intra-capsular** and **extra-capsular**

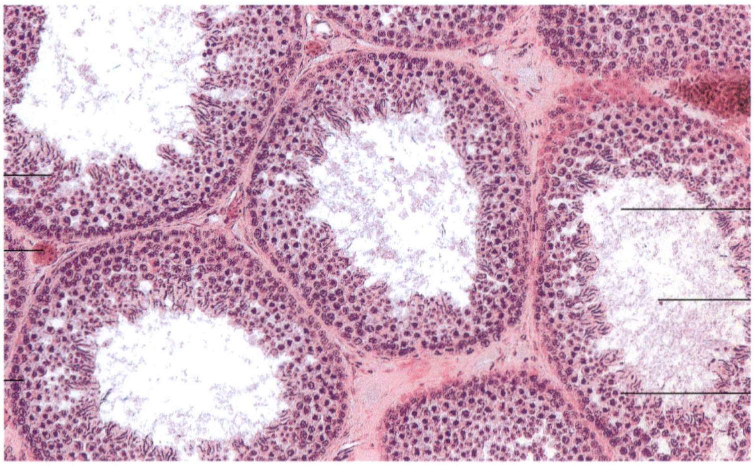

13.17 Testis (cock). Haematoxylin and eosin stain (x120).

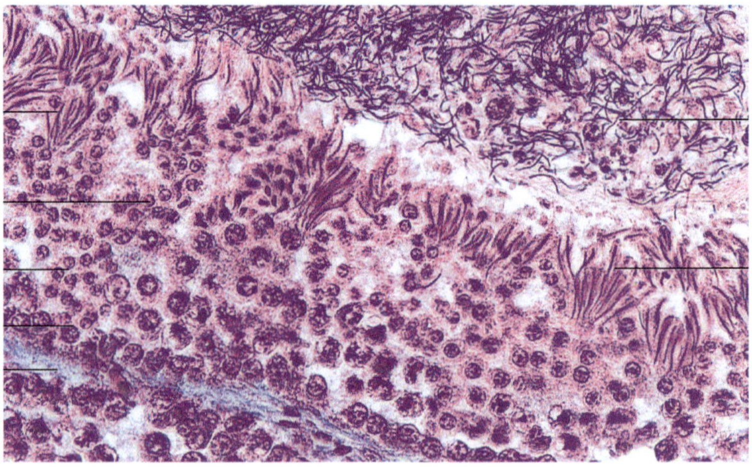

13.18 Testis (cock). Haematoxylin and eosin stain (x440).

components. The last of these opens into the **ductuli efferentes proximales** from which sperm are conducted into the epididymis.

Epididymis

The epididymis is firmly attached to the testis at the margo epididymalis. It has three macroscopically distinguishable components: the **head** (caput), **body** (corpus) and the **tail** (cauda).

The head of the epididymis (Figure 13.16) contains the ductuli efferentes testis and the initial segment of the ductus epididymidis (refer to *Veterinary Anatomy of Domestic Mammals: Textbook and Colour Atlas* for more information).

Epididymal duct (ductus epididymidis)

The epididymal duct is formed from the convergence of the ductuli efferentes testis. It is tremendously tortuous and varies considerably in length (stallion 72–81 m, bull 40–50 m, boar 17–18 m, dog 5–8 m). Despite this, the time taken for transport of spermatozoa through the duct is 10–15 days in all mammals.

Based on its morphological features, the ductus epididymidis can be divided into **segments** (1–6 in the bull and ram), each with distinctive functions. Segments 1–3 lie in the head of the epididymis, segments 4 and 5 are in the body and segment 6 is found in the tail.

The epithelium of the epididymal duct is **pseudostratified columnar** (**epithelium pseudostratificatum columnare**). Distally the height of the epithelium decreases. The epithelium is surrounded by **smooth muscle** which becomes distinctly thicker in the tail. Adjacent segments of the duct wall are connected by loose connective tissue containing macrophages, leucocytes and abundant vessels and nerves. The density of capillary bundles increases markedly in the tail.

The functions of the ductus epididymis include:

- maturation and storage of spermatozoa, and delivery of spermatozoa into the ductus deferens,
- absorption of fluid and
- secretion of metabolically active substances.

Particularly in segment 1 of the epididymal duct, proteins are released by the apocrine mode for maturation of spermatozoa. In segment 6, the environment facilitates survival of spermatozoa prior to ejaculation.

The **epithelium of the epididymal duct** contains principal and basal cells. **Principal cells** have an ovoid, heterochromatic nucleus. The cytoplasm is rich in metabolically active organelles, lysosomes and pinocytotic vesicles. The free surface is covered with **stereocilia** that are sometimes clumped together in bushels. Stereocilia **secrete enzymes** and **glycoproteins**, including phosphatases and glycosidases.

The apical cytoplasm contains pinocytotic invaginations and numerous multivesicular bodies, signifying a high capacity for **resorption of fluid**. Ninety percent of the luminal fluid is absorbed in the ductuli efferentes and the initial portion of the epididymal duct. Androgen-binding proteins and inhibin are also reabsorbed in the proximal part of the duct.

Polygonal **basal cells** have a small spherical nucleus. Their cytoplasm contains numerous fat vacuoles and few organelles. Basal cells are active in substance exchange. Intra-epithelial lymphocytes and macrophages are also present (Figures 13.19 and 13.20).

Maturation of spermatozoa is completed in the head and body of the epididymis. The tail is primarily a site of storage. In the epididymal duct, the spermatozoa acquire their **capacity for progressive motility** and their meta-

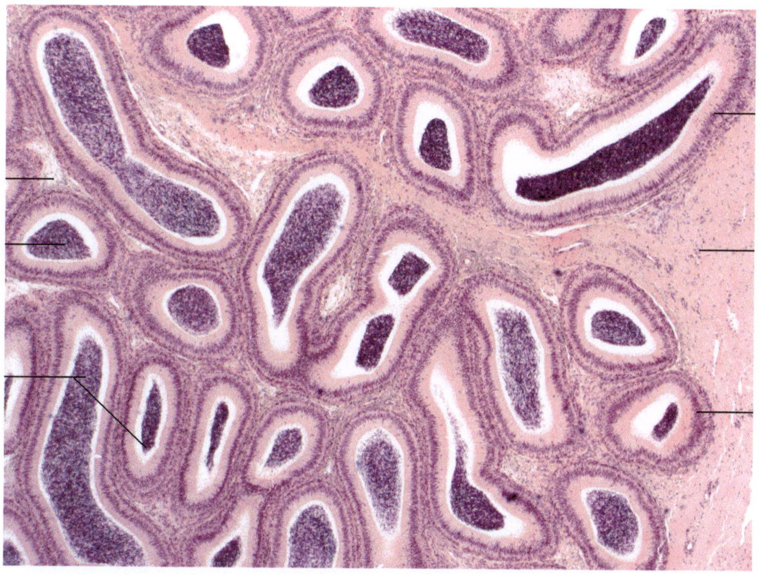

13.19 Ductus epididymidis (bull). Haematoxylin and eosin stain (x35).

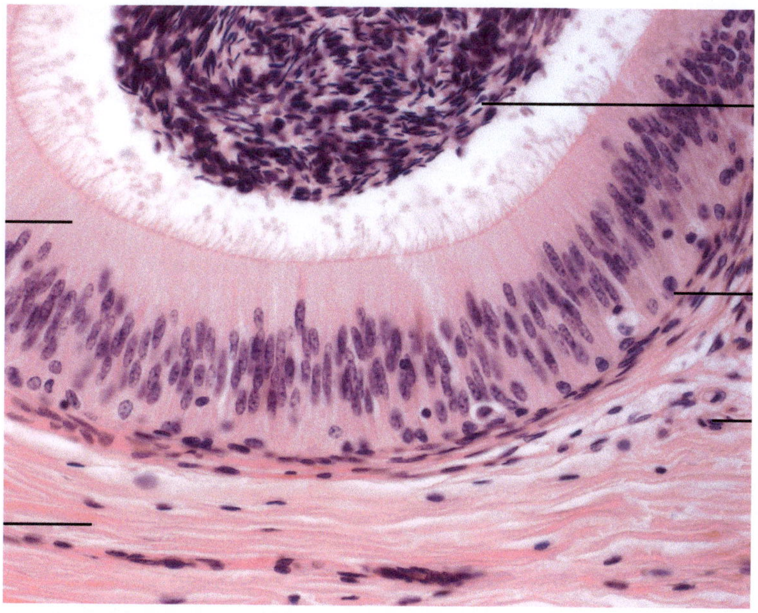

13.20 Ductus epididymidis (cross-section; bull). Haematoxylin and eosin stain (x275).

bolic activity changes. While they remain in the epididymal duct, however, motility of the spermatozoa is **limited** by the acid environment. Changes also occur on the surface of the cell membrane and there is an increase in negative charge. The localisation of **glycoprotein receptors** in the **post-acrosomal region** is important for facilitating contact between spermatozoa and the zona pellucida of the oocyte.

Towards the end of the maturation process, the spermatozoon loses the cytoplasmic droplet (remnant of spermiogenesis). Failure of this process renders spermatozoa infertile. Mature spermatozoa are subsequently stored for some time in the tail of the epididymis.

Pampiniform plexus

Through its histological structure, and its anatomical association with the loops of the testicular artery, the pampiniform plexus serves primarily to facilitate **heat exchange**. These features also promote the **diffusion** of gases, low-molecular weight substances, adrenalin, noradrenalin, serotonin and lipid-soluble substances such as prostaglandins and steroid hormones.

Anastomoses between the larger veins of the plexus markedly reduce the **rate of blood flow**. This vasoregulatory mechanism is augmented by adventitial and intramural portal systems in the centre of the plexus.

Epididymis of birds

The **epididymis of the chicken** lies against the dorsomedial surface of the testis. It extends along approximately two-thirds of the testicular border. Unlike the mammalian epididymis, which consists of a head, body and tail, the epididymis of birds has **no subdivisions**. **Ductuli efferentes** emerging from the testis enter the epididymis along its entire length. The epithelium of the ductules is simple columnar. The proximal efferent ductules narrow to form **distal efferent ductules** (ductuli efferentes distales) (approximately 70 in the cock). These empty via **connecting ductules** (ductuli conjugentes) into the **epididymal duct**.

The **epididymal duct** (**ductus epididymidis**) is lined by pseudostratified epithelium with stereocilia. It is surrounded by loose connective tissue invested with smooth muscle cells (Figures 13.21 and 13.22). Throughout its course, the epididymal duct gradually increases in thickness. At the caudal pole of the epididymis it opens into the deferent duct.

Ductus deferens

The ductus deferens extends from the epididymal duct to the pelvic urethra. The gently coiled initial portion lies on the medial side of the testis. From the testis, the ductus deferens passes within the spermatic cord (**funiculus spermaticus**), together with the testicular artery and vein, lymphatic vessels and sympathetic nerves. In the pelvic cavity, the left and right deferent ducts pass into the plica urogenitalis. The section within this fold comprises the **pars glandularis of the ductus deferens**. In the stallion, bull and dog, this portion is expanded to form an **ampulla** (**ampulla ductus deferentis**) (see below).

> **Species variation**
>
> **Horse and ox**: Shortly before the urethra, the ductus deferens merges with the **ductus excretorius** of the vesicular glands to form the **ductus ejaculatorius**.

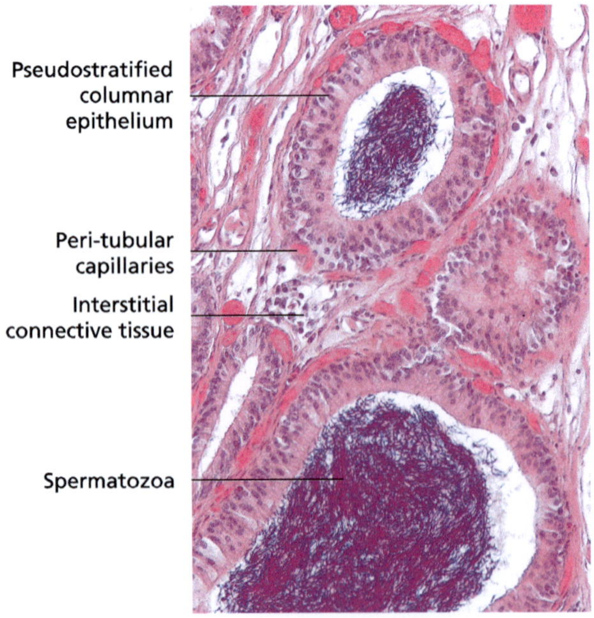

13.21 Ductus epididymidis (cock). Haematoxylin and eosin stain (x275).

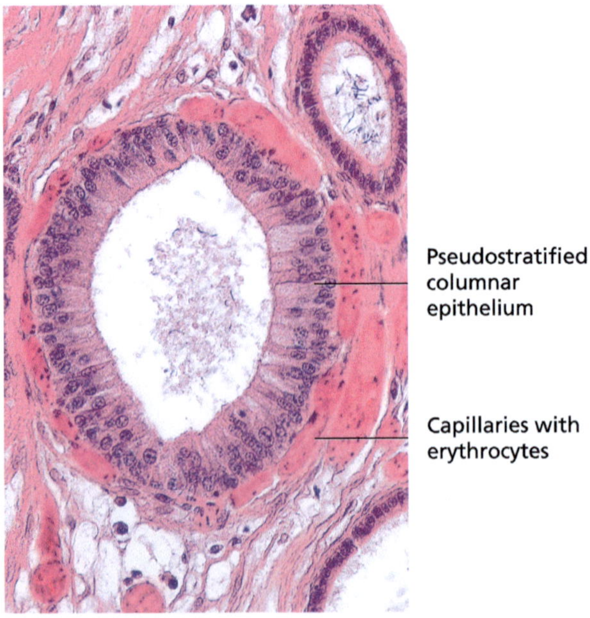

13.22 Ductus epididymidis (drake). Haematoxylin and eosin stain (x275).

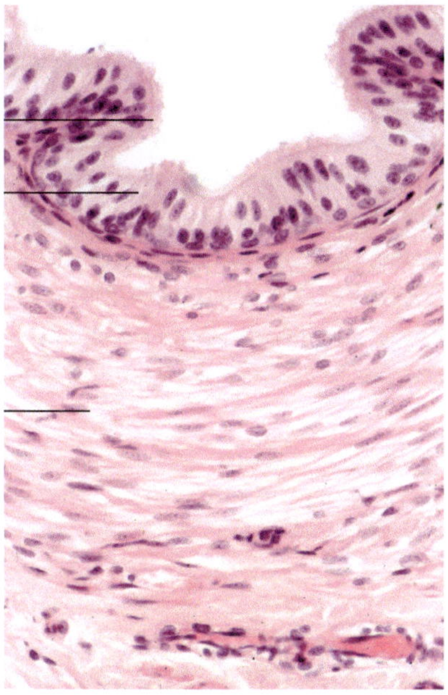

13.23 Ductus deferens with folded mucosa and circular smooth muscle layer (tomcat). Haematoxylin and eosin stain (x400).

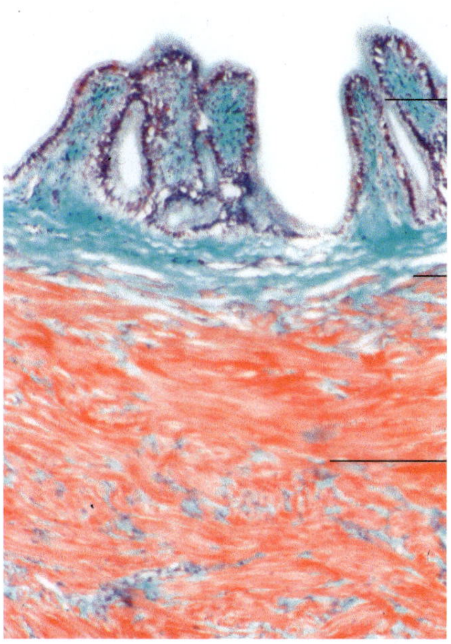

13.24 Distal segment of ductus deferens with deep longitudinal folds (bull). Goldner's Masson trichrome stain (x250).

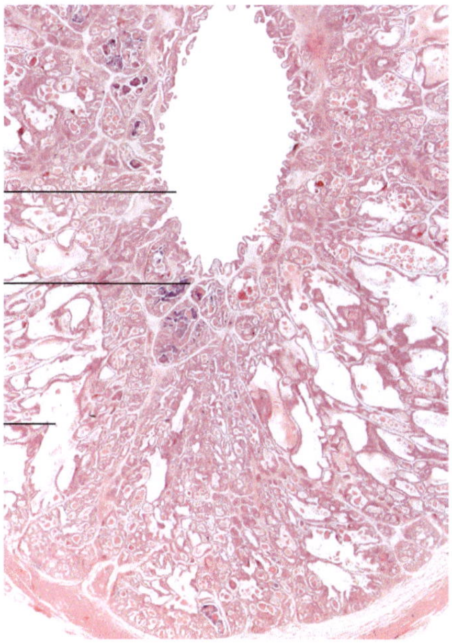

13.25 Ampulla of ductus deferens (bull). Haematoxylin and eosin stain (x20).

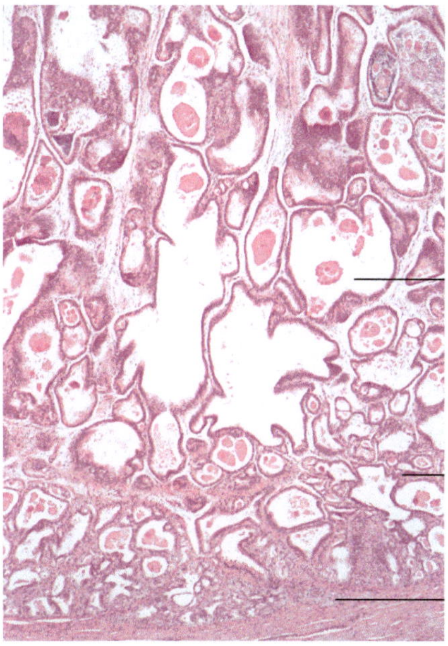

13.26 Ampulla of ductus deferens (bull). Haematoxylin and eosin stain (x40).

Pig: The ductus deferens and ductus excretorius open separately into the urethra.

Carnivores: The ductus deferens opens into the urethra independently as there are no vesicular glands.

The ductus deferens is composed of clearly discernible layers (Figures 13.23 to 13.26). The **mucosa** (**tunica mucosa**) has prominent **longitudinal folds** (**plicae mucosae**). Initially pseudostratified, the epithelium becomes simple columnar towards the end of the duct. Regions bearing short stereocilia may be seen on the epithelial surface. In the bull, the basal epithelial cells contain numerous lipid droplets.

A narrow **lamina propria** lies external to the mucosa. Up to the pars glandularis, the lamina propria is non-glandular and contains extensive networks of elastic fibres. The elastic fibres are contiguous externally with the smooth muscle of the thick **tunica muscularis**. In the stallion, bull and boar, muscle fibre bands of varying orientation (circular, oblique, longitudinal) are intermingled, whereas the tunica muscularis of the dog and tomcat consists mainly of inner circular and outer longitudinal layers.

The tunica muscularis is surrounded by a **tunica adventitia** or, within the peritoneal and pelvic cavities, a **tunica serosa**. The loose connective tissue of the tunica adventitia is extensively vascularised and rich in nerve plexuses.

Ductus deferens of birds

The ductus deferens of birds is lined by pseudostratified epithelium with few stereocilia and secretory cells. Near its opening into the cloaca, the ductus deferens straightens to become the pars recta ductus deferentis. This straight portion is continued by the ampulliform **receptaculum ductus deferentis**. This structure is not homologous with the ampulla ductus deferentis of mammals, as there are no secretory cells in its walls. The ductus deferens opens at the **ostium ductus deferentis**. The ostium is located on the conical **papilla ductus deferentis**, which projects into the lumen of the urodeum.

Within the wall of the urodeum, near the receptaculum, there is an **arterial network** (rete mirabile arteriosum) arising from the pudendal artery. This is referred to as the **vascular body of the phallus** (**corpus vasculare phalli**).

Accessory glands (glandulae genitales accessoriae)

The combined secretions of the accessory glands of the male reproductive system constitute the **seminal plasma**. Ejaculate is composed of seminal plasma and **spermatozoa**. The secretory activity of the accessory glands is controlled largely by the reproductive cycle, particularly in non-domesticated animals with seasonal breeding cycles.

The primary function of accessory glands is to produce serous or mucous secretions that nourish, transport and activate spermatozoa, and to protect spermatozoa by neutralising the acid urine. The **accessory glands** are comprised of the:

- terminal (glandular) portion of the deferent ducts,
- vesicular glands (glandula vesicularis),
- prostate gland (glandula prostatica) and
- bulbourethral glands (glandula bulbourethralis).

Species variation

Horse, ox and pig: All accessory glands are present in the stallion, bull and boar. The pars glandularis of the ductus deferens is ampulliform in the stallion and bull (see above) (Figures 13.25 and 13.26).

Carnivores: Vesicular glands are absent.

Dog: The pars glandularis of the ductus deferens is ampulliform. There are no bulbourethral glands.

Structural features of the accessory glands are summarised in Table 13.1.

Pars glandularis of the ductus deferens

The lamina propria of the glandular portion of the ductus deferens is densely packed with branched tubular glands. The end pieces may have vesicular expansions.

The **pseudostratified columnar glandular epithelium** varies in height depending on the degree of secretory activity. Release of the acidophilic secretion into the typically dilated glandular lumen is primarily by the **apocrine mode**. The adluminal region of the wall of the glandular portion of the ductus deferens may contain a mixture of seminal plasma and spermatozoa. Recent findings suggest that the ampulla of the ductus deferens may act as a storage area in which maturation processes occur at the cell membrane of the spermatozoa.

During ejaculation, the secretory product is released via dilated collecting ducts into the ductus ejaculatorius (stallion, bull) or the lumen of the ductus deferens (dog, boar). In the bull, lipid droplets may be present in the basal cells of the epithelium. The glands are divided into lobules by connective tissue septa containing numerous capillaries. In the stallion and bull, the septa are reinforced by thin slips of smooth muscle cells.

Vesicular glands (glandula vesicularis)

The paired vesicular glands are **compound tubulo-alveolar glands** lined by pseudostratified columnar epithelium (Figures 13.27 and 13.28). The columnar cells vary in density, depending on the functional state of the gland. Modified microvilli are present on the surface. The cells are rich in organelles associated with secretory activity (endoplasmic reticulum, Golgi apparatus, peroxisomes). Secretory product is released by the **apocrine mode**. The epithelium contains solitary small, dark basal cells. Within the glandular lobules, the tubular segments are expanded to form **reservoirs for glandular secretions**. These portions, and the main excretory ducts, are lined by simple **cuboidal epithelium**.

In the lamina propria, individual tubulo-alveolar units are interconnected by highly vascular loose connective tissue. Dense collagenous septa divide the glandular tissue into lobules of varying size. The glands are surrounded by a tunica muscularis composed of smooth muscle and a tunica adventitia.

The vesicular glands produce a white to yellowish gel-like secretion rich in **fructose** and **citric acid**. The alkaline conditions produced by the secretion promote the **motility of spermatozoa**, with fructose acting as an energy source. Inositol and ergothioneine have been detected in vesicular gland secretions in boars. There is also evidence that the vesicular glands synthesise prostaglandins.

The columnar epithelial cells are **highly active secretory cells**. In addition to glycogen, they contain **peroxisomes** and **lipid droplets**. Larger lipid droplets are seen in basal cells ('**dwarf cells**'). The lipid material consists of

Table 13.1 Structural features of the accessory glands of the male reproductive system of mammals.

Organ	Structure	Cells	Features
Pars glandularis of the ductus deferens	Simple branched, tubular glands in the lamina propria; ampulla (ampulla ductus deferentis) present in stallion, bull and dog, absent in tomcat and boar; smooth muscle in stallion and bull	Pseudostratified columnar epithelium with spherical basally located nuclei; apocrine mode of secretion; expanded glandular lumen	Acts as storage area where maturation processes occur at the surface membrane of spermatozoa; presence of basal cells containing coalesced fat droplets (bulls)
Vesicular gland (glandula vesicularis)	Compound tubulo-alveolar within lamina propria; tubular portions expanded into collecting ducts; collagenous connective tissue septa divide the gland into lobules	Pseudostratified columnar epithelium with organelles indicative of secretory activity; apocrine mode of secretion; fructose- and citric acid-rich secretory products promote motility of spermatozoa	Energy source for spermatozoa; stallion – markedly vesicular morphology and expanded excretory duct lined with cuboidal epithelium; bull – central excretory duct, lipid droplets and peroxisomes in secretory epithelium; high secretory activity
Prostate gland (glandula prostatica)	Compound tubulo-alveolar gland composed of two layers: an outer portion (corpus prostatae) and an inner portion (pars disseminata); the glandular tissue is divided into distinct lobules by connective tissue septa in the lamina propria and tunica submucosa; a stratum myoelasticum is present in the glandular tissue, the capsule consists of a stratum musculare and a stratum fibrosum; the excretory ducts are typically dilated and contain secretion	Cuboidal to columnar epithelium with principal cells that produce a serous to seromucous secretion (released by apocrine mode)	The usually mixed secretion includes electrolytes, citric acid and glucuronic acid, which promote motility of spermatozoa and initiate forward progression of ejaculated spermatozoa; secretion is weakly alkaline, high fructose content in bull; pars disseminata absent in stallion
Bulbourethral gland (glandula bulbourethralis)	Compound tubular gland in the tomcat, boar and billy goat, branched tubulo-alveolar in the stallion, bull and ram. Expanded collecting ducts are surrounded by smooth muscle cells and fibro-elastic tissue; skeletal muscle present peripherally	Simple epithelium, usually columnar, with spherical basally located nucleus; mucous secretion; in the excretory duct system the epithelium gradually transforms into pseudostratified, becoming transitional at the end of the bulbourethral duct	The stringy, mucous secretion acts as a pre-ejaculate (not in pigs), serving to neutralise the internal urethral environment and moisten the vagina; particularly well developed in the boar; in the cat, in which vesicular glands are absent, the secretory product contains glycogen as an energy source; 6–8 excretory ducts open into the urethra in the stallion

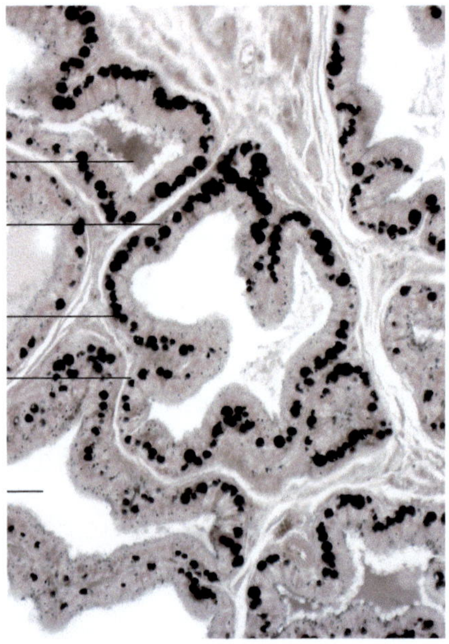

13.27 Alveolar end pieces of the vesicular gland with basal cells containing large lipid droplets (bull). Osmium impregnation (x250).

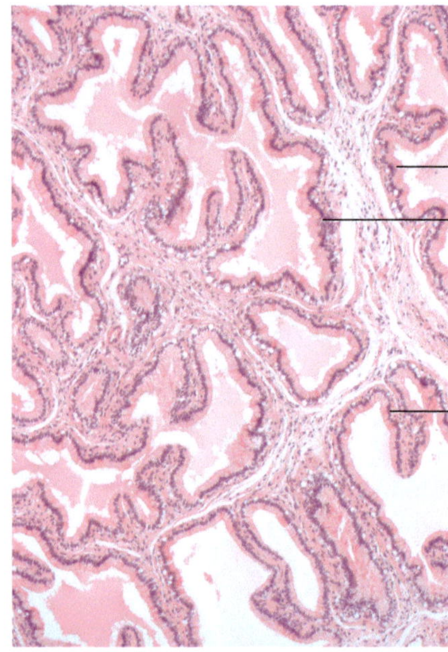

13.28 Alveolar end pieces of the vesicular gland (bull). Haematoxylin and eosin stain (x30).

cholesterol and its esters, triglycerides and phospholipids. It may be involved in **prostaglandin** synthesis (Figures 13.27 and 13.28).

The vesicular glands are surrounded by a **thick layer of smooth muscle** that sends prominent muscular septa into the interlobular connective tissue. The tunica adventitia consists of dense layers of collagen fibres with isolated smooth muscle fibres.

Species variation

Horse: The mucosa is **deeply folded**. The tubular portions of the glands form **expanded vesicles**. Secretions produced by the tubulo-alveolar glands pass through short branches into a **large excretory duct**. Smooth muscle cells are interspersed throughout the loose interstitial connective tissue. The excretory duct joins with the ductus deferens to form a communal passage, the ductus ejaculatorius, which opens into the urethra at the **colliculus seminalis**.

Ox: A central excretory duct passes through each vesicular gland. Along the course of the duct, towards the periphery of the gland, there are increasing numbers of short irregular branches and outpouchings (small bulges to well-developed alveoli). In cross-section, the tubular segments are usually larger than the alveoli. In the bull and the billy goat, the basal cells may contain massive accumulations of lipid.

Pig: The tubular lumina form **expanded collection chambers** for storage of large volumes of secretion. The epithelium has prominent folds. Lobulation of the gland is marked. There is little smooth muscle.

Prostate gland (glandula prostatica)

In most domestic mammals, the prostate gland is a **compound tubulo-alveolar gland** with excretory ducts that empty into the pelvic urethra (Figures 13.29 and 13.30). In the bull, the glandular tissue is tubular. Macroscopically, the gland may be divided into the **corpus prostatae** (pars externa), which surrounds the initial portion of the urethra, and the **pars disseminata** (pars interna), located in the lamina propria and tela submucosa of the urethra. The pars disseminata is particularly well developed dorsally and extends around the lateral and ventral walls. Histologically, the two portions of the gland are similar.

The secretory units and intraglandular ducts of the prostate gland are lined with **cuboidal** to **columnar epithelium** with **high secretory activity**. Basal cells are occasionally seen. The **principal cells** contain abundant protein-synthesising organelles, rough ER, Golgi apparatus, mitochondria, acidophilic secretory vacuoles and lipid droplets. The cells are characterised by **extensive enzyme activity**. A small proportion of the principal cells produce **mucous secretion**, while the majority **secretes a protein-rich serous** product. Vacuolar evaginations seen at the surface of active epithelial cells are indicative of **apocrine secretion**.

The lumen of the secretory end pieces and the **excretory duct system** sometimes contains small, concentrically layered concretions of secretions. Before reaching the wall of the urethra, the columnar epithelium of the excretory duct transforms into **transitional epithelium**.

The glandular tissue is surrounded by a loose network of collagen and elastic fibres in which smooth muscle fibres are

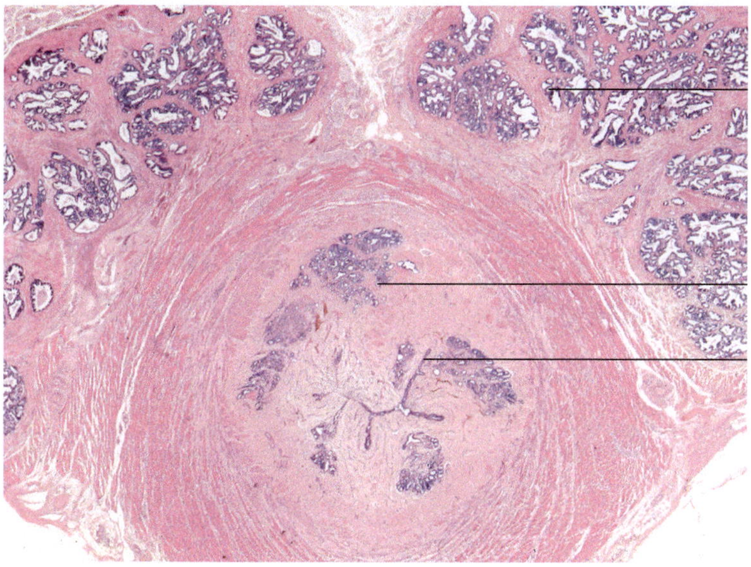

13.29 Prostate gland (dog). Haematoxylin and eosin stain (x32).

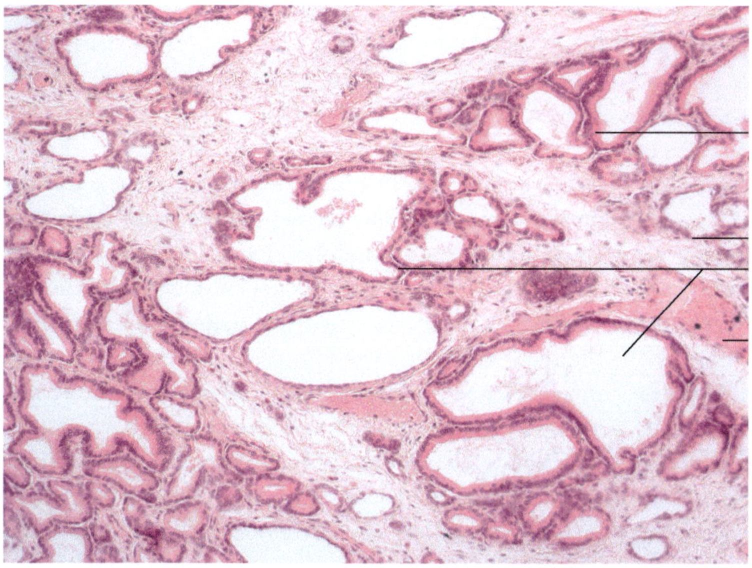

13.30 Actively secreting end pieces of the prostate gland with interstitial connective tissue containing smooth muscle (dog). Haematoxylin and eosin stain (x480).

enmeshed (**stroma myoelasticum**). Smooth muscle cells are particularly well developed in the corpus prostatae. The prostate gland is surrounded by a **capsule** (capsula prostatae) that includes connective tissue and muscular elements (**stratum musculare** and **stratum fibrosum**). Prominent connective tissue septa extend from the capsule and subdivide the two components of the gland into lobules.

Species variation

Horse: The corpus prostatae consists of two lateral lobes joined dorsally by the isthmus prostatae. A pars disseminata is lacking. The tubular glandular segments are typically dilated and filled with secretion. Smooth muscle cells are widespread throughout the connective tissue capsule and stroma.

Ox and pig: A flattened corpus prostatae lies dorsal to the urethra. Together with the m. urethralis, the distinct pars disseminata forms a sleeve around the urethra. The tubular components of the pars disseminata are arranged radially.

Small ruminants: Only the pars disseminata is present in the ram and billy goat. It contains numerous expanded secretion-filled chambers.

Carnivores: The corpus prostatae is particularly prominent, while the pars disseminata is scant.

The secretion is typically **mixed** (seromucous), with the serous component predominating. In dogs it is purely serous. The secretory product is high in electrolytes (e.g. sodium, potassium, calcium, bicarbonate), citric acid, glucuronidase and acid phosphatases, as well as fibrolysin and prostaglandins. While the secretion of the vesicular glands promotes motility of spermatozoa by its alkaline nature, the secretory product of the prostate gland initiates active progressive movement of ejaculated spermatozoa. The weakly alkaline secretion neutralises the acid environment of the vagina.

Bulbourethral gland (glandula bulbourethralis)

The paired bulbourethral glands lie on the dorsolateral aspect of the pelvic urethra at the level of the proximal bulbus penis. In the tomcat, boar and billy goat, the gland is compound and predominantly tubular. The glandular morphology in the bull, ram and stallion is **branched tubulo-alveolar**. Bulbourethral glands are absent in the dog.

The gland contains lobules of varying size. Alveolar and tubular end pieces open into well-developed **collecting ducts** from which the secretion travels through a main excretory (bulbourethral) duct into the urethra (Figure 13.31). The glandular tissue is surrounded by loose connective tissue incorporating solitary **smooth muscle cells.** Denser fibrous trabeculae connect the connective tissue with a superficial **fibro-elastic capsule**. As well as smooth muscle, the capsule encloses **striated muscle** tissue or merges with adjoining skeletal muscles (e.g. m. bulboglandularis, m. bulbospongiosus).

The secretory portion of the gland is lined by **simple columnar epithelium** with isolated basal cells. The basophilic cytoplasm houses a spherical nucleus. Secretory product is released into collecting ducts lined with cuboidal to columnar epithelium. In the larger intraglandular portions of the duct system, the epithelium gradually becomes **pseudostratified**. At the end of the bulbourethral duct (ductus glandulae bulbourethralis) the lining transforms into **transitional epithelium**.

The secretory product of the bulbourethral gland is **mucous**, **gelatinous** and **stringy**. It is discharged **prior to ejaculation** serving to **neutralise** the urethra and lubricate the vagina (in the pig, bulbourethral gland secretion is part of the ejaculate).

Species variation

Horse: The gland is surrounded by striated muscle (m. bulboglandularis); six to eight ductus glandulae bulbourethrales open into the urethra.

Ox and sheep: Short intermediate segments connect expanded collecting ducts with secretory end pieces.

Pig: The glandula bulbourethralis is particularly well developed. The m. bulboglandularis forms a cuff around the cylindrical gland.

Cat: The ducts are expanded into sinus-like chambers. These are connected by short, unbranched portions to the glandular end pieces. Due to its high glycogen content, the glandular secretion (pre-ejaculate) may act as a source of energy for the spermatozoa (fructose-producing vesicular glands are absent in the tomcat).

Urethra

The male urethra commences at the internal opening of the neck of the bladder (ostium urethrae internum). It passes along the floor of the pelvis to the ischial arch and enters the penis. The urethra ends at the ostium urethrum externae. In the boar and carnivore, the ostium is near the tip of the penis. In the stallion, bull, ram and billy goat, the external urethral opening is located at the end of the processus urethrae. The urethra is divided into a **pelvic portion** (**pars pelvina urethrae**) composed of a pars praeprostatica, pars prostatica and a pars membranacea, and a cavernous **penile portion** (**pars spongiosa urethrae, pars externa urethrae**).

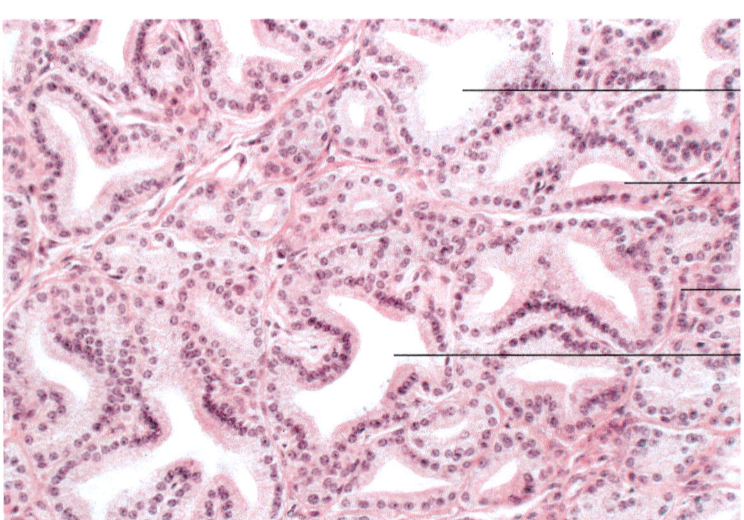

13.31 Lobule of bulbourethral gland (bull). Haematoxylin and eosin stain (x200).

Until it is joined by the ductus deferens, the urethra exclusively **carries urine** (pars praeprostatica). Beyond this point, it assumes the additional function of **transporting semen**.

The urethra is a **musculomembranous tube** (Figures 13.32 to 13.34). Longitudinal mucosal folds are evident throughout its length. These are lost during ejaculation and urination. Most of the urethra is lined with **transitional epithelium**. Isolated regions of simple stratified columnar epithelium may be present. Near the glans penis or processus urethrae the mucosal lining transforms into stratified squamous epithelium.

In the **pelvic urethra**, the lamina propria is composed of fibro-elastic tissue containing smooth muscle cells and, in some cases, lymphocytic infiltrates. Mucous tubular glands (glandulae urethrales) are present in the stallion and tomcat. At the end of the pelvic portion, the lamina propria contains numerous thin-walled veins (caverns) that form a subepithelial **vascular stratum** (stratum cavernosum or vasculare). The extent of the vascular stratum varies considerably. In the penile urethra it becomes markedly enlarged, forming the corpus spongiosum penis. The innermost cavernous spaces are small, becoming larger towards the periphery. The caverns are particularly prominent in the stallion.

The tunica muscularis begins at the neck of the bladder as a three-layered muscular mantle. It continues as striated muscle (outer and inner layer of the m. urethralis). The circularly oriented fibres form a complete layer in the stallion, carnivore and billy goat. In the bull, boar and ram the dorsal component of this layer is missing. The tunica muscularis is surrounded by a tunica adventitia which radiates into the capsule of the penis.

Penis

The penis consists of the **body** (corpus penis) with its **paired erectile bodies** (corpora cavernosa penis), and the urethra and its associated **unpaired erectile tissue** (corpus

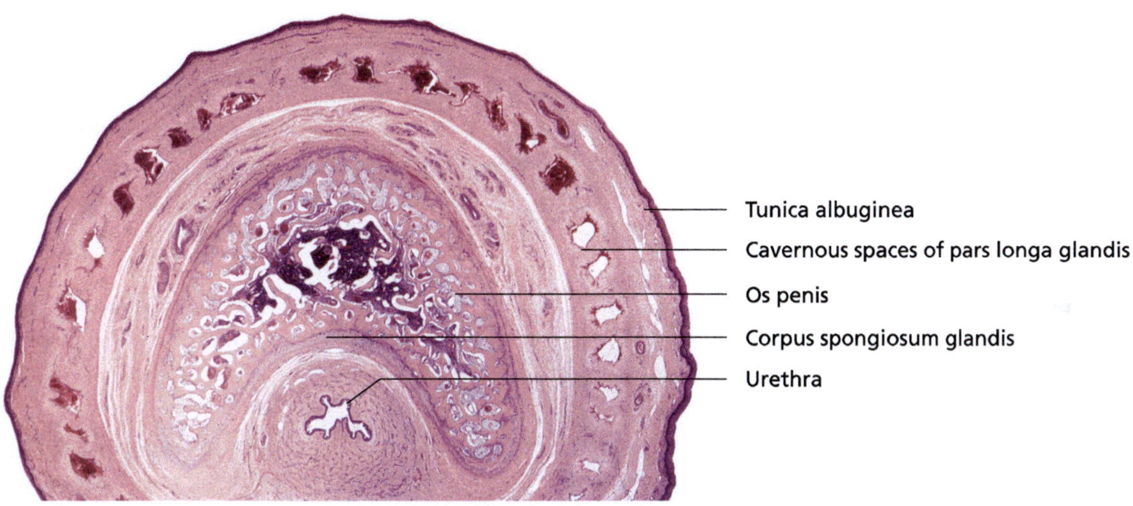

13.32 Cross-section of penis at the level of the glans (dog). Haematoxylin and eosin stain (x7).

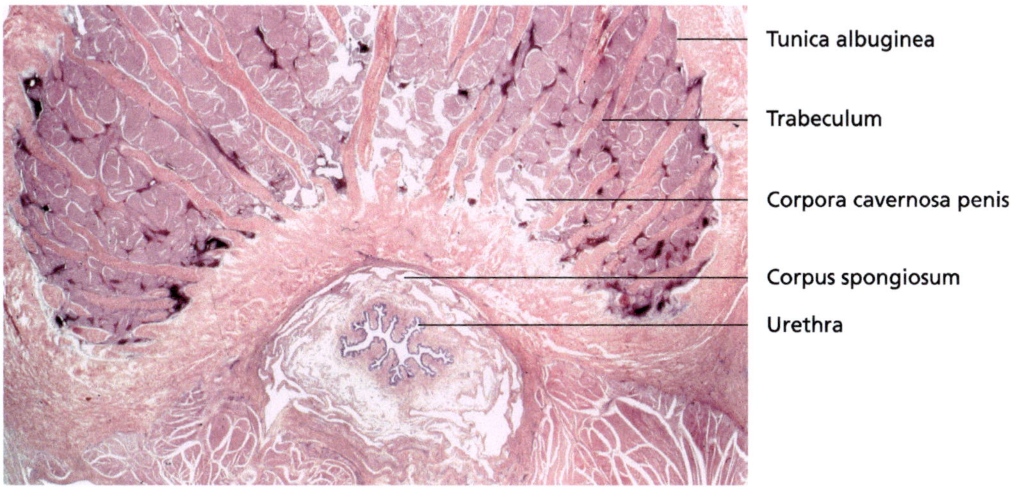

13.33 Cross-section of penis (stallion). Haematoxylin and eosin stain (x5).

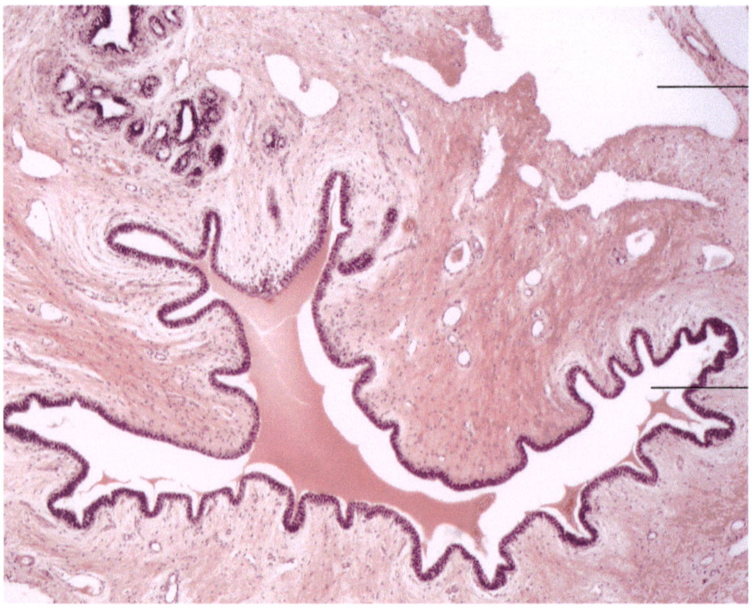

13.34 Corpus spongiosum (boar). Haematoxylin and eosin stain (x175).

spongiosum penis) (Figures 13.32 to 13.34). The unpaired erectile body begins as the **bulbus penis** and continues as the **corpus spongiosum penis** and the terminal **corpus spongiosum glandis**. The last of these forms the basis of the glans penis.

Other components of the penis include dense connective tissue layers, smooth and striated muscle, blood and lymph vessels and nerve plexuses.

The **body** of the penis incorporating the **paired corpora cavernosa penis** is enclosed in a densely woven mesh of collagen and elastic fibres (**tunica albuginea**). Connective tissue septa and trabeculae project into the erectile tissue, surrounding this to a varying extent. In the dog, a complete median **septum** (septum penis) is formed throughout, maintaining the paired arrangement. In the stallion, bull, boar and tomcat, a complete septum is present only towards the root of the penis.

The paired corpora cavernosa form an integrated **erectile structure** (Figures 13.32 and 13.33). The **erectile tissue**, located between the trabeculae, consists of expanded **cavernous vascular spaces** and **fibromuscular tissue**.

The vascular spaces of the **corpora cavernosa penis** are supplied by the **helicine arteries** (aa. helicinae). The tunica interna (intima) of the arteries contains smooth muscle cells that reduce the size of the lumen. Anastomoses connect the arteries with veins. Relaxation of the smooth musculature promotes filling of the cavernous spaces, leading to erection of the penis. This is facilitated by compression of venous drainage by the tunica albuginea and the musculature of the penis. Thus, erection is regulated by increased arterial supply and reduced venous outflow.

The unpaired **corpus spongiosum penis** is surrounded by a thin tunica albuginea incorporating elastic fibres. Connective tissue trabeculae emanate from the tunica albuginea. In the stallion and dog, the trabeculae are invested with smooth muscle fibres. The fibrous trabeculae provide the structural foundation for cavernous vascular spaces resembling a longitudinally oriented venous network. During erection, the **caverns** receive blood from the a. bulbi penis, resulting in enlargement of the urethra. Towards the tip of the penis, the corpus spongiosum is continued by the corpus spongiosum glandis. During erection this connection results in enlargement of the glans.

Species variation

Horse: The fibres of the connective tissue sheaths are arranged in a lattice, surrounded by bundles of fibres. The erectile tissue is composed largely of longitudinally oriented smooth muscle. In the non-erect penis, the muscle reduces the cavernous spaces to narrow slits. Connective tissue in the erectile body is relatively sparse.

Horse and dog: The **penis** is of the **musculocavernous type**. The arrangement of connective tissue fibres permits limited expansion of the tunica albuginea during erection. The erect penis is firm and elastic. The well-developed erectile tissue of the glans penis is continuous with the corpus spongiosum (via deep veins of the glans in the dog). The loose connective tissue between the vascular spaces contains numerous elastic fibres and smooth muscle cells.

Carnivores: The erectile tissue is surrounded by smooth muscle; connective tissue is relatively meagre. An os penis is present (Figure 13.32).

Ox: The outer collagen fibre bundles have a mainly longitudinal orientation. They send trabeculae and septa into the erectile body.

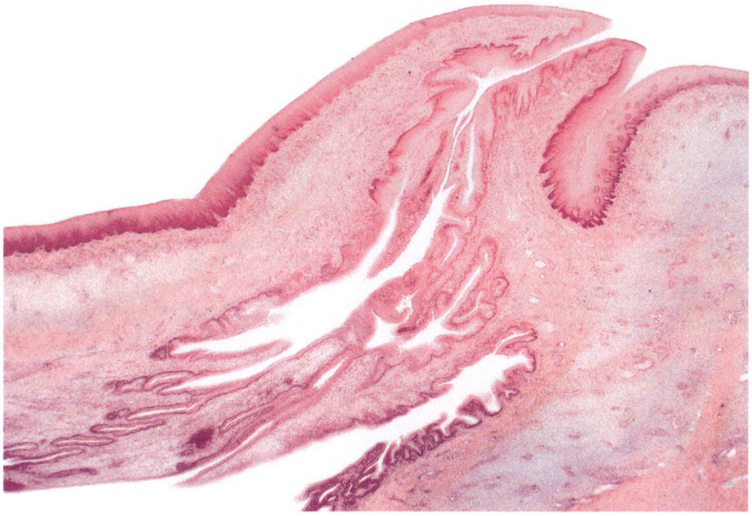

13.35 Longitudinal section of the glans penis and external urethral orifice (ostium urethrae externum) (dog). Haematoxylin and eosin stain (x15).

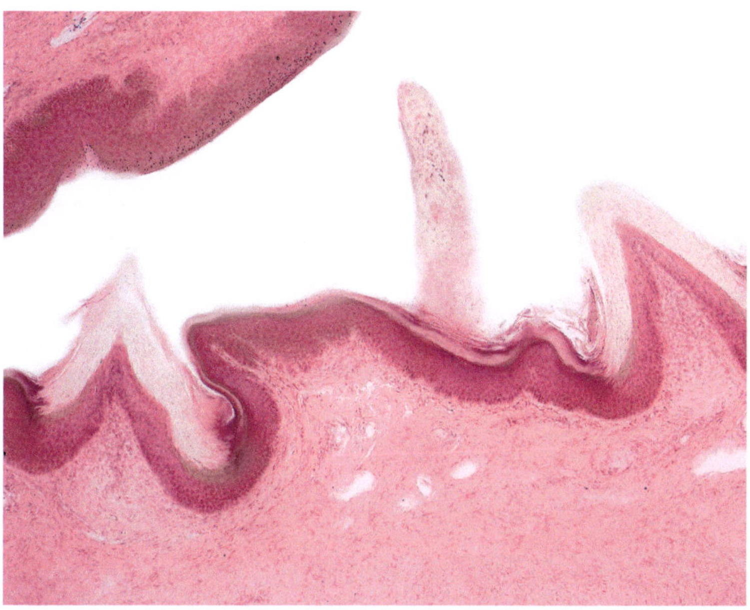

13.36 Glans with keratinised papillae (tomcat). Haematoxylin and eosin stain (x250).

Ox and pig: The **penis** is of the **fibro-elastic type**. Elongation of the penis results primarily from straightening of the sigmoid flexure. The tissue between the vascular spaces consists mainly of fibro-elastic networks with few smooth muscle cells. The glans penis contains a modestly developed subepithelial stratum cavernosum that does not bring about enlargement of the glans (Figures 13.35 and 13.36).

Prepuce (praeputium)

The prepuce is a fold of skin composed of an outer layer (lamina externa) and an inner or parietal layer (lamina interna). The inner layer is continuous with skin of the free end of the penis.

The **lamina externa** has the typical structure of skin. It has a light covering of hair and, particularly towards the ostium praeputiale, contains sebaceous glands. The **lamina interna** is lined by stratified squamous epithelium. In most domestic species, the internal layer incorporates sebaceous and sweat glands and is mostly hairless. Together with the secretory product of the sebaceous glands, vacuolar lipid degeneration in the epithelial cells gives rise to a fatty secretion (smegma praeputii). The lamina interna contains numerous sensory receptors and abundant free nerve endings.

Species variation

Ox, pig and dog: Lymphatic nodules are frequently observed throughout the inner layer.

Cat: The mucosal covering of the glans penis has small keratinised barbs (Figure 13.36).

Pig: The **preputial diverticulum** (diverticulum praeputiale) is lined by a deeply folded non-glandular mucosa. The contents of the diverticulum (cell debris and urine) produces a characteristic odour.

Penis of birds

In birds with a protrusible phallus, the penis arises as the **basis phalli** in the ventral wall of the cloaca, where it rests in a trough-like plate of fibrocartilage, the corpus fibrocartilagineum. It incorporates a **lymphatic cistern** (cisterna lymphatica basis phalli) that is partly divided into left and right components. The cistern continues as a narrow chamber (cisterna lymphatica corporis phalli) that extends around the **cutaneous** and **glandular phallic sacs** (saccus cutaneous phalli and saccus glandularis phalli). These sacs form the hollow interior of the body (corpus) of the phallus. The more proximal cutaneous sac leads into the glandular sac. In the non-tumescent phallus, the body is completely invaginated and the junction between the cutaneous and glandular phallic sacs, the **flexura phalli**, is curved.

During intumescence, **lymph** derived from the vascular body of the phallus (see below) fills the lymphatic cisterns to bring about erection. This results in eversion of the cutaneous phallic sac. The glandular sac is not everted (it comes to lie within the cutaneous sac). As a result, the exteriorised flexura phalli becomes the tip (apex) of the erect phallus. A **phallic sulcus** (sulcus phalli) spirals around the free part of the erect phallus.

In species with a non-protrusible phallus, erection also occurs due to engorgement with lymph, although in these species the erect phallus protrudes only slightly, if at all, from the cloaca.

Accessory structures of the phallus

The **vascular body of the phallus** consists of a capillary tuft (originating from the **pudendal artery**) that is intricately intermingled with lymphatic vessels. Fluid passes from blood capillaries into the interstitium, from which it enters the lymph vessels. The lymph passes through two ducts into the lymphatic cisterns of the phallus. Filling of these cisterns is responsible for erection, aided by contraction of the m. sphincter cloacae.

During detumescence, the phallus is returned to its invaginated state by the action of the typically striated **m. retractor phalli** in the ventral wall of the cloaca, with assistance from the elastic ligament of the phallus. In waterfowl, lymph is pumped from the phallus by two lymph hearts (cor lymphatica), each located above the transverse process of the first free caudal vertebra.

Female reproductive system (organa genitalia feminina)

14

The female reproductive organs of domestic mammals are comprised of the:

- paired ovaries (ovaria),
- paired uterine tubes (tubae uterinae),
- uterus and cervix
- vagina and vestibule (vestibulum vaginae) and
- vulva.

The **ovaries** are the site of development and maturation of female germ cells. In addition, the ovaries function as endocrine glands, synthesising several sex hormones including oestrogen, progesterone, testosterone and other androgens. At certain stages of the reproductive cycle, and during pregnancy, a hormone-producing corpus luteum (or several corpora lutea, in multi-ovulatory species) is (are) formed in the ovary.

The **uterine tubes** transport germ cells, including the ova of the female and the spermatozoa of the male. Union of the two haploid germ cells (**fertilisation**) occurs in the proximal segment of the **uterine tubes** (**ampulla tubae uterinae**). This gives rise to the zygote from which the embryo forms. The newly formed embryo passes through the uterine tube into the uterus, where it becomes implanted in the mucosa (**nidation**, **implantation**) and continues its embryonic and fetal development. During pregnancy, the mucosa of the uterus undergoes species-dependent modifications and contributes to the formation of the placenta (refer to embryology texts).

The **cervix**, **vagina**, **vestibule** and **vulva** constitute the birth canal. The vagina and labia of the vulva represent the external genitalia and copulatory organs.

In sexually mature animals, the organs of the female reproductive tract undergo cyclic changes in structure. These are most pronounced in the **parenchyma of the ovary** and in the **mucosa** of individual organs.

Ovary (ovar, ovarium)

In sexually mature domestic mammals, the ovaries have two main functions: **production of mature oocytes** and **synthesis of reproductive hormones** (Figure 14.1). Both are subject to cyclic influences, mediated by feedback

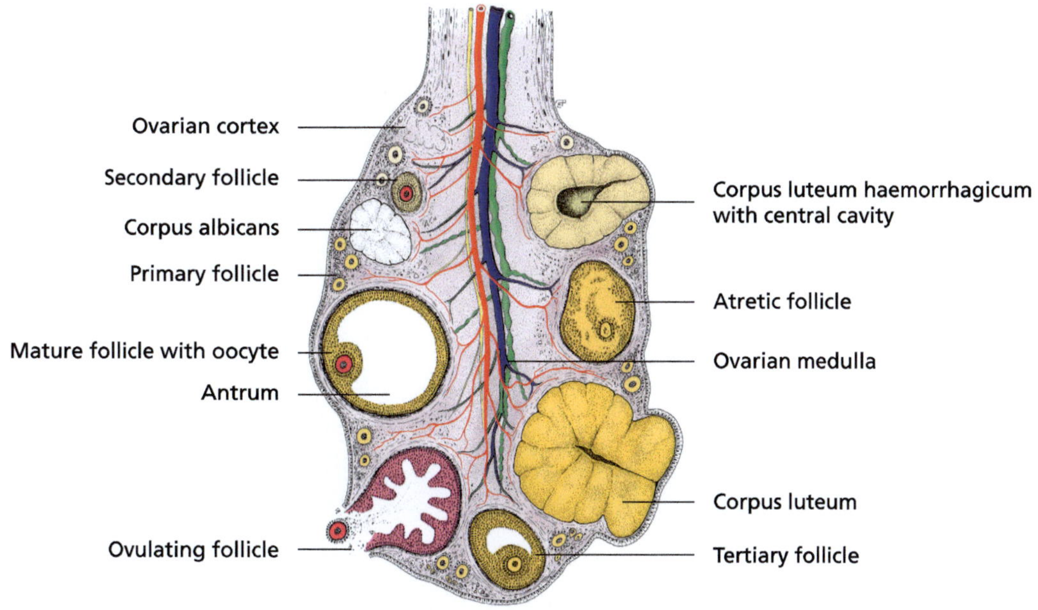

14.1 Ovary of the cow depicting various stages of follicular development (schematic; König and Liebich, 2009).

mechanisms involving hormones of the hypothalamus and hypophysis.

In the female gonad, germ cell maturation and hormone production are both associated with the same structure, the **ovarian follicle**. This differs from males, in which development of spermatozoa occurs in the seminiferous tubules and hormones are synthesised separately by interstitial cells (see below). The macroscopic appearance of the ovary varies widely among the domestic mammals (see *Veterinary Anatomy of Domestic Mammals: Textbook and Colour Atlas*). In contrast, the basic microscopic structure of the ovary is relatively consistent, varying primarily with the reproductive cycle and the age of the animal.

Structure of the ovary

From exterior to interior, the ovary is composed of:

- mesovarium (ligamentum latum uteri) – part of the supportive apparatus of the female reproductive organs,
- germinal epithelium – simple cuboidal epithelium,
- tunica albuginea surrounding the:
  - cortex (cortex ovarii, zona parenchymatosa) – connective tissue stroma enclosing follicles and the corpus luteum/corpora lutea and
  - medulla (medulla ovarii, zona vasculosa) containing blood vessels, lymph vessels and nerves.

The **surface** of the ovary is rendered irregular by various features including mature follicles, ovulation fossae (mare), corpora lutea and scar tissue.

The ovaries are covered by a **single layer** of flattened yet usually still **cuboidal surface epithelium** (epithelium superficiale). This layer is continuous with the serosal epithelium of the peritoneum. The ovarian epithelium, also referred to as **germinal epithelium**, is a specialised form of surface epithelium derived from the mesoderm.

Species variation

Horse: The surface epithelium is present only at the **ovulation fossa**. Elsewhere the ovary is covered by a tunica serosa.

Beneath the epithelium is a thick **tunica albuginea** (up to 100 μm thick). This sparsely vascularised connective tissue layer is contiguous with the stroma of the ovarian cortex.

Cortex (cortex ovarii, zona parenchymatosa)

In species other than the horse, the cortex lies external to the inner medulla of the ovary. The structural core of the cortex is formed by **metabolically active cells** in a connective tissue stroma (**spinocellular connective tissue**). Resembling fibrocytes, the stromal cells are characterised by a high regenerative capacity, a propensity for multiplication and phagocytic ability. In the corpus luteum, stromal cells transform into hormone-producing epithelioid cells, synthesising progesterone, oestrogens and possibly oxytocin. After involution of the corpus luteum, these cells transform back into stromal cells.

The stromal connective tissue is pervaded by a delicate network of capillaries that provides the vascular supply for developing follicles (see below) and contributes to the transformation of the collapsed follicle into the corpus luteum following ovulation.

In sexually mature animals, the cortex contains **follicles** (primary oocytes and follicular cells) in various **stages of development** (primordial, primary, secondary, tertiary, mature) and **corpora lutea**. During embryonic development, primordial germ cells (oogonia) become arranged in cords and later clusters, in which they are brought into contact with somatic cells.

Multiplication of germ cells ceases before birth. **Oogonia** differentiate into **oocytes**. These enter **meiosis I** and become arrested in the diplotene (dictyotene) stage of prophase until ovulation (see Chapter 1, 'The cell' under 'Meiosis', and embryology texts).

Somatic cells differentiate into **follicular cells** during embryogenesis. These cells provide metabolic support for the developing germ cell. In this sense, they resemble sustentacular cells in the seminiferous tubules of males. Follicular cells surround the oocyte in single or multiple layers, depending on the stage of follicular development.

OVARIAN FOLLICLE

In the sexually mature female, **primary oocytes** in the ovarian cortex remain in **late prophase of meiosis I**. Together with their surrounding **follicular cells** they form a structural and functional unit referred to as an **ovarian follicle**. Follicles are separated from surrounding stromal cells by a basal lamina.

The **follicles** in the ovarian cortex are at different **developmental stages** (Table 14.1), in which the number and arrangement of follicular cells vary (Figures 14.2 to 14.9). Follicles are classified as:

- primordial (folliculus ovaricus primordialis),
- primary (folliculus ovaricus primarius),
- secondary (folliculus ovaricus secundarius),
- tertiary (folliculus ovaricus tertiarius) and
- mature (preovulatory).

Primordial and primary follicles

Primordial follicles are composed of a primary oocyte (diameter ca. 30 μm) surrounded by a layer of **flattened undifferentiated follicular cells**. The oocyte contains an eccentric nucleus with a nucleolus, an expanded Golgi complex, mitochondria, ribosomes and ER. Externally, the

Table 14.1 Structure of ovarian follicles of domestic mammals at different stages of development.

Follicle type	Oocyte	Associated glandular activity	Special features
Primordial follicle	Primary oocyte surrounded by a single layer of flattened follicular cells	None	Arranged in rosettes in carnivores, evenly distributed throughout the cortex in ungulates
Primary follicle	Slight increase in volume of primary oocyte; oocyte surrounded by single layer of cuboidal follicular cells	Gradual increase in FSH secreted by adenohypophysis	In some species, release of FSH induces a synchronous wave of follicular development; the last two waves are ovulatory
Secondary follicle	Substantial increase in size of primary oocyte (80 μm), mitotic division results in multilaminar follicular cell stratum (5–10 layers); differentiation of stromal cells into theca follicularis; development of zona pellucida	Rise in FSH	Beginning of antrum (antrum folliculare) formation through widening of intercellular spaces
Tertiary follicle	Oocyte reaches 130–300 μm; follicular cells differentiate into basal, intermediate and granulosa cells; formation of cumulus oophorus and corona radiata (single layer of columnar follicular cells)	Falling FSH, rising oestrogens (from granulosa cells)	Filling of antrum (diameter 0.3 mm) with protein-rich liquor follicularis; theca interna forms from stromal cells (steroid hormone synthesis) and spinocellular connective tissue differentiates into fibrous theca externa
Mature follicle	Preovulatory follicle; follicle and oocyte reach maximum size; follicle lies immediately under tunica albuginea, avascular stigma forms; cumulus oophorus floats freely in antrum; follicle and stigma begin to degenerate	Oestrogens rise, FSH decreases, secretion of LH and prostaglandins, collagenase activity	Completion of meiosis I in primary oocyte (does not occur until after ovulation in the horse and dog)
Corpus luteum	Initial formation of corpus haemorrhagicum (after rupture of stigma, collapse of follicle lumen and release of oocyte); formation of corpus luteum cyclicum or, if pregnancy occurs, the corpus luteum graviditatis; regression of corpus luteum leads to formation of scar-like corpus albicans, corpus nigrescens and corpus rubrum	Rise in progesterone during luteal cell activity; progesterone decreases late in the oestrous cycle; FSH eventually rises	Transformation of granulosa cells of follicle into large granulosa luteal cells and stromal cells of theca interna into theca luteal cells; accumulation of yellowish pigments (lipochromes; not in pigs and ruminants)

follicle is surrounded by loose spinocellular connective tissue. Primordial follicles represent a quiescent stage that becomes reactivated to form primary follicles (Figures 14.3 to 14.5 and Table 14.1).

In **primary follicles**, the follicular cells comprise a **single layer of cuboidal cells**. The cytoplasm of the oocyte gradually increases in volume (Figures 14.1 and 14.3 to 14.5).

Secondary follicles

Mitotic division of the follicular cells of a primary follicle leads to formation of the secondary follicle. Features of secondary follicles (Table 14.1) include:

- an increase in the volume of the oocyte (relative to primary follicles),
- the zona pellucida,
- layering of the follicular cells and
- differentiation of stromal cells to form the theca follicularis.

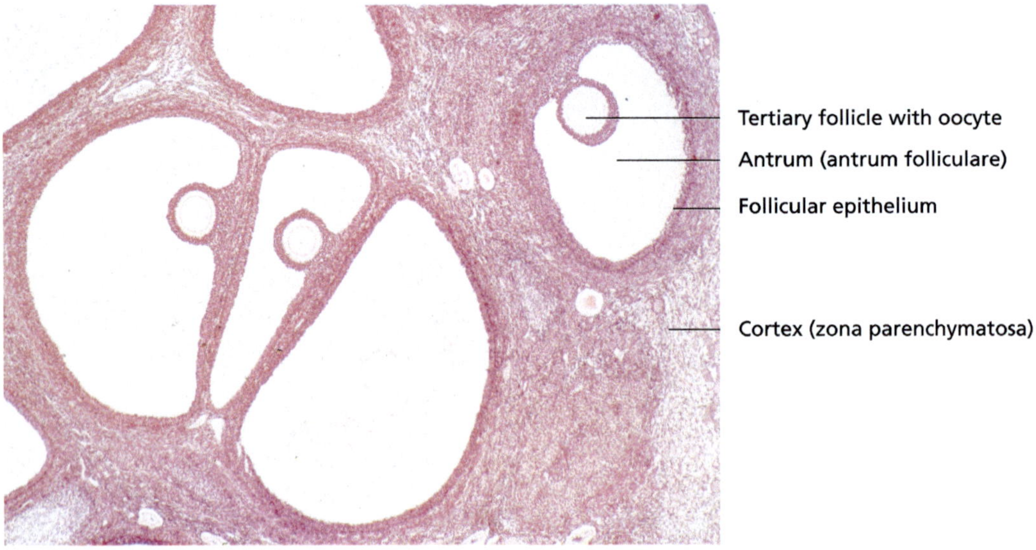

14.2 Ovary sectioned through a tertiary follicle (cat). Haematoxylin and eosin stain (x18).

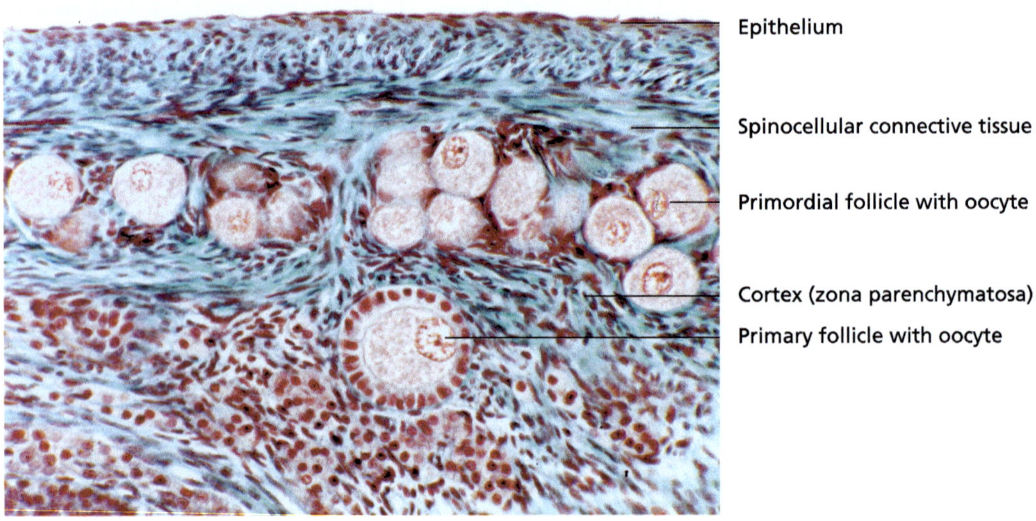

14.3 Cortex of ovary (cat). Goldner's Masson trichrome stain (x120).

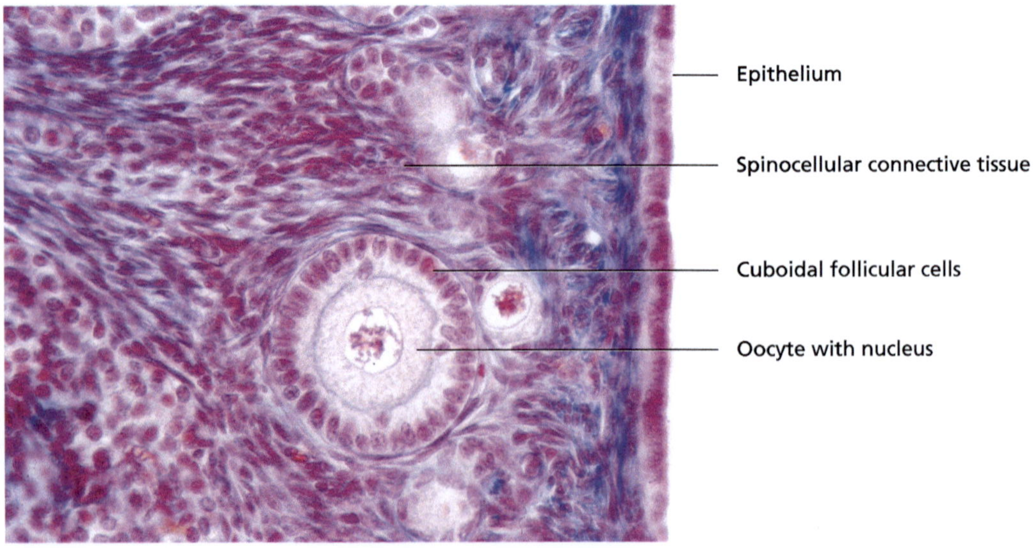

14.4 Cortex of ovary with primary follicle (cat). Azan stain (x250).

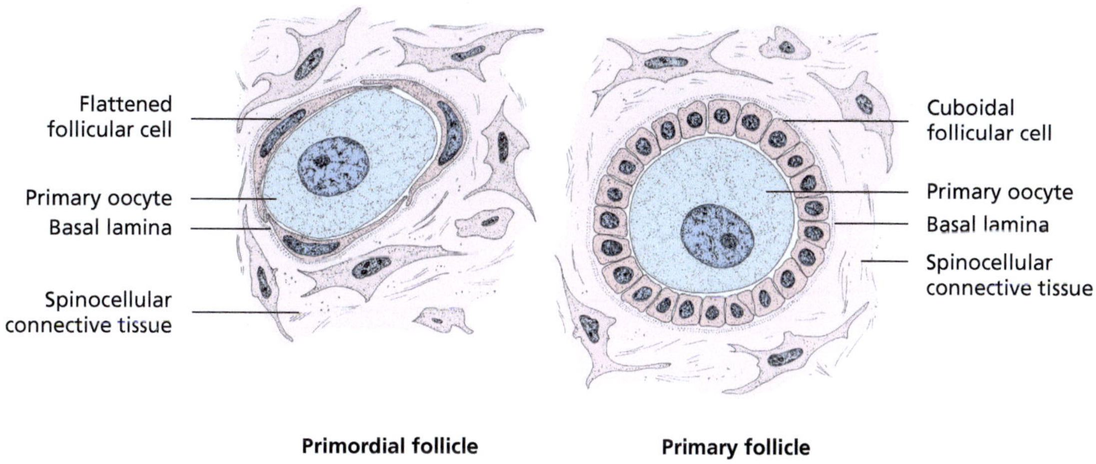

14.5 Primordial and primary follicles (schematic).

In secondary follicles, the oocyte grows to 80 µm in diameter. Concurrently, the cytoplasm undergoes structural differentiation with an increase in protein-synthesising organelles (ER and ribosomes) and enlargement of the Golgi complex.

> **Species variation**
>
> **Ruminants**: The oocytes contain vacuolar lipid granules.

Cortical granules accumulate under the plasmalemma of the oocyte and the cell surface is irregularly studded with minute cellular processes. The whole oocyte increases in size (this continues until the early tertiary follicle stage) (Figure 14.6).

The **zona pellucida** is a fibrillar glycoprotein layer (12–13 µm thick) that forms in the **perivitelline space** between the surface of the oocyte and the adjacent follicular cells (Figure 14.6). The zona pellucida is penetrated by follicular cell processes that are connected to the oocyte by desmosomes and, later, by gap junctions. The primary function of these intercellular connections is to provide metabolic support to the oocyte (Figures 14.6 and 14.7).

The zona pellucida:

- can be penetrated only by spermatozoa originating from organisms of the same species,
- prevents the penetration of multiple spermatozoa (polyspermy),
- counteracts premature implantation of the blastomeres in the uterine tube,
- supports the structural integrity of the oocyte and
- regulates the uptake of nutrients.

Secondary follicles are characterised by the **proliferation of follicular cells**. Mitotic cell division gives rise

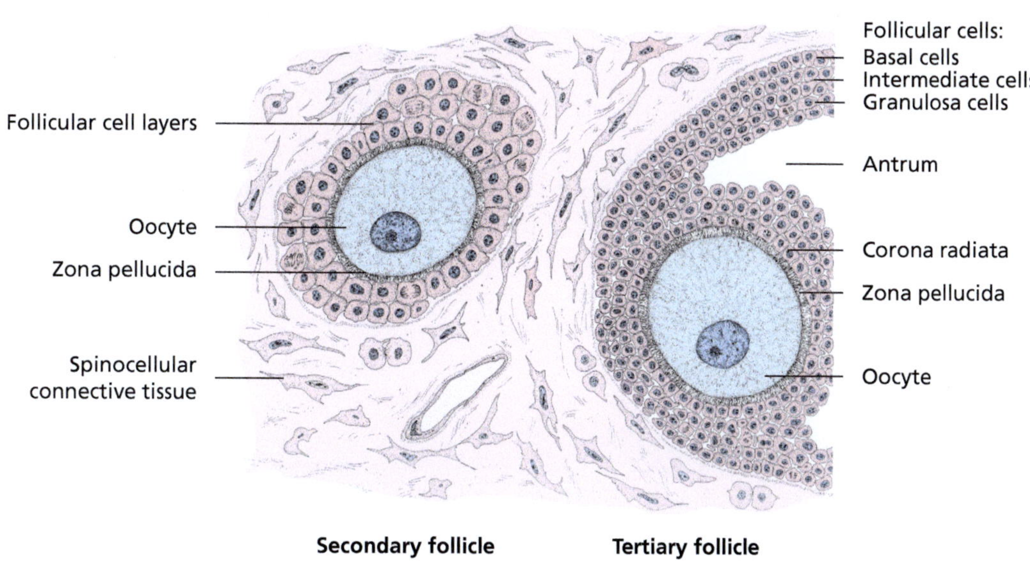

14.6 Secondary and tertiary follicles (schematic).

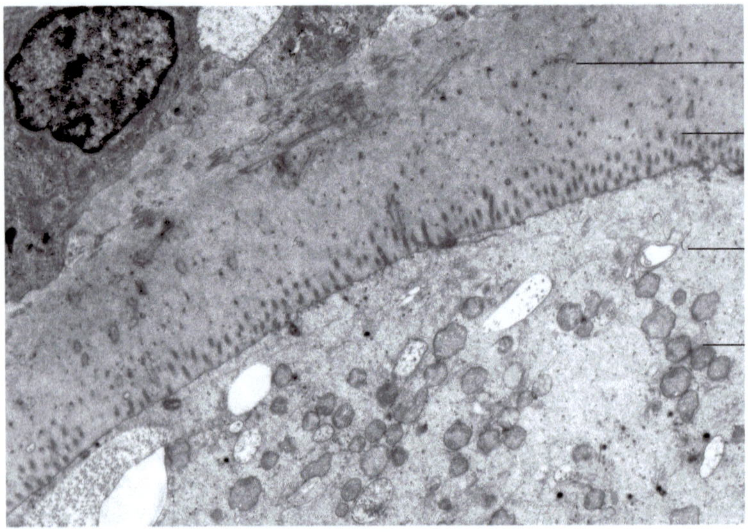

14.7 Fine structure of the zona pellucida and adjacent oocyte (sheep; x9000).

to **several cell layers** that encircle the oocyte (typically five layers, up to ten in ruminants). Due to irregular polar cell division, secondary follicles often appear oval. Individual cells are polygonal and contain few organelles. Differentiation of follicular cells into an inner granulosa cell layer, middle intermediate cell layer and outer basal cell layer (see below) commences in the secondary follicle stage. Stromal cells surrounding the follicle become organised into a circular layer. The cells enlarge and form a thin connective tissue sheath termed the **theca follicularis**.

In late secondary follicles, the follicular cells are loosely bound together. Expansion of intercellular spaces between intermediate cells results in clefts that coalesce to form a larger **cavity**, the antrum folliculare. This marks the transition from a secondary to a tertiary follicle.

Tertiary follicles

Characteristic features of tertiary follicles include:

- the presence of a large fluid-filled cavity (antrum folliculare),
- differentiation of follicular cells within the wall of the follicle,
- development of the cumulus oophorus and
- stratification of the theca follicularis to form the theca interna and theca externa.

Spaces between the follicular cells can be detected with the light microscope when the follicle reaches a diameter of approximately 0.3 mm. These clefts merge to form the **antrum** (antrum folliculare). The **fluid** in the antrum (liquor follicularis) is rich in hyaluronic acid and protein. Expansion of the antral cavity results in displacement of follicular cells to the periphery of the follicle. The follicular cells form a multi-layered lining.

According to their location in the multilaminar wall of the follicle (Figures 14.6, 14.8 and 14.9), the follicular cells are designated as:

- basal cells,
- intermediate cells and
- granulosa cells.

Basal cells are in close contact with the basal lamina of the follicle. Their functions include transport of metabolites for nourishment of the oocyte and production of follicular fluid. In the endoplasmic reticulum, **oestrogens** are formed from androgens (testosterone) synthesised by the epithelioid stromal cells of the theca interna.

Intermediate cells form the middle layer of the follicular wall. These cells are involved in the transport of substances between cells and contribute to follicular fluid production.

Granulosa cells constitute the inner layer of the wall of the follicle, surrounding the antrum and the cumulus oophorus (see below). These modified follicular cells synthesise protein-rich, hormone-containing antral fluid. In tertiary follicles, many granulosa cells enclose PAS-positive granules (**Call–Exner bodies**) which are considered precursors of follicular fluid.

The oocyte is located eccentrically in the antrum and is surrounded by a cluster of cells (cumulus oophorus) that contacts the follicle wall. The cumulus oophorus comprises basal cells, intermediate cells and an inner layer of (granulosa) cells, the corona radiata. The oocyte lies centrally within the cumulus oophorus (Figures 14.8 and 14.9).

The **corona radiata**, comprising a simple layer of **columnar follicular cells**, lies immediately external to the zona pellucida. Small processes extending from the cells of the corona radiata project radially through the zona

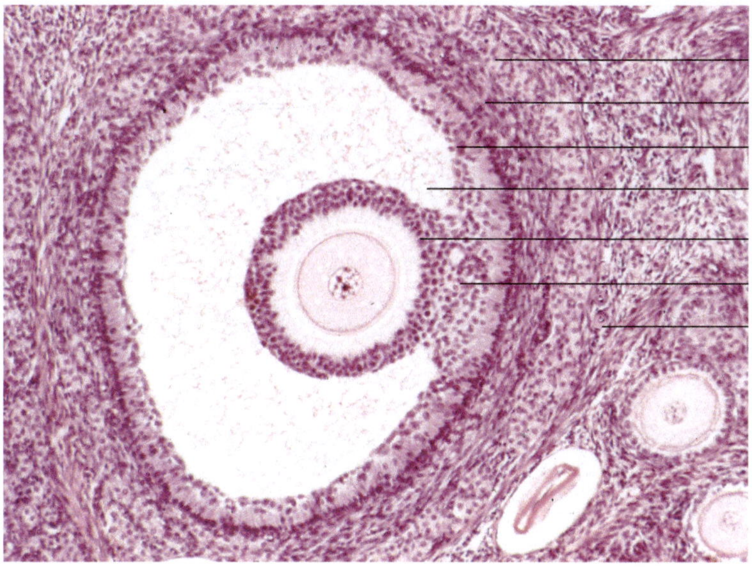

14.8 Tertiary follicle (cat). Haematoxylin and eosin stain (x120).

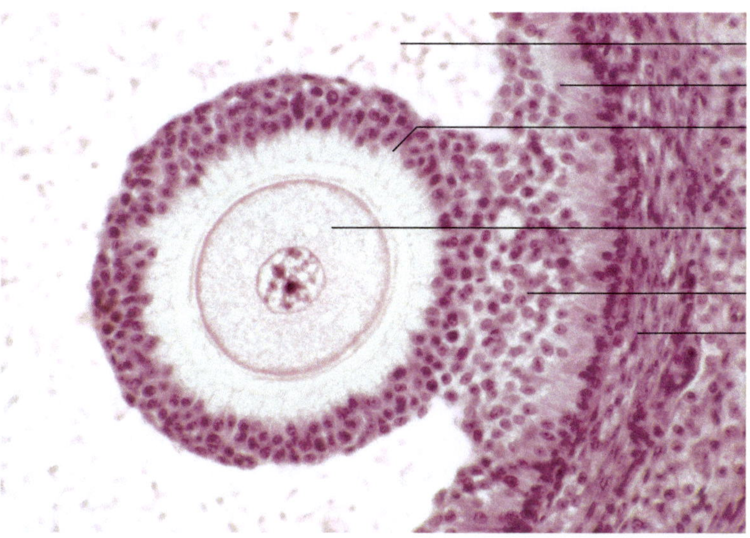

14.9 Oocyte, cumulus oophorus and adjacent structures (cat). Haematoxylin and eosin stain (x300).

pellucida and contact the oocyte, providing the germ cell with nutritional support.

In the tertiary stage, the oocyte ceases to grow, having reached a **size of 130–300 μm** in domestic mammals. The structure of the oocyte of the tertiary follicle differs little from that of the secondary follicle (Figures 14.8 and 14.9).

The loose connective tissue surrounding tertiary follicles is differentiated into two layers, an inner theca interna and an outer theca externa. In the **theca interna**, stromal cells are transformed into **epithelioid cells** that synthesise **steroid hormones** (androgens). This endocrine function is indicated in the cytoplasm by the presence of mitochondria with tubular cristae, smooth endoplasmic reticulum and lipid vacuoles. The theca interna is extensively vascularised with a dense capillary network surrounding the epithelioid cells.

The theca interna merges with the outer **theca externa**, which is composed largely of spindle-shaped stromal cells (spinocellular connective tissue). The cell layers, which are typically oriented parallel to the follicular surface, are interspersed with reticular fibres, small blood vessels and lymph channels.

Mature follicles

The **mature preovulatory follicle** (Table 14.1) forms a macroscopically visible bulge on the surface of the ovary. The follicles measure 2 mm in the **dog**, over 1 cm in the **pig**, 17–18 mm in the **ox** and 3–6 cm in the **horse**. The initially broad-based cumulus oophorus contracts to form a stem and peripheral follicular cells become detached. Surrounded by the **zona pellucida**, **cells of the corona radiata** and individual **follicular cells**, the **oocyte** separates from the follicular wall and **floats freely** in the **follicular fluid**. In most domestic mammals, the **primary oocyte** (ovocytus primarius) completes meiosis I prior to ovulation. In the **horse** and **dog**, this occurs after ovulation has taken place. During the completion of meiosis I, **genetic information** is distributed evenly among the two resulting nuclei, while the cytoplasm is unequally apportioned. This gives rise to a **secondary oocyte** (ovocytus secundarius) and a non-viable **polar body** (polocytus primarius). Immediately after completion of the first meiotic division (reduction division), meiosis II (equatorial division) commences in the secondary oocyte. This is completed only after penetration of the oocyte by a spermatozoon within the uterine tube. This division is also uneven, resulting in a **haploid ovum**, which is capable of being fertilised, and a small, non-functional **polar body**.

Follicular atresia

Most primordial and primary follicles, and many follicles that reach later stages of development, undergo regression (**follicular atresia**). This is a normal, continuously occurring process. Only a small minority of oocytes develop to the point of ovulation. Further development into a mature ovum only occurs after penetration of a spermatozoon.

In **primary follicles**, atresia begins with degeneration of the **oocyte**, followed by breakdown of the follicular wall. The products of follicular disintegration are phagocytosed by macrophages. The process of atresia is similar in **secondary follicles**, though the zona pellucida prevents rapid and complete lysis. In **tertiary follicles**, degenerative changes are first observed in the **follicle wall**. Follicular cells increase in size and become detached from the cellular stratum. Disintegrating cells enter the follicular fluid, which also becomes partly vascularised. Breakdown of the oocyte occurs as a secondary process. Morphologically, atretic follicles are characterised by shrinking and condensation of the nucleus, and hyalinisation of the basal lamina.

Ovulation

Ovulation involves **rupture of the mature follicle** and **release of the oocyte**. This process is brought about primarily by hormonally mediated changes in the microvasculature and enzymatic lysis of loose connective tissue at the **predetermined site of follicular rupture** (**stigma folliculare**) (Figure 14.11).

Rupture of the follicle wall is preceded by a brief period of hyperaemia and subsequent **narrowing of the capillaries of the theca interna**. Interruption of the blood supply to the stigma is followed by **complete degeneration of the capillary network**. This is accompanied by **enzymatic breakdown** (collagenases, proteases) of the tunica albuginea and the theca, and a reduction in the number of follicular cells. Breakdown of the follicle wall is mediated by hormones, primarily luteinising hormone (LH), oestrogens and prostaglandins (PGE_2 and $PGF_{2\alpha}$). Fragmentation of cellular and fibrous components of the follicle wall results in leucocyte activation and histamine release.

Rupture occurs roughly at the middle of the stigma. The **oocyte**, surrounded by the **zona pellucida**, **cells** of the **corona radiata** and a few additional follicular cells (Figure 14.10), is flushed from the follicle within the follicular fluid and taken up into the infundibulum of the uterine tube. In the **cow**, the oocyte is released **together with the zona pellucida**, but without follicular cells. The wall of the follicle collapses and becomes folded, partially sealing the rent in the stigma.

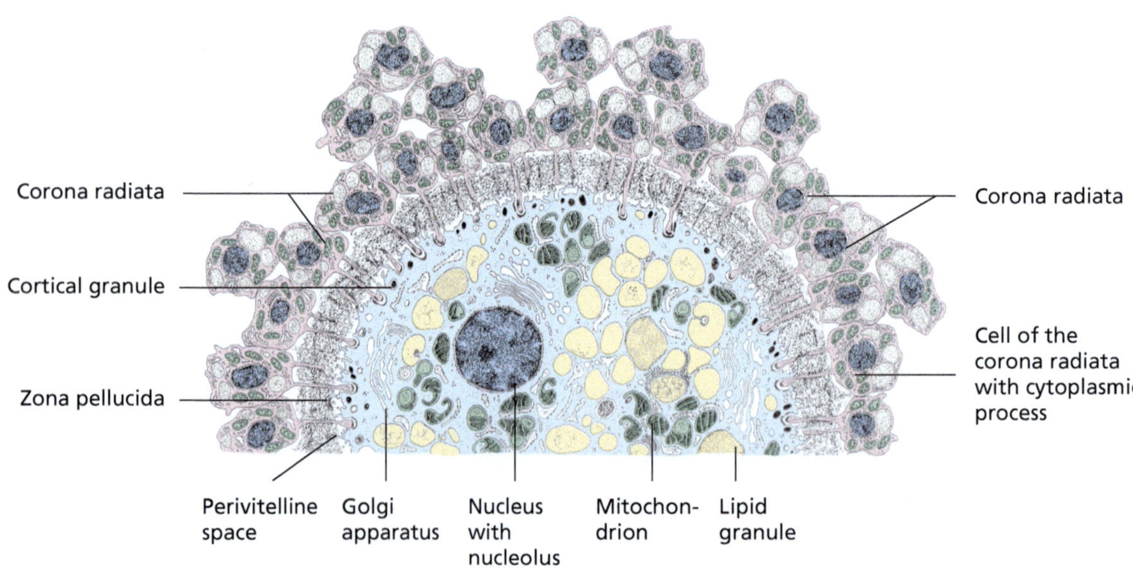

14.10 Structure of the postovulatory oocyte of the ewe (schematic; adapted from Rüsse, 1983).

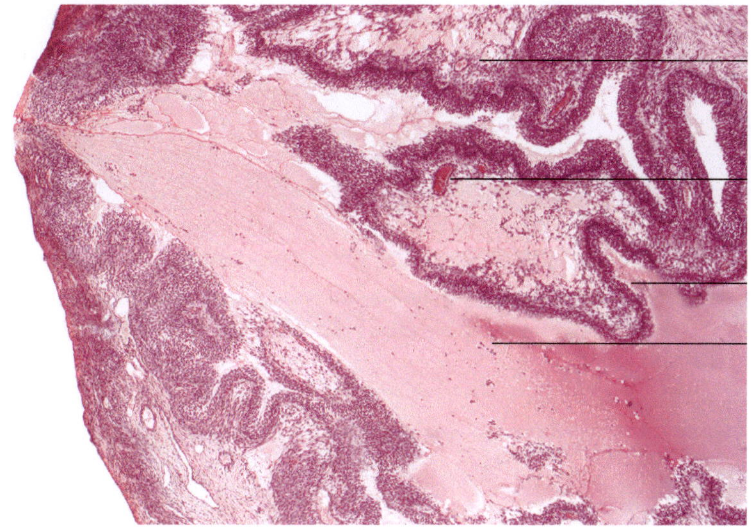

14.11 Stigma following rupture of the follicle with folding and fragmentation of the follicle wall. Haematoxylin and eosin stain (x14).

CORPUS LUTEUM

The corpus luteum (Figures 14.12 to 14.14) is a **transient endocrine gland** that forms after ovulation from the remaining cells of the follicle wall and stromal cells of the theca. Hormones synthesised by the corpus luteum include **progesterone**, **oestrogens** and possibly **oxytocin**. If **fertilisation** does not occur, the corpus luteum undergoes further development before regressing (**corpus luteum cyclicum**). In the event that fertilisation takes place, the corpus luteum persists for the duration of pregnancy (**corpus luteum graviditatis**). When the corpus luteum regresses, it is replaced by fibrous scar tissue (**corpus albicans**). Development and regression of the corpus luteum involves reorganisation of cellular, vascular and connective tissue of the follicle and surrounding theca.

FORMATION OF THE CORPUS LUTEUM

Formation of the corpus luteum commences with **tearing of the basal lamina** between the basal cells and theca interna. This is followed immediately by ingrowth of capillaries into the avascular follicle wall. Together with hairpin-like arterioles of the theca externa, the capillaries sprout into the former cavity of the follicle.

Species variation

Horse, ox, pig and dog: In the mare, cow, sow and, to a lesser extent, the bitch, the lumen of the postovulatory follicle is filled with serum, coagulated blood and remnants of follicular fluid (**corpus haemorrhagicum**). Vessels growing into the former antrum are accompanied by stromal cells, fibroblasts and macrophages. Within the first 5 days after ovulation, these cells begin to reorganise the corpus haemorrhagicum. Remnants of blood components and follicle fragments are phagocytosed by macrophages. Vascularisation of the interior of the follicle leads to formation of the **corpus luteum**.

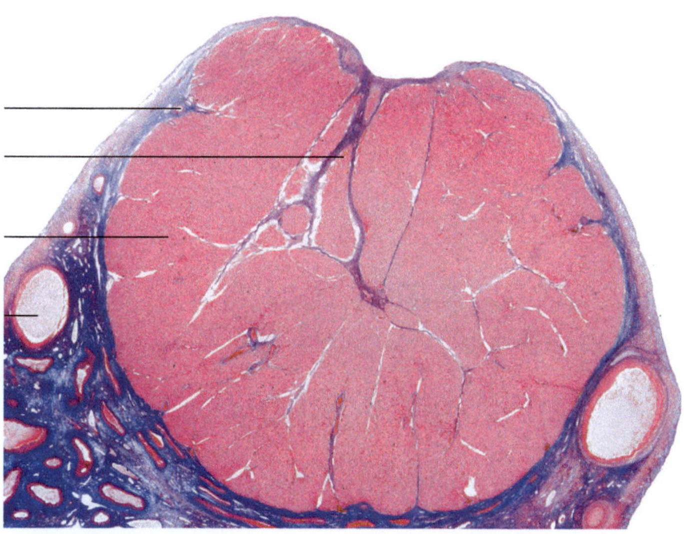

14.12 Corpus luteum (sheep). Azan stain (x15).

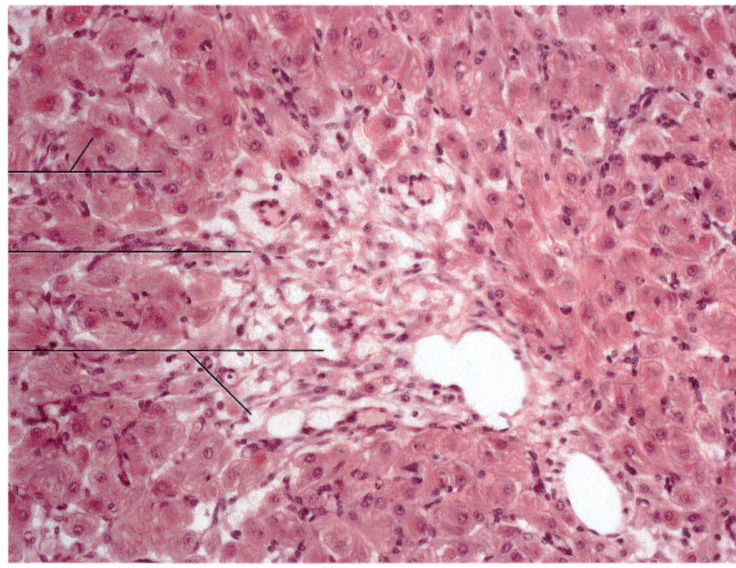

14.13 Developing corpus luteum with budding capillaries (pig). Haematoxylin and eosin stain (x250).

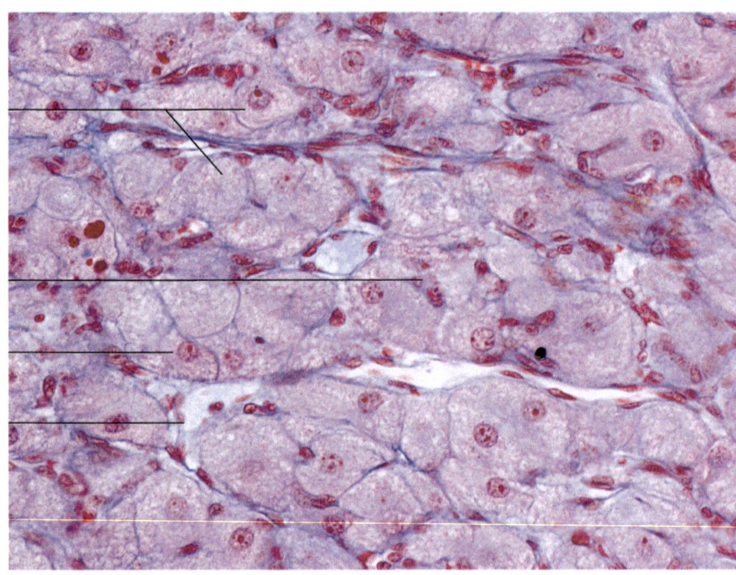

14.14 Corpus luteum (cat). Azan stain (x400).

Changes associated with development of the corpus luteum are first seen in the follicular cells (granulosa cells) and stromal cells of the theca interna in the late preovulatory phase. These become considerably more pronounced after ovulation. Transformation of the follicular and theca cells into luteal cells occurs through functional hypertrophy (increase in the volume of the cytoplasm) and hyperplasia (cell proliferation). Numerous yellow pigments (lipochromes) appear in the cytoplasm (not observed in sows and small ruminants). This process is referred to as luteinisation. There are two types of luteal cells:

- granulosa luteal cells and
- theca luteal cells.

Granulosa luteal cells develop from the cells of the **follicle wall**. These are highly mitotically active and contribute substantially to the size of the corpus luteum. Granulosa luteal cells are polyhedral (diameter 40 μm) with a large, ovoid nucleus. Characteristic features include mitochondria with tubular cristae, smooth endoplasmic reticulum and abundant small lipid inclusions (phospholipids, triglycerides, cholesterol and its esters). These steroid-synthesising organelles primarily produce **progesterone** (also oestrogens and possibly oxytocin).

Theca luteal cells are derived from **stromal cells of the theca interna**. They are smaller (diameter up to 15 μm) and **less numerous** than granulosa luteal cells. Theca luteal cells have a similar function to granulosa luteal cells but contain more lipochromes. In the cow and ewe, theca luteal cells are difficult to distinguish from granulosa luteal cells.

From early in its formation, the corpus luteum is pervaded by a dense **capillary network**. The capillaries and hairpin arteries contribute to **lobulation** of the corpus luteum. Connective tissue septa that subdivide the corpus luteum arise from the theca externa and, to a lesser degree, the theca interna. When the corpus luteum is actively secreting hormones, the capillary loops are in close contact with the luteal cells, facilitating the uptake of progesterone into the blood circulation.

Regression of the corpus luteum

Regression of the corpus luteum is initiated by **prostaglandin** (**PGF$_{2\alpha}$**) secreted by the uterine mucosa. Hypertrophy of blood vessel walls eventually results in blockage of the lumen and degeneration of the capillary network. This is accompanied by an increase in the amount of lipochrome pigments in the luteal cells and merging and enlargement of lipid vacuoles. The luteal cells undergo **fatty degeneration**, with associated karyolysis, and are broken down by macrophages. There is concurrent fibrosis (increase in collagen fibres).

In the ox, **regression** begins from about 15 days after ovulation and becomes more rapid between days 18 and 21. Complete replacement of the corpus luteum with the **corpus albicans** can take considerable time. Thus, a developing corpus luteum may appear alongside structures from previous ovarian cycles. Other changes associated with regression include the appearance of pigments (**corpus nigrescens**) or carotenoids (**corpus rubrum**).

Medulla (medulla ovarii, zona vasculosa)

In most species, the medulla is the **inner portion** of the ovary enclosing blood vessels and nerves. Arteries enter at the hilus and are arranged in coils within the medulla. At the junction with the cortex, they form a plexus that supplies the cortical tissue. These capillary networks are subject to cyclic structural changes regulated by specialised arteries ('barrier arteries') and arteriovenous anastomoses. Medullary lymph vessels and veins leave the ovary at the hilus. Predominantly autonomic nerve fibres innervate the follicles and smooth muscle cells of the blood vessel walls.

Species variation

Ruminants: **Rete ovarii** originating from the mesonephros are commonly present near the hilus. This is observed less frequently in other species. The rete ovarii consists of anastomosing cords and channels. These are composed of epithelium-like cells and are surrounded by a basal lamina.

Horse: In the mare, the cortex lies internally, surrounded by the medulla. Cortical tissue is only present on the surface of the ovary at the **ovulation fossa**.

Ovary of birds

In the juvenile and non-laying mature female chicken, the ovary is a compact, roughly triangular structure, measuring approximately 15–20 × 10 mm and weighing around 0.5 g. Its surface has a finely granular appearance. **During the laying period**, follicular development takes place only in the **left ovary**. Through the enlargement of the follicles,

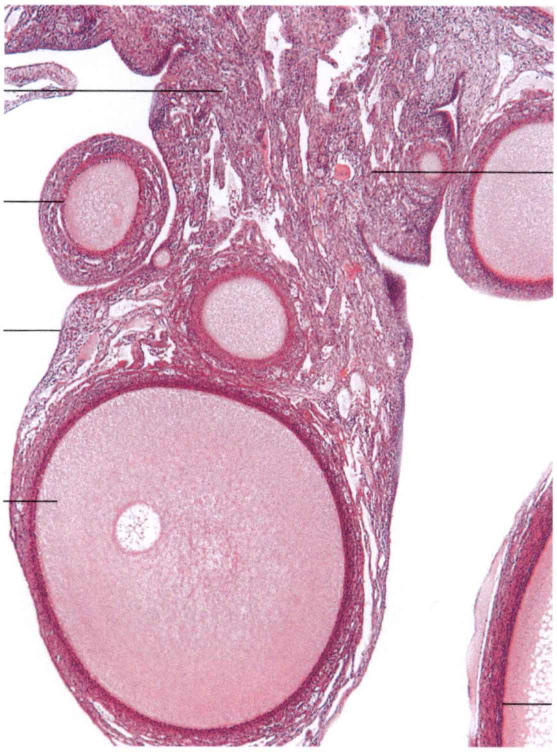

14.15 Ovary (chicken). Haematoxylin and eosin stain (x5).

the ovary increases to a size of 110 × 70 mm and reaches a weight of approximately 60 g.

In the newly hatched chick, the ovary consists of a **cortex** (**cortex ovarii**) and an inner **medulla** (**medulla ovarii**). The cortex contains the ovarian follicles, comprising oocytes surrounded by follicular epithelial cells. At sexual maturity, the macroscopic distinction between the cortex and medulla is lost.

The **mature oocyte of birds** is the **largest female gamete in the animal kingdom** (Figure 14.15). At the preovulatory stage, the surrounding follicular wall consists of several cell layers. The follicle is connected to the ovary by a peduncle containing blood vessels, nerves and smooth muscle. The richly vascularised and innervated follicle wall also contains smooth muscle cells. Positioned meridionally in the follicle is a pale and relatively poorly vascularised region, the **stigma**. Endoscopic visualisation of ovarian follicles can be used for sex determination in monomorphic avian species.

OOGENESIS

Development and maturation of the avian oocyte begins early in embryogenesis. Primordial germ cells migrate from the embryonic yolk sac to the gonadal area and differentiate into **oogonia**. Mitotic division of oogonia gives rise to **primary oocytes**. These remain in the diplotene state of prophase until shortly before ovulation.

During this phase, the oocyte increases in size through the uptake of large amounts of yolk into its cytoplasm (**vitellogenesis**). The gel-like yolk (**vitellus**) consists of lipids and soluble proteins.

Yolk formation takes place in three phases of different length. During the first phase, which may take several years, the oocytes undergo a modest increase in size. In the subsequent phase, the volume of the oocyte grows markedly over a period of 8–10 months (oocyte reaches 4 mm). The third phase is associated with a substantial accumulation of yolk, with the oocyte reaching its typical final size of around 40 mm in the chicken and 20 mm in the pigeon. This stage takes approximately 14 days.

Completion of the **first meiotic division** occurs just a few hours before ovulation, resulting in a **secondary oocyte** and production of the first polar body. An additional division of this polar body has not been observed in birds.

Ovulation occurs under the influence of luteinising hormone. The **secondary oocyte** is released by rupture of the follicular wall along the **stigma**. Spermatozoa, if present, penetrate the oocyte around 15 minutes after ovulation. This is followed, within the infundibulum of the oviduct, by the **second meiotic division** (resulting in a mature female gamete and a second polar body) and **fertilisation**. In contrast to mammals, **polyspermy** (penetration of the oocyte by more than one spermatozoon) may occur but only one spermatozoon fuses with the nucleus of the ovum.

In birds, the female is **heterogametic**. The oocyte contains either a Z or a W chromosome, whereas only the Z chromosome is present in avian spermatozoa. Sex is thus determined **prior to fertilisation**.

Each subsequent ovulation takes place about **half an hour after an egg is laid**. Not all oocytes enter the infundibulum. At the beginning and end of the laying period, some ovulated oocytes pass into the coelomic cavity where they are quickly resorbed. Occasionally these may undergo concretion and persist for some time.

Immediately **after ovulation**, the wall of the follicle regresses. Only an insignificant vestige remains after 6 days and this disappears altogether after 1 month. A corpus luteum resembling that of mammals is **not formed**. **Oestrogens** are produced by endocrine cells of the **theca**, while androgens are synthesised by interstitial cells. It is unclear whether the postovulatory follicle produces progesterone. Oestrogens are responsible for stimulating production of the yolk by the liver. The yolk is transported by the blood stream to the ovarian follicles.

Uterine tube (tuba uterina)

The uterine tube is a paired tubular organ that extends from its opening into the abdomen near the ovary (ostium abdominale) to the horn of the uterus. The internal lining of the uterine tube undergoes cyclic changes that ensure **optimal metabolic conditions** for the oocyte, spermatozoa, zygote and early stages of embryonic development (blastomeres). The uterine tubes contribute to:

- transport of the gametes,
- **final maturation** of the female oocyte (completion of meiosis II upon fertilisation) and
- **final maturation** of the spermatozoa (capacitation).

After fertilisation in the ampulla tubae uterinae (see below), the zygote and developing blastomeres are conveyed by the uterine tubes to the uterus. Throughout this passage, the mucosa of the uterine tube provides nutrition for, and facilitates forward progression of, the embryo. The uterine tube thus plays a **crucial role** in the **reproductive process**.

The initial portion of the uterine tube (**infundibulum tubae uterinae**) gathers up the oocyte with its coating of zona pellucida and (in some species) follicular cells.

Fertilisation takes place in the subsequent segment, the expanded **ampulla tubae uterinae** (Figures 14.16 to 14.18). Folds of varying height and density (longitudinal, secondary and tertiary folds) increase the metabolically active surface area of the mucosa, facilitating the provision of a suitable environment for the gametes. The oocyte inserts itself within mucosal niches where it is nourished by mucosal secretions (see below) for up to 24 hours.

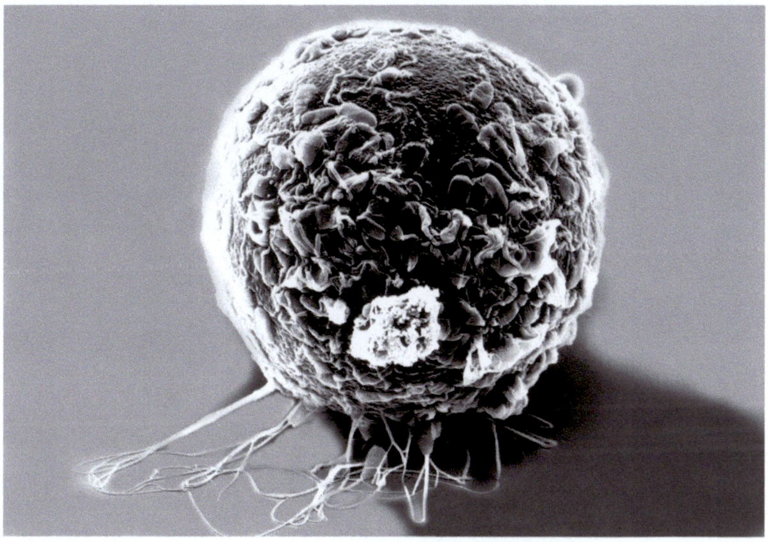

14.16 Scanning electron microscope image of the surface of the oocyte of a cow with spermatozoa.

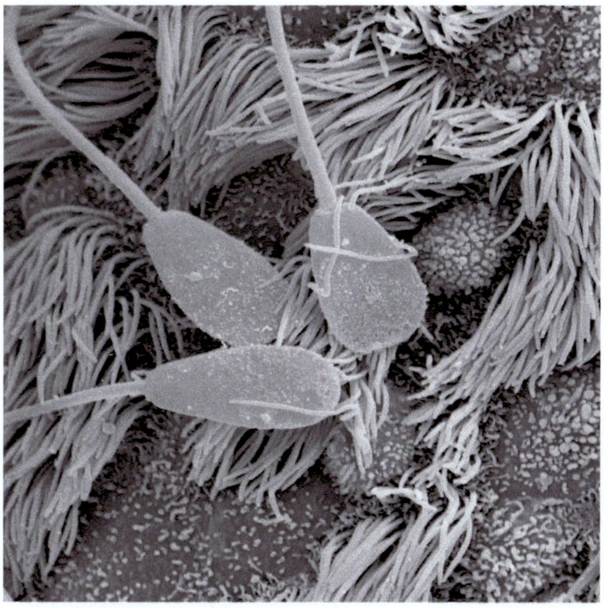

14.17 Scanning electron microscope image of the surface of ciliated epithelial cells of the ampulla tubae uterinae (cow in oestrus; x3200).

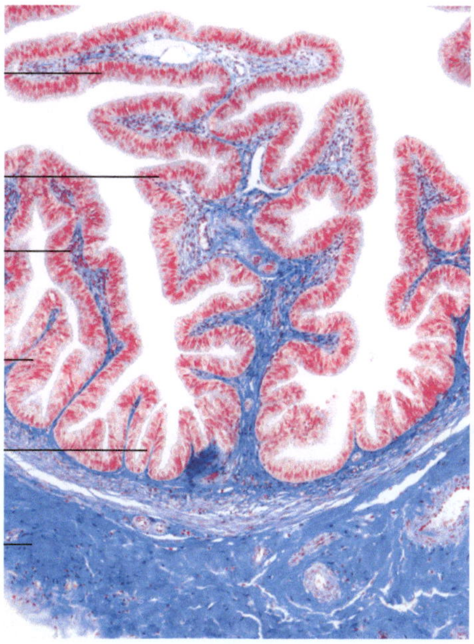

14.18 Mucosal folds in the ampulla of the uterine tube (cat). Azan stain (x40).

The mucosal folds diminish along the length of the narrow terminal section of the uterine tube (**isthmus tubae uterinae**), eventually disappearing before the junction with the uterine mucosa. Concomitantly, the thickness of the muscular tunic increases. Nutritional support for the embryo is provided by increasing volumes of mucus. The role of the zona pellucida is described above under 'Secondary follicles'.

Structure of the uterine tube

The wall of the uterine tube consists of the:

- **tunica mucosa:**
  - ciliated simple or pseudostratified columnar epithelium with secretory cells, peg cells and basal cells,
  - lamina propria mucosae,
- **tunica muscularis:**
  - stratum circulare,
  - stratum longitudinale,
- **tela subserosa and**
- **tunica serosa.**

Tunica mucosa

The tunica mucosa (Figures 14.18 and 14.19) is an important functional component of the uterine tube. It is lined with simple or pseudostratified columnar epithelium containing two main cell types:

- ciliated cells and
- secretory cells.

The **ciliated cells** have motile cilia. Following ovulation, the secondary oocyte enters the ampulla and, in the early phase of metoestrus, is sustained by the products of secretory cells. Flow of fluid towards the uterus establishes 'negative rheotactic' movement of the spermatozoa, promoting their movement towards the ampulla. After fertilisation, the secretory capacity of the epithelium is maintained towards the uterus, ensuring sustained nourishment of the developing embryo.

Rhythmic movement of the cilia facilitates the movement of fluid and, thereby, the progression of the zygote towards the uterus (during gestational dioestrus). Following implantation of the blastocyst in the uterine mucosa, secretion by the cells of the uterine tube is suspended. If pregnancy does not occur, secretory activity resumes in subsequent pro-oestrus and oestrus.

Secretory cells release weakly acidic mucus and nutrients (particularly proteins) that provide support for the gametes. Secretion is by the merocrine mode. In addition, secretory cells produce electrolytes, enzymes, albumins, glucose and amino acids required for final differentiation and maturation of the gametes. Both cell types undergo marked cyclic changes.

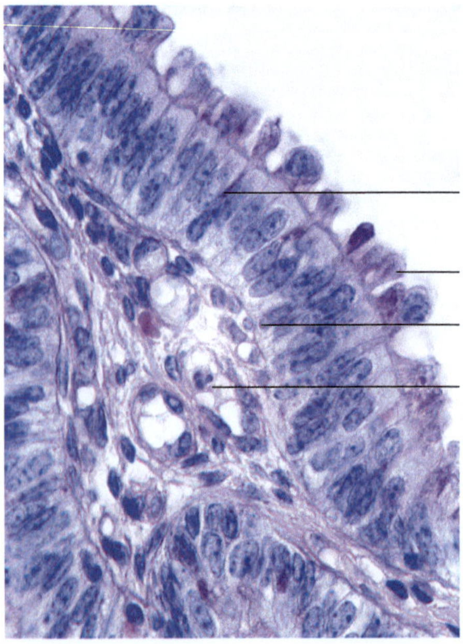

14.19 Primary mucosal fold in the ampulla of the uterine tube (cow; 18 days after implantation). PAS stain (x1000).

The epithelium also contains **peg cells**. These are thought to be cells that have become inactive after a secretory phase, or those that represent a transitional type. They are characterised by a typically pyknotic nucleus and little cytoplasm. **Basal cells** lying close to the basal lamina serve as reserve cells.

Tunica muscularis

The thickness of the tunica muscularis **varies along the length of the uterine tube**. In the infundibulum and ampulla, the smooth muscle layers are thin. Circular and isolated longitudinal or oblique muscle bundles are present without consistently discernible layering. The muscle layer is markedly thicker in the isthmus and the fibre orientation is predominantly oblique. The inner component is continuous with the circular muscle layer of the uterus. Outer longitudinal muscle bundles radiate into the muscle of the tela subserosa of the uterus.

Tela subserosa and tunica serosa

Longitudinal muscle fibres extend through the **tela subserosa** of the isthmus tubae uterinae (lamina muscularis serosae). Blood vessels are present beneath the tela subserosa. A **tunica serosa** surrounds the uterine tube along its entire length.

Uterus

The uterus consists of a **body** (**corpus uteri**) connected to the uterine tubes by the **uterine horns** (**cornua uteri**). The neck of the uterus, or **cervix** (**cervix uteri**), separates the uterine body from the vagina (refer to *Veterinary Anatomy of Domestic Mammals: Textbook and Colour Atlas*). The uterus and cervix are an integrated functional unit, and both are subject to cyclic hormonal influences (refer to endocrinology texts). The various functions of the uterus all serve to support the reproductive process. Cyclic changes in uterine structure (proliferation, secretion, involution) are mediated by **endocrine regulatory mechanisms** and form part of the overall reproductive cycle (see below, under 'Oestrous cycle'; refer also to endocrinology texts).

The surface epithelium and smooth muscle of the uterus facilitate **transport of spermatozoa** towards the **uterine tubes**. This is also influenced by cyclic events. Uterine secretions contribute to **capacitation** (**final maturation**) **of spermatozoa** which enables spermatozoa to penetrate the cells of the corona radiata and the zona pellucida, allowing fertilisation to occur.

The uterus supports the developing embryo and serves to expel the placenta at the end of pregnancy. Cyclic modifications of the uterine mucosa are necessary to provide optimal conditions for implantation and formation of the placenta.

During pregnancy, areas of contact between the uterine mucosa and the fetal membranes develop into the placenta. This is a temporary endocrine gland that produces progesterone for the duration of pregnancy.

The muscle of the uterine wall adapts throughout gestation to the increasing size and weight of the fetus. At the end of pregnancy, wave-like contractions of the musculature bring about fetal expulsion.

The uterine mucosa synthesises prostaglandin ($PGF_{2\alpha}$) which induces lysis of the **corpus luteum**.

Structure of the uterus

The wall of the uterus consists of:

- endometrium (tunica mucosa):
  - simple columnar/pseudostratified columnar, epithelium
  - lamina propria mucosae (stroma endometrialis),
- myometrium (tunica muscularis),
- perimetrium:
  - stratum musculare longitudinale and
  - tela subserosa and tunica serosa.

Endometrium

The mucosa of the endometrium is composed of surface epithelium and a lamina propria mucosae (stroma endometrialis). The lamina propria lies adjacent to the muscular tunic; a distinct tela submucosa is lacking. Both mucosal components experience cyclic structural variations (Figures 14.20 to 14.22).

The **surface epithelium** is simple columnar (epithelium simplex columnare) in the mare and bitch. In ruminants and in the sow, there may be areas of pseudostratified columnar epithelium (epithelium pseudostratificatum columnare). The cells may bear cilia and usually have microvilli (secretory cells). The secretory activity of the epithelial cells is under hormonal control. During the proliferative phase, secretions are given off by the merocrine mode under the influence of oestrogen. Towards the end of the secretory phase the epithelial cells disintegrate and are shed as part of the vaginal discharge.

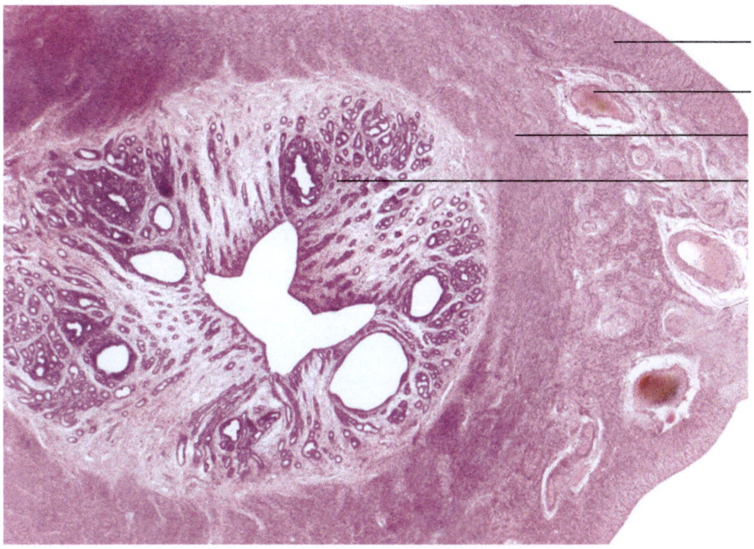

14.20 Low-power view of uterus (cat). Haematoxylin and eosin stain (x20).

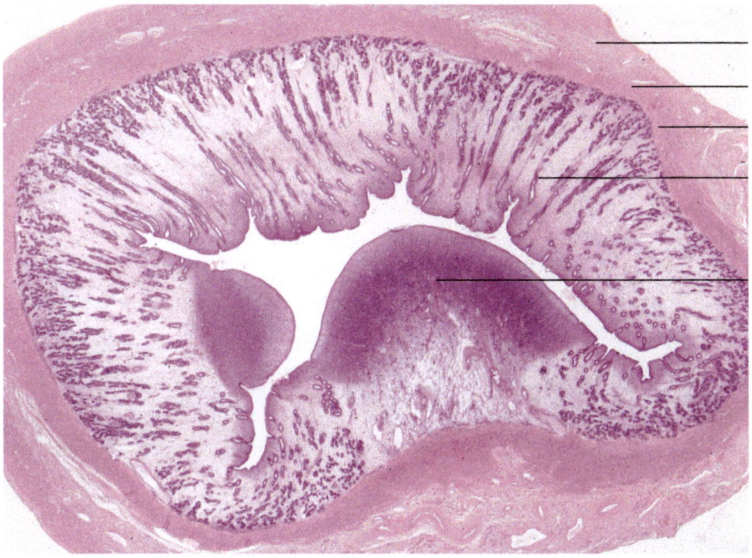

14.21 Low-power view of uterus (sheep). Haematoxylin and eosin stain (x6).

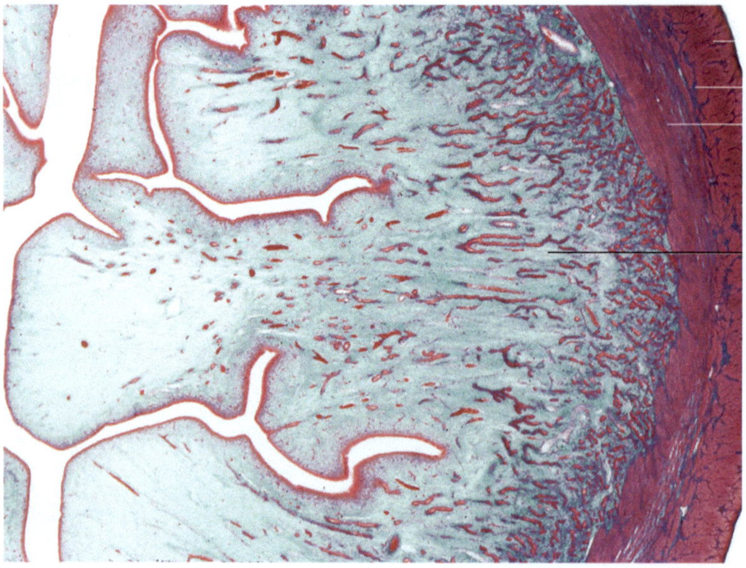

14.22 Low-power view of uterus (pig). Goldner's Masson trichrome stain (x13).

Spinocellular connective tissue forms the structural framework for the lamina propria (stroma endometrialis), which contains a multitude of branched, tubular uterine glands. Terminal portions of the glands may extend into the tunica muscularis. The connective tissue scaffolding has a high capacity for structural and functional adaptation and supports the metabolic role of the uterine mucosa during pregnancy and placental development. This is facilitated by the presence, beneath the epithelium, of cells of the innate and adaptive immune system (macrophages, lymphocytes, plasma cells, mast cells).

All components of the stroma endometrialis – the connective tissue, glands and vessels – exhibit cyclic morphological variation.

During the **proliferation phase** (pro-oestrus, oestrus), when the hormonal milieu is dominated by oestrogen, the uterine glands are elongated. The gland lumina are narrowed and epithelial cells are numerous. The intercellular spaces expand; they contain interstitial fluid and are densely vascularised. Production of collagen fibres by the cells of the spinocellular connective tissue increases. As ovulation approaches, high oestrogen levels cause the tissue to swell through uptake of intercellular fluid. The entire mucosa thickens. Towards the end of the proliferation phase, high molecular weight ground substance components are broken down into smaller molecules and the tissue becomes oedematous. The microvasculature increases.

In the **secretory phase**, under the influence of **progesterone** produced by the corpus luteum, the uterine glands become shortened and tightly coiled. The lumina of the glands expand and fill with secretion. The cells of the simple cuboidal glandular epithelium bulge into the lumen. Their secretory product is mucoid. Branching of the tubular glands is less apparent in bitches and queens than in mares.

> **Species variation**
>
> **Ruminants**: Knob-like elevations of the lamina propria, termed **caruncles**, are present in the cow. Similar structures are present in the ewe but have a concave central depression. The spinocellular connective tissue that forms the structural core of the caruncles (Figure 14.21) contains numerous fibroblasts and blood vessels. There are no glands in the caruncles. In the cow, caruncles are arranged in four rows. Caruncles form the maternal mucosal attachment site for the **cotyledons** of the fetal membranes. Together, the caruncles and cotyledons form the **placentome**.

Myometrium

The tunica muscularis consists of **smooth muscle fibre bundles** that continue from the muscular layer of the uterine tube and extend into the wall of the cervix (Figure 14.20). In the body and horns of the uterus, the muscle layer is **circular** (**stratum circulare**) with predominantly spiralling fibres that cross over one another. In addition to smooth muscle fibres, the outer muscle layer contains modified fibroblasts (contractile myofibroblasts) that support the smooth muscle layers. Particularly during pregnancy, these transform into muscle cells. After parturition they regress and synthesise collagen fibres.

During gestation, the smooth muscle cells adapt to the changing demands of the fetus. The amount of muscle increases through **hypertrophy** (expansion of the sarcoplasm) and **hyperplasia** (cell proliferation). Smooth muscle cells may reach 800 μm in length. The circular-spiral muscle layer is surrounded by a prominent **vascular layer** (**stratum vasculosum**) containing substantial arteries, veins and lymph vessels (Figures 14.20 to 14.22). Vessels and accompanying nerve fibres (myelinated and non-myelinated) extend from the stratum vasculosum into the endometrium to supply the glands and the epithelium.

Perimetrium

The perimetrium surrounds the myometrium. It consists of an outer **tunica serosa**, comprising a single layer of mesothelium, underlaid by a **tela subserosa** and a well-developed layer of longitudinally oriented smooth muscle fibres (**stratum musculare longitudinale**). The muscle radiates into the broad ligament of the uterus and is continuous with the muscle of the cervix.

Cervix (cervix uteri)

The cervix is the distal continuation of the body of the uterus. To perform its functions, the cervix must open temporarily and close again. Dilation of the cervix during oestrus facilitates the passage of spermatozoa to the uterine tubes. Considerable amounts of mucus are produced at this time. The cervix closes during dioestrus (**corpus luteum cyclicum** and **corpus luteum graviditatis**) under the influence of progesterone. A mucous seal forms at its distal end, providing additional protection against entry by spermatozoa and foreign agents (e.g. bacteria). During parturition, the cervix dilates markedly to allow the passage of the fetus. The structure of the cervix includes special features that accommodate these diverse functions.

The cervix is composed of **layers**. These are thick in ruminants (Figures 14.23 and 14.24), and relatively thin in the pig.

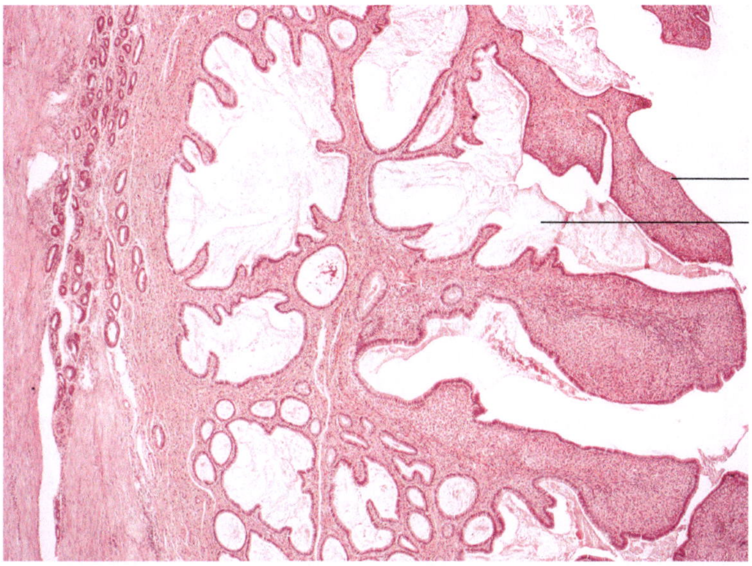

14.23 Low-power view of cervix (cow). Haematoxylin and eosin stain (x15).

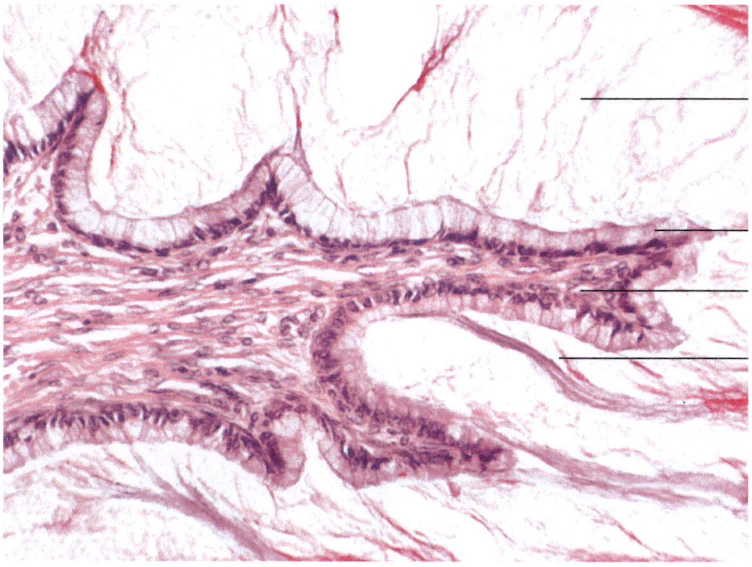

14.24 Mucosal fold of cervix (cow). Mucus production by the columnar epithelium varies throughout the oestrous cycle. Haematoxylin and eosin stain (x275).

The **mucosa-submucosa** is thrown into primary **folds** with secondary and tertiary folds. The arrangement of the connective tissue fibres in the folds allows them to flatten out during parturition. In addition, the folds enlarge the secretory surface area and reinforce the seal formed by the closed cervix (refer to *Veterinary Anatomy of Domestic Mammals: Textbook and Colour Atlas*).

The **mucosal epithelium** is simple **columnar**. It contains cells that produce **mucus** composed of acid and neutral proteoglycans. Ciliated cells also occur in isolated areas in the cow. The mucus-secreting cells are concentrated on the sides and ridges of the mucosal folds (Figure 14.24). In the presence of high progesterone levels (dioestrus), the mucus thickens to form a seal. Under the influence of oestrogen it becomes thin.

In actively secreting cells, the supranuclear region bulges towards the lumen. During oestrus the cells become smaller.

The **lamina propria mucosae** consists of loose connective tissue that becomes highly oedematous under the influence of oestrogen. Lattices of dense connective tissue fibre bundles form the core of the cervical folds. Networks of branching fibres extend between the externally adjacent muscle cells.

Species variation

Cat and goat: While the lamina propria contains no glands in most species, tubular cervical glands may be present in the queen and doe.

The **tunica muscularis** consists of a thick inner circular layer and a thinner outer longitudinal layer. The circular layer incorporates elastic fibres that aid in closing the cervix after passage of the fetus.

Vagina

The vagina and vestibule form the female copulatory organ. In ruminants, the ejaculate is deposited in the vagina. In other species the seminal plasma and spermatozoa are ejaculated into the uterus (horse, dog) or cervix (pig). The structure of the vaginal wall varies with species and, in some instances, exhibits marked cyclic changes. Except during mating and parturition, the lumen of this musculomembranous tubular organ is reduced to a potential space.

Structure of the vagina

The vagina has a typical layered structure comprised of the:

- tunica mucosa:
  - stratified squamous epithelium,
  - lamina propria mucosae with loose connective tissue,
- tunica muscularis incorporating:
  - smooth muscle cells,
  - elastic fibres and
- tunica adventitia or tunica serosa.

Tunica mucosa

The **tunica mucosa** is mostly non-glandular and has flat longitudinal folds that quickly disappear when the mucosa is distended. The epithelium is **stratified squamous** and, depending on species, may be **keratinised**.

Species variation

Ox: Columnar mucus-producing cells are present in the mucosal folds, particularly near the cervix.

Dog: Solitary intra-epithelial secretory cells may be present during oestrus.

In the bitch, cyclic changes in the vaginal epithelium can be used to **determine the stage of the oestrous cycle**. During **pro-oestrus** and oestrus the epithelium thickens, surface cells become keratinised and the cell nuclei become pyknotic and gradually disappear. Erythrocytes from the underlying connective tissue traverse the epithelium via diapedesis and enter the vaginal lumen. During **oestrus** the epithelial cells become completely keratinised and anuclear, and the number of free erythrocytes decreases. The epithelial lining becomes disrupted and superficial cells disintegrate. In the subsequent, longer phase of the oestrous cycle, **metoestrus**, the epithelium continues to thin through **desquamation** and new, non-keratinised cells form the surface layer. Neutrophils enter the epithelium, and erythrocytes and cell fragments disappear.

The connective tissue framework of the **lamina propria mucosae** consists of an array of collagen fibres. With the aid of elastic fibre bundles, this arrangement of fibres allows the vagina to expand and contract during and after parturition. Depending on the stage of the cycle, this subepithelial tissue contains leucocytes and plasma cells. Particularly during pro-oestrus and oestrus these are found in the cervical mucus.

Tunica muscularis

The inner layer of the **tunica muscularis** consists of smooth muscle cells in a circular orientation. This layer is surrounded by longitudinal muscle fibres. The muscle cell layers are connected by a network of collagen and elastic fibres that supports the mechanical strength, plasticity and contractility of the vaginal wall.

Tunica serosa and tunica adventitia

Within the peritoneal cavity, the vagina is surrounded by a loose **tunica serosa**. This is replaced by a **tunica adventitia** over the retroperitoneal portion of the organ (Figure 14.25).

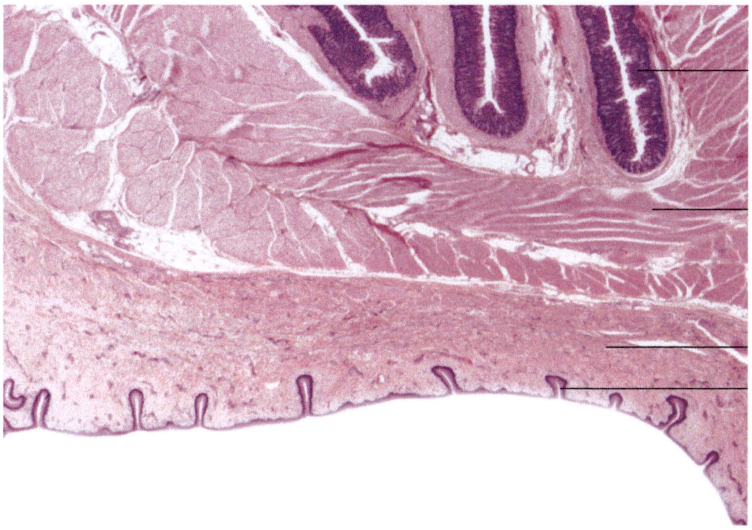

14.25 Low-power view of the dorsal wall of the vagina (sheep). Haematoxylin and eosin stain (x9).

Vulva

The vulva consists of the:

- vestibule (vestibulum vaginae):
  - non-keratinised stratified squamous epithelium,
  - vestibular glands (glandulae vestibulares),
- labia (labia vulvae) and
- clitoris.

As the caudal continuation of the vagina, the **vestibule** forms part of the copulatory organ and the birth canal. It is also a component of the urinary tract, as the urethra opens into the floor of the vestibule. The epithelium is **non-keratinised stratified squamous** and contains numerous subepithelial lymphocytic infiltrates. The extensively papillated epithelium rests upon loose connective tissue incorporating elastic fibres. Papillation lends strength to the surface layer. **Vestibular glands** (**glandulae vestibulares**) are located beneath the epithelium. The thick mucous secretions of these branched, tubular glands serve to lubricate the copulatory organ.

Species variation

Dog, pig, sheep and horse: Minor vestibular glands (glandulae vestibulares minores) are present in the bitch, sow, ewe and mare.

Ox and cat: These species have compound major vestibular glands (glandulae vestibulares majores).

The **musculature** of the vestibule is a continuation of the smooth muscle of the vagina. The outer layers are interspersed with striated muscle fibres of the mm. constrictores vestibuli.

A small portion of the **labia vulvae** is lined with non-glandular mucosa (stratified squamous epithelium). The bulk of the labia is covered by external skin (integumentum commune) containing sweat glands and sebaceous glands. Bundles of smooth and striated muscle fibres are found deep within the connective tissue (collagen and elastic fibres) that forms the core of the labia.

The **clitoris** consists of the two crura clitoridis, the corpus clitoridis containing the corpus cavernosum clitoridis and the glans clitoridis. It contains numerous free nerve endings and sensory receptors (end-bulbs of Krause, genital corpuscles).

Species variation

Horse: The erectile tissue of the clitoris is particularly well developed in the mare. It incorporates smooth muscle cells. The glans clitoridis contains cavernous tissue.

Ruminants and pig: Erectile tissue is sparsely developed.

Dog: As in the horse, the glans clitoridis has a cavernous structure. In other species the glans is composed of loosely organised, extensively vascular tissue.

Oestrous cycle

In sexually mature females, the reproductive organs are subject to cyclic hormonal influences that bring about changes in the structure and function of individual segments of the genital tract (**oestrous cycle**). The ovaries are stimulated to produce mature follicles and the uterine mucosa is prepared for the transport of spermatozoa and potential implantation of a blastocyst. Cyclic modifications also occur in the uterine tubes, cervix and vagina. In addition, hormones regulate the receptiveness of the female to the male (e.g. standing reflex, increased arousal, agitation). Clinically, the onset of oestrus is signalled by changes in the external genitalia (e.g. swelling of the vulva).

All cyclic changes in the reproductive organs are regulated by the hypothalamus and the hypophysis (see Chapter

9, 'Endocrine System'). Neurosecretory cells located in hypothalamic nuclei periodically secrete releasing and inhibiting hormones that are transported by the hypophyseal portal system to the adenohypophysis, where they stimulate or inhibit the release of gonadotrophic hormones.

Ovarian function is regulated by the **gonadotropins** follicle-stimulating hormone (FSH), luteinising hormone (LH) and prolactin. Luteinising hormone stimulates the production of androgens (testosterone, androstenedione) by thecal cells. Follicle-stimulating hormone activates the aromatase enzyme system of the granulosa cells for conversion of androgens to oestrogens. The ratio of FSH:LH determines the timing of ovulation. Production of progesterone by the corpus luteum is mediated by prolactin. Feedback loops regulate the release of gonadotropins from the adenohypophysis.

The **oestrous cycle** is divided into the following phases:

- pro-oestrus,
- oestrus,
- metoestrus and
- dioestrus.

In theriogenology, metoestrus, dioestrus and pro-oestrus are also combined under the term **interoestrus**, representing the period between oestrous phases of the cycle. Anoestrus, the period in which oestrus does not occur, is observed in monoestrous species (bitch, see below) at the end of a prolonged metoestrus, or after conception.

Division of the oestrous cycle into phases is based on **structural changes** in the reproductive organs and associated fluctuations in circulating hormone concentrations. Cyclic changes in FSH, oestrogens, progesterone, LH and prolactin vary among species. Hormone levels measured in the blood do not necessarily indicate the **sensitivity of hormone receptors** on the target cells (refer to veterinary endocrinology and physiology texts).

The **length** of the oestrous cycle varies considerably among domestic mammals. Based on **cycle frequency**, a distinction is made between:

- polyoestrous species (e.g. mare, cow, sow) and
- monoestrous species (e.g. bitch).

In monoestrous animals, an extended period of metoestrus (50–70 days) is followed by anoestrus. In polyoestrous species, the corpus luteum regresses and the animal enters pro-oestrus and then oestrus (see endocrinology and theriogenology texts).

Cyclic changes in the ovary

During **pro-oestrus**, release of FSH from the adenohypophysis brings about follicular maturation. Oestrogen secretion increases.

In the **oestrous** phase, the follicle develops to full maturity and blood oestrogen levels peak. Levels of LH rise rapidly while FSH secretion begins to decline. In most species, a surge in LH is followed by ovulation (**spontaneous ovulation**). Ovulation in cats occurs in response to mating (**induced ovulation**). Depending on species, ovulation occurs at the end of oestrus or at various timepoints during metoestrus.

In **metoestrus**, the corpus haemorrhagicum transforms into the corpus luteum, which begins to synthesise progesterone.

The corpus luteum reaches maximum activity in **dioestrus**. Regression of the corpus luteum is triggered by prostaglandins ($PGF_{2\alpha}$) produced by the uterine mucosa (corpus luteum cyclicum). If conception occurs, progesterone production is maintained (corpus luteum graviditatis) and prostaglandin-induced retrogression of the corpus luteum is delayed until the end of pregnancy. Regression is followed by development of the **corpus albicans**.

Hormonal effects on the uterine tubes

The uterine tubes are quiescent in **pro-oestrus**. During **oestrus**, rising **oestrogen levels** lead to increased activity of the secretory epithelial cells.

The greatest volumes of secretion are produced during **metoestrus** when the oocyte is in the ampulla tubae uterinae. This is accompanied by increased beating of the cilia.

In the subsequent phase, **dioestrus**, the activity of the uterine tube epithelium rapidly declines. The cells become shorter and partly degenerate.

Cyclic changes in the uterus

During **pro-oestrus**, the uterine epithelium grows, the glands enlarge but remain straight and vascularisation increases (**proliferative phase**).

Uterine changes reach their peak during **oestrus**. Under the influence of oestrogen, epithelial cells and uterine glands release secretions (**uterine milk**), the spinocellular subepithelial connective tissue thickens and intercellular spaces become expanded and oedematous.

Hyperplasia of the uterine glands continues into **metoestrus**. During this phase, the connective tissue layer thins and oedema decreases.

In **dioestrus**, the glands become extensively coiled and shortened. Progesterone brings about maximal glandular secretion, which is sustained if pregnancy occurs. If implantation does not take place, secretory activity gradually decreases, the blood supply decreases and the glands revert to their tubular morphology (**involution**).

Changes in the **cervix** are closely linked with those occurring in the uterus. Under the influence of oestrogens, the cervical epithelium secretes increasing amounts of thin, clear **mucus**. During dioestrus, the mucus becomes more viscous.

Oviduct of birds

The oviduct of birds incorporates the organs responsible for transport of eggs and formation of the egg shell (Figures 14.26 to 14.30):

- infundibulum,
- magnum,
- isthmus,
- uterus and
- vagina.

Structure

In common with other hollow organs, the wall of the oviduct, from interior to exterior, comprises the:

- tunica mucosa:
  - epithelium mucosae,
  - lamina propria mucosae,
- tela submucosa,
- tunica muscularis:
  - stratum circulare,

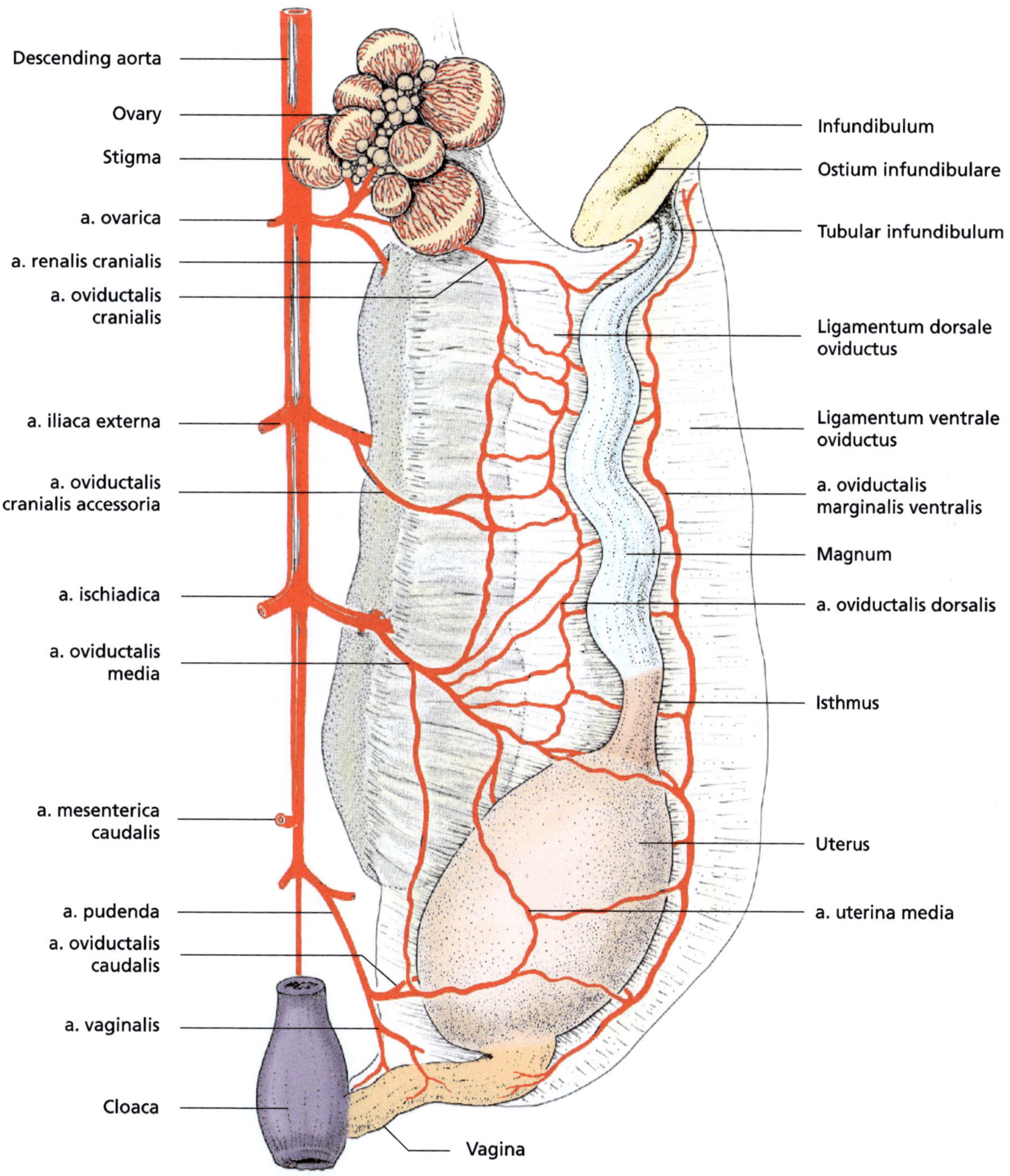

14.26 Ovary and segments of the oviduct of the hen with vascular supply (schematic; ventral view; König and Liebich, 2009).

  - stratum longitudinale,
- tunica serosa:
  - epithelium serosae and
  - lamina propria serosae.

The **epithelium mucosae** is initially simple and flat, then transitions through cuboidal to pseudostratified columnar. The columnar cells consist of intra-epithelial gland cells, ciliated surface cells and basal cells. The distal segments contain regions of pseudostratified columnar epithelium that subsequently become reduced in thickness.

The **lamina propria mucosae** contains glands along most of its length. These vary considerably in structure, number and density in different segments of the oviduct.

Mucosal folds are present to a greater or lesser degree throughout the oviduct. The height and thickness of the folds vary from one segment of the oviduct to another (Figures 14.27 to 14.29). The arrangement of the folds in a gentle spiral causes the egg to turn slowly around its longitudinal axis as it travels through the oviduct.

The circular and longitudinal muscle layers of the **tunica muscularis** bring about peristaltic contractions that assist in transporting the egg, and antiperistaltic contractions that facilitate swift passage of spermatozoa.

Infundibulum

The infundibulum (Figures 14.26 and 14.27) consists of a **funnel-shaped** proximal section and a **tubular** distal portion. Its **opening** (**ostium infundibulare**) is approximately 80 mm wide and has relatively few **fimbriae** (**fimbriae infundibulares**). The thin wall of the funnel is thrown into shallow primary and secondary folds. Initially the infundibulum is **non-glandular** (Figure 14.27). Towards the caudal portion of the funnel, alveolar invaginations (**fossae glandulares infundibuli**) appear in the lamina propria.

In the subsequent tubular segment, these infundibular glands increase in size and complexity forming **glandulae tubi infundibulares**. These produce a protein-rich secretion that surrounds the oocyte.

The wall of the funnel contains smooth muscle, giving it contractile properties that aid in the uptake of oocytes after ovulation. In the **tubular section**, the wall of the infundibulum is thicker and features more prominent primary and secondary folds. **Fertilisation** of the oocyte by spermatozoa occurs in this tubular portion.

Transit of the egg through the infundibulum takes around 15–20 minutes. During its passage, the egg becomes surrounded by **glycoproteins** secreted by the glands. These form the **inner dense layer of albumen** which later gives rise to the twisted **chalazae** that suspend the yolk as it rotates about its longitudinal axis.

Magnum

The magnum is the longest segment of the oviduct. In the chicken, it reaches 34 cm. The magnum follows a looping course, resembling that of the jejunum. Within this segment, the epithelium transitions from pseudostratified columnar to a single layer of mostly columnar cells (Figures 14.26 and 14.28). The mucosa is arranged in **folds** up to 22 mm high (there are **no secondary** folds). The lamina propria of the mucosal folds contains coiled **tubular glands** (**glandulae magni**), forming a **substantial secretory apparatus**. The glands produce ovalbumin,

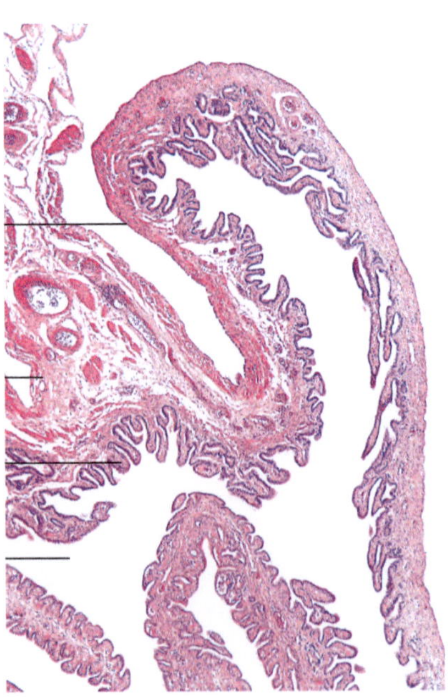

14.27 Infundibulum of the uterine tube (hen). Haematoxylin and eosin stain (x120).

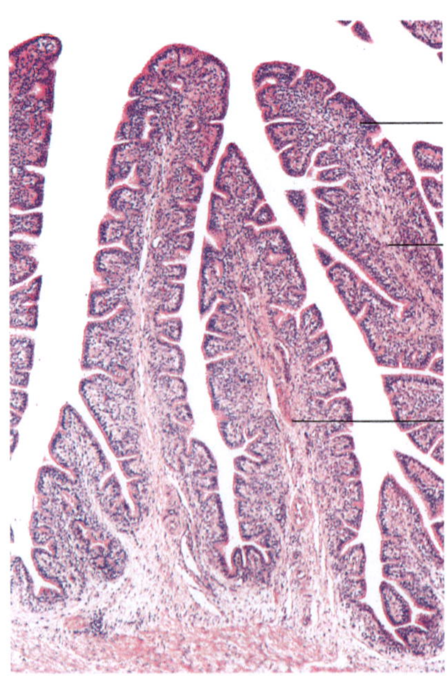

14.28 Magnum of the oviduct (hen). Haematoxylin and eosin stain (x300).

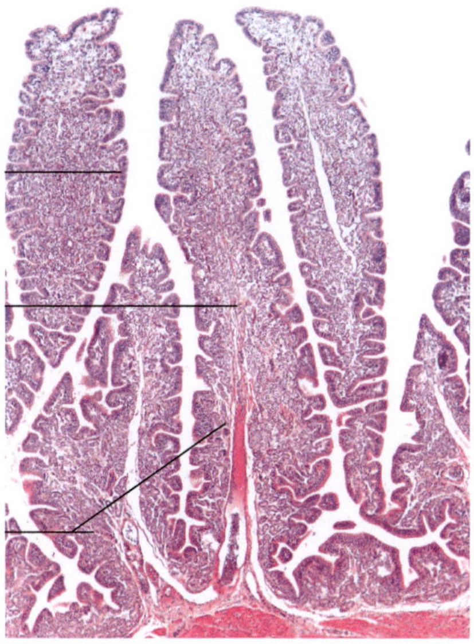

14.29 Isthmus of the oviduct (hen). Haematoxylin and eosin stain (x300).

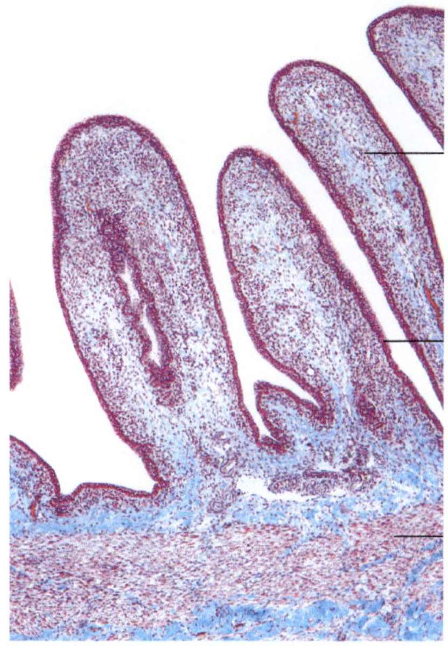

14.30 Uterus (hen). Haematoxylin and eosin stain (x240).

ovotransferrin and ovomucoid. These proteins form the **main component of albumen** (**egg white**), to which water is added in the uterus. The time spent by the egg in the magnum is approximately 3 hours.

Isthmus

The isthmus is approximately 10 cm long (Figures 14.26 and 14.29). The beginning of the isthmus is marked by the translucent, non-glandular **pars translucens isthmi**, in which the mucosa is devoid of folds. The epithelium is simple columnar.

Further distally, the mucosa becomes thicker, is thrown into folds and contains numerous **tubular glands** (**glandulae isthmi**) (Figure 14.29). The mucosal folds are shallower than those of the magnum and are endowed with secondary folds.

The egg passes through the isthmus in around 1.5 hours. The glands of the isthmus resemble those of the magnum. Their sulfur-containing secretion, which is unique to this segment of the oviduct, forms the **inner and outer shell membranes** that surround the albumen. The **air cell** later forms in the space between these membranes, at the blunt end of the egg. More albumen is also added in the isthmus.

Uterus

The uterus is sometimes also referred to as the '**shell gland**'. It continues from the isthmus **with no clearly visible demarcation**. The uterus is 8 cm long. Initially tubular, the uterus expands into a pouch-like portion. The muscular tunic is well developed. Longitudinal mucosal folds are intersected by circular folds, giving rise to leaf-like lamellae (Figure 14.30).

The branched tubular **uterine glands** (**glandulae uterinae**) are similar to those of the isthmus, though they are packed more tightly within the lamina propria. The final component of the albumen is laid down in the uterus and a large amount of water is added, 'plumping up' the egg white.

The egg spends around 20 hours in the uterus. Most of this time is occupied by formation of the **calcareous shell**.

The organic matrix of the shell is produced from secretions of the columnar epithelial cells.

The thin, organic outermost layer of the egg, known as the **cuticle**, is also derived from the uterus.

Vagina

At the junction between the uterus and the vagina, the circular muscle thickens to form the **m. sphincter vaginae**. The vagina is approximately 8 cm long, has a well-developed muscular tunic and is folded upon itself into a sigmoid shape.

The vaginal mucosa has a ciliated pseudostratified epithelium and is arranged in narrow primary and secondary folds. Near the m. sphincter vaginae the lamina propria contains the branching **tubular utero-vaginal sperm host glands** (**fossulae spermatici** or **tubulae spermatici**) that serve as storage sites for spermatozoa. These reservoirs are remarkable in that they can house viable spermatozoa for some weeks, allowing a female chicken to lay a fertilised egg for **up to 2 weeks after copulation**. Passage of the egg through the vagina takes 5–10 minutes.

15

Common integument (integumentum commune)

The common integument constitutes the external surface of the body. It protects the animal from the environment while also presenting a large surface area over which interactions with the exterior can occur. These roles are supported by other sensory and regulatory organs; in this capacity, the nervous system (via sensory organs) and the immune system (via innate and adaptive immune cell populations) are significant components of the skin.

The common integument has **numerous functions**. It forms a **protective barrier** against mechanical, thermal, chemical and biological influences and prevents dehydration. By means of its well-developed vascular supply, the common integument contributes to **thermo-** and **hydroregulation**. Skin glands have multiple functions that are under autonomic control. Fat deposits in the subcutaneous tissue serve as **energy stores** and participate in thermoregulation and mechanical cushioning. As indicated above, the skin also serves as a **sensory organ** and as an **immunoprotective layer**.

The **external layer of the skin**, the **epidermis**, incorporates several **modifications**. Epithelial cells differentiate through various stages into **hair** or, with extensive keratinisation, into the cornified layer of the **hoof**, **nail**, **claw** and **horn**. In the deeper layers of the skin, epithelial cells undergo transformation to form **skin glands** (sweat and sebaceous glands). In specific locations, further modification of apocrine sweat glands gives rise to the **mammary glands**. These specialisations of the epidermis are accompanied by structural changes in the deeper layers of the skin (Figure 15.1).

The structure of the skin varies with species and with body region. Various factors (e.g. external mechanical or thermal insult) bring about adaptations in skin thickness, hair cover or the number and distribution of skin glands. The epidermis is thin in regions with a thick hair coat, becoming thicker in areas in which hair is sparse or absent.

Structure of the skin

While it performs a diverse range of functions, and exhibits its regional structural modifications, the basic structure of the common integument is consistent, comprising the following layers:

- **cutis:**
  - epidermis (epithelial layer),
  - dermis (corium) and
- **subcutis (tela subcutanea).**

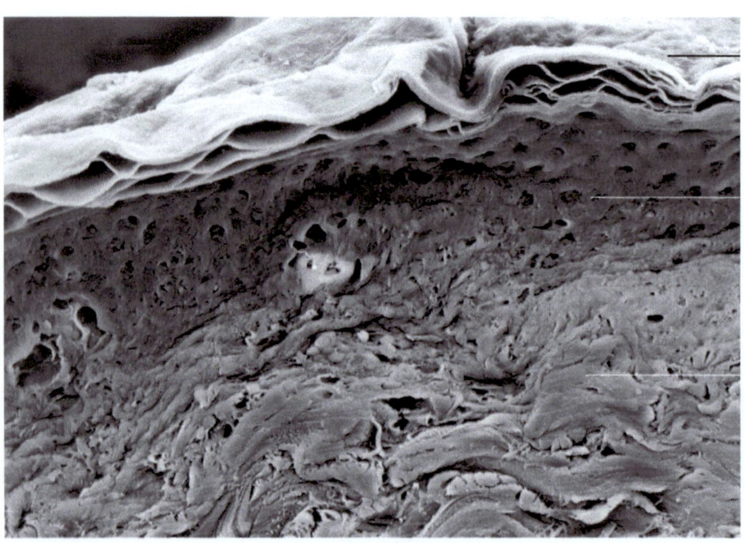

15.1 Scanning electron microscope image of the layers of the skin (cut surface) (pig; x30).

In a stricter sense, the epidermis and dermis may be considered to constitute the skin, which is underlaid by the **subcutis**. The layers of the skin are further subdivided as follows:

- **epidermis:**
  - stratum corneum (keratinised layer),
  - stratum lucidum (eleidin layer),
  - stratum granulosum (formation of keratohyalin granules),
  - stratum spinosum (keratinocytes),
  - stratum basale (keratinocytes),
- **dermis (corium):**
  - stratum papillare and
  - stratum reticulare.

Skin as a protective organ

Epidermis

As the most superficial layer of the skin, the epidermis protects the organism against damage caused by mechanical, thermal, chemical and biological influences (Figures 15.2 to 15.8). It consists of **stratified squamous epithelium** that exhibits regional variation in cornification, as determined by prevailing mechanical forces (see also Chapter 2, 'Epithelial tissue'). Approximately 85% of the cells of the epidermis are keratinocytes that move from the base to the surface of the epithelium. As they progress to the surface, the cells undergo **multiple stages of differentiation** associated with the process of **keratinisation**, culminating in the formation of dead, keratinised cells.

The various layers each perform important functions in the continuous process of formation, keratinisation and ultimately removal (desquamation) of keratinocytes. The **stratum basale** serves as a germinal layer in which new keratinocytes are constantly produced. For this reason, it is also referred to as the **stratum germinativum**. The newly formed cells move into the **stratum spinosum** (Figure 15.3), where changes associated with keratinisation begin to occur. Keratinisation takes place in the transition from the **stratum granulosum** to (in some cases) the **stratum lucidum** and to the **stratum corneum**. In the stratum corneum, the keratinocytes are packed together to form a dense cornified band that serves as the protective epidermal barrier of the skin.

The **stratum basale** consists of a single layer of cuboidal to columnar cells that rests on a basal lamina. The cells are connected to the basal lamina by **hemidesmosomes**, firmly anchoring the epidermis to the dermis. This mechanical connection is reinforced by tight interdigitations between dermal papillae and complementary epidermal invaginations (epidermal pegs). Formation of new keratinocytes in the stratum basale occurs by mitosis. The rate of cell division is influenced by the rate of desquamation and by mechanical wear and tear of the cornified cells at the surface of the epithelium. A full cycle

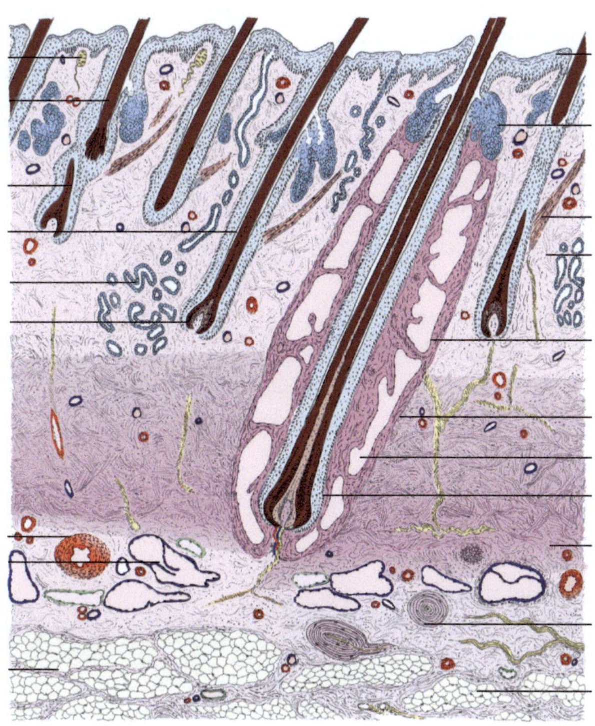

15.2 Skin incorporating a sinus hair (schematic).

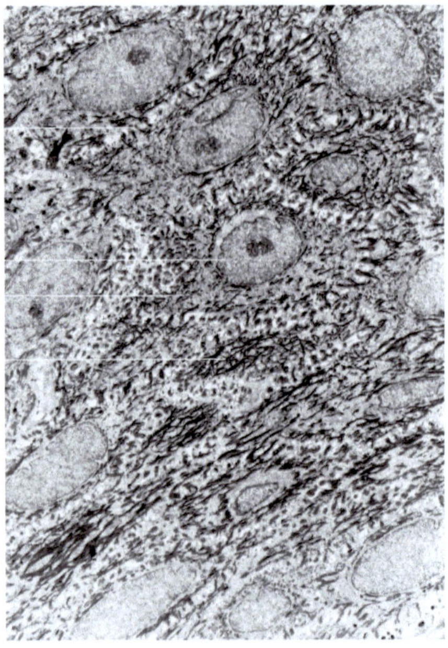

15.3 Stratum spinosum of the epidermis (pig). Note the narrow intercellular spaces (x4000).

of keratinocyte replacement takes between 20 and 30 days, depending upon species.

The cells of the **stratum spinosum** are predominantly polygonal with a round nucleus. More superficially, towards the stratum granulosum, they become flattened. Short cytoplasmic processes span the intercellular spaces visible with the light microscope. Processes of neighbouring cells are connected by desmosomes, giving rise to the term '**prickle cell layer**', sometimes used to describe this stratum. The cytoplasm contains bundles of **intermediate filaments** (**tonofilaments**, **cytokeratin filaments**) that extend into the cell processes and insert on the desmosomes. In this way, the filamentous skeleton of one cell extends into the neighbouring cell without the filaments penetrating the adjacent cell. The forces of tension and pressure acting upon the epithelium influence the intracellular arrangement and number of the tonofilament bundles.

Processes of cellular differentiation associated with keratinisation become evident in the stratum spinosum. These include:

- increased prominence of cytokeratins (tonofilaments) and
- formation of membrane-coating granules (MCG).

Cytokeratins are sulfur-rich filamentous proteins that form part of the cytoskeleton. The basic unit of epidermal keratin filaments is a pre-keratin molecule consisting of numerous polypeptide chains arranged in α-helices. The presence of various cytokeratins, of which at least 20 (CK 1–20) have been recognised, is used as a marker in the identification of epithelial tissue and its stage of differentiation in the diagnosis of neoplasia. Cytokeratins are assembled in a specific manner, depending upon the functional demands on the epithelium. Accordingly, epidermal regions and structures such as hairy skin, digital pads and the claws each exhibit a characteristic cytokeratin pattern.

Membrane-coating granules (**MCG**) are small organelles (diameter 0.1–0.3 μm) filled with membrane-coating material (MCM) containing 40% phospholipids – in a bilipid layer arranged in membrane stacks – and enzymes (e.g. acid phosphatase). Membrane-coating granules are formed in the stratum spinosum, probably by the Golgi apparatus. In the upper layers of the epidermis, the contents of the granules (MCM) are released into the intercellular space by exocytosis (Figure 15.4).

The **stratum granulosum** is characterised by the presence of flattened keratinocytes containing basophilic **keratohyalin granules**. These granules contain **profillagrins**, the precursors of **filaggrins**. Filaggrins are histidine-rich proteins that aggregate keratin filaments into a **filament–matrix complex**. The stratum granulosum is present in tissues in which soft keratin is formed (e.g. skin, digital pads). In comparison to the epidermis of the pads, the stratum granulosum of hairy skin is very thin, consisting of one to two cell layers, and is frequently discontinuous. In epidermal tissue in which hard keratin is formed (e.g. hoof, nail), the stratum granulosum is indistinct or absent, as the filaggrin precursors are not stored in keratohyalin granules.

As keratinisation progresses, **cytokeratin filaments** are joined with each other, and with **filaggrins**, via disulfide

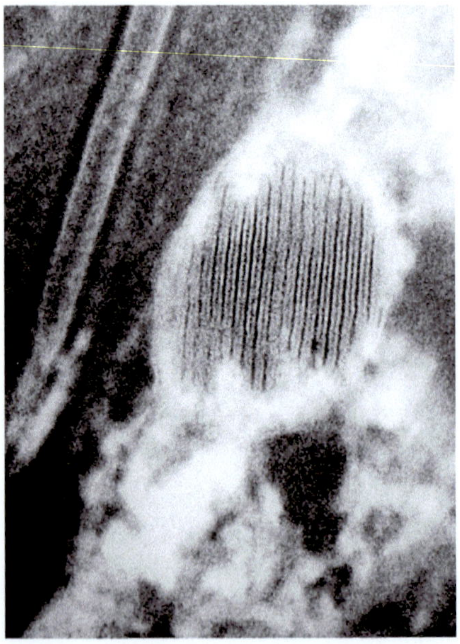

15.4 Membrane-coating material (MCM, intercellular lipid-rich matrix) of the stratum corneum in the skin (horse; x70,000). (Courtesy of H. Bragulla).

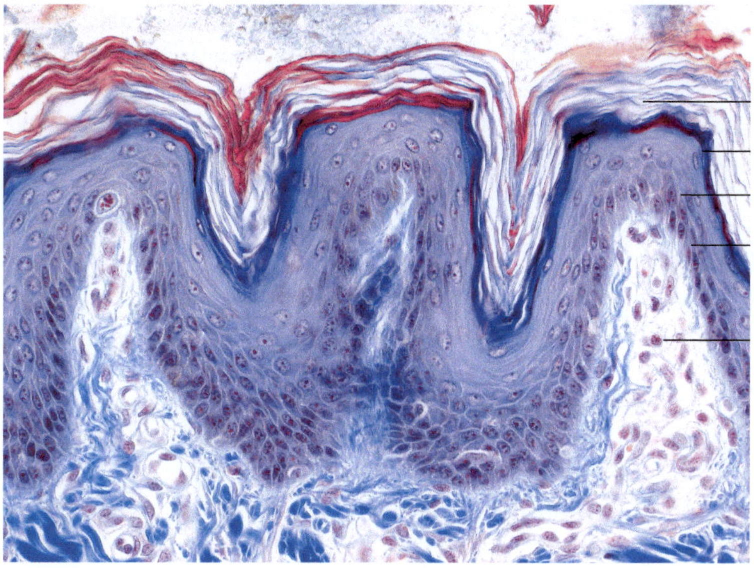

15.5 Epidermis (horse). Azan stain (x400).

bonds to form aggregates. Concurrently, proteins (e.g. involucrin, keratolinin) are synthesised and deposited on the cytoplasmic surface of the cell membrane forming the **cornified envelope**. This plays an important role in the barrier function of the stratum corneum.

In addition, the keratinocytes undergo a process of necrobiosis, in which the cellular organelles degenerate, and the nucleus breaks down into fragments.

Aggregation of keratin filaments and condensation of the filament–matrix complex continues in the stratum corneum (Figure 15.5). Consequently, newly keratinised cells can be distinguished from those located more superficially by their histochemical and mechanical characteristics. In the epidermis of particularly thick skin and hairless regions (e.g. nasal plane and foot pads), the deeper layer of recently keratinised cells is strongly acidophilic and is termed the stratum lucidum.

The keratinised cells of the **stratum corneum** are held together primarily by:

- MCM and
- cellular junctions (desmosomes).

Within the epidermis, the **MCM** consists primarily of acylglucosylceramides that establish a stable connection between the membrane stacks of the MCM and the cell membrane of the keratinocytes. In addition to its mechanical function, the MCM serves as a crucial barrier protecting the organism against loss of fluid through the epidermis. It also prevents transcutaneous ingress of water-soluble and hydrophilic chemicals and microorganisms.

At the outer surface of the **stratum corneum**, enzyme-induced weakening of the intercellular lipid matrix results in desquamation of superficial keratinised cells. This layer of constantly shedding cells is also referred to as the **stratum disjunctum**. In the hard coronary horn of the digital organs, the MCM is composed largely of glycoproteins that strengthen the cornified tissue. These glycoproteins are not enzymatically degraded and the superficial layer of horny tissue does not desquamate. In the absence of sufficient natural wear and tear, this layer must be trimmed (e.g. hoof trimming).

In the stratum spinosum and stratum granulosum, keratinocytes are held together by **desmosomes**. As the cells move towards the surface of the stratum corneum, the function of the desmosomes is gradually replaced by the intercellular substance.

The ordered process of keratinisation and the integrity of the resulting cornified tissue are dependent upon the availability of an adequate supply of **nutrients** and **energy**, derived by diffusion from vessels in the dermal papillae (see below). The surface area across which diffusion can occur is greater on the sides of the papillae (**peripapillary**) than at the tips (**suprapapillary**) or the regions between the papillae (**interpapillary**). Accordingly, keratinised epithelium formed in the peripapillary region is structurally distinguishable and mechanically superior to that arising from the supra- and interpapillary zones. Compromise of the nutrient supply to the epidermis due to local vascular derangement or general nutritional deficiency causes a reduction in the quantity and quality of keratinised tissue. A notable example is the development of circular depressions in the hard keratin (horn) of cattle during pregnancy (pregnancy grooves).

In addition to keratinocytes, the epidermis contains other cell types that perform a variety of roles and contribute to the function of the outer skin. These cells, considered **specialised epidermal structures**, include:

- melanocytes (pigment cells), protective function,
- Langerhans cells (macrophages), immune function and
- Merkel cells, sensory (tactile) function.

Dermis (corium)

The dermis is the connective tissue layer that underlies the epidermis (Figures 15.2 and 15.5 to 15.10). Based upon variations in density and the arrangement of its scaffold of **collagen** and **elastic fibres**, the dermis is divided into two layers:

- **stratum papillare (papillary layer)** with:
  - dermal papillae,
  - connective tissue fibres, hair, sebaceous and sweat glands,
  - microvasculature (capillary loops),
  - autonomic innervation and
- **stratum reticulare (reticular layer)** containing a lattice of connective tissue fibres.

Papillary layer (stratum papillare)

As the most superficial layer of the dermis, the papillary layer is in contact with the epidermis. The papillary layer interdigitates with the epidermis via finger-like dermal projections (**dermal papillae**). Depending on region and species, these projections may also manifest as tongue-shaped or strip-like protrusions. The papillary layer performs mechanical, nutritional and immune functions and contributes to cardiovascular regulation and sensation. Accordingly, the **microvasculature** and **autonomic innervation** are well developed (see below). It is particularly in this layer that epidermal appendages such as **hairs,** and **sebaceous** and **sweat glands** are embedded (see below).

The **papillary layer** is composed of loose connective tissue, comprising a lattice of collagen fibres interwoven with elastic fibres, the latter condensing to form a strong subepithelial layer. (Figure 15.7). Type III collagen fibres interweave with the basal lamina, forming a **functional** connection with the network of tonofibrils within the epithelial keratinocytes. This close association between the papillary layer and the basal cells of the epidermis imparts considerable **mechanical strength** to the outer layers of the skin.

Hairpin-shaped **capillary loops** sprout into the dermal papillae, supplying blood to the epidermis (Figure 15.8). Interdigitation of the papillary layer with the epidermis facilitates **diffusion of nutrients** into the epidermis in general, and the regenerative capacity of the stratum germinativum in particular.

The loose connective tissue of the papillary layer is interspersed with lymphocytes, plasma cells, macrophages and mast cells. The presence of considerable numbers of these cells is indicative of adaptive and innate immune responses that occur continuously within the skin.

Reticular layer (stratum reticulare)

The reticular layer (Figure 15.9) is a taut layer of connective tissue in which fibres are plentiful and cells are sparse. Collagen fibres (type I), accompanied by bundles of elastic fibres, predominantly run parallel to the surface. The fibre bundles are arranged in a **lattice**, forming rhomboid loops that allow even displacement of the skin for accommodation of the tensile forces imposed upon it.

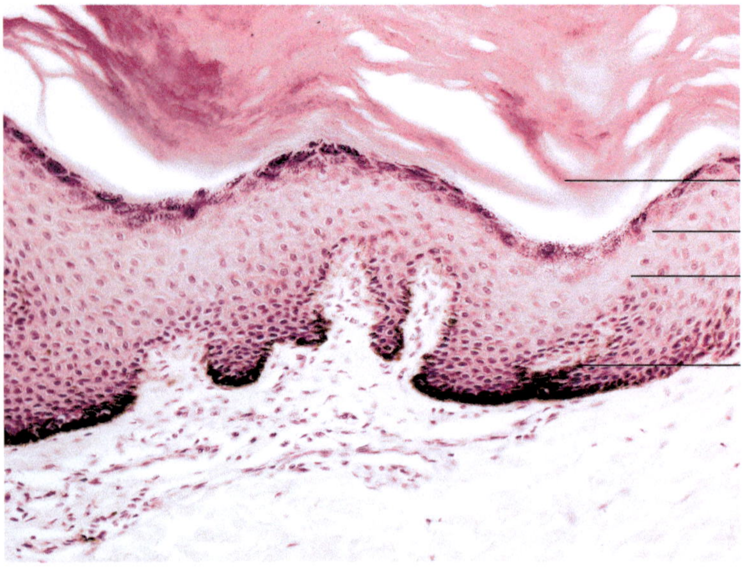

15.6 Strongly pigmented skin (horse). Note the well-developed keratinised layer and distinct dermal papillae. Haematoxylin and eosin stain (x360).

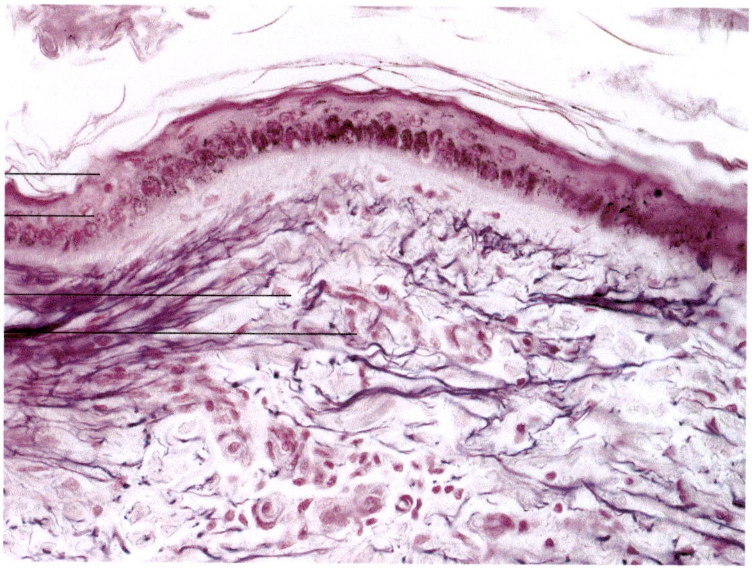

15.7 Stratum papillare of the dermis (horse). Numerous elastic fibres contribute to the considerable strength of this layer. Haematoxylin and eosin stain (x280).

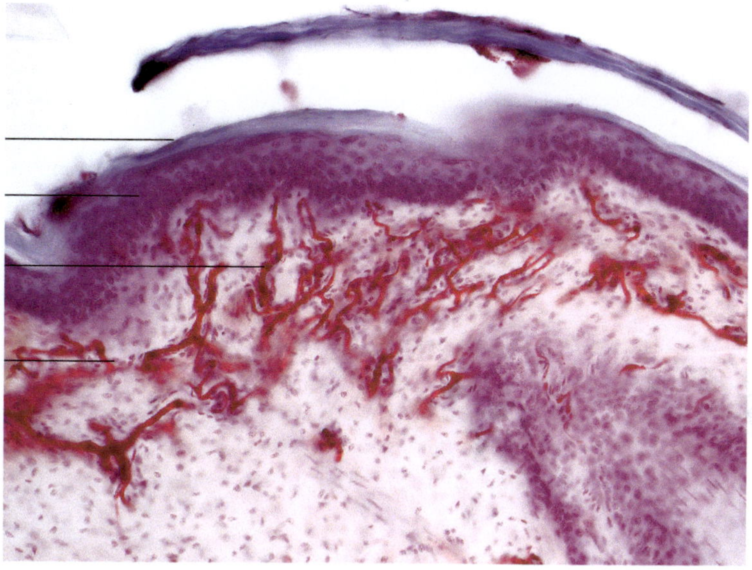

15.8 Subepidermal capillary network in the skin (dog). Injection specimen (x280).

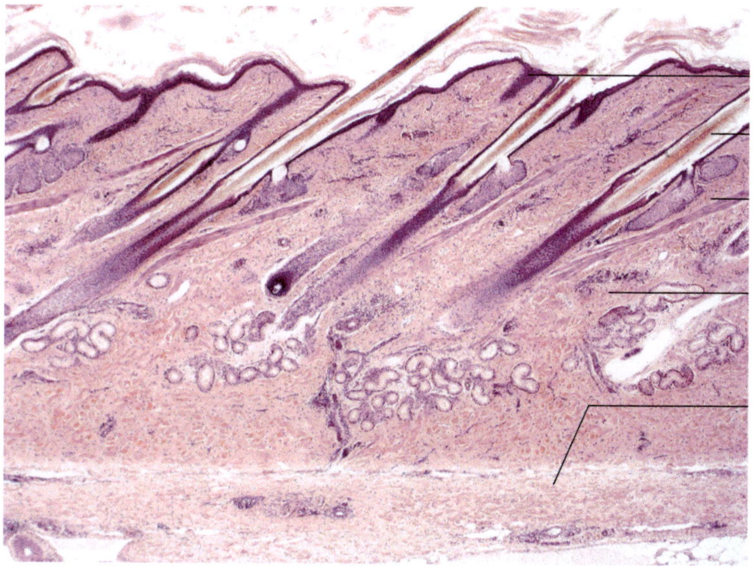

15.9 Low-magnification view of hairy skin (horse). Haematoxylin and eosin stain (x16).

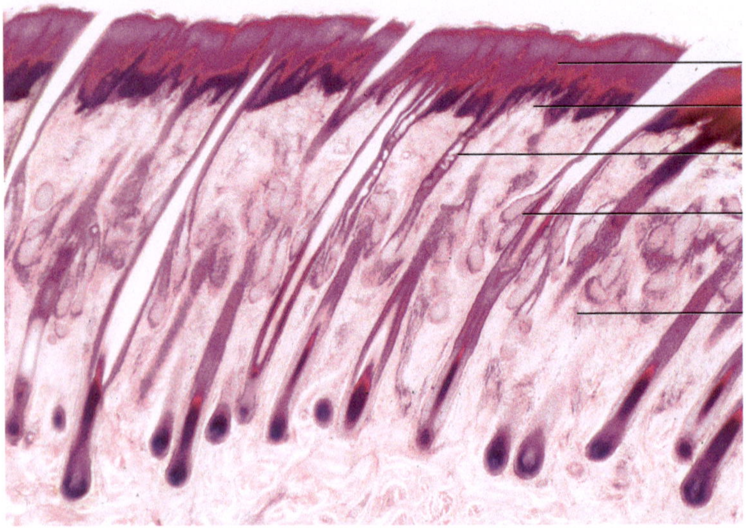

15.10 Epidermis and stratum papillare of the skin (horse). Haematoxylin and eosin stain (x32).

The **plasticity and deformability** of the skin is attributable largely to the abundance of elastic fibres that enable the collagen lamellae to resume their original arrangement after stretching. The reticular layer is relatively poorly vascularised. It is populated primarily by small arteries and veins passing to and from more superficial layers.

The dermis exhibits considerable regional and species-related **variation in thickness**. Additional factors affecting the development of the dermis include functional load, climate and breed. Among domestic mammals, the dermis is thickest in cattle. In leather production (tanning), the elastic skin of young animals is more suitable than that of older animals.

Hypodermis (subcutis)

The hypodermis is composed of loose, irregularly arranged connective tissue. It forms a mobile connection between the skin and the fascia or muscles (Figure 15.11). Distinguishing features include:

- a network of blood vessels,
- variable quantities of adipose tissue and
- embedded striated muscle tissue.

The subcutis is vascular and rich in adipose tissue. The degree of fat accumulation in this layer varies with species, gender and body region. Fat deposits act as energy reserves and provide thermal insulation. In parts of the body

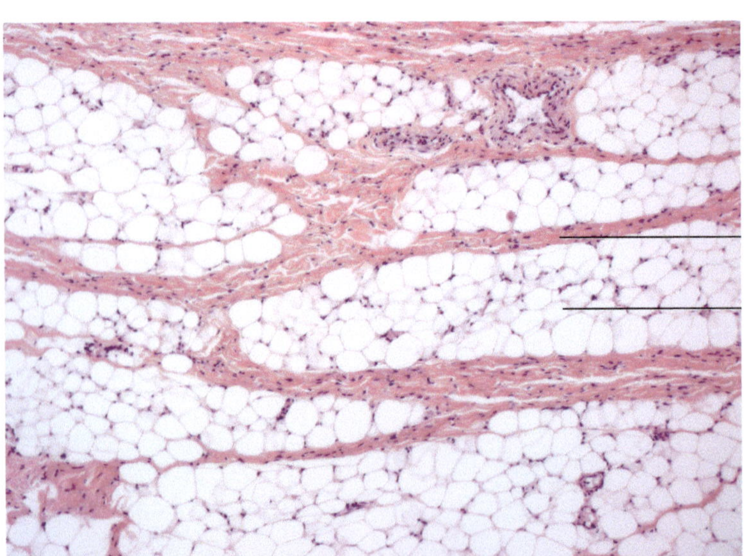

15.11 Deep layers of the skin (horse). Haematoxylin and eosin stain (x16).

subjected to mechanical stress (e.g. digital pads), the fatty tissue is divided into compartments by connective tissue septa, increasing its resilience. The subcutis incorporates local striated muscle tissue that serves to tauten the skin.

Skin glands (glandulae cutis)

The glands of the skin are divided into **two types** (Table 15.1). Embryologically, both are considered derivatives of the epidermis. The types of glands, and their features and functions, are as follows:

- **sweat glands (glandulae sudoriferi):**
  - exocrine, extra-epithelial,
  - tubular, simple or branched,
  - single layer of secretory cells, apocrine or merocrine,
  - participate in thermoregulation, serve as scent glands, occur in modified forms (e.g. glands of the nasolabial plane, glands of the anal sacs),
- **sebaceous glands (glandulae sebaceae):**
  - exocrine, extra-epithelial,
  - alveolar, simple or compound,
  - secretion formed by mass of cells, holocrine and
  - produce sebum, which forms the bulk of the epidermal surface lipid layer.

Sweat glands (glandulae sudoriferi)

Sweat glands are exocrine, extra-epithelial, tubular (sometimes saccular) glands (Figure 15.12). Their secretory product is released by the apocrine or merocrine (eccrine) modes.

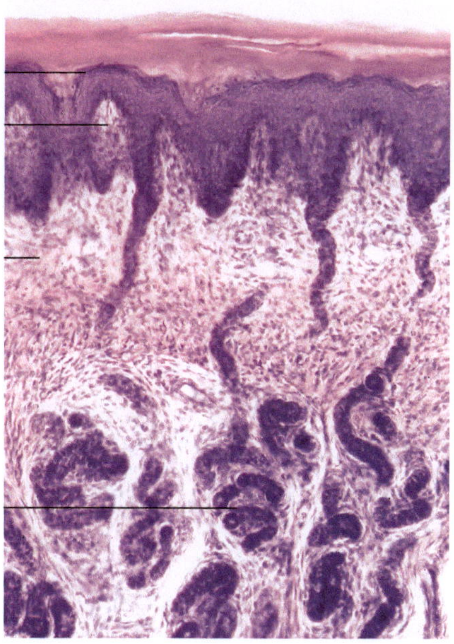

15.12 Coiled tubular sweat glands in a foot pad (cat). Haematoxylin and eosin stain (x40).

Apocrine glands, the most numerous type of sweat gland in domestic mammals, are associated with hair follicles (Figure 15.15). Their secretory product encloses components of the apical cytoplasm and incorporates **scents** that are specific to the individual animal of origin. The secretory portion is coiled and the duct opens into the hair follicle.

Merocrine glands occur less frequently in domestic mammalian species and are limited to hairless areas such as the foot pads of carnivores. They are unbranched coiled

Table 15.1 Structural differences between sweat and sebaceous glands.

Gland	Structure	Location	Mode of secretion	Special features
Sweat glands (glandulae sudoriferi)	Exocrine, extra-epithelial, tubular, single layer of secretory cells	Distributed across the entire skin surface, apocrine type usually closely associated with hair follicles	Apocrine secretion directly into the hair follicle, eccrine (merocrine) secretion directly onto the skin surface; secretion comprises proteolytic enzymes, electrolytes, water and albuminoid substances	Contribute to thermoregulation and excretion of soluble waste products, source of species-specific scents including pheromonones (apocrine type)
Sebaceous glands (glandulae sebaceae)	Exocrine, extra-epithelial, alveolar, mass of cells gives rise to secretory product	Closely associated with the external root sheath of hair follicles	Holocrine secretion; sebum, composed of various fats and oils	Occur independently of hair in some locations (e.g. eyelids [Meibomian glands], on the penis and in the external acoustic meatus); increase suppleness and reduce dehydration of the skin; secretion has antibacterial properties

tubular glands (Figure 15.12). The epithelial lining of the tubular secretory portion is cuboidal to columnar, depending on secretory activity. The ducts open independently of hair follicles directly onto the surface of the skin. Release of secretory products into the tubular lumen is facilitated by **myoepithelial cells** that lie on the deep aspect of the secretory units. These are modified epithelial cells that have acquired the ability to contract.

Sweat glands have **several functions**. They contribute to thermoregulation through evaporation of sweat and provide a means of eliminating products of metabolism. Their secretions mix with those of sebaceous glands forming a film on the surface of the skin. In domestic mammals this layer is only weakly acidic, becoming alkaline with increased output from the apocrine sweat glands. In contrast to the hairless skin of humans, this layer does not provide protection in the form of an acidic environment. The antimicrobial effect of the layer coating the skin surface is probably related to free fatty acids, formed during the decomposition of epidermal surface lipids.

Sebaceous glands (glandulae sebaceae)

Sebaceous glands are exocrine, extra-epithelial, alveolar glands (Figure 15.13). Their mode of secretion is holocrine. In the main, sebaceous glands are associated with hair follicles (Figure 15.10), their secretion (**sebum**) passing via short ducts into the follicle, giving rise to the pilosebaceous canal. Synthesis of sebum begins at the base of the alveolar secretory unit, within undifferentiated rapidly dividing epithelial cells. Fatty acids, cholesterol and triglycerides accumulate in intracellular lipid droplets that eventually fill the cytoplasm of the cells. The nucleus becomes pyknotic and the organelles degenerate. As production of new cells continues, older cells are forced into the lumen of the alveolar gland where they break down. The cell debris and secretory product together form **sebum**. Sebaceous glands may be simple or compound. They also occur independently of hair follicles, e.g. in the eyelid (Meibomian glands), in the prepuce and penis, and in the external ear canal.

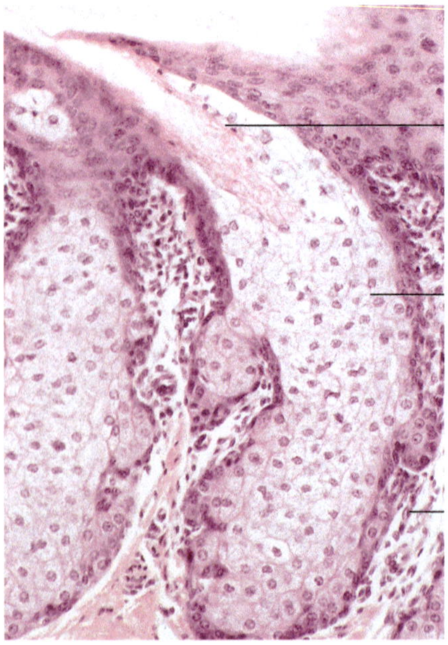

15.13 Alveolar sebaceous gland (horse). Haematoxylin and eosin stain (x400).

The secretory product of sebaceous glands spreads over the surface of the skin, covering the entire epidermis with a thin layer of lipid. It serves as a waterproofing agent, has an antimicrobial function and lubricates the stratum corneum of the epidermis and the hair.

Numerous **modified sweat** and **sebaceous glands** are found in domestic mammals. The structure of the glands of the planum nasolabiale of ruminants, glands of the anal sacs of carnivores and the circumanal glands of dogs is described in Chapter 10, 'Digestive system'.

Pigmentation

Even in densely haired regions, the presence of pigments in the skin plays a role in protecting against intense exposure to light. Pigmentation also occurs in hairless regions.

Pigment is produced by **melanocytes**. Originating from the neural crest, these cells come to lie between the keratinocytes of the basal layer of the epidermis. Their cytoplasm contains melanin pigment (**melanosomes**), the precursors of which develop within **premelanosomes** from 3,4-dihydroxyphenylalanine (DOPA) in the Golgi apparatus. Melanosomes pass from melanocytes to adjacent keratinocytes in the stratum basale (Figure 15.6).

Skin as an organ of thermoregulation

Maintenance of constant body temperature is of considerable importance for warm-blooded animals. In domestic mammals, the vessels of the skin together with the dense hair coat form the key organ of thermoregulation. The hairs can become erect (via the **m. arrector pili**), thus trapping a layer of air that contributes to thermal insulation.

Vessels of the skin

The skin incorporates deep (subcutaneous), cutaneous and subepithelial vascular networks. Arterioles extend from the subcutaneous vessels through the layers of the dermis and ramify superficially into a **cutaneous network**. This empties into an extensive **subepithelial venous plexus** that serves as a means of transferring heat to the epidermis. The microcirculation of the skin and associated thermoregulation is controlled autonomically via arteriovenous anastomoses. Capillaries extend from the cutaneous vascular network into the papillary region forming hairpin loops, particularly in the dermal papillae (Figure 15.8). The walls of the capillaries are located close to the epidermis, without penetrating this layer. Nourishment of the epidermis results from diffusion of nutrients across the intercellular space. The capillaries drain into venules and veins that ultimately join the subcutaneous venous network.

Hair (pili) and hair follicles

Hairs are thin, tension-resistant strands of keratin that develop from invaginations of the epidermis known as hair follicles. During embryonic development, localised thickenings extend as cone-shaped structures into the loose connective tissue of the future dermis. At the end of this hair-anlage, the downgrowth expands to form the **epithelial hair bulb**, which becomes invaginated by a **connective tissue** (**dermal**) **papilla**. Mitotic division of epithelial cells in the central portion of the hair bulb gives rise to the cylindrical hair. The outer components of the bulb differentiate into the **epithelial root sheath**. Superficially, the root sheath is continuous with the stratum basale of the epidermis (Figure 15.14).

The exterior of the hair anlage is surrounded by a **connective tissue** (**dermal**) **sheath** that forms a sleeve around the differentiated epidermal root sheath. Structures found in association with the hair follicle include smooth muscle cells (mm. arretores pili), a delicate capillary network and an extensively elaborated system of sensory nerves.

Sebaceous and sweat glands arise together with hair follicles from the epidermal anlage and become embedded in the tissue beneath. Thus, a 'triad' of epidermal structures – hair, sweat glands and sebaceous glands – is formed.

In certain regions of the body, elements of the triad may be missing or extensively modified. This phenomenon is usually associated with specialisation of epidermal cells (e.g. mammary gland, horns, hooves and claws). These components of the integument are referred to as modified skin.

Hair structure

Individual hairs are comprised of the following components:

- root (radix pili) and bulb (bulbus pili) and
- shaft (scapus pili) and tip (apex pili).

  A further distinction is made between the:
- medulla (medulla pili) and the
- cortex (cortex pili) and cuticle.

The proximal portion of the hair is termed the root (radix pili). At the terminal part of the root is an onion-shaped structure, the bulb. The distal component of the hair is

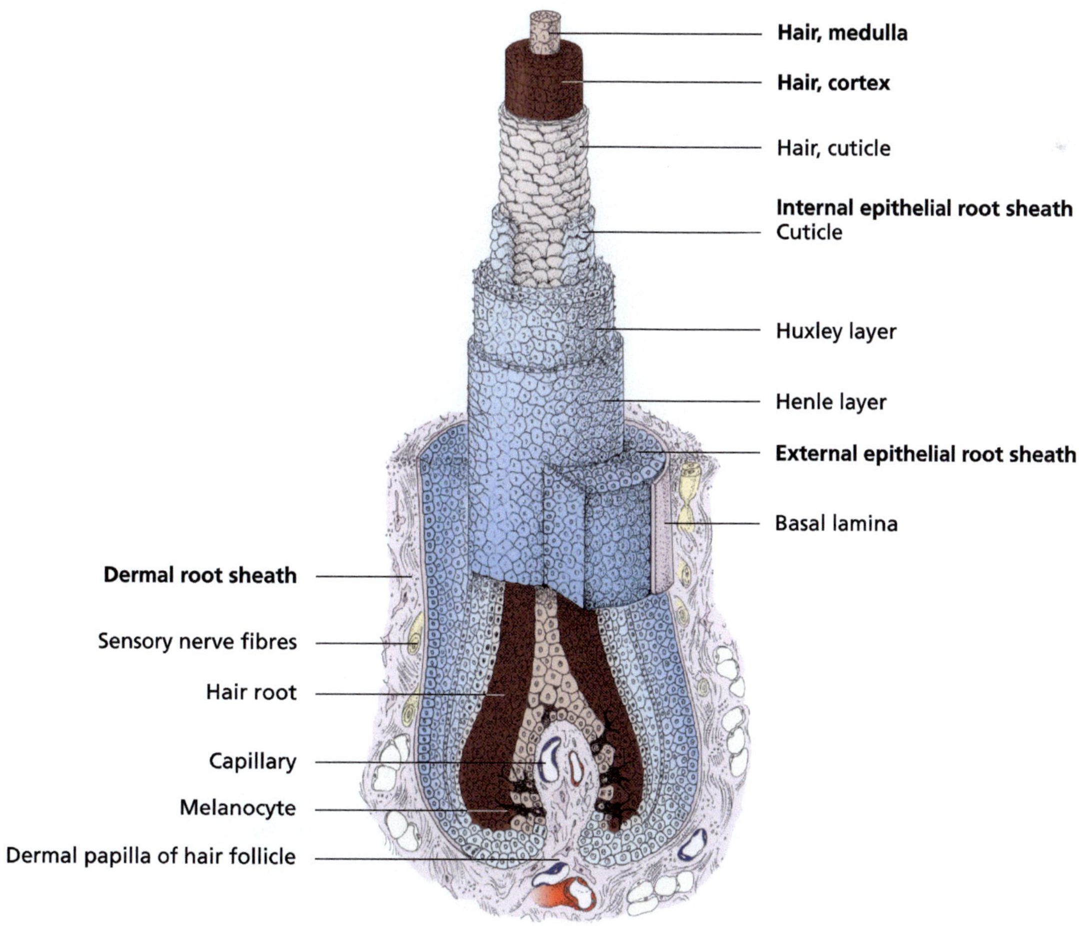

15.14 Strucure of a hair, the root sheaths and adjacent dermal root sheath and papilla (schematic).

composed of the shaft (scapus pili) and its free tip (apex pili).

The medulla (medulla pili) arises from the deep layers of the stratum basale overlying the tip of the dermal papilla (suprapapillar) (Figure 15.14). These epithelial cells are constantly dividing, are vacuolated and are minimally keratinised. Production of new medullary cells pushes older cells towards the exterior. The latter lose their pigmentation, their nuclei become pyknotic and trichohyalin granules appear within them. Degenerated medullary cells may contain gas bubbles that, together with lack of pigmentation, result in greying of the hair. The medulla is absent in wool fibres.

The cortex (cortex pili) develops from epithelial cells located at the margins of the papilla (peripapillar). It forms a densely cellular, strongly keratinised mantle around the medulla. Some of its cells contain melanin pigment granules. The density of melanosomes determines the colour of the hair. Cortical keratinocytes are flattened and are reinforced by longitudinal tonofilaments that impart mechanical strength, flexibility and elasticity to the hairs.

The **external surface** of the hair is lined by a single layer of flattened keratinised cells termed the **cuticle** (**cuticula pili**). The cells partially overlap in a manner resembling roof tiles, with their free edges directed towards the hair tip (Figure 15.19). Interlocking of these cells with oppositely oriented superficial cells of the internal epithelial root sheath (see below) serves to secure the hair *in situ*.

The structure of the medulla and cuticle is highly species-specific and can thus be used for forensic purposes. Distinguishing characteristics include the structure of the medullary cells, the thickness and number of the medullary layers, the relative thickness of the medulla and cortex and the surface profile of the cells of the cuticle.

Root sheath structure

The root sheaths surrounding the hair are comprised of the:

- **epithelial root sheath:**
  - internal epithelial root sheath,
  - external epithelial root sheath,
  - basal lamina (glassy membrane),
- **dermal root sheath:**
  - internal dermal root sheath,
  - external dermal root sheath and
- **dermal papilla.**

EPITHELIAL ROOT SHEATH

Proximally, the epithelial root sheath forms a sleeve around the hair, accompanying it as far as the follicular orifice at the skin surface. It is divided into internal and external layers (Figure 15.14).

The **internal root sheath** is composed of three layers. The **cuticle of the internal root sheath** consists of a single layer of flattened cells that lies adjacent to the surface of the hair. These keratinised cells are arranged in a shingle-like pattern with their free margins directed towards the bulb. The interlocking of these cells with those of the hair cuticle holds the hair in place.

The cuticle of the root sheath is surrounded by one to three layers of nucleated cells (Huxley layer) that may contain trichohyalin in places. A usually single layer of non-nucleated cells (Henle layer) forms the outermost layer of the internal root sheath (Figure 15.16).

The **external epithelial root sheath** represents the continuation of the layers of the epidermal stratum basale, which it largely resembles in structure.

On the outside of the external root sheath is a clearly developed **basal lamina** (**glassy membrane**). This separates the epidermal portions of the hair from the surrounding connective tissue (mesodermal) layers.

Free sensory nerve endings penetrate the basal lamina and arborise in the outer root sheath, particularly near the follicular orifice. These nerve endings terminate in receptors that detect touch, pressure and vibration, forming part of the superficial sensory apparatus.

DERMAL ROOT SHEATH

During embryonic development, the downgrowth of epidermal tissue into the underlying connective tissue gives rise to a mantle termed the dermal root sheath (Figures 15.14 to 15.16). This is typically composed of two layers: an **internal layer** comprising collagen and elastic fibre bundles arranged in a predominantly circular orientation, and an **external layer** in which the fibre bundles are mostly

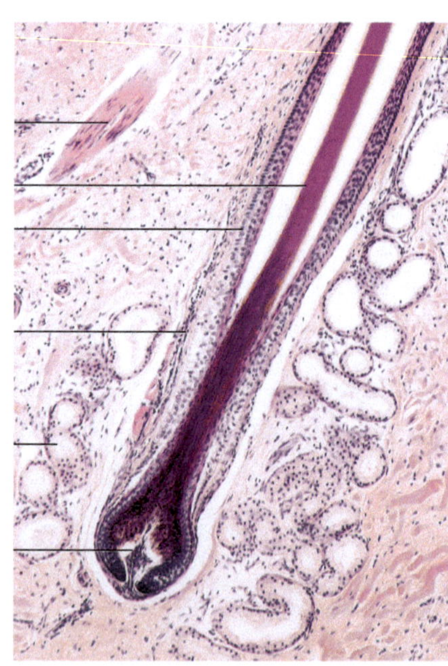

15.15 Longitudinal section of a hair and sweat glands (dog). Haematoxylin and eosin stain (x100).

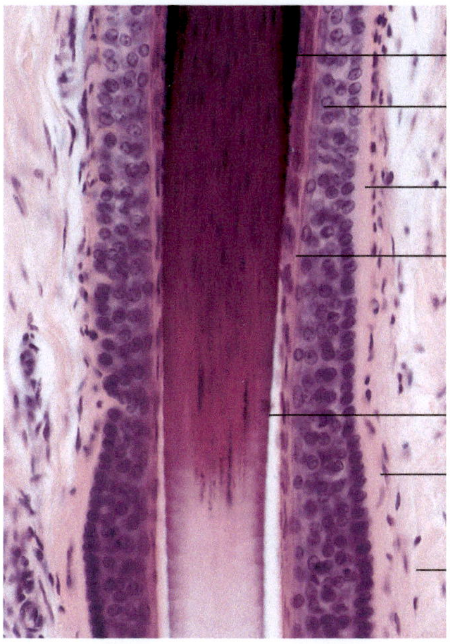

15.16 Hair and epidermal and dermal root sheaths (horse). Haematoxylin and eosin stain (x250).

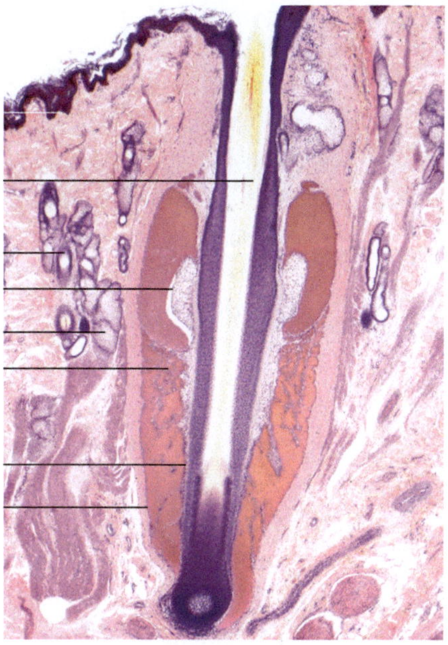

15.17 Skin and sinus hair (sinusoidal type, dog). Haematoxylin and eosin stain (x30).

aligned parallel to the longitudinal axis of the hair. This fibrous sheath contains blood vessels and myelinated nerve fibres, the latter passing into the external root sheath as free nerve endings.

The dermal root sheath gives rise to the **dermal papilla**, which manifests as a cone-shaped protrusion into the hair bulb (Figure 15.14). The dermal papilla contains dense capillary loops that supply the metabolically active cells of the stratum basale, thereby supporting the growth and development of new hairs.

Types of hair

Domestic mammals exhibit great diversity in the development of the hair coat including variation in length, thickness, distribution and arrangement (see *Veterinary Anatomy of Domestic Mammals: Textbook and Colour Atlas*). Specialised hair types include cilia, eyelashes and tactile hairs. Tactile hairs, closely associated with the sense of touch, are also referred to as **sinus hairs**.

SINUS HAIR (PILUS TACTILIS)

Sinus hairs are characterised by their pronounced thickness and length. They are embedded deep in the dermis, almost reaching the subcutis. There, they are in direct contact with striated muscle, which enables their movement.

The dermal root sheath exhibits characteristic modification comprising separation of the **internal** and **external layers** by an endothelium-lined **blood sinus**.

Species variation

Horse and ruminants: The entire blood sinus is traversed by delicate connective tissue trabeculae, dividing the sinus into irregular compartments (**cavernous type**) (Figure 15.18).

Carnivores and pigs: The distal portion of the sinus, nearest the epidermis, is annular and free of trabeculae (**sinusoid type**) (Figure 15.17). Here the internal dermal root sheath bulges into the lumen of the sinus (sinus pad).

The connective tissue walls and the trabeculae of the blood sinus contain a fine meshwork of **sensory nerve fibres**. Free nerve endings extend from these fibres as far as the external root sheath of the sinus hairs, where they arborise. These nerve processes are **specialised pressure receptors** that detect and transmit amplified signals generated by perturbation of the sinus hairs and impulse waves in the blood sinus.

Skin as a sensory organ

The epidermis and the nervous system are both derived from ectodermal tissue. While the epidermal layer serves primarily to insulate the body against external influences, the nervous tissue within the skin infiltrates this barrier and allows various stimuli to be detected and transmitted to central sensory centres in the brain.

Receptive fields and their corresponding neurons occur in various layers of the skin. The epithelium contains **free nerve endings** and **Merkel cells**. Non-encapsulated or encapsulated tactile corpuscles are present in the subepithelial layers. The deeper the level at which a sensation is detected, the more complex the structure of the receptor (a detailed description of skin receptors is provided in Chapter 16, 'Receptors and sense organs').

Skin as an immunological barrier

Like the lungs and the gastrointestinal tract, the skin is an organ that presents a particularly large surface area and is

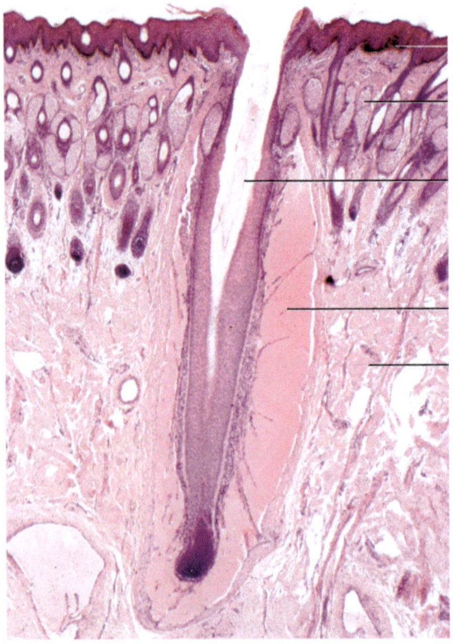

15.18 Skin and sinus hair (cavernous type, horse). Haematoxylin and eosin stain (x16).

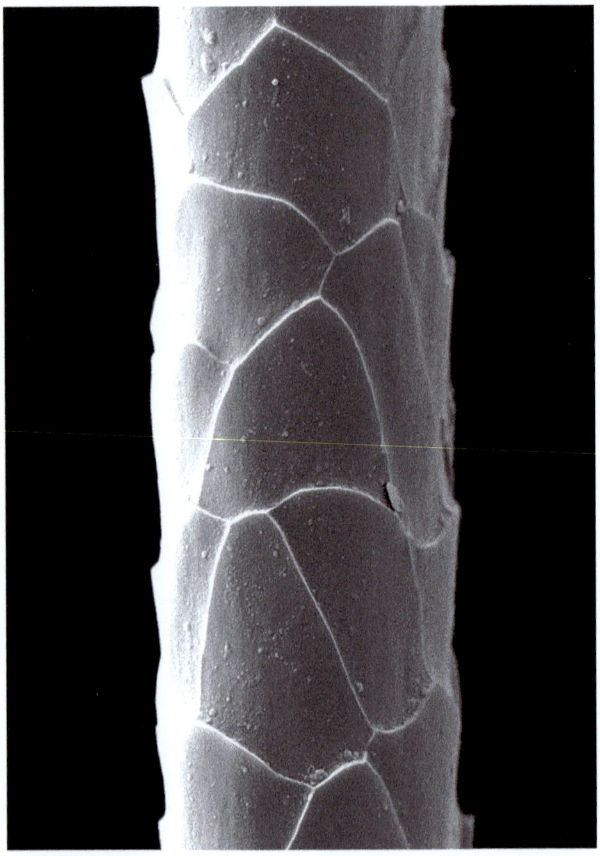

15.19 Scanning electron micrograph of the hair cuticle in a cat (x1500).

in close contact with the environment. Accordingly, the skin contains specialised components of the innate and adaptive immune systems.

The skin is covered with a thin, **poorly viscous film** that aids in protecting the epidermis against biological insult. Its **lipid components**, produced by the sebaceous glands (see above), prevent the ingress of water and associated derangement of intradermal ion balance. Free fatty acids formed during decomposition of surface lipid exert antimicrobial effects. Both of these features serve as **non-specific protective barriers**.

The epithelium incorporates **Langerhans cells**. These cells are components of the mononuclear phagocytic system. They develop from macrophages and migrate into the epidermis. Langerhans cells are **antigen-presenting** cells. Antigens that have penetrated the layers of the epidermis (e.g. bacteria) are processed within the cell and displayed on the cell surface.

Within local lymph nodes, these antigens are presented by Langerhans cells to T lymphocytes, which then undergo activation and proliferation as part of the adaptive immune response (see Chapter 8, 'Immune system and lymphatic organs'). The cascade of events involved in the immune response to foreign antigens thus commences in the epidermis. Morphologically, immune processes occurring in the skin are reflected by the presence of various immune cells (including T lymphocytes, B lymphocytes, macrophages, histiocytes and mast cells) near the vessels of the skin.

Skin modifications

Like the epidermis and associated skin glands, the modified structures of the skin are derivatives of the ectodermal germ layer. The **mammary gland** is a modified **apocrine sweat gland** with a specialised secretory function. The **hooves, claws** and (in ruminants) the **horns** are superficial sheets of cornified tissue formed by massive proliferation of keratinocytes and extensive keratinisation.

Mammary gland (udder, mamma, glandula mammaria)

The mammary gland is a compound organ composed of:

- glandular tissue (glandular parenchyma) and an associated duct system that empties peripherally into the teat, and
- connective tissue septa (interstitium) incorporating autonomic nerve fibres, vessels and loose connective tissue.

Superficially, the mammary gland is covered in skin. The body of the gland is supported by a capsule of connective tissue that extends from the fascia of the trunk. Considerable species variation exists in the number, macroscopic anatomy and vascular supply of the mammary glands (see *Veterinary Anatomy of Domestic Mammals: Textbook and Colour Atlas*). Microscopically, the structure of the mammary gland is relatively consistent.

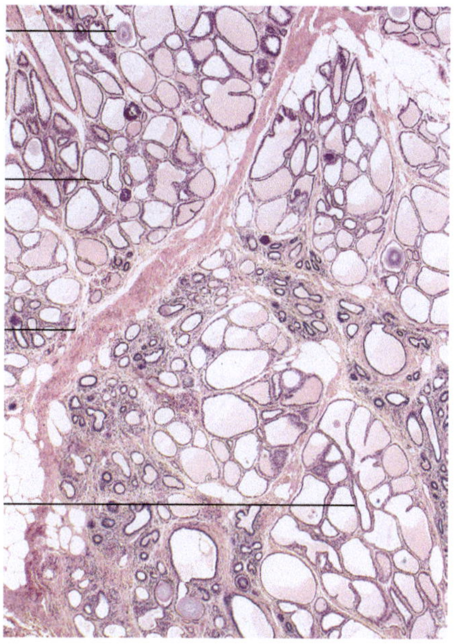

15.20 Lactating udder with tubulo-alveolar glands (cow). Haematoxylin and eosin stain (x120).

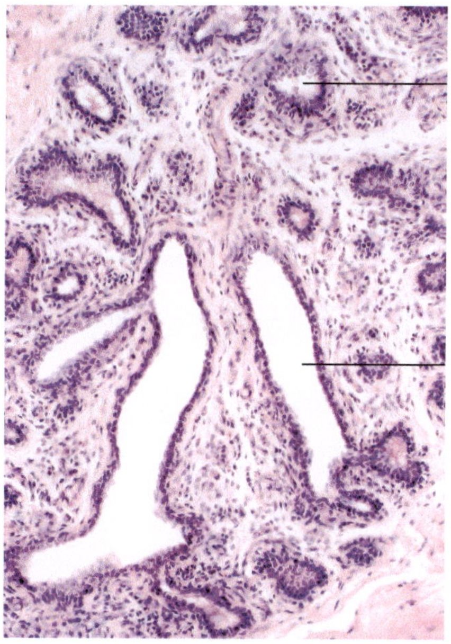

15.21 Juvenile udder with limited glandular tissue (calf). Haematoxylin and eosin stain (x320).

The glandular tissue of the mammary gland of domestic mammals is arranged in a variable number of lobules. The smallest individual unit comprises an organ-specific secretory tubule and alveolar end piece, enclosed in a layer of connective tissue.

Based on the arrangement of these components, the mammary gland is classified as a **compound tubulo-alveolar gland** with branching alveoli (Figures 15.20 and 15.21). The secretory units within the lobules represent a series of interconnected complexes, in which the secretory product, milk, can be stored temporarily in the lumen.

Structure of lactating mammary gland

The glandular parenchyma has three main components, each with a separate function:

- **alveoli**: milk production and ejection,
- **ductus lactiferi**: transport of milk and
- **sinus lactifer**: milk cistern, collection chamber.

ALVEOLI (ACINI)

The alveoli are lined by a **simple glandular epithelium** that varies in height and in the degree of development of the organelles, according to the functional state of the gland. During the **secretory phase** (Figure 15.20) the cells develop from cuboidal to columnar (Figure 15.22). The shape of the nucleus alters accordingly, from flattened to spherical to oval. In alveoli filled with secretory product, the height of the epithelial cells is once again relatively low.

The **organelles** of the glandular epithelium undergo considerable changes throughout the secretory cycle. During the synthetic phase, the endoplasmic reticulum (ER) and Golgi apparatus develop in size, and finely vacuolated lipid droplets form. In the **secretory phase**, dense stacks of ER appear in the basal region of the cells while the apical cytoplasm bulges into the lumen of the alveolus. The apical region encloses an extensively developed Golgi apparatus and usually a lipid droplet (Figure 15.22).

The **components of milk** include:

- **milk fat**, released with involvement of the Golgi apparatus by the apocrine mode of secretion,
- **milk proteins**, product of the rough ER, released by the merocrine mode of secretion (exocytosis),
- **immunoglobulin** (**IgA**) produced by plasma cells, locally produced or derived from blood,
- **lactose**, product of Golgi apparatus and
- **electrolytes**, taken up from the blood.

The lipids found in milk, predominantly triglycerides, arise as droplets. These coalesce to form larger droplets that are released by the **apocrine mode of secretion**, in which the droplet becomes surrounded by a membrane originating from the apical cell membrane. Lipoproteins and albumin-bound fatty acids used in the synthesis of milk lipids are taken up from the blood.

Milk proteins (e.g. casein, lactalbumin) are produced in the basal region of the cell in the membrane stacks of the rough ER. Through the usual protein biosynthetic pathways, these proteins are processed by the Golgi apparatus for vesicular transport to the cell surface. The milk proteins are released into the lumen of the alveolus by exocytosis (**merocrine secretion**).

Immunoglobulins (**IgA**), particuarly abundant in colostrum, are produced by **plasma cells**. These antibodies circulate in the **blood** or are produced **locally in the**

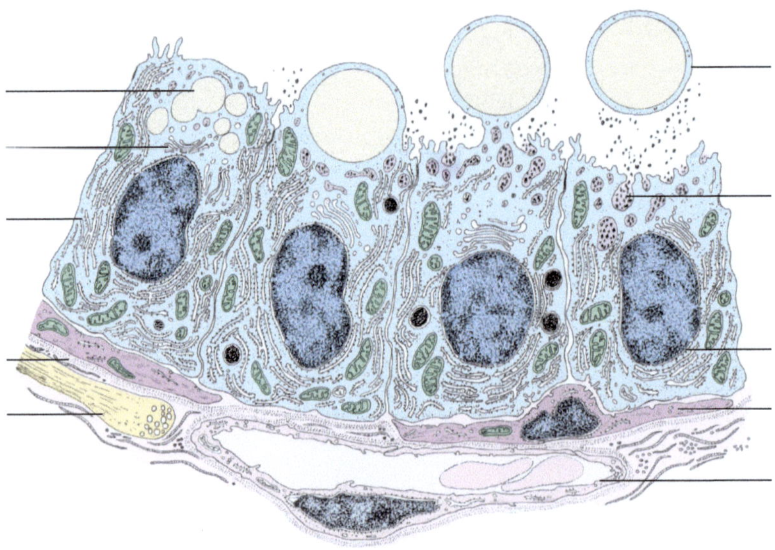

15.22 Secretion of milk components by the columnar epithelium of the mammary gland (schematic).

mammary gland by plasma cells in the interstitial connective tissue, and reach the milk via trans-epithelial transport. They provide **passive immunity**. Early intake of immunoglobulins by the neonate is important for immune protection of domestic mammals with an epitheliochorial type of placenta (horse, ruminant, pig).

Lactose (glucose and galactose) and most of the **enzymes** present in milk are produced locally in the secretory epithelium of the mammary gland. A product of the Golgi apparatus, lactose is synthesised exclusively in the mammary gland.

Other milk components, particularly **electrolytes** (calcium, potassium, chloride, phosphate, iron), enter the epithelial cells from underlying capilllaries and are transported into the milk.

The non-luminal surface of the epithelial cells of the alveoli is surrounded by **myoepithelial cells**. These ectodermal derivatives have become modified to include contractile filaments and thus perform a similar function to smooth muscle cells. Myoepithelial cells carry **oxytocin receptors** on their surface. Activation of these receptors results in contraction of the cell and narrowing of the alveolar lumen (**milk let-down reflex**, **milk ejection reflex**). The myoepithelial cells are lined externally by the basal lamina.

DUCTS (DUCTUS LACTIFERI)

The duct system begins as small excretory passages within the intralobular connective tissue (Figure 15.20). These converge to form larger interlobular ducts, which join to give rise to a **lactiferous duct** that drains a mammary lobe. The proximal portions of this duct system are lined by a simple cuboidal to columnar epithelium. More distally the epithelium becomes bi-layered. The initial portion of the duct epithelium is capable of secretory activity. The ducts are surrounded by a loose network of myoepithelial cells that facilitate the ejection of milk.

LACTIFEROUS SINUS (SINUS LACTIFER)

Larger ducts empty into expanded chambers referred to as lactiferous sinuses. These are lined with a bi-layered cuboidal to columnar epithelium. The number of sinuses corresponds with the number of teat canals (two in the horse, one in the cow and two to three in the sow).

INTERSTITIUM OF THE LACTATING MAMMARY GLAND

The interstitial connective tissue of the mammary gland (Figure 15.20) is composed predominantly of collagen fibre bundles. Particularly near alveoli and proximal lactiferous ducts, these bundles incorporate smooth muscle cells. Delicate elastic fibres form basket-like investments around the terminal alveoli. The connective tissue houses a dense capillary network, arterioles, venules, lymph vessels and autonomic nerve fibres. The cell population includes immune cells (lymphocytes and plasma cells) and mast cells.

Structure of the quiescent mammary gland

When the gland becomes inactive, during the dry period or after a sudden cessation of milking, secretion accumulates in the alveoli, the epithelium reduces in height and the organelles contributing to secretion become largely inactive. Adjacent alveoli often become disrupted, forming larger terminal sections. There is an increase in the population of macrophages, partial degeneration of the parenchyma and involution of alveoli. The loose connective tissue becomes partially infiltrated with fat.

Hormonal regulation of the mammary gland

Development of the mammary gland and secretion of milk is largely under hormonal control. **Oestrogens** induce **development of the duct system**. Development and growth of the **secretory end pieces** (**alveoli**) occurs under the influence of progesterone. During pregnancy, the inhibitory effect of oestrogen on **prolactin** suppresses the activity of the mammary gland.

Following parturition, blood oestrogen levels decrease and prolactin concentrations increase, leading to the induction of parturition. **Milk let-down** is facilitated by oxytocin. This hormone, originating from the neurohypophysis (see Chapter 9, 'Endocrine system'), promotes contraction of myoepithelial cells that surround the alveoli and parts of the excretory duct system. Hormones that regulate metabolism (e.g. thyroxin, growth hormone) also have a stimulatory effect on the mammary gland.

Sructure of the teat (papilla mammae)

Teats are classified as being of the proliferation type (ruminants, horse) or the eversion type (pig, carnivores). Within the teat is the **teat sinus** (the papillary component of the

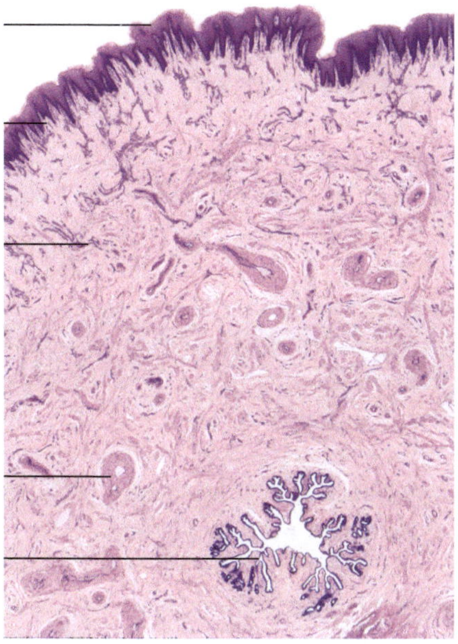

15.23 Cross-section of the wall of a teat (cow). Hamatoxylin and eosin stain (x20).

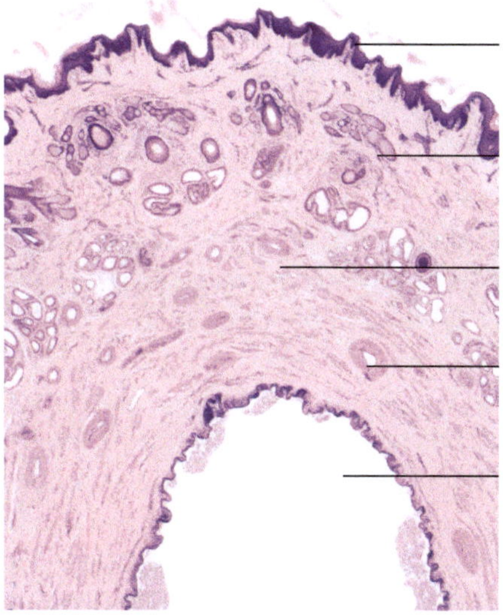

15.24 Cross-section of the mid-section of the wall of a teat (mid-section; ewe). Haematoxylin and eosin stain (x16).

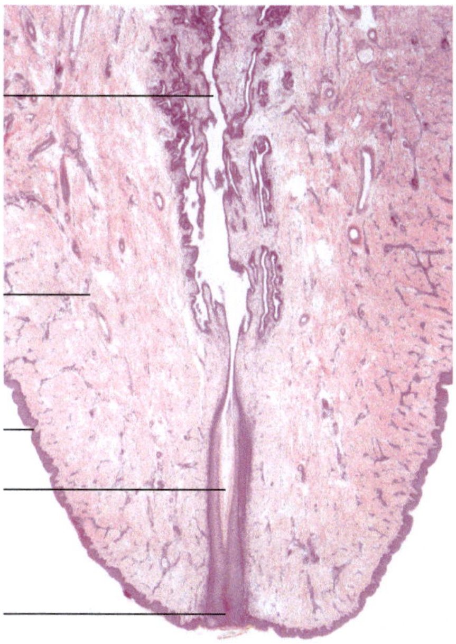

15.25 Longitudinal section of a teat (calf). Haematoxylin and eosin stain (x20).

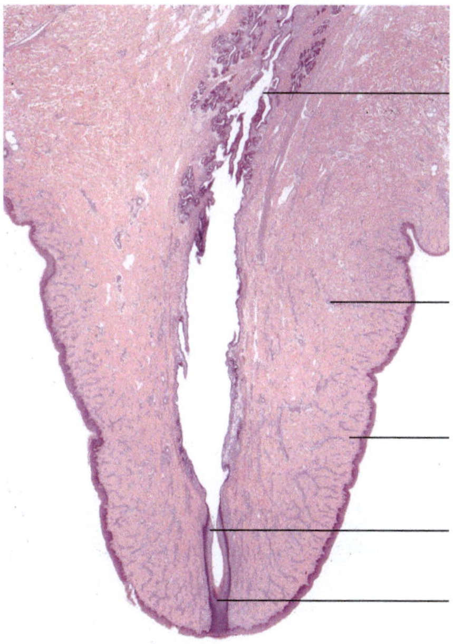

15.26 Longitudinal section of a teat (sow). Haematoxylin and eosin stain (x14).

lactiferous sinus). The milk exits the teat sinus through the **teat canal** (streak canal, ductus papillaris). The wall of the teat contains connective tissue (including elastic fibres) and smooth muscle. Proximally, the teat wall contains large-calibre, thick-walled veins (venae myotypicae). The inner surface of the teat is lined with mucosa. Externally, it is covered with variably modified skin (see below) (Figures 15.23 to 15.26).

Within the **teat sinus** the epithelium transitions from **bi-layered cuboidal epithelium** to the keratinised stratified squamous epithelium of the teat canal. In ruminants and cats this transition is abrupt, while in other species it is more gradual.

The teat wall contains a network of **collagen** and **elastic fibres** with embedded smooth muscle cells. From inside to outside, the orientation of muscle cells exhibits characteristic variation. Closest to the teat sinus, abundant smooth muscle cells are arranged in a circular fashion. In the middle of the teat wall, the muscle fibres are oriented parallel to the lengthwise axis of the teat. From there they radiate towards the teat surface.

As the number of muscle cells decreases towards the exterior, the amount of elastic fibres markedly increases. Near the teat opening (ostium papillare), the radial fibres give rise to a rosette that projects into the teat canal. At this location, muscle fibres concentrate to form the m. sphincter papillaris that aids in sealing the canal.

At the ostium papillare, the epithelium turns into the teat lumen to form a stratified keratinised mucosa. Desquamated keratin may temporarily obstruct the teat canal (Figures 15.25 and 15.26).

The skin on the **external surface of the teat** is hairless in the cow. In the sheep, the skin may contain hairs and sebaceous and sweat glands. In the horse, the skin of the teat bears fine hairs and is pigmented and rich in sebaceous glands.

Digital organs and horn

In certain body regions, the external skin undergoes **extreme modification**. Massive proliferation of the epidermis and permanent cornification of this external skin layer gives rise to **species-specific digital organs** (the equine hoof, the ruminant and swine hoof, the claw, or nail, of carnivores) and the horn of ruminants. In some cases, these modifications are accompanied by considerable structural alteration of the dermis in the form of papillae and dermal laminae, and accumulation of subcutaneous tissue to form pads and cushions. The structure of the layers of the wall of the digital organs varies considerably between species (see *Veterinary Anatomy of Domestic Mammals: Textbook and Colour Atlas*).

At the microscopic level the individual layers of the skin are also modified, reflecting the functional requirements of the tissue. The exposed location of the digital organs, in which they are subjected to **constant mechanical stress** and **wear**, necessitates continuous generation of horn-producing keratinocytes by the stratum germinativum. This is supported by specialised microvasculature in the form of capillary networks that facilitate the requisite metabolic processes. The digital organs also have sensory functions, and therefore contain abundant mechanoreceptors and nerve fibres.

The species-specific differentiation of the dermis into dermal papillae and laminae serves to increase considerably the strength of the horn by enabling the development of tubular and lamellar horn. Mechanical strength is conferred both by the quantity of horn and organisation of the lamellae.

At the tip of a papilla, the surface area over which the epidermis receives nutrients by diffusion from the capillaries of the underlying dermis (corium) is comparatively small. The keratinocytes become removed from their source of nutrition relatively quickly as they are pushed towards the surface. The resulting degree of cornification is limited. Cornified cells originating from the suprapapillar region are large, soft and relatively loosely packed. They form the **medulla** of the **tubular horn**.

In contrast, the epidermis overlying the sides of the **papillae** is amply supplied with nutrients across a relatively large surface area. Cornification of these cells is optimised, giving rise to a strong, dense band of cells. This **peripapillar cylinder of cornified cells** forms the cortex of the tubular horn, and contributes significantly to the overall strength of the cornified tissue.

Horn arising from between two papillae is termed **intertubular horn**. It lacks the hardness and strength of tubular horn.

Equine hoof (ungula)

The hoof is a complex epidermal organ in which the layers of the skin exhibit particularly marked modification. Accumulation of collagen-rich connective tissue and, in some locations, abundant fatty tissue in the subcutis gives rise to perioplic, coronary and digital cushions (Figures 15.27 to 15.29). Tubular glands, adipose tissue and elastic fibres present in this region support the mechanical function of the hoof and provide shock absorption. There is no subcutis in the wall and sole segments of the hoof.

In the perioplic and coronary segments, and in the sole, frog and bulbs, the corium is studded with papillae. These are particularly long (4–8 mm) in the coronary dermis. In the wall segment and in the bars, the dermis is arranged into longitudinally oriented laminae that give off secondary laminae from their surface. The dermis contains a dense vascular network (plexus venosus ungulae) and a large number of sensory nerve fibre plexuses and mechanoreceptors.

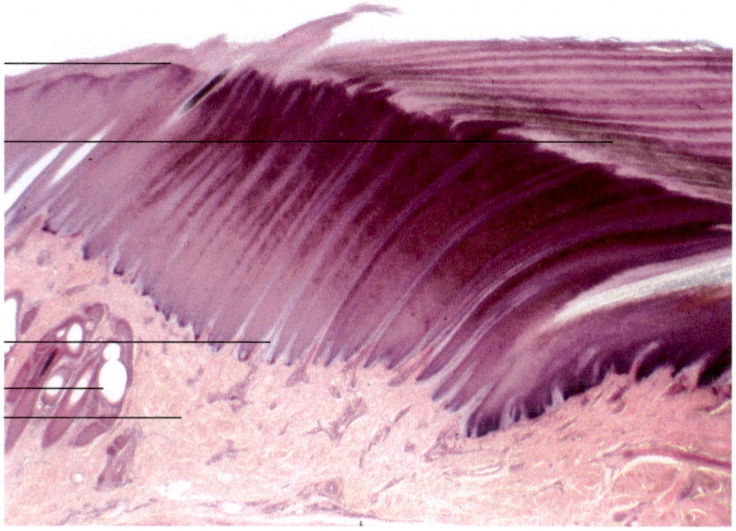

15.27 Longitudinal section of the coronary segment (horse). Haematoxylin and eosin stain (x17).

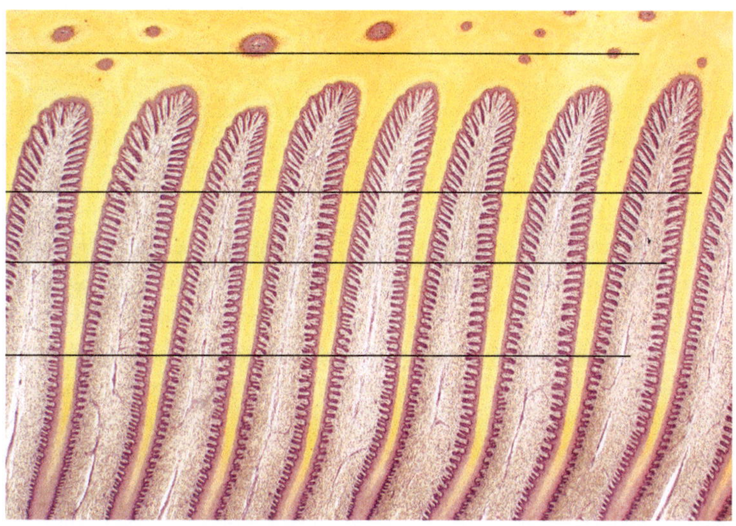

15.28 Wall segment of the hoof (horse). Picric acid stain (x40).

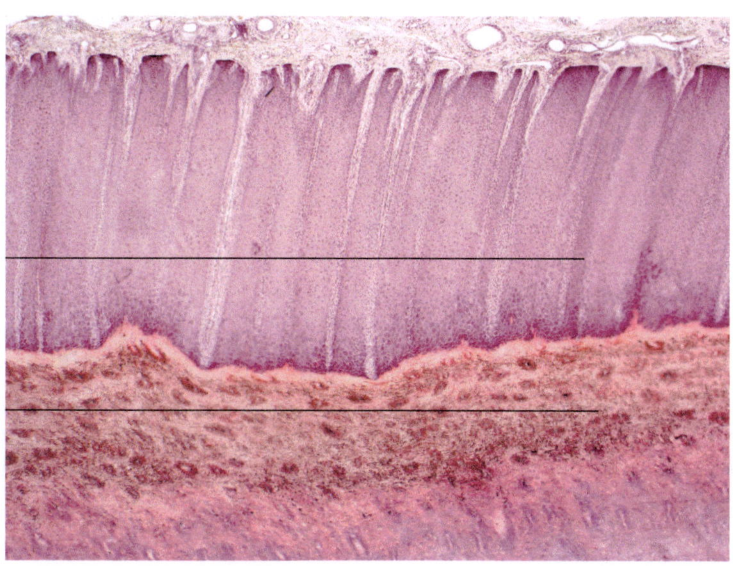

15.29 Chestnut (horse). Haematoxylin and eosin stain (x33).

The epidermis makes up the cornified hoof capsule. As determined by the surface architecture of the dermis, the horn of the perioplic and coronary segments, sole, frog and bulbs is tubular in form. The tubules run parallel to the surface of the hoof. Comprising horn of suprapapillar and peripapillar origin, these are firmly connected by intertubular horn arising between adjacent papillae. The tubules extend distally from the coronary segment over the lamellar horn of the walls and bars of the hoof. The perioplic horn forms a thin, shiny layer on the external surface of the hoof.

The cortex of the tubules comprises concentric layers in which inner, middle and outer zones can be distinguished. The individual layers are reinforced by tonofibrils arranged in oppositely oriented spirals.

Corresponding to its dermal template, the cornified epidermis of the walls and bars is laminar in form. The epidermis that interdigitates with the secondary dermal laminae is not cornified (see *Veterinary Anatomy of Domestic Mammals: Textbook and Colour Atlas*).

Ruminant and swine hoof (ungula)

The structure of the hoofs of ruminants and pigs exhibits species-specific modifications of the periople, coronary segment, walls, sole and bulbs. Cushions formed by accumulation of connective tissue in the subcutis protrude to a varying degree in the perioplic and coronary segment and in the bulbs. Particularly in the bulbs, the cushions are reinforced with aggregates of adipose tissue. In the wall and sole segments, the dermis lies directly adjacent to the phalanx, without a subcutis.

The **corium** bears tufts of numerous short papillae. In the perioplic segment these measure 1–2 mm in length. A characteristic feature of the hoof of ruminants is the absence of **secondary laminae** in the wall segment. (Figure 15.30). The **epidermal hoof capsule** is composed of a dorsal border, abaxial and axial walls, the sole and digital pad (bulb segment). In accordance with the mechanical forces experienced by the hoof, the tubular horn is most prominent at the perioplic and coronary segments. Laminar horn is present at the bearing edge, where the wall segment transitions to the sole.

The **structure of the tubular horn** differs markedly from the layered arrangement of equines. Instead, the tubules are arranged around the medulla in concave segments, resembling the structure of a pine cone. The bundles of tonofibrils are arranged in a circular fashion.

Claw (unguicula)

The **epidermal modifications** that constitute the claw, or nail, are **relatively simple**. The perioplic and coronary segments (Figure 15.31), located within the sulcus unguicularis, are underlain by a thin subcutis. The wall and sole segments and their associated corium directly overlie the **unguicular process** of the distal phalanx. The perioplic segment, located adjacent to the internal surface of the bony ungual crest, gives rise to the external layer of claw horn. This lacks tubular horn and is relatively soft, becoming worn away well before reaching the distal tip of the nail.

The horn that develops over the papilla-studded dermis of the coronary segment is tubular and makes up the bulk of the wall of the nail (claw plate) (Figure 15.31). In the wall segment, the corium carries very short laminae that interdigitate with uncornified epidermal laminae. Thus, the horn of the wall **does not have a laminar structure**. The narrow sole segment lines the plantar surface of the unguicular process. The epidermis of the sole is soft and non-tubular.

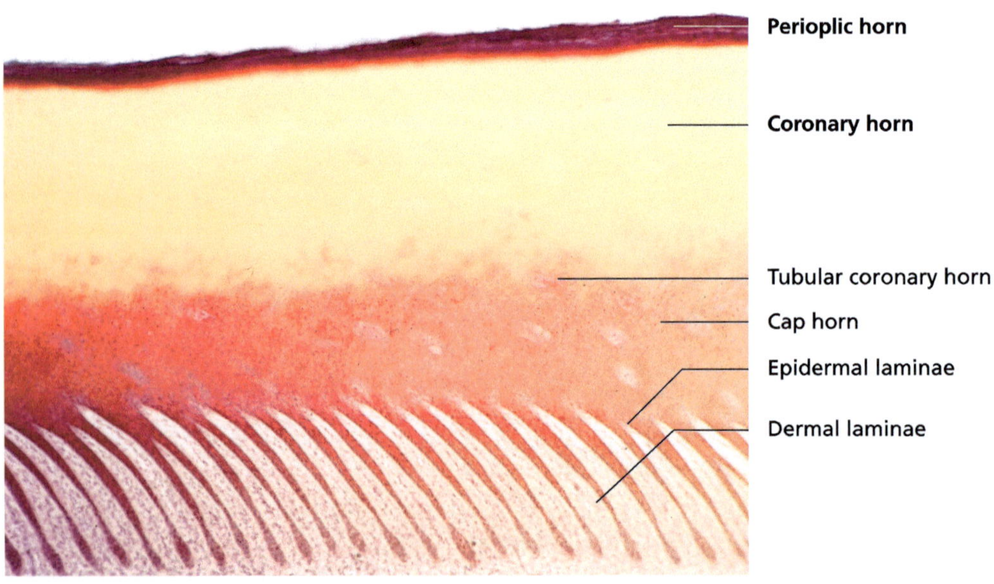

15.30 Hoof (young sheep). Picric acid stain (x80).

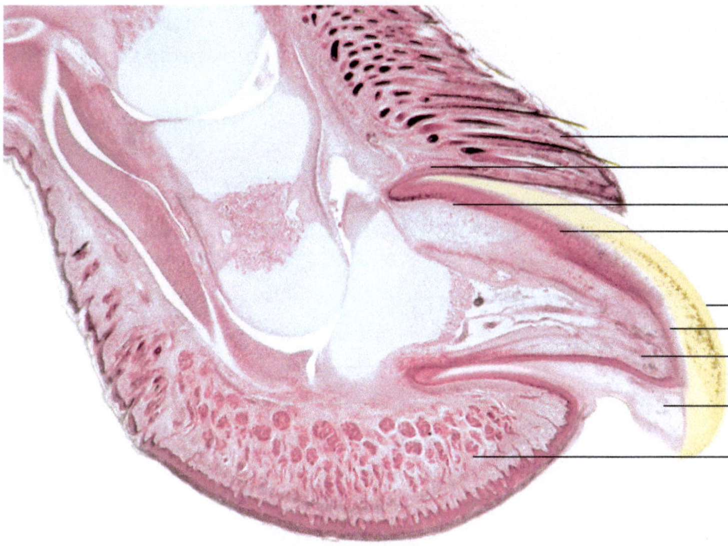

15.31 Longitudinal section of a claw (young dog). Haematoxylin and eosin stain (x32).

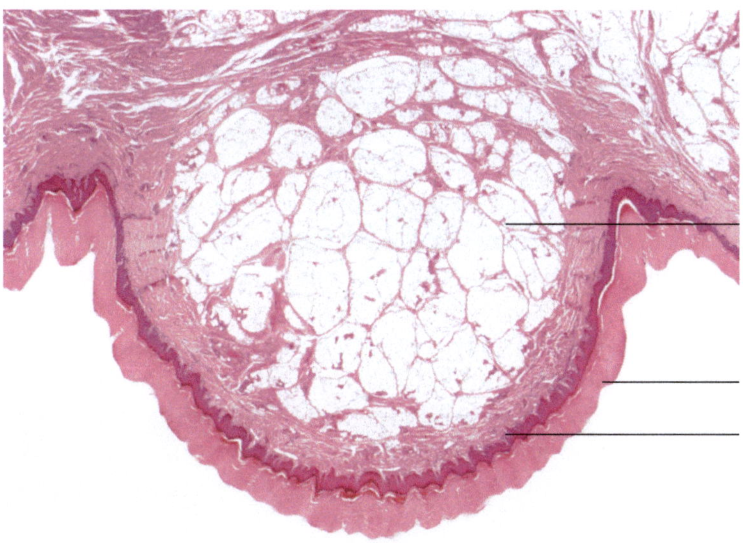

15.32 Digital pad (cat). Haematoxylin and eosin stain (x25).

The **digital pad** is characterised by a thickened, modified subcutis that is reinforced with strands of connective tissue fibres and encloses pockets of adipose tissue (Figure 15.32). Eccrine sweat glands are present within the connective tissue cushion. The epidermis is extensively keratinised. In the cat, it contains numerous pressure sensitive lamellar bodies.

Horn

Like the digital organs, the horn of ruminants is a modification of the external skin in which the layered structure is largely preserved. The horn covers the **hollow cone of bone** (cornual process) projecting from the frontal bone of the skull. The tough periosteum of the bone is continuous with the thin subcutis of the horn. The papillated dermis adheres tightly to the subcutis, forming the template for the horny epidermis. In the epidermis, the keratinocytes are transformed into predominantly **tubular horn** that gives rise to the characteristic shape of the horn casing.

Intertubular horn is minimal in cattle and more developed in small ruminants. Fluctuation in the nutritional supply of the basal cells of the stratum germinativum results in the **formation of rings** that manifest as irregularities in the surface of the horn (e.g. during and after pregnancy and disease).

Skin of birds

The majority of the avian body is covered with **feathers** (**pennae**). Originating from the epidermis, these structures are a characteristic and unique feature of the class Aves.

The feather coat of birds performs many functions for which hairy skin is responsible in mammals, including:

- provision of a barrier against irradiation and mechanical, thermal, chemical and biological influences,
- thermoregulation and
- communication.

In addition, the feathers are fundamental in enabling flight.

Where **feathers are present**, the skin is relatively thin. Feathered skin consists of an epidermis and dermis (corium) underlaid by the subcutis (hypodermis) (Figure 15.33). While the structure of the avian **epidermis** is homologous with that of mammals (Figure 15.34), differences are apparent in the layers of the **dermis**. In birds, the dermis comprises the:

- **stratum superficiale,**
- **stratum profundum:**
  - stratum compactum and
  - stratum laxum.

The superficial layer (**stratum superficiale**) is composed of loose connective tissue. Discrete dermal papillae are present only in association with feather follicles. The **stratum compactum** of the deep layer contains dense connective tissue that gives the dermis its mechanical strength. Smooth muscle cells in the **stratum laxum** tense the skin and connect the feather follicles, thus contributing to the movement of the feathers.

The subcutis serves as a mobile layer of tissue connecting the skin to the underlying structures. It contains adipose tissue concentrated into localised fat bodies (corpora adiposa).

In chickens and turkeys, a **bursa** (**bursa sterni**) is located within the subcutis over the cranial aspect of the sternum. This frequently becomes pathologically enlarged in broilers and laying hens housed under inappropriate conditions.

The lack of nerves in feathered skin, except in the vicinity of feather follicles, renders this tissue relatively insensitive.

During incubation, many bird species develop a median ventrosternal **brood patch** (**area incubationis**). Feathers are lost in this region and the vascularity of the dermis increases to facilitate the transfer of body heat to the eggs. Waterfowl, such as ducks and geese, do not develop brood patches. Instead, they warm their eggs with plucked down feathers.

Featherless body regions

The stratum corneum of the epidermis is thicker in featherless regions, corresponding with the mechanical forces to which these parts of the body are subjected. Various epidermal modifications are also present, including:

- the horny beak (rhamphotheca) with the cere (cera),
- scales (scuta) and small scales (scutella),
- pads (pulvini),
- claws (ungues) and
- the spur (calcar metatarsale).

The horn is particularly hard at the edges of the beak, in the scales and spur and on the dorsum of the claws. Soft horn is found at the cere, between the scales and on the plantar surface of the claws. Additional specialisations associated with the avian integument include:

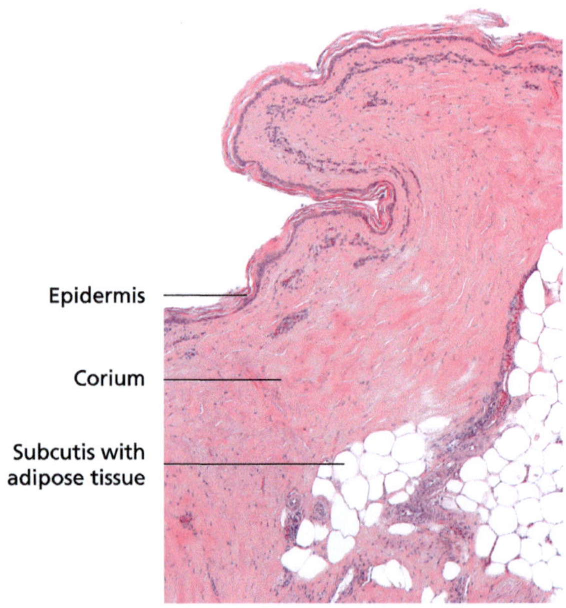

15.33 Skin of the thigh (chicken). Haematoxylin and eosin stain (x30).

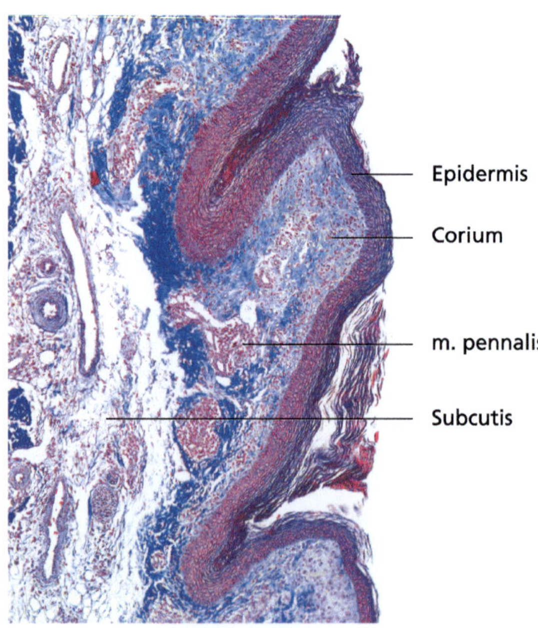

15.34 Skin of the lateral trunk (chicken). Azan stain (x45).

- skin glands (glandulae cutis),
- accessory skin structures (appendices integumenti),
- the skin folds of the wings (patagia) and
- interdigital webs (telae interdigitales).

Skin glands

Birds **do not have sweat glands. Sebaceous glands** are found in only three locations:

- above the tail: uropygial gland (glandula uropygialis),
- in the external acoustic meatus: auricular glands (glandulae auriculares) and
- in the cloaca: the vent glands (glandulae venti).

The **uropygial gland** is consistently present in chickens and water birds, but may be absent in psittacids and pigeons. It consists of two bilaterally symmetrical lobes, each with an excretory duct. The ducts open on the unpaired median **uropygial papilla (papilla uropygialis)**, upon which a tuft of small down feathers (circulus uropygialis) is often present. The oily holocrine secretory product is used in preening to cover the feathers in a fatty waterproof film. It is thought that the uropygial gland may also play a role in the storage of vitamin D, allowing this nutrient to be taken up by the beak during grooming.

The **glands of the external acoustic meatus** produce a waxy secretion containing numerous sloughed cells. A mucoid substance is secreted by the **glandulae venti** located on the labia of the cloaca.

Feathered body regions

Feathers

Related phylogenetically to the scales of reptiles, feathers are the distinguishing feature of all birds. Through their many specialised characteristics (e.g. lightweight construction, interlocking of the vanes, compliance and conformability), feathers confer upon birds the capacity for flight. Particularly in males, feathers are often brightly and characteristically coloured.

FEATHER STRUCTURE

The following description is based on the structure of a mature contour feather, consisting of the:

- shaft (scapus),
  - calamus,
  - rachis (rhachis) and
- internal and external vexillum.

The **shaft** is divided into the calamus and the rachis. A small opening, the **distal umbilicus (umbilicus distalis)** is located at the junction between these segments. The calamus is embedded in the skin; the rachis forms the visible portion of the feather. Located at the tip of the calamus is a round opening, the **proximal umbilicus (umbilicus proximalis)**, into which the dermal papilla projects. The papilla is covered by a layer of living epidermal cells, from which the new feathers are formed after moulting.

The calamus is round in cross-section and, in the mature feather, predominantly hollow. During feather development, the calamus is filled with pulp consisting of a loose mesenchymal reticulum surrounding a central artery and vein. During maturation, the pulp recedes leaving behind a series of air-filled compartments.

The rachis contains pith formed from epithelial cells. Its upper surface is convex, while the ventral side (facing the body) bears a groove (sulcus ventralis). The rachis carries two rows of slender, rigid **barbs (rami)**. Arising from each barb are two rows of fine **barbules (radii, barbulae)**. Barbulae of adjacent barbs cross one another at right angles. The **distally directed barbulae (radii distales)** possess tiny **hooklets (hamuli)** that interlock with the **proximally directed barbulae (radii proximalis)** (Figure 15.37). Disruption of this interlocking arrangement by external mechanical forces is corrected during preening, whereby the hooklets and barbules are reconnected ('zipping the feathers').

Together, the interconnected barbs form the **vane (vexillum)**. The vexillae of neighbouring feathers overlap in a shingle-like arrangement such that one is covered (vexillum internum) while the other is exposed (vexillum externum).

A small afterfeather (hypopenna) projects from the distal umbilicus. This may consist of just a tuft of umbilical barbs (barbae umbilicales) or may – as is typical of covert feathers – have an aftershaft (hyporhachis) with two hypovexillae. The calamus is set within a cylindrical cutaneous pit known as the feather follicle. A close fit is formed between the calamus and the follicle, resembling the relationship between the hair and the hair follicle in mammals.

The feather follicle has an inner epidermal and outer dermal wall (Figures 15.35 to 15.37). The epidermis of the follicle is continuous with the calamus at the proximal umbilicus. Here, the living epithelial cells of the follicle give way to the dead keratinised cells of the calamus. At the base of the feather follicle the small **dermal papilla** projects into the proximal umbilicus (Figure 15.36) and blends with the mesenchymal pulp within the calamus of the developing feather. In the young, growing feather, the dermal papilla is well vascularised to provide adequate nutrition to the epidermis for the processes involved in feather development.

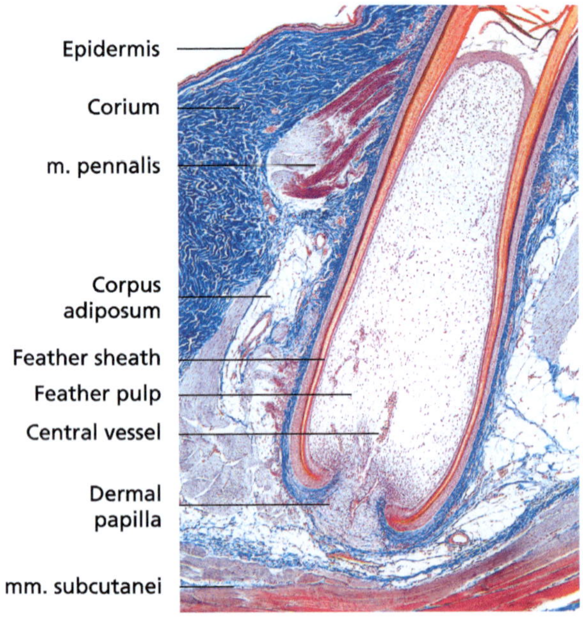

15.35 Feather (penna) with surrounding skin and subcutis. Azan stain (x25).

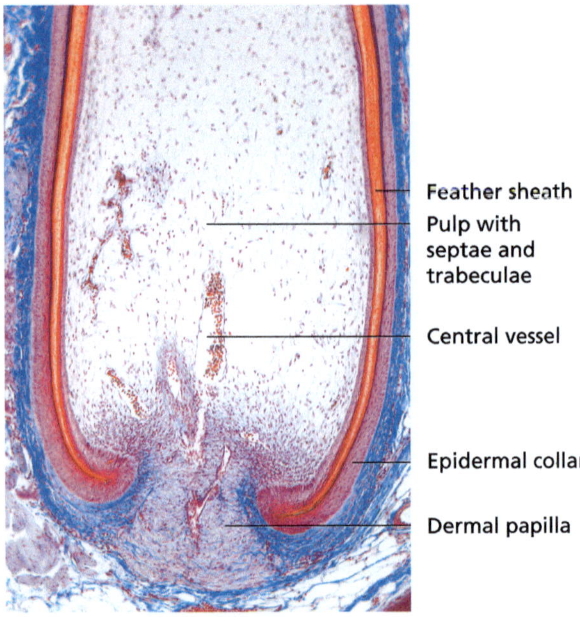

15.36 Feather follicle. Azan stain (x40).

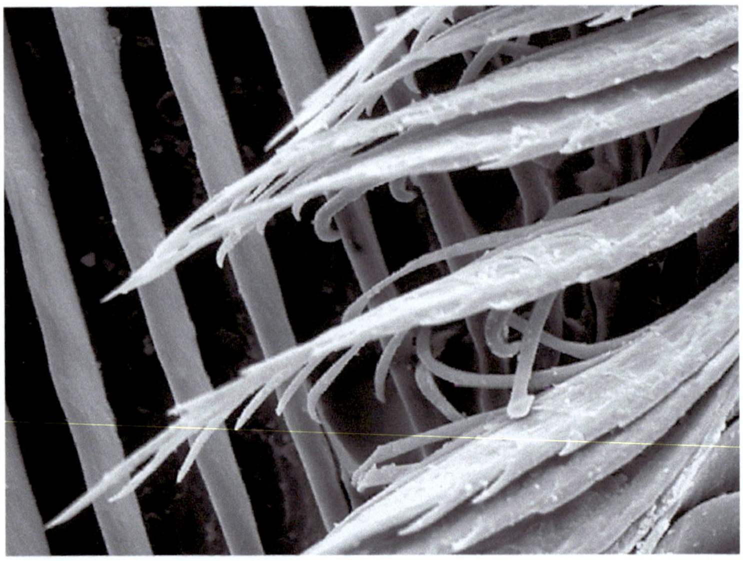

15.37 Scanning electron microscope image illustrating interlocking of hooklets and barbules.

Receptors and sense organs (organa sensuum)

16

Living cells are characterised by the ability to detect, transmit, store and, in some cases, respond to stimuli. Through evolution, mammals have developed a highly differentiated system of receptors and sense organs that allows the organism as a whole to adapt to environmental influences. This sensory system continuously receives external physical and chemical inputs and transmits these to the central nervous system. The components of the sensory system include **receptor organs**, neural **transmission pathways** and **processing centres** within the grey matter of the brain.

Superficially located receptor organs, or exteroreceptors, permit detection of stimuli by the skin and other external surfaces. In the broadest sense, the sensory cells of the eye, ear, taste buds and olfactory tissues can be included in this group.

Receptor cells that detect movement and changes in tension in muscle, tendons and joint capsules are referred to as proprioceptors. These include sensory cells that regulate balance.

Enteroreceptors convey stimuli from the internal organs.

Based on morphological and functional criteria, sensory receptors can be described as primary or secondary.

Primary receptors are nerve cells in which stimuli are detected by dendrites. Alteration of the potential difference at the cell membrane elicits an action potential that is transmitted to the central nervous system (e.g. neurosensory cells of the olfactory epithelium, photoreceptors of the retina, unmyelinated free nerve endings in the epidermis).

Secondary receptors are modified epithelial cells that synapse with dendritic processes of afferent neurons. They are activated by mechanical, thermal, chemical and acoustic stimuli (e.g. taste buds, hair cells of inner ear).

Exteroreceptors

External sensory stimuli include touch, pressure, vibration, pain and changes in temperature. Reflecting the diverse nature of these inputs, the morphology of exteroreceptors varies widely from simple nerve endings to complex receptor organs. Particular physiological stimuli are not necessarily associated with a specific type of receptor structure. While many receptors have a high specificity for a particular kind of stimulus, sensory perception occurs elsewhere, at the level of the central nervous system. Morphologically, exteroreceptors are divided into:

- free nerve endings,
- simple receptors and
- lamellar receptors.

Free nerve endings

Free nerve endings are terminal dendritic branches of neuronal axons. They lose their Schwann cell sheath as they penetrate the basal lamina and come to lie in the epithelium (Figure 16.1). The nerve fibre receives metabolic support from adjacent epithelial cells. In this sense, epithelial cells perform a similar function to glial cells. The axon penetrates the deeper layers of the epithelium, branches extensively and ends near the surface. Free nerve endings are found in various locations, including the epidermis, non-glandular mucosa, corneal epithelium and in the epithelial layers of the external root sheath of hair follicles. They convey stimuli associated with **touch** and **pain**.

Some free nerve endings are closely associated with specialised tactile epithelial cells (**Merkel cells**) located primarily in the basal layer of the epithelium. These nerve–epithelial cell complexes (Merkel's corpuscles) are particularly numerous in the external root sheath of hair follicles and in the planum rostrale of the nose of the pig. Merkel's corpuscles are pressure-sensing mechanoreceptors.

Simple receptors

Simple receptors are found in connective tissue. They consist of a thin outer connective tissue layer encircling an irregularly bundled or branched free nerve ending (Figures 16.2 and 16.3). The nerve endings frequently have a bulbous terminal expansion. Their Schwann cell coating ends as they enter the connective tissue sheath.

Simple receptors are numerous in the papillary layer of the dermis and around hair follicles.

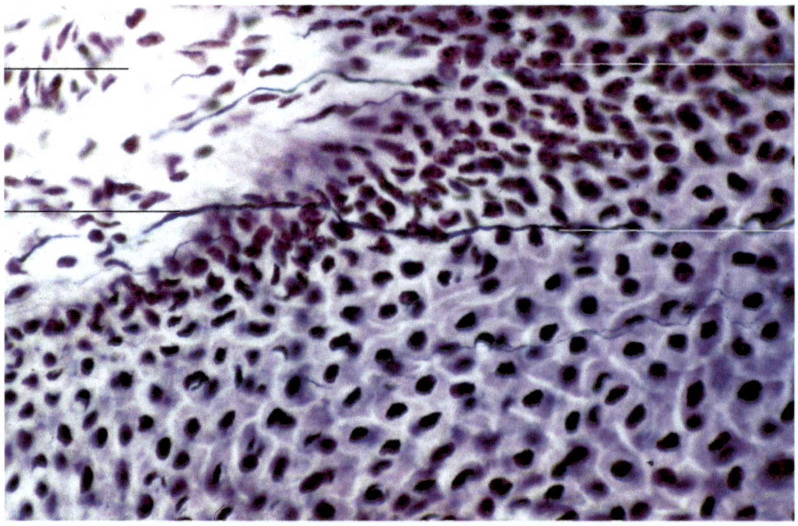

16.1 Intra-epithelial free nerve endings (nasolabial plate, ox). Preparation according to Schefthaler–Mayet (x480).

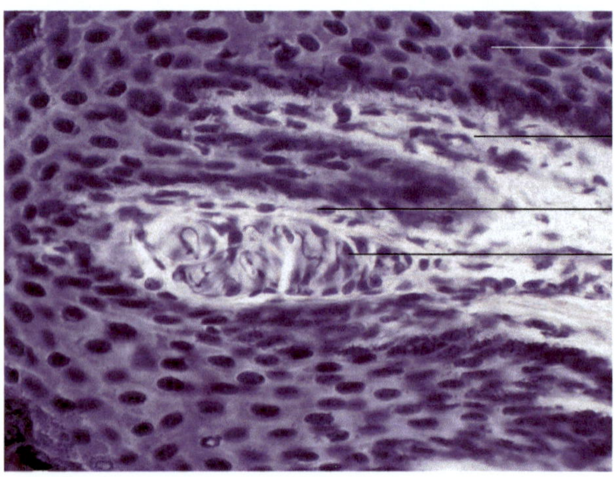

16.2 Subepithelial Meissner's corpuscle (nasolabial plate, ox). Preparation according to Schefthaler–Mayet (x480).

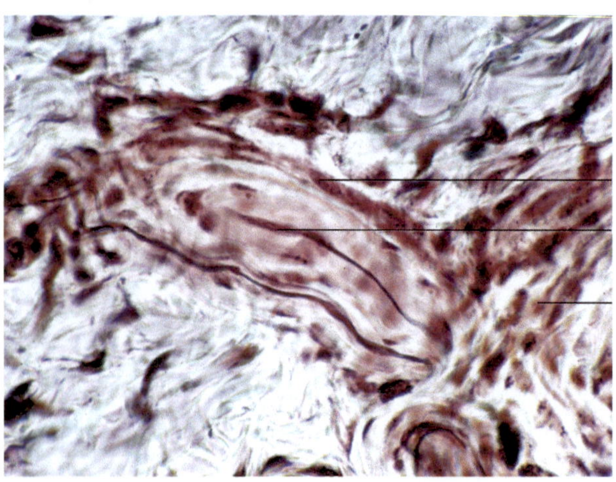

16.3 Ruffini's corpuscle (hypodermis, ox). Preparation according to Schefthaler–Mayet (x480).

Meissner's corpuscles (120 × 70 μm) have an incomplete connective tissue capsule. The central neural component comprises extensively branched axons. Sheets of modified Schwann cells lie between the axons, with which they are in direct contact. Meissner's corpuscles are **touch receptors** found in the stratum papillare of the dermis.

Ruffini corpuscles (0.25–1.5 mm long) are completely encapsulated. The associated axon loses its myelin sheath upon entering the capsule, before arborising into branches that terminate in small bulbs. Ruffini corpuscles are **mechanoreceptors** and are located in the joint capsules, in the hypodermis, along vessels, in the digital pads and in the corium of the hoof. They may also function as **cold** and **pain receptors**.

Lamellar receptors

Lamellar receptors (**Vater's corpuscles, Pacinian corpuscles**) consist of an axon surrounded by 10–60 concentric lamellae that resemble the layers of an onion (Figure 16.4). The inner lamellae are composed of flattened Schwann cells; the outer layers are formed by **fibrocytes**. Spaces between the lamellae contain **interstitial fluid**. Capillaries and collagen fibre bundles may penetrate the interlamellar gaps.

These types of receptors are visible macroscopically, reaching up to 4 mm in diameter. They occur in the deeper layers of the hypodermis, the corium of the hoof and claw, the metacarpal pads of carnivores, the mesenteries, the nasolabial plate of the ox and the pancreas of the cat. Lamellar receptors detect stimuli associated with **pressure** and **vibration**.

Proprioceptors

Proprioceptors contribute to fine tuning of movement involving **joints**, **tendons** and **muscles** by conveying information about **position** and **movement**.

In **joints**, proprioceptive stimuli are detected primarily by free nerve endings, Ruffini corpuscles and modified lamellar corpuscles within the joint capsule.

Golgi tendon organ

Golgi tendon organs are found in tendons, towards the muscle belly. They are stretch receptors that monitor tension within the musculotendinous apparatus. Golgi tendon organs (1.0 × 0.1 mm) are enclosed in a connective tissue capsule that merges with the perineurium of the associated neuron. At their centre, bundles of collagen fibres are closely associated with a branching network of non-myelinated nerve endings. Muscle contraction increases the pressure on the receptor, generating an action potential.

Muscle spindle

Muscle spindles are large (2–10 × 0.2 mm) proprioceptors located in **striated muscle**. Their outer connective tissue capsule is continuous with the perimysium. A second, internal capsule surrounds a fluid-filled cavity containing two types of modified muscle fibres: **nuclear bag** and **nuclear chain fibres**. These fibres are supplied by motor and sensory neurons. The sensory nerve endings serve as **stretch receptors**. The impulses they generate are transmitted to the central nervous system, which regulates the activity of the motor neurons supplying the muscle.

Enteroreceptors

Free sympathetic and parasympathetic nerve endings ramify within various layers of the viscera to provide **autonomic regulation of organ function**. Within the walls of arteries near the heart (carotid body, aortic arch), these receptors modulate blood pressure. Enteroreceptors in the walls of the atria monitor and control filling of the heart; others detect stretching within the lungs. In the gastrointestinal tract, free nerve endings convey impulses generated by stretching of smooth muscle and organ capsules. These signals are interpreted as pain.

Gustatory organs (organa gustus)

Gustation is mediated by **chemoreceptors** located within **taste buds** (gemmae gustatoriae). Taste buds are found primarily on the surface of the tongue and in the pharynx. They are abundant on the side walls of vallate, foliate and, in young animals, fungiform papillae. Taste buds contain **secondary sensory cells** that develop by **modification of epithelial cells**.

Taste buds

Taste buds (50–70 μm) consist of intra-epithelial clusters of 20–30 individual cells (Figures 16.5 and 16.6). They

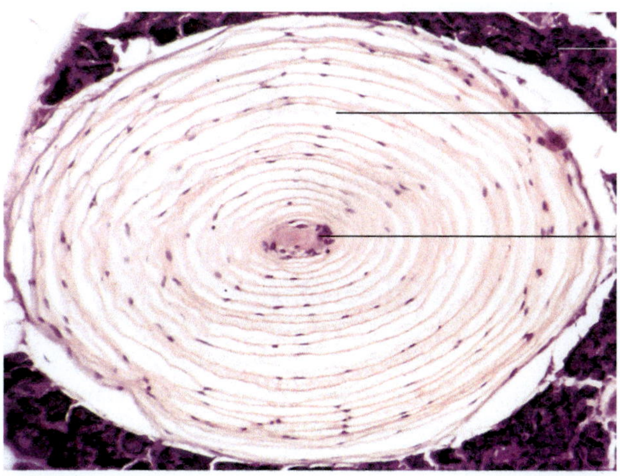

16.4 Multilaminar Pacinian corpuscle (pancreas, cat). Haematoxylin and eosin stain (x100).

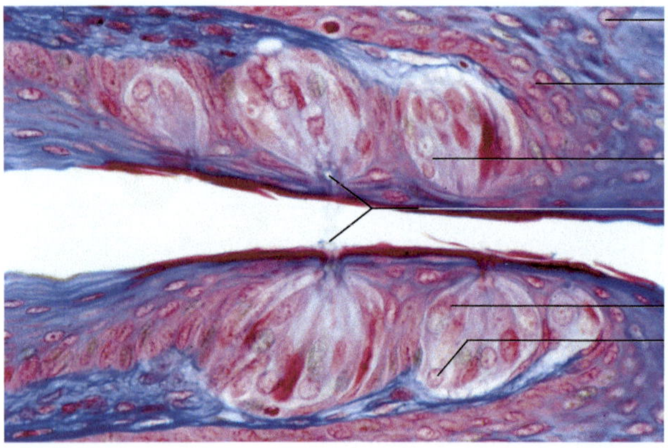

16.5 Taste buds in the wall of foliate papillae at the base of the tongue (horse). Azan stain (x250).

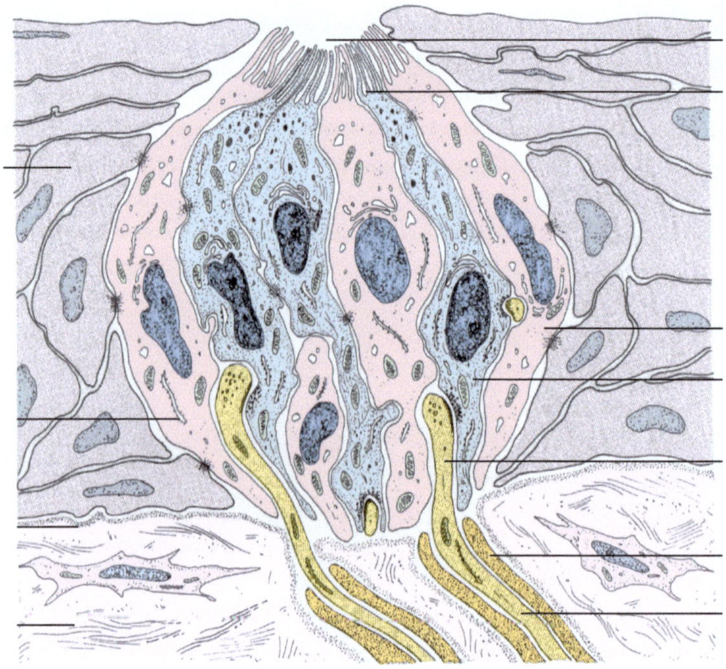

16.6 Taste bud (schematic).

extend from the basal lamina to a small **taste pore** at the surface of the epithelium. Within the taste pore, dissolved substances stimulate chemoreceptors on sensory cells in the taste bud (see below). Numerous (up to 50) free nerve endings located at the basolateral aspect of the taste bud direct the stimulus to the central nervous system. The **lifespan** of taste bud cells is approximately 10 days. They are replaced by basal cells (see below).

The cell types found in taste buds are comprised of:

- sensory cells,
- supporting (sustentacular) cells and
- basal cells.

The pillar-like **sensory cells** (chemoreceptor cells) are situated between sustentacular cells. **Microvilli** extending from the luminal surface of the sensory cells serve as the site of excitation. Basolaterally, the receptor cells synapse with axons that constitute the initial fibres of the gustatory neural pathway. Sensory cells can be distinguished with the light microscope. They are rich in organelles.

Supporting cells also extend through the full thickness of the epithelium. These contain abundant enzyme-forming organelles and a dense ER. Glycosaminoglycans synthesised by supporting cells are released into the taste pore to facilitate taste perception. Supporting cells are thought to be capable of differentiating into sensory cells.

Basal cells are undifferentiated cells that undergo mitotic division to provide continuous replacement of sensory and supporting cells. They have relatively few organelles and are situated around the nerve fibres.

In some regions, the **lamina propria mucosae** contains **serous, tubulo-acinar glands** (**gustatory glands**). The secretory product empties via excretory ducts into the sulcus of vallate papillae and sometimes into the spaces between foliate papillae. The watery secretion rinses the taste buds, permitting the detection of new stimuli. The number of glands increases with the number of taste buds.

Olfactory organs (organa olfactus)

In animals, the olfactory sense plays an important role in acquisition of food, identification of conspecifics and sexual behaviour. Domestic mammals are considered macro-osmatic animals (those with highly developed organs of smell). Olfactory stimuli are detected in the **olfactory mucosa** (tunica mucosa olfactoria). The mucosa is composed of the **olfactory epithelium** (epithelium olfactorium) and underlying **lamina propria mucosae**.

The olfactory epithelium contains several cell types. Of primary importance for olfaction are the **bipolar neurons** (**neurosensory cells**) (Figures 16.7 to 16.10). The olfactory **chemoreceptors** lie on the surface of the sensory cell (see below). Olfactory epithelium is present in circumscribed areas of the nasal mucosa and in the vomeronasal organ.

The **olfactory epithelium** is pseudostratified and contains three cell types:

- neurosensory cells,
- supporting cells and
- basal cells.

The perikarya of the **neurosensory cells** (**bipolar neurons**) are located in the epithelium, the cell nuclei lying approximately at mid-epithelial level. The cells are pear- to bottle-shaped and are flanked by supporting cells. At the epithelial surface, the dendritic process of the neurosensory cell ends in a club-shaped expansion (**dendritic bulb**) (Figure 16.9). A number of cilia (generally 8–20, considerably more in the dog) extend from the surface of the dendritic bulb.

Chemoreceptors for **odorant substances** are located on the ciliary membrane. The cilia consist of a thick initial portion with a typical tubular ultrastructure (9×2+2 pattern) and a distal portion containing only two micro-

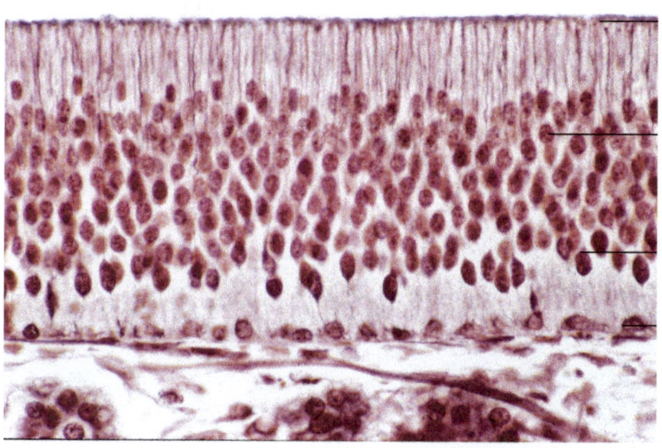

16.7 Olfactory epithelium (goat). Preparation according to Bodian (x480).

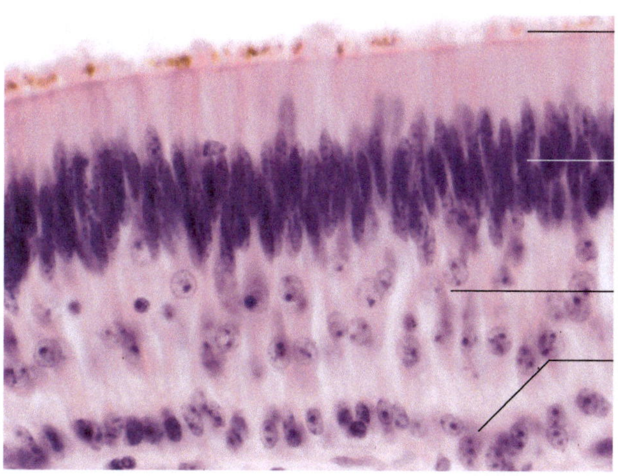

16.8 Olfactory epithelium (calf). Haematoxylin and eosin stain (x480).

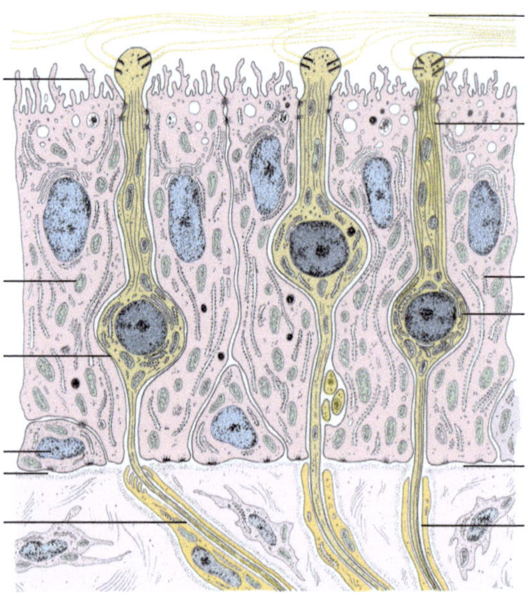

16.9 Olfactory epithelium (schematic).

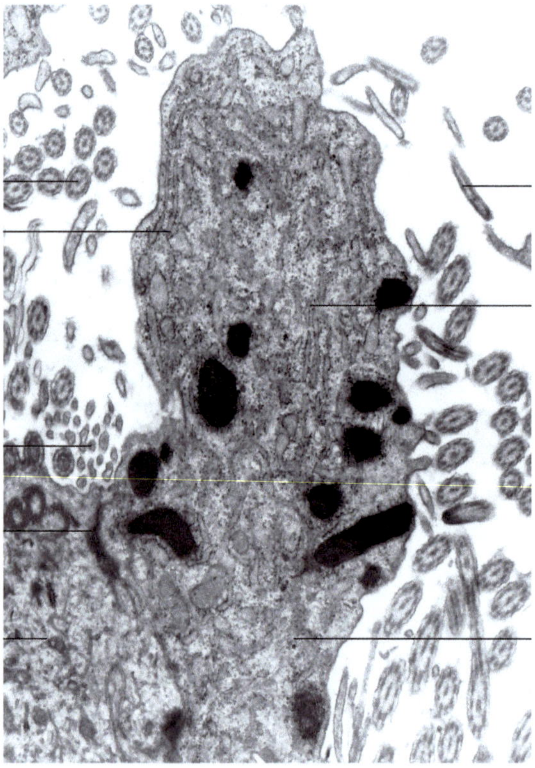

16.10 Fine structure of the dendritic bulb on the free surface of a neurosensory cell of the olfactory mucosa (ruminant; x14,000).

tubules. These cellular processes (50–100 µm) are bathed in a layer of thin mucus that is secreted in part by the supporting cells (see below), and to a greater extent by glands of the olfactory mucosa. Odoriferous chemicals diffuse into the mucous layer and interact with chemoreceptors on the ciliary membrane. The resulting action potential is transmitted across the perikaryon to the efferent arm of the axon. The axon extends from the basal aspect of the cell body and penetrates the basal lamina. Axons combine to form bundles of myelinated nerve fibres (**fila olfactoria**) that course to the lamina cribrosa of the ethmoid bone, terminating in the olfactory bulb at the olfactory glomerulus.

Supporting cells extend from the basal lamina to the epithelial surface. Numerous irregularly branching microvilli project from the surface of the cell. In the olfactory epithelium, supporting cells perform a role equivalent to that of glial cells. In addition, these organelle-rich cells exocytose mucoid substances. Intracellular pigments give the mucus its characteristic colour.

Basal cells are small cells lying adjacent to the basal lamina. These undergo mitotic division and differentiate into supporting cells.

The olfactory epithelium rests on loose connective tissue containing myelinated nerve fibres, vessels and **tubulo-acinar olfactory glands** (glandulae olfactoriae). The extremely watery protein- and enzyme-rich product of these serous glands passes through long excretory ducts to reach the epithelial surface. The secretion binds odorant chemicals to facilitate detection of olfactory stimuli, and also contributes to the breakdown of these molecules to prevent their accumulation.

Eye (organum visus)

The eye consists of a receptor organ, the eyeball or bulb (bulbus oculi) and associated supportive and protective structures (vessels, nerves, fat, ocular muscles, eyelids and lacrimal apparatus). Neural impulses generated in the bulb are conveyed by the **optic nerves** (nn. optici) and the **central visual pathways** to the **visual cortex** of the brain, where interpretation of visual stimuli takes place.

Bulb (bulbus oculi)

The bulb is a spheroid structure that **receives light** stimuli. The resulting nerve impulses are transmitted by neural pathways to the grey matter of the brain. The receptors within the eye and the associated neural tracts are formed from the diencephalon during embryonic development.

Structure

The wall of the bulb consists of three layers:

- **fibrous (outer) tunic** (tunica fibrosa or externa bulbi):
  - sclera,
  - cornea,
- **vascular (middle) tunic** (uvea, tunica vasculosa or media bulbi):
  - choroid,
  - ciliary body (corpus ciliare),
  - iris,
- **nervous (inner) tunic** (neuro-epithelial tunic, retina, tunica interna bulbi):
  - pars optica retinae and
  - pars caeca retinae.

Fibrous tunic (tunica fibrosa or externa bulbi)

The outer tunic of the eye is a tough fibro-elastic layer composed of an opaque posterior component, the **sclera**, and a transparent anterior portion, the **cornea** (Figure 16.11). At the corneoscleral junction, a shallow groove (sulcus sclerae) is present on the external surface of the eye.

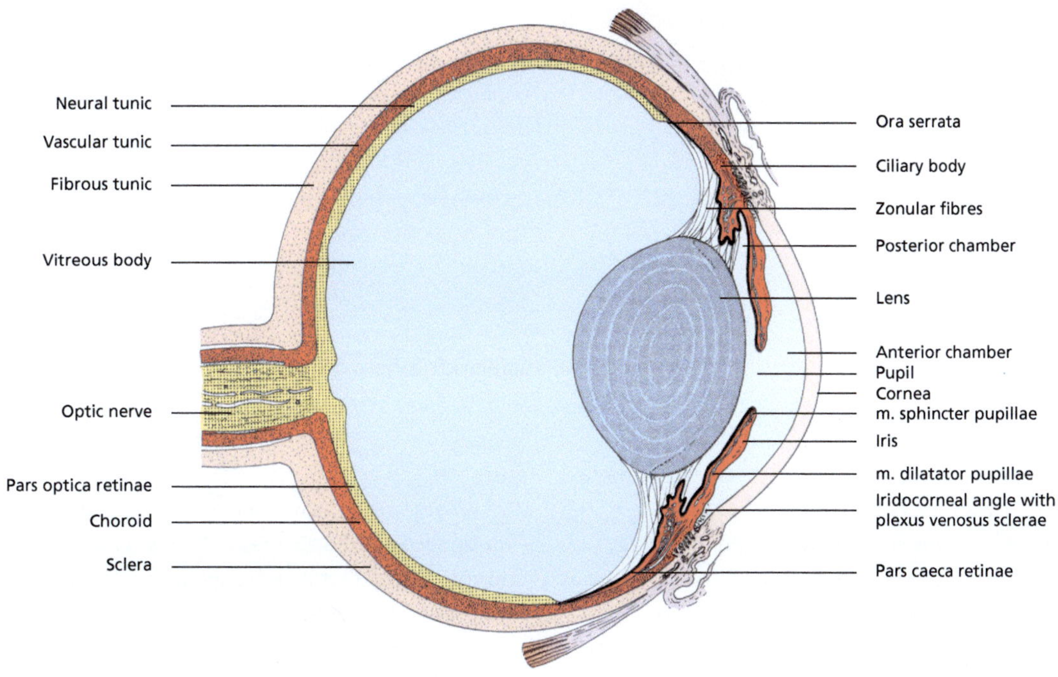

16.11 Bulb (schematic).

SCLERA

The sclera consists predominantly of interwoven layers of collagen fibres. Most fibres are oriented parallel to the surface of the bulb. In some regions, elastic fibres are interspersed among the collagen fibre bundles. The shape of this fibro-elastic layer is determined by intraocular pressure, and by tension exerted by the ocular muscles.

The space between the collagen fibres contains scant quantities of ground substance, solitary fibrocytes and, in ruminants, numerous pigmented cells. Few blood vessels are present in the sclera. The thickness of the sclera gradually increases from the equator of the bulb towards the posterior pole. At the sieve-like **area cribrosa sclerae**, the sclera is perforated by vessels and by nerve fibres that form the optic nerve. The posterior portion of the sclera is surrounded by a loose network of collagen fibres (**lamina episcleralis**).

Anteriorly, the sclera is covered by the conjunctiva. At the corneoscleral junction, the sclera thickens (particularly in carnivores) and is associated internally with a ring of fibro-elastic tissue, the annulus sclerae. The **plexus venosus sclerae**, located adjacent to the annulus sclerae, drains the aqueous humour and thus participates in regulation of intraocular pressure.

Species variation

Birds: Embedded within the connective tissue of the sclera is a lamina of hyaline cartilage (**lamina cartilaginea sclerae**) and an osseous scleral ring (**annulus ossicularis sclerae**). The cartilaginous lamina (Figures 16.18 and 16.19) reinforces the posterior wall of the bulb. It may become ossified near the point of exit of the optic nerve, forming the horseshoe-shaped os nervi optici. The osseous scleral ring confers mechanical stability upon the concave annular portion of the eyeball. It also serves as a buttress during accommodation which, in contrast to mammals, involves active compression of the lens. The scleral ring consists of 10–18 (usually 15) individual ossicles (ossicula sclerae) that overlap in a manner resembling fish scales.

CORNEA

Towards the anterior pole of the bulb, the sclera is continued by the transparent cornea. The corneoscleral junction is termed the **limbus corneae**. The bulk of the cornea is formed by lamellae of parallel collagen fibres (**substantia propria corneae**) (see below).

The cornea consists of five layers (Figures 16.15 and 16.16):

- anterior epithelium (epithelium anterius),
- subepithelial basement membrane,
- stroma (substantia propria corneae),
- posterior limiting lamina (Descemet's membrane, lamina limitans posterior) and
- posterior epithelium (epithelium posterius).

The **anterior epithelium** (epithelium anterius corneae) is non-keratinised stratified squamous in type. It is continuous with the conjunctiva at the limbus. The surface of the corneal epithelium is protected by the thin precorneal tear film, a complex fluid layer consisting of mucous, aqueous and lipid components.

The **subepithelial basement membrane** (Bowman's membrane in primates, humans and birds) lies deep to the anterior epithelium. It is composed of delicate fibrils and dense ground substance. The membrane serves as a barrier against the entry of water into the corneal stroma.

The **stroma** (substantia propria corneae) consists of perpendicularly oriented collagen fibre lamellae (ca. 10%) and largely watery ground substance (ca. 90%). In addition, the cornea contains insoluble collagen, glycosaminoglycans and ions. Present between the fibrous layers are flattened fibroblasts and a dense network of non-myelinated sensory and autonomic nerve fibres, most of which extend into the epithelium. The stroma is avascular. Nutritional support is provided to the cornea by diffusion from peripherally located arteries, the precorneal tear film and from the aqueous humour.

Corneal transparency is dependent upon optimal hydration of the stroma (72–78% water) and maintenance of the regular arrangement of collagen fibrils. These factors minimise the scattering of incident light. Excessive hydration of the cornea results in gaps between collagen fibrils and loss of corneal transparency. This occurs post-mortem and as a consequence of corneal damage. The surface layers of the cornea and the anterior and posterior epithelia also play an important role in maintaining the optical clarity of the cornea.

The **posterior limiting lamina** (Descemet's membrane) lies internally adjacent to the corneal stroma. It consists of a thick basement membrane incorporating hexagonally interwoven microfilaments. Descemet's membrane contains collagen type VIII, which is unusual in other basement membranes.

The simple squamous **posterior epithelium** (epithelium posterius corneae) lines the posterior aspect of the cornea. It also serves as the endothelial lining of the anterior chamber (Figure 16.12). This single-cell layer aids in maintaining corneal transparency by actively removing water from the corneal stroma (ATPase and carbonic anhydrase pumps). It also produces proteins used in the formation of Descemet's membrane.

Species variation

Birds: Except in water birds and several diurnal birds of prey, the avian cornea is relatively thin. Compared with mammals, its relative diameter is also small. In contrast, the radius of curvature exhibits considerable species variation. In water birds, the cornea is comparatively flat whereas in owls it is strongly curved with a correspondingly deep anterior chamber. The corneoscleral junction is marked by an annular depression. At the periphery of the cornea, the corneoscleral junction contains pigment deposits that can be differentiated gonioscopically into an inner and outer pigment band (annulus corneae). The cornea is extremely sensitive due to the presence of abundant **sensory nerve fibres**. Blood vessels – that would compromise the transparency of the cornea – are absent. The cornea is nourished by diffusion from the aqueous humour and the precorneal tear film. In contrast to mammals, birds have a thick Bowman's membrane that contributes substantially to the structural integrity of the cornea. Descemet's membrane is relatively thin and is not present in all bird species. The corneal stroma is composed of collagen fibrils and abundant hydrophilic chondroitin sulfate-rich ground substance. Corneal transparency results from the arrangement of the collagen fibrils and regulation of water content in the stroma.

Vascular tunic (uvea, tunica vasculosa or media bulbi)

The middle tunic of the bulb is a loosely arranged layer containing pigmented cells, collagen and elastic fibres, muscle, nerve fibres and abundant vessels (Figures 16.16 and 16.17).

The vascular tunic consists of a posterior portion, the **choroid** (choroidea), and two anterior components, the **ciliary body** (corpus ciliare) and the **iris**. The free edge of the iris forms the boundary of the **pupil**.

CHOROID (CHOROIDEA)

The choroid extends posteriorly from the ciliary body at the ora serrata (anterior limit of the sensory retina, see below). It is extensively vascularised. Choroidal vessels are embedded in loose connective tissue incorporating fibrocytes, melanocytes, networks of elastic fibres and lymphoid cells. The layers of the choroid (Figures 16.20, 16.23, 16.24 and 16.29), from outermost to innermost, are the:

- suprachoroid layer (lamina suprachoroidea, lamina fusca sclerae),
- vascular layer (lamina vasculosa),
- choriocapillary layer (lamina choriocapillaris) and
- basal complex (lamina vitrea).

The **suprachoroid layer** establishes a loose connection between the choroid and the sclera. It consists of connective tissue incorporating numerous pigmented cells. The **vascular layer** is the thickest layer of the choroid. Like the suprachoroid layer, it is composed of lamellae of pigmented connective tissue. Relatively large vessels coursing through the vascular layer supply the inner layers of the retina (e.g. aa. ciliares, vv. vorticosae). These vascular loops extend into the **choriocapillary layer** where they give rise to a dense, inner capillary network. This supplies the outer retinal layers (rods and cones).

The **basal complex** (**Bruch's membrane**) lies between the choriocapillary layer and the outermost layer of the retina (retinal pigment epithelium). It is relatively thick (1–3 μm). The basal complex contains a central layer of elastic fibres inserted between layers of collagen fibres. These collagen layers lie adjacent to the capillaries of the choriocapillary layer (externally) and the basal lamina of the retinal pigment epithelium (internally). The basal complex is firmly attached to the retinal pigment epithelium.

Species variation

Horse, ruminants and carnivores: Dorsal to the optic nerve head, a crescent-shaped reflective layer, the **tapetum lucidum**, is incorporated into the choroid, between the vascular and choriocapillary layers (Figures 16.21 and 16.24). In carnivores, the tapetum lucidum consists of 10–15 layers of cells (**tapetum cellulosum**). Herbivores have a tapetum lucidum consisting of concentrically oriented fibres (**tapetum fibrosum**). In the region occupied by the tapetum lucidum, the retinal pigment epithelium is non-pigmented and translucent, permitting light to fall directly on the tapetal layer. Reflection of light from the tapetum lucidum results in additional retinal stimulation, improving vision in low light conditions.

Birds: Diurnal birds have a heavily pigmented choroid, whereas little if any pigment is present in crepuscular species (Figure 16.29). A **tapetum lucidum choroideae**, present in several species of crepuscular mammals, has not been observed in birds. A white reflective area (tapetum lucidum retinae) is present in the dorsal fundus of the European nightjar, but this is associated with the retinal pigment epithelium and is not the equivalent of the choroidal tapetum of mammals.

Sinuses containing mucous substances are present within the choroid of woodpeckers. These act as shock absorbers that dampen the impact of pecking.

CILIARY BODY (CORPUS CILIARE)

The mammalian ciliary body is comprised of the following components:

- epithelial lining (pars ciliaris retinae),
- anterior region (pars plicata) with ciliary processes (processus ciliares),
- posterior region (pars plana, orbiculus ciliaris) and
- ciliary muscle.

The ciliary body extends anteriorly from the ora serrata (anterior limit of the choroid) to the base of the iris (margo ciliaris iridis). It is situated at the level of the lens, to which it is connected by the zonular fibres. The ciliary body forms the peripheral boundary of the posterior chamber of the eye and is in contact with the vitreous body (Figures 16.13 and 16.16). It is covered externally by the sclera.

The surface of the ciliary body is lined with a double layer of epithelium, the **pars ciliaris retinae**, consisting of an inner non-pigmented layer and an outer **pigmented layer**. The pars ciliaris retinae, together with the pars iridica retinae (see below) constitutes the non-sensory portion of the retina (pars caeca retinae) (Figure 16.11).

The anterior portion of the ciliary body (pars plicata, corona radialis), has numerous meridional folds (70–80 in the dog, over 100 in the ox and horse). These extend towards the lens equator as the **ciliary processes** (**processus ciliares**). The core of the ciliary processes comprises loose connective tissue and dense capillary networks. **Aqueous humour** is secreted by the ciliary processes into the posterior chamber (Figure 16.13).

In the posterior region of the ciliary body (pars plana, orbiculus ciliaris) the meridional folds are reduced in height. The zonular fibres that suspend the lens originate from ciliary epithelium of the pars plicata and pars plana.

The connective tissue stroma of the ciliary body contains elastic fibres, melanocytes, vessels and the smooth **ciliary muscle**. The m. ciliaris is responsible for **accommodation**. It is relatively weak in the horse, and comparatively well developed in carnivores.

In mammals, the ciliary muscle consists of circular, meridional and radial components intermingled with elastic fibres. Contraction of the various components of the muscle alters the tension in the zonular fibres, thus changing the shape of the lens. An increase in convexity of the lens, particularly on its anterior surface, facilitates near vision; flattening of the lens permits focusing for distant vision. The ciliary muscle receives parasympathetic (from the ciliary ganglion) and sympathetic innervation via the ciliary nerves.

Species variation

Birds: The ciliary body is anchored externally to the osseous **scleral ring** (**annulus ossicularis sclerae**). As in mammals, the anterior portion of the ciliary body is covered in numerous meridionally oriented folds (**pars plicata**, **corona radialis**) that taper off posteriorly to form the **pars plana** (**pars plana**, **orbiculus ciliaris**). In contrast to mammals, the ciliary processes attach to the periphery of the lens, their tips fusing with the lens capsule (Figure 16.14). The surface of the ciliary body is lined by the double-layered **pars ciliaris retinae** (outer layer of pigmented cells, inner layer of columnar epithelial cells; Figure 16.27).

In most bird species, the inner layer of the pars ciliaris retinae is non-pigmented. **Nocturnal owls** are an exception. In this species, the cells of the inner layer contain large granules filled with **lipofuscin** (Figure 16.28). This additional pigment aids in the absorption of scattered light by the long, tubular ciliary body and prevents peripheral illumination of the sclera, which is incompletely covered by the orbit. The zonular fibres arise from the basal lamina of the inner epithelial layer and pass to the lens capsule. Their role in attaching the ciliary body to the lens is considerably less significant than in mammals (Figure 16.14).

In contrast to mammals, the ciliary muscle is striated. It is embedded within the stroma of the ciliary body. The ciliary muscle consists of two parts: the m. ciliaris anterior and the m. ciliaris posterior. Both muscles arise from the sclera deep to the scleral ring. The m. ciliaris anterior passes in an anterior direction to attach to the corneal stroma. The posterior muscle extends posteriorly to join the base of the ciliary body (Figure 16.14).

The main action of the m. ciliaris anterior is to alter the curvature of the cornea (**corneal accommodation**) (Figure 16.14). Contraction of the **m. ciliaris posterior** draws the ring-shaped ciliary body forward, thus also reducing its diameter as the scleral ring narrows anteriorly. Constriction of the ciliary body alters the shape of the lens, increasing its convexity (**lenticular accommodation**) (Figure 16.14). In nocturnal birds, such as owls, accommodation is predominantly corneal. The m. ciliaris anterior is well developed in these birds, while the m. ciliaris posterior is a rudimentary structure. In diving birds, which rely almost exclusively on lenticular accommodation, the relative degree of muscle development is reversed.

The **cilioscleral sinus** (**sinus cilioscleralis**) divides the ciliary body into **inner** and **outer sections**. The two sections are connected only at the posterior aspect of the pars plana. At the level of the iris base, the cilioscleral sinus communicates with the anterior chamber at the iridocorneal angle (angulus iridocornealis). The cilioscleral sinus is traversed by a mesh of delicate connective tissue fibres (**reticulum trabeculare**), enclosing the **spaces of Fontana** (**spatia anguli iridocornealis**) (Figure 16.14). The transition to the iridocorneal angle is demarcated by strong, straight fibre bundles that anchor the base of the iris to the sclera (**ligamentum pectinatum**) (Figure 16.14). The cilioscleral sinus permits the inner section of the ciliary body and its associated folds to become displaced, thus serving to underpin the avian mechanism of lenticular accommodation. For this reason, the cilioscleral sinus of diving birds (in which extreme compression of the lens results in a particularly wide range of accommodation) is relatively deep.

IRIS

The iris is the most anterior portion of the vascular layer. It projects into the interior of the eye from the base of the ciliary body, partially covering the lens. The circular free edge of the iris (margo pupillaris) surrounds a central opening, the **pupil** (Figure 16.11). The iris is an opaque diaphragm that separates the aqueous chamber of the eye into an anterior chamber (camera anterior bulbi) and a posterior chamber (camera posterior bulbi). The anterior and posterior chambers communicate via the pupil.

The **anterior surface of the iris** forms the posterior boundary of the anterior chamber. A continuous epithelium is lacking, the surface layer being comprised of flattened fibroblasts, melanocytes and connective tissue fibres of the iris stroma (Figure 16.17). Irregular grooves and crypts on the anterior surface result in an intimate association between the aqueous humour and the stroma.

The iris stroma consists of a loose mesh of collagen fibres in an amorphous matrix. It is highly vascularised and contains smooth muscle cells, melanocytes and nerve fibres.

The **collagen bundles** are arranged in arcades, allowing them to adapt to the narrowing (miosis) and dilation (mydriasis) of the pupil. The extensive stromal **vascular supply** provides nutritional and mechanical support. Collagen fibres form cuffs around the vessel walls, preventing interruption of the microcirculation during contraction and relaxation of the iris.

The iris stroma incorporates two **smooth muscle elements** that regulate the size of the pupil: the m. sphincter pupillae and the m. dilatator pupillae (Figure 16.11).

The circular fibres of the **m. sphincter pupillae** form a ring at the free edge of the iris. In species with a non-circular pupil (cat, sheep, ox), these muscle fibres are reinforced peripherally by a sharply angled muscle fibre lattice. The interweaving of these muscle fibres produces a slit-like or oval (transverse or longitudinal) pupil. The m. sphincter pupillae receives parasympathetic (cholinergic) innervation. A loose association exists between the fibres of the m. sphincter pupillae and m. dilatator pupillae.

The **m. dilatator pupillae** (Figures 16.11 and 16.17) is formed by myoepithelial cells that make up the anterior layer of the posterior iris epithelium (pars iridica retinae; see below). Contractile, non-pigmented processes project radially from the basal portion of the cells. This layer is supplied by sympathetic (adrenergic) nerve fibres. Contraction of the m. dilatator pupillae results in dilation of the pupil.

Pigmented cells found in the iris originate from the neural crest (stromal melanocytes) and neuroectoderm (pigmented iris epithelium; see below). Melanin protects the retina from excessive incident light and from scattered light by acting as a neutral-density filter. The degree of pigmentation (number and size of melanosomes) determines the **colour of the iris**. Iris colour is encoded in several nondominant genes, resulting in a range of hues.

A blue iris indicates an absence of stromal melanocytes. The blue colour arises from light falling on collagen fibres lying anterior to the pigmented layer of the epithelium. Condensation of the collagen fibres produces a blue-grey to grey tone (pig, goat). A thin stroma and large melanocyte population results in a dark brown iris (horse, ox). The light-brown to yellowish iris colour seen in dogs, pigs and small ruminants is associated with a relative paucity of melanin granules. Ocular albinism results from a lack of pigmentation.

The **posterior surface** of the iris is lined by a double layer of epithelium (pars iridica retinae) derived from the leaves of the anterior rim of the optic cup. The inner leaf becomes the pigmented continuation of the non-pigmented epithelial layer of the ciliary body. This layer is **simple columnar**. At the free edge of the iris, the inner layer of the embryonic optic cup reflects on itself to become the outer layer. This develops into a single layer of apically **pigmented epithelial cells** with non-pigmented basal extensions containing filamentous contractile elements (Figure 16.17). These pigmented **myoepithelial cells** constitute the m. dilatator pupillae. The **pars iridica retinae** is part of the nonsensory retina. Only the pars optica retinae develops into a multi-layered photosensitive organ.

Species variation

Horse and ruminants: **Iridic granules (granula iridica)** are found at the dorsal and ventral pupillary margin. These are formed by proliferation of the pigmented epithelium and increased vascularisation of the iris stroma. Particularly in small ruminants, iridic granules contain isolated cystic cavities. Iridic granules secrete aqueous humour.

Birds: The iris forms an 'aperture ring' that surrounds the usually round, occasionally transversely ovoid, pupil. As in mammals, it separates the anterior chamber (between the iris and cornea) from the shallow posterior chamber (between the iris and the lens). The **colour of the iris** varies with species and, in some cases, with sex and age. In some sexually monomorphic species, such as cockatoos, iris colour may thus be utilised for sex determination. Nutritional and seasonal factors can also influence the colour of the iris. A feature unique to pigeons is the presence of a tapetum lucidum iridis consisting of reflective iridocytes.

Also particular to pigeons is the annulus iridis, a non-pigmented region with few blood vessels. This region appears dark because of the underlying pigmented posterior portion of the iris. Referred to by pigeon breeders as the 'circle of correlation', it has no significance with respect to vision or flying ability. In female blue-footed boobies, the portion of the iris adjacent to the pupil contains dark pigment deposits. The resulting contrast with the yellow of the remainder of the iris makes the pupil appear deceptively large.

The width of the iris, and thus the diameter of the pupil, is controlled by the m. sphincter and m. dilatator pupillae. In birds, these muscles are predominantly striated, permitting faster adjustment to changes in light exposure compared with mammals.

The striated pupillary muscle of birds is under voluntary control and, in contrast to mammals, is not responsive to commonly used ophthalmic drugs. Thus, while parasympatholytics are routinely used in mammalian patients to achieve mydriasis for ophthalmoscopic examination of the fundus, this practice is ineffective in birds. In several diving birds, including penguins and cormorants, the m. sphincter pupillae is particularly well developed and the lens protrudes through the pupil during accommodation. This increases the refractive capacity of the lens, compensating for reduced corneal refraction under water.

INNERVATION OF THE IRIS AND CILIARY BODY

The muscular and vascular components of the mammalian iris are controlled by neural and endocrine mechanisms. The iris and ciliary body receive sympathetic and parasympathetic innervation from the short and long ciliary nerves. **Postganglionic sympathetic fibres** supply the **m. dilatator pupillae**, the blood vessels of the iris and ciliary processes, stromal melanocytes, fibroblasts and, in some species, also the iris sphincter muscle. **Parasympathetic impulses** originating primarily from the oculomotor nerve are conveyed by postganglionic fibres to the m. sphincter pupillae and the ciliary muscle. The effects of parasympathetic stimulation include pupillary constriction and contraction of the ciliary muscle for accommodation.

Parasympathetic signals are transmitted by **acetylcholine** secreted at the neuro-effector junction. Cholinergic agents (e.g. pilocarpine, carbachol) activate muscarinic receptors, resulting in constriction of the pupil and contraction of the ciliary muscle. Blockage of these nerve impulses by the plant alkaloids atropine and hyoscine causes passive mydriasis and disruption of accommodation.

The **sympathetic** (**adrenergic**) **system** is activated by noradrenaline, serving as a neurotransmitter, and by circulating adrenaline. The effect of these molecules, which bind with α- and β-receptors, can be modified by catecholamine-depleting agents (e.g. reserpine).

Other substances that act as neurotransmitters in the regulation of iris and ciliary muscle function include the neuropeptides substance P, vasoactive intestinal peptide (VIP) and neuropeptide Y (NPY).

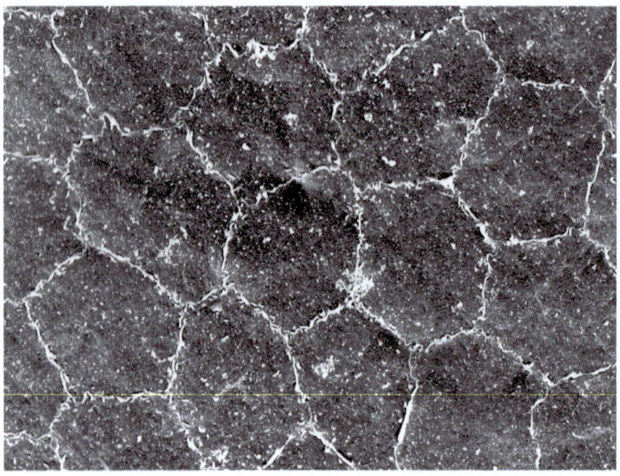

16.12 Scanning electron microscope image of the posterior epithelium of the cornea (horse; x5000).

Neural tunic (retina, tunica interna bulbi)

The retina is divided into an anterior portion devoid of photoreceptors, the pars caeca retinae, and a posterior photosensitive portion, the pars optica retinae (Figure 16.11). Both portions consist of an inner and outer layer, reflecting their embryonic origin.

In the **pars caeca retinae**, the two leaves of the optic cup remain largely undifferentiated, each forming a simple layer of epithelium. The two layers are closely apposed but remain separate. Based on its relationship to the ciliary body and iris, the **pars caeca retinae** is subdivided into the:

- pars ciliaris retinae,
- pars iridica retinae and
- ora serrata (ora serrata retinae).

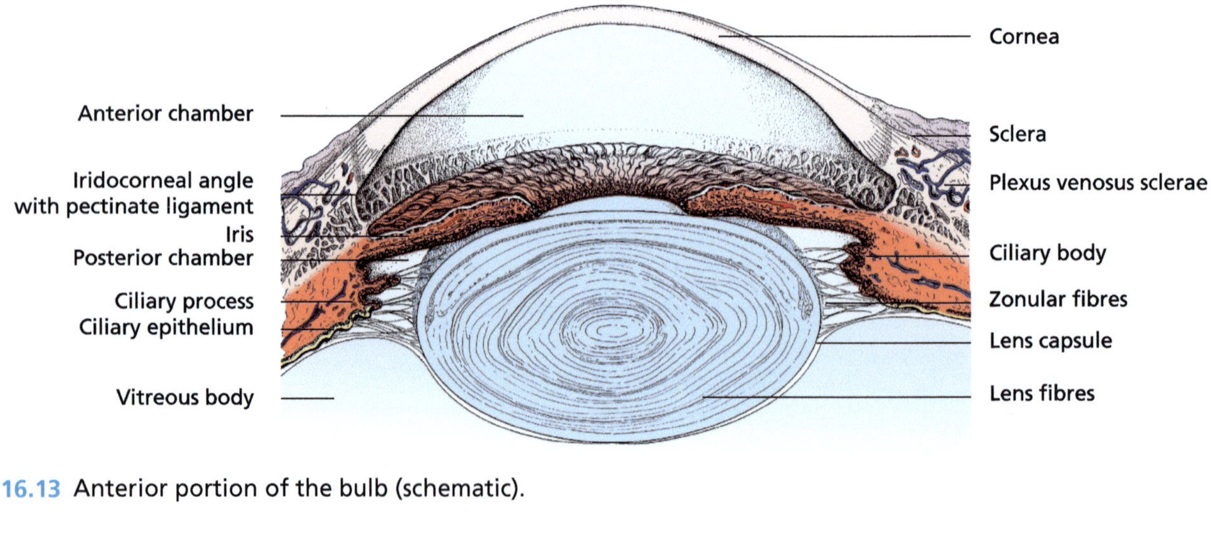

16.13 Anterior portion of the bulb (schematic).

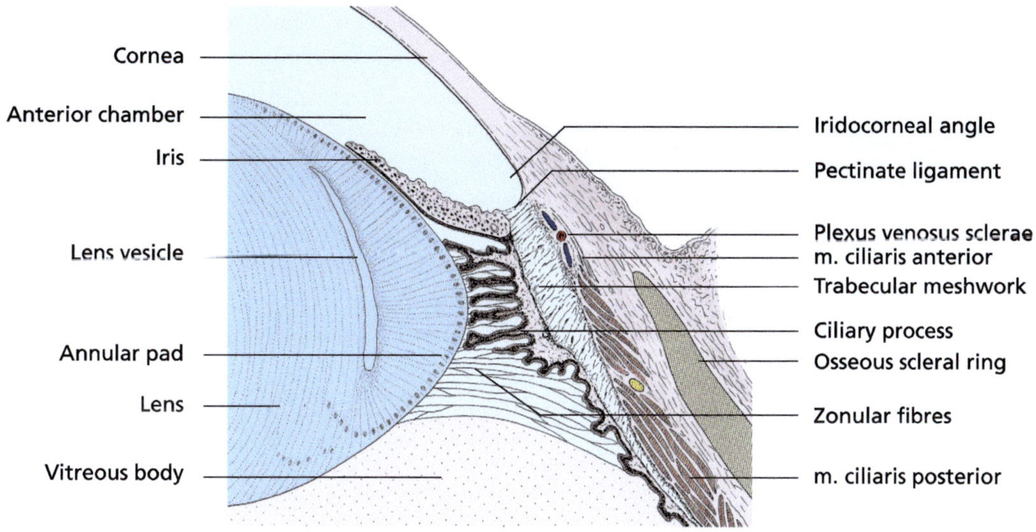

16.14 Ciliary body and iridocorneal angle (pigeon; meridional section, schematic).

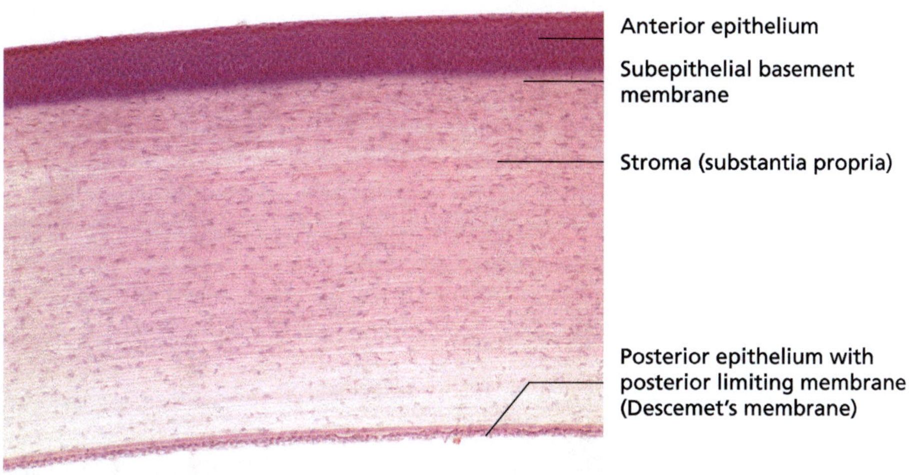

16.15 Cornea (ox). Haematoxylin and eosin stain (x75).

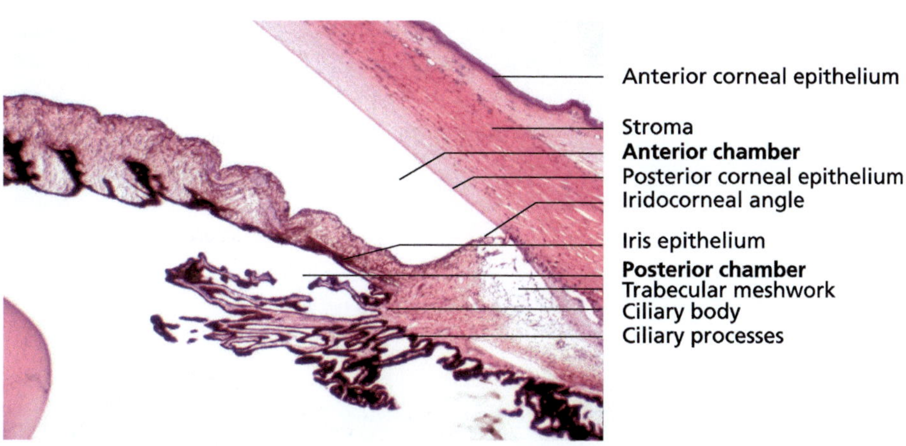

16.16 Iridocorneal angle (ox). Haematoxylin and eosin stain (x20).

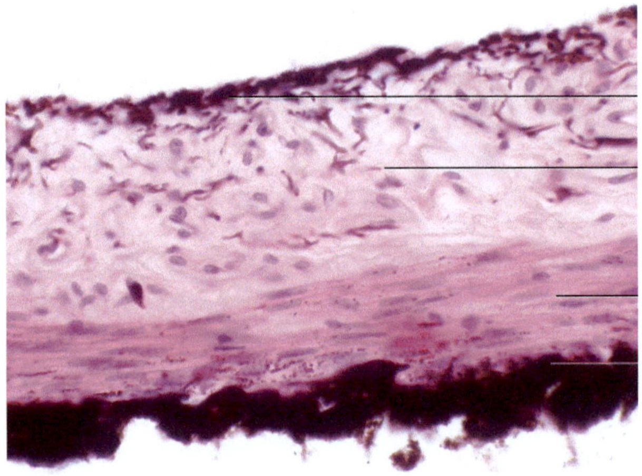

16.17 Iris (ox). Haematoxylin and eosin stain (x120).

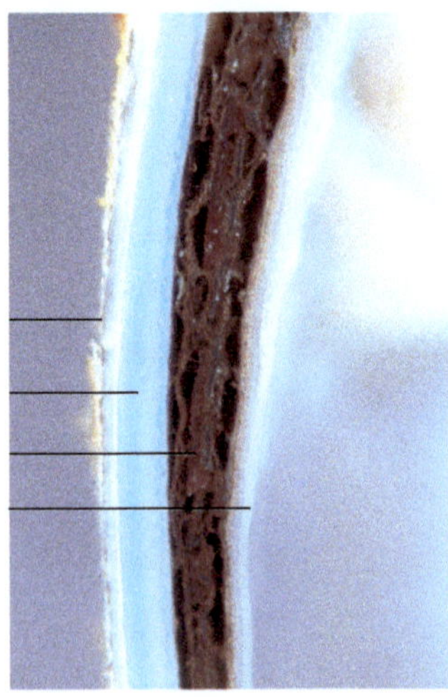

16.18 Fundus oculi (chicken; meridional section). Methylene blue stain (x7).

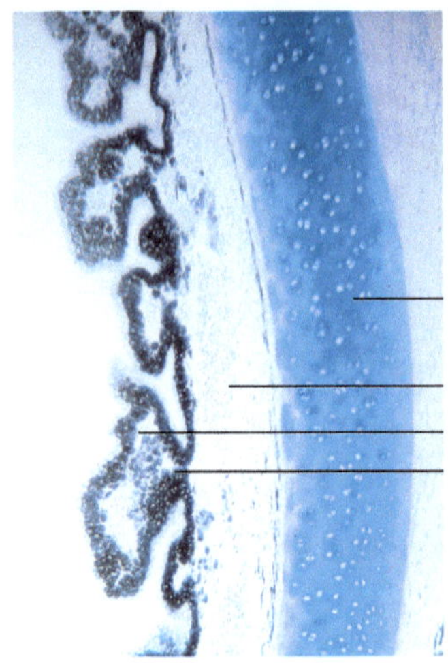

16.19 Pars plicata ciliaris (chicken; meridional section). Methylene blue stain (x18).

The structure of the pars ciliaris retinae and pars iridica retinae is described under the headings 'Ciliary body' and 'Iris'. The ora **serrata** is the boundary between the pars caeca retinae and the pars optica retinae.

The layers of the **pars optica retinae** are the:

- outer retinal pigment epithelium (stratum pigmentosum retinae) and
- inner, neurosensory layer of the retina (stratum nervosum retinae).

RETINAL PIGMENT EPITHELIUM (STRATUM PIGMENTOSUM RETINAE)

The retinal pigment epithelium develops from the outer leaf of the optic cup (Figures 16.20 to 16.22). This layer lies between the basal complex of the choroid and the outer segment of the photoreceptors (rods and cones of the stratum nervosum retinae, see below). A firm connection between the retinal pigment epithelium and the stratum nervosum retinae exists only at two locations: at the ora serrata and at the optic nerve head (**discus n. optici**, **papilla optica**). The epithelium consists of a single layer of hexagonal cells.

The cells of the **retinal pigment epithelium** have an eccentric nucleus, abundant mitochondria, a dense endoplasmic reticulum and a well-developed Golgi apparatus. The supranuclear region contains numerous melanosomes, lysosomes, residual bodies and phagolysosomes. Microvilli and finger-like evaginations project from the apical surface. These extend between and around the outer segments of the rods and cones.

Under intense illumination, **melanosomes** (**pigments**) accumulate in the cellular processes surrounding the rods and cones. This improves the resolution capacity of the eye and prevents scattering of light onto adjacent receptors. In dark conditions, the pigments recede, the light sensitivity of the retina increases and the resolving power declines. In the region where the tapetum lucidum is present, pigmentation of the retinal pigment epithelium is markedly reduced or absent.

Additional functions performed by the retinal pigment epithelium include:

- nutritional support for the retina,
- transport of metabolites between the choroid and the outer layers of the sensory retina,
- uptake and digestion of phagocytosed material from the outer segments (membranous discs) of the photoreceptors,
- replenishment of rhodopsin through esterification of vitamin A and
- synthesis of melanin.

NEUROSENSORY RETINA (STRATUM NERVOSUM RETINAE)

The neurosensory retina, derived from the inner leaf of the embryonic optic cup, consists of several layers (Figures 16.20 to 16.23). As a component of the diencephalon, this part of the retina contains **glial cells** (**Müller cells**, **radial glial cells**) and **nerve cells** (neurons).

Müller cells (Figures 16.23 and 16.26) support all layers of the neurosensory retina except the rods and cones. They also form the internal and external limiting membranes (stratum limitans gliae internum and externum).

The **neurons** are arranged in structurally distinct layers that are connected in series to form a three-neuron pathway. From outside (most external) to inside (most internal) (Figures 16. 20 to 16.23) the pathway consists of:

- **neuron 1:**
  - rod and cone layer (stratum neuro-epitheliale),
  - outer nuclear layer (stratum nucleare externum),
  - outer plexiform layer (stratum plexiforme externum),

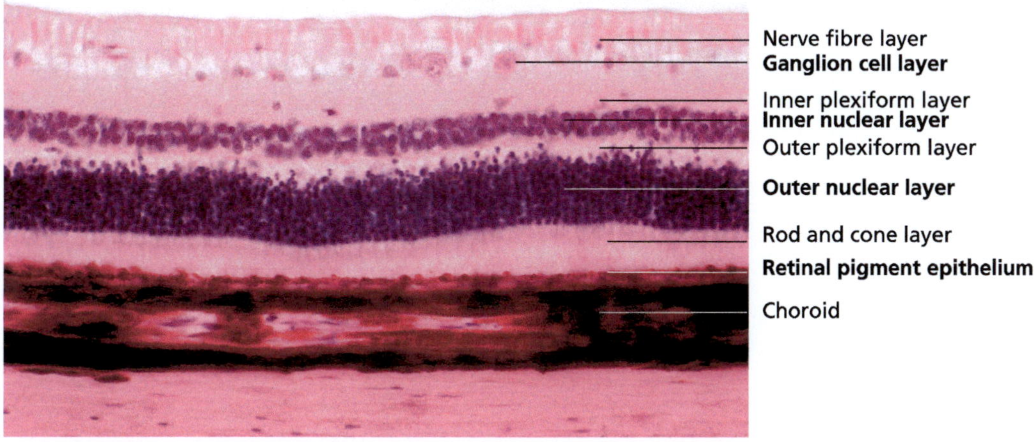

16.20 Pars optica retinae (fundus, horse). Haematoxylin and eosin stain (x250).

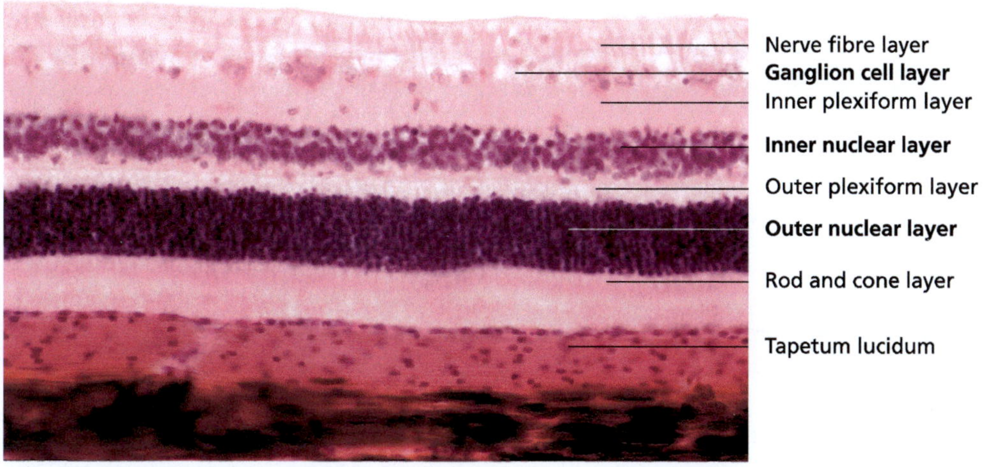

16.21 Pars optica retinae in region of tapetum lucidum (fundus, horse). Haematoxylin and eosin stain (x250).

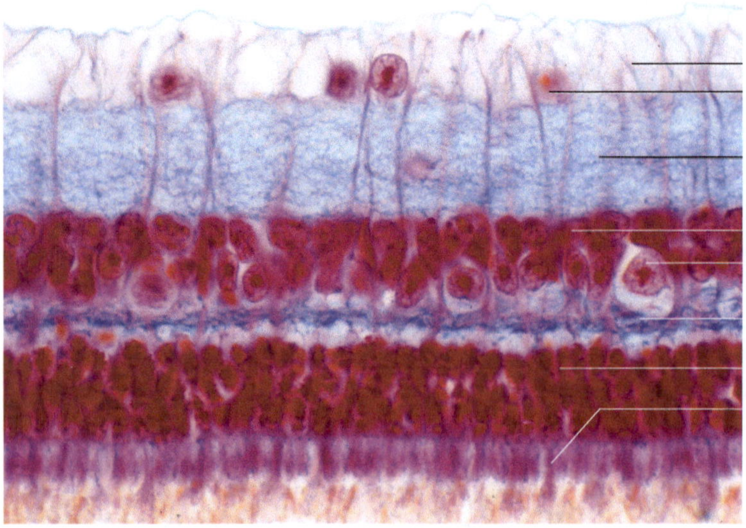

16.22 High power view of pars optica retinae (fundus, cat). Azan stain (x1000).

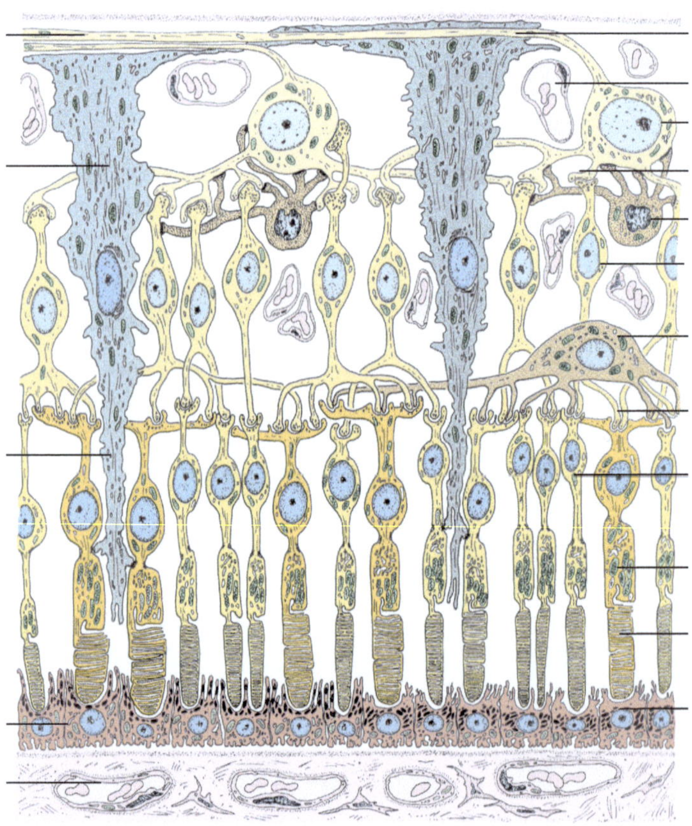

16.23 Layers of the neurosensory retina (schematic).

- **neuron 2:**
  - inner nuclear layer (stratum nucleare internum),
  - inner plexiform layer (stratum plexiforme internum),
- **neuron 3:**
  - ganglion cell layer (stratum ganglionare nervi optici) and
  - nerve fibre layer (stratum neurofibrarum).

During embryonic development, the light-sensitive receptor layer comes to lie furthest from the incoming light signal, while the nerve layer that conducts the resulting impulse faces the interior of the eye.

The **photosensory layer** (stratum neuro-epitheliale, rod and cone layer) comprises the processes of cells (epitheliocyti neurosensorii) that have their perikarya in the outer nuclear layer. These processes constitute the photoreceptors of the eye and are divided into inner and outer segments (see below). There are two types of photoreceptors (Figures 16.23 and 16.24):

- **rods** – highly sensitive light-dark sensors and
- **cones** – colour receptors.

The perikarya of the cells of the first neuronal layer constitute the **outer nuclear layer** (stratum nucleare externum). Axons of first-layer neurons and dendrites of second layer neurons (bipolar nerve cells) form the **outer plexiform layer** (stratum plexiforme externum). The **inner nuclear layer** (stratum nucleare internum) is composed of the cell bodies of bipolar nerve cells and adjacent horizontal cells. Axons of the bipolar cells are interwoven with dendrites of the third layer of neurons (ganglion cell layer), forming the **inner plexiform layer** (stratum plexiforme internum). An additional cell type (amacrine cell) is found at the outer aspect of the inner plexiform layer (Figure 16.23).

The **ganglion cell layer** (stratum ganglionare nervi optici) consists of the cell bodies of large multipolar and smaller autonomic nerve cells. Considerably fewer neurons are present in this layer than in the bipolar cell layer. The axons of the ganglion cells course towards the optic nerve head as the **nerve fibre layer** (stratum neurofibrarum). At the optic nerve head, they leave the bulb as the **optic nerve**. In this region, the sclera contains numerous perforations for passage of the nerve fibres (**area cribrosa**) (Figure 16.30).

Rods and cones: These form the photosensitive outermost layer of the neurosensory retina that lies internally adjacent to the retinal pigment epithelium (Figures 16.23 to 16.25).

The **outer segment** of **rods** contains dense stacks of **membranous discs** containing **rhodopsin** ('**visual purple**'). The discs are formed from regular folding of the plasma membrane. The double lipoprotein layer is constructed from precursors produced by organelles in the inner segment.

Continuous production of discs pushes the older discs towards the periphery of the outer segment. From there, the discs are shed and phagocytosed by the retinal pigment epithelium. Membrane remnants are digested by lysosomes. Chemical reactions occurring in these membrane systems trigger visual signals under low light conditions. The outer segment is connected to the inner segment by a modified cilium.

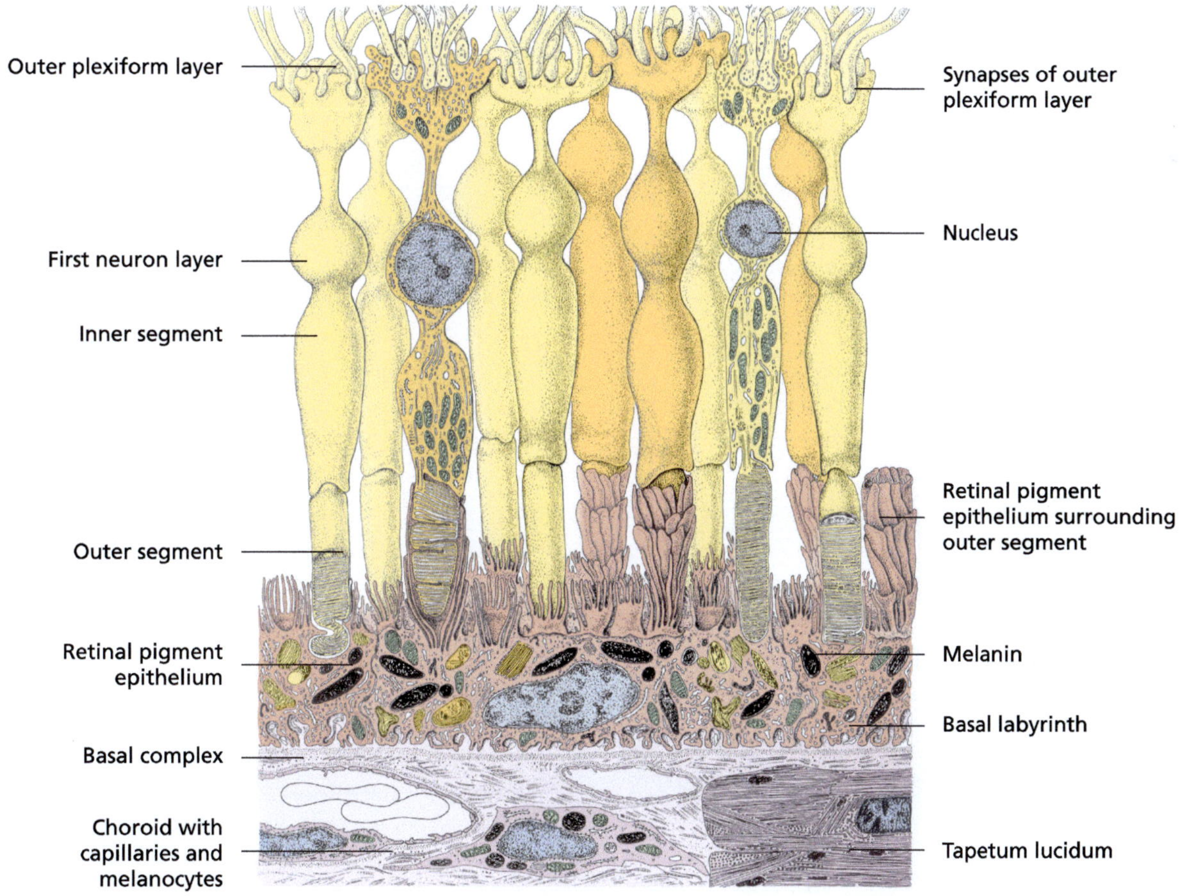

16.24 Layers of the retina (rod and cone layer and retinal pigment epithelium) and inner layers of the choroid (schematic).

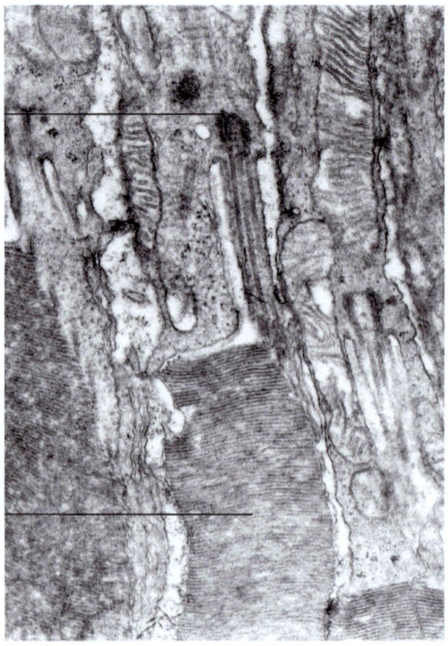

16.25 Fine structure of the outer and inner segments of rods in the stratum neuro-epitheliale (dog; x16,000).

The **inner segment** consists of a glycogen-rich outer ellipsoid, containing numerous mitochondria and a centriole, and an inner region, or myoid, which encloses the Golgi apparatus, endoplasmic reticulum and microtubules. The inner segment acts as a metabolic centre, producing energy for the photoreceptor layer and synthesising proteins for the membranous discs of the outer segment.

The size and structure of **cones** is similar to that of rods. The expanded, club-shaped **outer segment** is filled with membranous discs containing **iodopsin**. The **inner segment** is larger than that of rods and contains an elliptical nucleus.

Horizontal cell (neurocytus horizontalis): These cells lie in the outer region of the inner nuclear layer. The expanded cell body is rich in organelles. Dendritic processes synapse with rods, cones and bipolar cells. Through this intermingling, horizontal cells modify communication between photoreceptor cells and bipolar cells of the second neuron layer (Figure 16.23).

Amacrine cell (neurocytus amacrinus): Amacrine cells are found on the internal aspect of the inner nuclear layer. They have no axons. The dendrites of amacrine cells synapse with axons of the bipolar nerve cells and with dendrites of the ganglion cells. Amacrine cells serve as interneurons (Figure 16.23).

Müller cell (radial glial cell, gliocytus radialis): Müller cells are modified fibrous astrocytes (Figure 16.23 and 16.26). At the internal surface of the retina, processes extend from the expanded cytoplasmic portion of Müller cells to form the internal limiting membrane (stratum limitans gliae internum) (Figure 16.26). The internal limiting membrane constitutes the boundary between the retina and the vitreous body.

Müller cells extend perpendicularly through the retina. Their nuclei form part of the inner nuclear layer. In the outer portion of the cell, the cytoplasm narrows and extends between the photoreceptors to the outer extremity of the inner segment. Zonulae adherentes between the Müller cells give rise to the **external limiting membrane** (stratum limitans gliae externum). Lying at the outer aspect of the outer nucler layer (Figures 16.26 and 16.29), the external limiting membrane forms an important metabolic barrier between the rods and cones and the inner layers of the retina. The more internal layers are supplied by the retinal vessels, while nourishment of the photoreceptors occurs by diffusion of molecules across the retinal pigment epithelium.

Area centralis rotunda: In primates, the area of greatest visual acuity is a well-circumscribed yellowish region of the retina, the macula lutea, and the associated fovea centralis. In domestic mammals, the yellow pigmentation is lacking, and the corresponding area is referred to as the area centralis rotunda. This region is characterised by an increased number of cones and ganglion cells. The area centralis rotunda is important for binocular vision.

Area centralis striaeformis: In the horse, ruminant and pig, pale striations are found dorsal to the optic nerve head. Termed the area centralis striaeformis, this region contains increased numbers of cones and bipolar nerve cells. The area centralis striaeformis contributes to monocular vision and motion detection.

NUTRITIONAL SUPPORT OF THE RETINA

The outer and inner segments of the rods and cones are supplied by the **capillary network** of the choroid. Molecules diffuse through the basal complex of the choroid and the retinal pigment epithelium to reach the photoreceptors. This is facilitated by the close contact between the retinal pigment epithelium and the rods and cones. The epithelial cells also have a regulatory function. The external limiting membrane restricts diffusion to the inner retinal layers.

Separation of the neural layers of the retina from the retinal pigment epithelium (retinal detachment) interrupts the nutritional supply to the rods and cones, resulting in degeneration of affected photoreceptors. The **central layers of the retina**, between the internal and external limiting membranes, are supplied by capillaries arising from the **central retinal artery**. The artery enters the bulb at the optic nerve head and comes to lie on the inner surface of the retina. It gives off branches (rami centrales) in a species-dependent pattern. The branches are distributed to the layers of the retina. Veins returning from the retinal layers combine to form the central retinal vein.

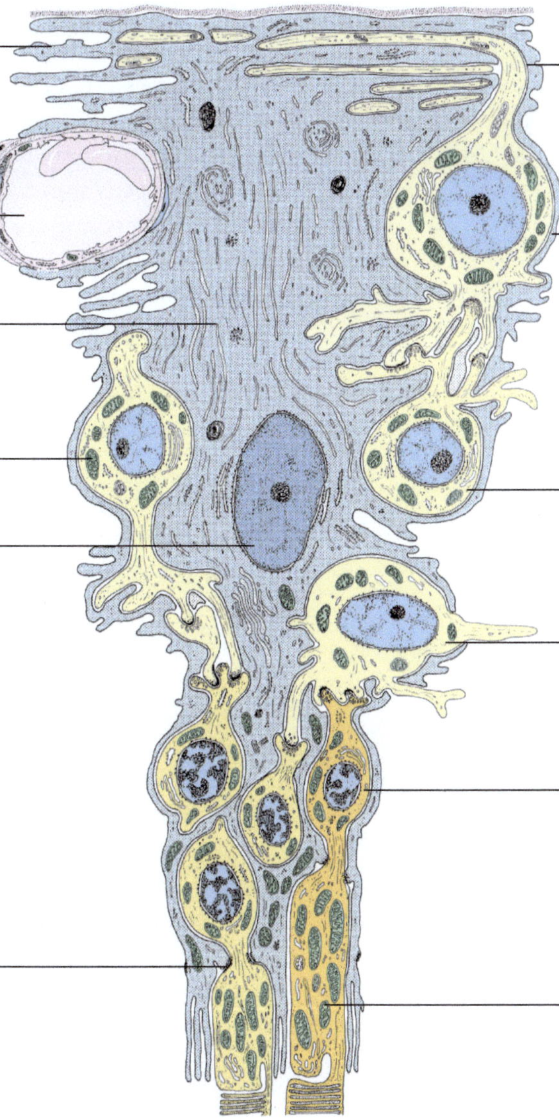

16.26 Müller (radial glial) cell with adjacent retinal neurons (schematic).

NEUROSENSORY RETINA OF BIRDS

The **retinal pigment epithelium** is firmly attached to the choroid. In diurnal birds, it contains large quantities of melanin granules. These absorb light that has passed through the light-sensitive retina, thus preventing interference by scattered light. In parrots, pigeons and diurnal raptors, the fundus oculi is particularly heavily pigmented, making ophthalmoscopic examination more difficult. The degree of pigmentation varies considerably, however, between individuals and species and is correlated with the colour of the feather coat. In crepuscular and nocturnal avian species, the retinal pigment epithelium is less developed. As a result, the underlying choroidal vessels give the fundus a striated, so-called 'tigroid' appearance on ophthalmoscopic examination.

The **pars optica retinae** consists of three layers of dense neuronal networks. While this arrangement is similar to the retina of other vertebrates, the retina of birds has specific features that contribute to the exceptional visual capacity of many avian species.

The avian retina contains a large number of neuronal connections that, in mammals, are established in higher neural centres. Thus, the pars optica retinae of birds is comparatively thick. The retina of pigeons, for example, with its well-developed inner nuclear and plexiform layers, is twice as thick as that of humans (Figures 16.27 to 16.29).

In birds, the visible light spectrum ranges from 320 to 680 nm. A particular feature of avian cone cells is the presence of oil droplets containing **carotenoid pigments**. At least five types of pigment have been identified, each with a different absorption spectrum. These are believed to act as intraocular chromatic filters. A sixth, colourless type of droplet has been linked with perception of **ultraviolet light**. Rods are considerably more light-sensitive and responsible for non-colour-dependent vision at low light intensity. They contain **rhodopsin**, a pigment with an absorption maximum in the range of 490–506 nm.

Cone cells predominate in the retina of diurnal birds, rods being far fewer in number and restricted to the periphery. In many diurnal birds of prey, the density of cones is greater than in humans. Moreover, there are only very few cone cells per efferent nerve cell (**low convergence**), resulting in a high degree of visual resolution. In contrast, the high light sensitivity of the retina of owls results from a large number of densely packed rods (representing up to 90% of photoreceptors) and the connection of more than 1000 rods with each bipolar nerve cell (**high convergence**).

The term **area retinae** is used to describe well-defined slightly thickened regions of the retina in which the density of cone cells is especially pronounced, resulting in particularly high resolution. In these regions, the ratio of photoreceptors to efferent neurons can reach the optimal value of 1:1. Visual resolution associated with these areas is further enhanced by the peripheral displacement of overlying neurons, resulting in a central depression known as the **fovea retinae**.

The position and shape of the areas and foveae vary considerably with species. Most bird species have a central round area centralis rotunda with a fovea centralis (absent

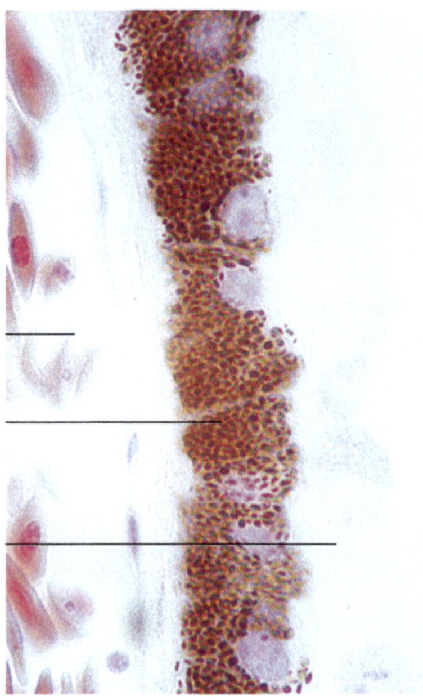

16.27 Pars ciliaris retinae (common buzzard, *Buteo buteo*). Haematoxylin and eosin stain (x480).

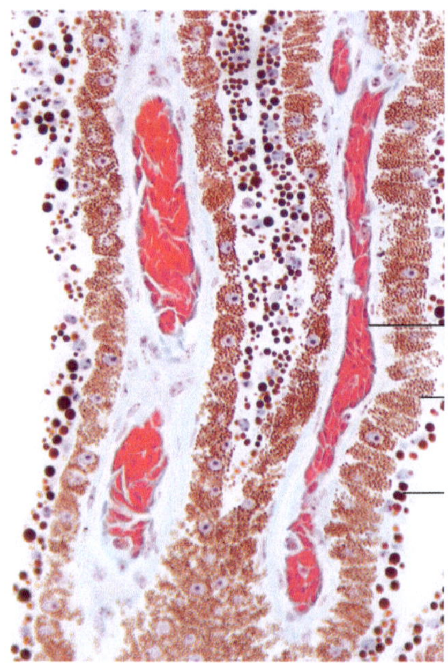

16.28 Pars ciliaris retinae (tawny owl, *Strix aluco*) with pigment in inner epithelial layer. Haematoxylin and eosin stain (x360).

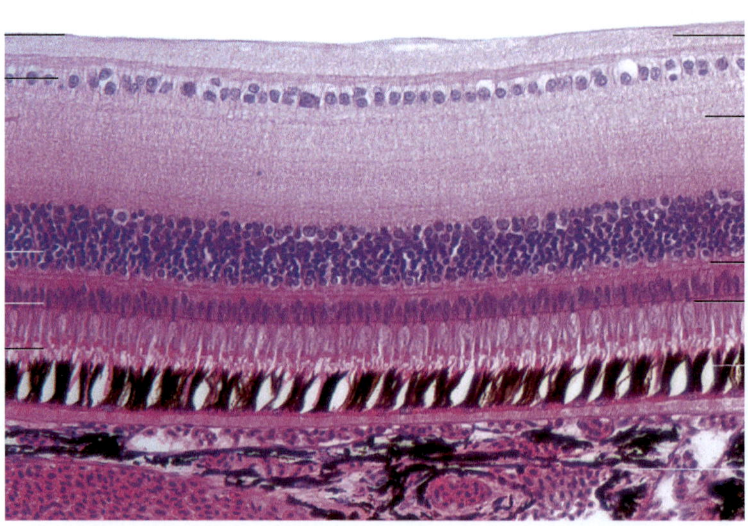

16.29 Pars optica retinae (chicken). Haematoxylin and eosin stain (x250).

in the chicken), representing the site of highest monocular visual resolution. In many water- and shore-birds, the central area is linear (termed the **area centralis horizontalis**) and contains a **fovea centralis**.

Several diurnal raptors also possess an area temporalis with a **fovea temporalis**, which contributes to binocular, stereoscopic vision. Owls have only an area temporalis.

In contrast to the retina of most mammals, the avian retina is **avascular**. It receives its nutrition by diffusion from the capillary network of the lamina choriocapillaris and from the richly vascularised **pecten oculi** (Figures 16.31 and 16.32).

OPTIC NERVE (NERVUS OPTICUS)

The optic nerve (cranial nerve II) is an afferent tract of the brain. The nerve is composed of axons of the multipolar ganglion cells that initially form the nerve fibre layer of the retina. The axons pass to the main visual relay centre of the brain, the lateral geniculate body. From there, nerve fibres of the visual pathway project to the visual cerebral cortex in the occipital lobe. Autonomic fibres in the optic nerve pass to the hypothalamus forming the retinohypothalamic tracts (suprachiasmatic nucleus).

Within the nerve fibre layer, the fibres are non-myelinated. After penetrating the area cribrosa of the sclera, the axons are surrounded by oligodendrocytes, through which they become myelinated (Figure 16.30). The autonomic fibres are poorly myelinated.

As a component of the brain, the optic nerve is ensheathed by pia mater, arachnoid and dura mater. Distinct subdural and subarachnoid spaces are evident. At the area cribrosa, the meningeal layers merge with the sclera. Numerous connective tissue septa extending from the pia, accompanied by capillaries, project between the

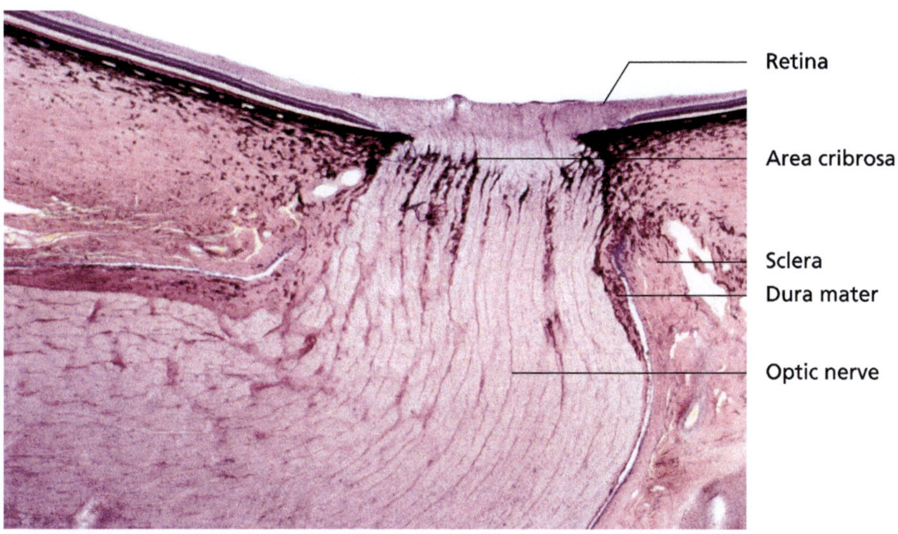

16.30 Optic nerve and area cribrosa (goat). Haematoxylin and eosin stain (x30).

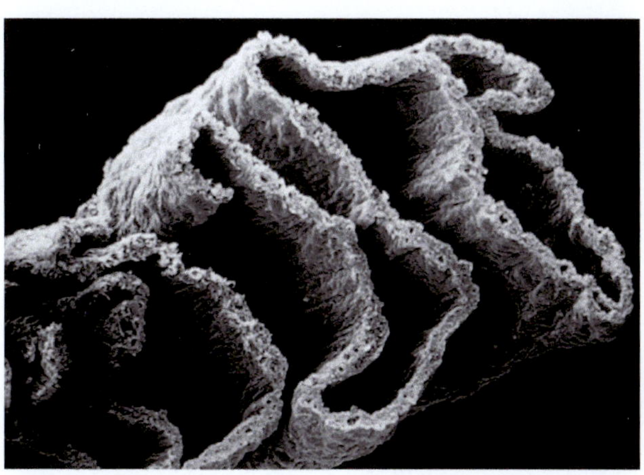

16.31 Scanning electron microscope image of the folds of a pleated pecten (common buzzard, *Buteo buteo*; x50).

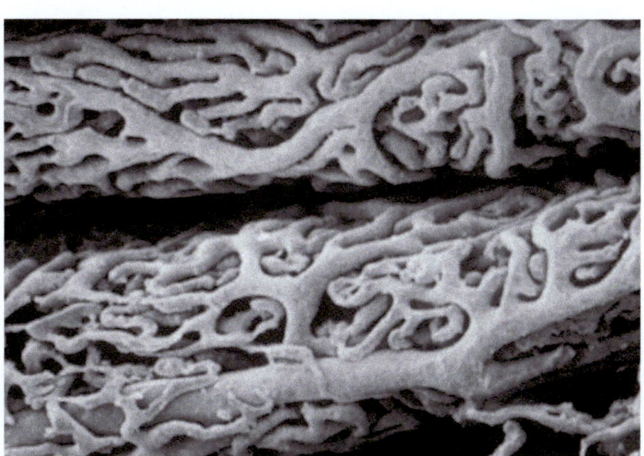

16.32 Scanning electron microscope image of the capillary network in a pleated pecten oculi (domestic pigeon; corrosion cast; x50).

nerve fibre bundles, separating these into individual fibres. Fibrous astrocytes located at the interface with the axon provide nutritional support.

Species variation

Birds: In most birds, all of the nerve fibres within each optic nerve decussate at the optic chiasm. Thus, a true consensual pupillary light response does not occur. Throughout its extracranial course, the optic nerve is surrounded by pia and dura mater. It incorporates very little slack in most avian species, and none at all in birds with minimal eye movement (e.g. owls).

A further peculiarity of the avian optic nerve is the presence of efferent nerve fibres originating from the isthmo-optic nucleus in the mesencephalon. These are responsible for further enhancing visual acuity. The point at which the optic nerve leaves the retina is oval in birds and is largely covered by the **pecten oculi** (Figures 16.31 and 16.32). The heavily vascularised connective tissue core of the pecten arises directly from the optic nerve. Consequently, the ovoid area that represents the equivalent of the optic nerve head in mammals is visible ophthalmoscopically only as a narrow, whitish-yellow margin at the base of the pecten. According to ontogenic studies, the pecten is derived from the **retina**. From its origin, the pecten extends into the vitreous body. Three **structural forms** of pecten have been described: pleated, vaned and conical.

The **pleated type** is characterised by closely apposed vertical folds that are joined at their tip by a bridge, the pons pectinis. This type is typical of carinate birds (Figure 16.31). In the **vaned type**, 25–30 vertical vanes are connected to a central lamina. A vaned pecten is found in ratites, such as the ostrich, emu and nandu. Only the kiwi is known to have the **conical type**, an undivided structure devoid of folds or laminae, resembling the conus papillaris of reptiles.

Despite extensive investigation, the function of the pecten remains unclear. The many hypothesised roles include protection of certain regions of the retina from glare, reduction of scattered light, immune functions, motion detection and sensing of magnetic fields to facilitate orientation. It is generally agreed that the pecten has a **nutritional role**, supplying the vitreous body and avascular retina, and that it contributes to **intraocular pressure** and **temperature regulation**. This is supported by the characteristics of the endothelium of the capillaries in the pecten, which indicate continuous, active trans-epithelial transport. The passage of substances from the capillaries to the vitreous body has been demonstrated using fluorescein angiography. Distribution of these substances throughout the vitreous body is facilitated by rhythmic contractions of the extrinsic muscle of the eye, which result in oscillatory eye movements and corresponding passive movement of the pecten.

Internal structures of the bulb

The interior of the bulb contains the **lens** and the **vitreous body** (corpus vitreum). In addition, three cavities can be distinguished within the eyeball (Figures 16.11 and 16.13):

- **anterior chamber** (camera anterior bulbi) between the cornea and the anterior surface of the iris,
- **posterior chamber** (camera posterior bulbi) between the posterior surface of the iris, the ciliary body, the zonular fibres and the lens and
- **vitreous chamber** (camera vitrea) posterior to the **lens**, surrounded by the retina.

LENS

The lens originates from the **ectoderm**. It arises embryologically from the **lens placode**, separating from the surface epithelium as the lens vesicle. Elongated cell processes extending from the posterior wall of the lens vesicle fill the internal cavity and differentiate into hexagonal lens fibres.

The lens is a transparent biconcave structure that is connected by zonular fibres to the ciliary body (Figures 16.11 and 16.13). The posterior surface, facing the vitreous body, is usually more convex than the anterior surface. Thickening of the lens during accommodation occurs mainly through an increase in curvature of the anterior surface. The lens is insensitive and avascular. It receives nutrition by diffusion from the aqueous humour. The lens has the following components:

- lens capsule (capsula lentis),
- lens epithelium (epithelium lentis) and
- lens fibres (fibrae lentis).

The lens is enclosed in a flexible, refractive **capsule** that is formed from secretions of the lens epithelium. The lens capsule comprises a broad basal lamina (anterior thickness 10–20 μm, posterior thickness 5 μm) composed of a dense network of type IV collagen microfilaments and embedded glycoproteins. The zonular fibres insert on the periphery of the lens capsule, merging with filaments of the capsule. The capsule forms a semipermeable barrier that is penetrable by metabolically active substances.

The **lens epithelium** lies on the anterior surface of the lens, beneath the lens capsule. It is simple cuboidal in type. The epithelial cells are the only cells of the lens that are capable of replication. Particularly at the lens equator (equator lentis), the cells divide and elongate, eventually differentiating into **lens fibres** (see below). The lens enlarges throughout life, as new lens fibres are laid upon existing ones. The posterior surface of the lens consists of lens fibres; there is no posterior epithelium.

The lens fibres, which form the bulk of the lens, are elongated prismatic cells (7–10 mm long, 5–12 μm wide,

2–4 μm thick). At the lens equator, the lens fibres contain a nucleus and numerous organelles. Towards the interior of the lens the nucleus is lost. The lens fibres form concentric layers that become condensed towards the centre, forming the lens nucleus. Individual lens fibres contact one another through zipper-like interdigitations. This contributes to the plasticity of the lens, which is required for accommodation.

Lens fibres contain water (70%), membrane proteins, cytoskeletal proteins, enzymes, crystallins and electrolytes. The shape of the lens is determined largely by its cytoskeletal elements. These include microfilaments such as fibronectin, vimentin and actin.

The lens fibres traverse the lens equator from the anterior to the posterior pole of the lens and vice versa. Where they meet at their end points, lens sutures (radii lentis) are formed. These join to form three-pointed **lens stars**. The orientation of the lens stars at the anterior and posterior aspects of the lens is offset by 60°.

Lens transparency is dependent upon the ordered structure and metabolic integrity of the lens fibres. Changes in these factors result in lens opacity.

Species variation

Birds: As in mammals, the lens is a transparent, biconvex structure of epithelial origin, positioned between the iris and the vitreous body (Figure 16.14). In altricial birds, the lens is opaque during the nestling stage, only becoming transparent after fledging. In diurnal birds, the lens is relatively flat, while in water birds and nocturnal species it is spheroid. Beneath the **lens capsule** (see below) is a layer of simple epithelium. Towards the lens equator, the epithelial cells become elongated, giving rise to radially oriented hexagonal **prisms** that combine to form the equatorial **annular pad** (**pulvinus anularis lentis**) (Figure 16.14).

The annular pad is a characteristic feature of the avian eye. It is marked by a row of indentations that correspond in number with the ciliary processes to which they are attached. The function of the annular pad is incompletely understood, although it is not considered to be part of the optical system. Instead, it is presumed to play an important role in the speed of **lenticular accommodation**, since the pad is particularly thick in fast fliers (especially diurnal birds of prey and pigeons) and less developed in diving birds. It is notably narrow in psittacines.

The annular pad may also have a **nutritional function**. Its cells secrete fluid, the **aqua vesiculae lentis**, into the cleft-shaped **lens vesicle** (**vesicula lentis**) (Figure 16.14) between the pad and the central **lens core** (**corpus centrale lentis**). The fluid is absorbed by the core. Lens stars, as seen in mammals, are not present in birds. The **lens capsule**, a derivative of basal lamina, forms a semipermeable barrier through which nutrients can diffuse from the aqueous humour. It also forms a permanent barrier separating the protein within the lens from the immune system. Protein released as a consequence of lens trauma may be recognised as foreign and can thus result in phacogenic uveitis (endophthalmitis phacoanaphylactica). In contrast to mammals, the **lens equator** is closely associated with the ciliary processes, the tips of the processes being tightly fused with the capsule. Fixation of the lens is supplemented by the ciliary zonule (zonula ciliaris), composed of the zonular fibres (fibrae zonulares).

The intimate association of the lens with the ciliary body and the relative pliability of the avian lens facilitate the process of active lenticular accommodation. Accordingly, the lens is relatively flexible in diving birds, in which lenticular accommodation predominates, and comparatively hard in owls, which rely almost exclusively on corneal accommodation. Age-related loss of lens pliability, seen in humans, dogs and cats, is not observed in birds.

VITREOUS BODY (CORPUS VITREUM)

The vitreous body is bounded by the lens, the ciliary body and the retina (Figure 16.11). It is tightly adherent to the ora serrata and the retinal vessels. The vitreous body is composed of a transparent, colourless hydrogel (**humor vitreus**) comprising 99% water. The fluid phase contains dissolved hydrophilic glycosaminoglycans (particularly hyaluronic acid polymers) bound with water.

The solid phase includes a relatively small population of cells, **hyalocytes**, that produce microfibrillar structural proteins and phagocytose free cells and fibril fragments. Type II collagen microfibrils form a scant structural framework. Optimal hydration of these collagen molecules is facilitated by the hyaluronidase system. Superficially, the collagen fibrils condense to form the **hyaloid membrane** that lies adjacent to the internal limiting lamina of the retina.

Species variation

Ox, pig and carnivore: A fluid-filled channel (**canalis hyaloideus**), a remnant of the embryonic **a. hyaloidea**, extends from the lens to the optic nerve head.

Ox, pig and sheep: The vitreous body is dense, giving it a firm consistency.

Horse: The vitreous body is amorphous and has a low optical density.

Carnivores: The vitreous has a dense core and a less structured outer portion.

As well as serving as a refractive medium, the vitreous body participates in retinal metabolism and homeostasis. By contributing to intraocular pressure, the vitreous body holds the retina in place against the retinal pigment epithelium. A reduction in pressure can lead to detachment of the retina (posterior to the ora serrata, where the corpus vitreum is firmly attached to the ciliary epithelium).

ANTERIOR AND POSTERIOR CHAMBERS

The **anterior chamber** (camera anterior bulbi) is an internal chamber of the bulb bounded by the posterior surface of the cornea and the anterior surface of the iris. It communicates with the **posterior chamber** (camera posterior bulbi) via the pupil (Figure 16.11 and 16.13). The walls of the posterior chamber are formed by the posterior surface of the iris, the ciliary body, the anterior surface of the vitreous body and the lens. The anterior and posterior chambers contain a clear watery fluid, aqueous humour, containing electrolytes, glucose, amino acids and ascorbic acid. The concentration of these substances in aqueous humour differs from that in plasma.

Production of **aqueous humour** is a complex process in which the blood–aqueous barrier (between the capillaries and epithelium of the ciliary processes) plays an important role. Aqueous humour is produced primarily by active transport of Na^+ ions across the ciliary epithelium and by osmotic transport of fluid into the posterior chamber. From the posterior chamber, aqueous humour flows through the pupil into the anterior chamber. At the **iridocorneal angle** (angulus iridocornealis) (Figures 16.16 and 16.33), the fluid drains through the spaces in the **ligamentum pectinatum** into the trabecular meshwork (within the ciliоscleral sinus) and then into the scleral venous sinus (plexus venosus sclerae). Certain plasma proteins are also reabsorbed by diffusion through capillary walls. Aqueous humour provides nutritional support for the avascular cornea and the lens.

Species variation

Birds: As in mammals, the anterior and posterior chambers contain aqueous humour, which is secreted continuously by the inner epithelial layer of the pars ciliaris retinae into the **posterior chamber**. Aqueous flows through the pupil into the **anterior chamber** (**camera anterior bulbi**) from whence it passes, at the iridocorneal angle, through the **pectinate ligament** into the **spaces of Fontana** of the **cilioscleral sinus** (Figure 16.14). From there it diffuses into the wide, usually bipartite **scleral venous sinus**, which is located more superficially in birds than in domestic mammals. In owls, the aqueous humour contains mucous substances secreted by the posterior corneal epithelium, making anterior chamber paracentesis more difficult in these birds.

Accessory organs of the eye

Eyelids (palpebrae)

The eyelids provide protection for the bulbs. In conjunction with the precorneal tear film, they cleanse the anterior surface of the eye and prevent it from desiccating. The palpebral reflex is an important component of this protective mechanism. In addition to an upper and lower eyelid (palpebra superior and inferior), domestic mammals have a conjunctival fold referred to as the third eyelid (palpebra tertia) (Figures 16.34 and 16.35).

UPPER AND LOWER EYELIDS (PALPEBRA SUPERIOR ET INFERIOR)

The upper and lower eyelids have a fibre-rich connective tissue core that is continued at the free eyelid margin by the **tarsal plate** (**tarsus palpebralis**) (Figure 16.34). At the base of the eyelids, circular bands of striated muscle (m. orbicularis oculi) extend through the connective tissue and merge with the tarsal plate and the m. tarsalis.

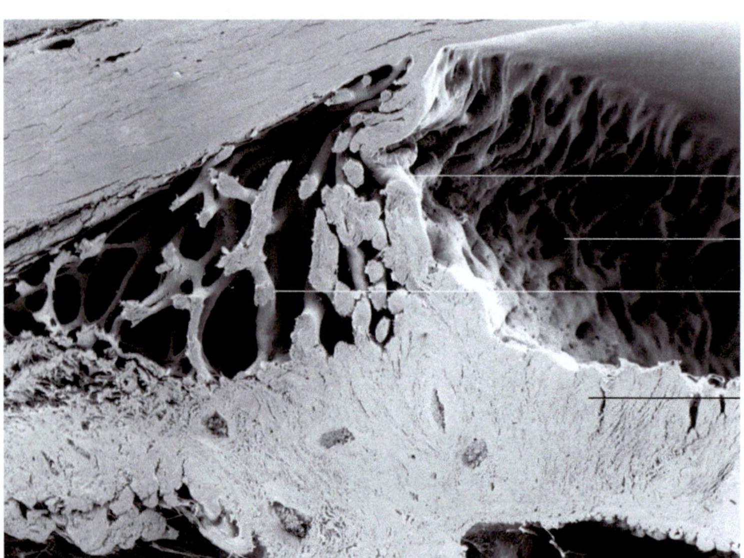

16.33 Scanning electron microscope image of the trabecular system in the iridocorneal angle (horse; x15).

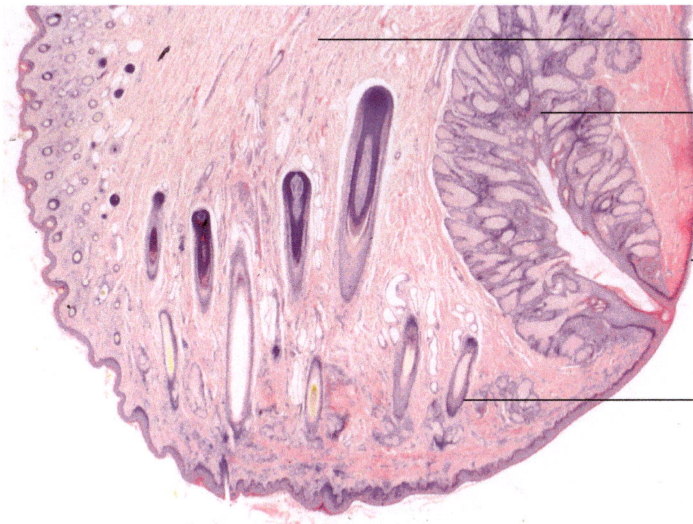

16.34 Eyelid (calf). Haematoxylin and eosin stain (x16).

Species variation

Birds: In most diurnal birds the **lower eyelid** (**palpebra ventralis**) is larger and more mobile than the **upper eyelid** (**palpebra dorsalis**). When closed, the lower lid almost completely covers the cornea. It is supported by a fibrous **tarsal plate**, which may be cartilaginous in birds of prey. In nocturnal species, such as owls, the upper eyelid is larger and more mobile. The upper eyelids of parrots are also comparatively moveable. A pit-like depression in the upper eyelid of domestic poultry is a common site of infestation with ectoparasites such as lice and fleas.

Tarsal plate (tarsus)

The tarsal plate comprises a taut layer of collagen fibres. It surrounds the **tarsal glands** (**glandulae tarsales, Meibomian glands**). Structurally, the tarsal glands (45–50 in the upper eyelid of the horse) are compound sebaceous glands (tubulo-alveolar; secretory units composed of multiple cell layers; secretion by holocrine mode). Their ducts open at the **inner eyelid margin** (limbus palpebrae posterior). The oily secretion of the tarsal glands lines the **free edge of the eyelid** (margo palpebrae) and hinders the overflow of tears.

The **external surface** of the eyelids consists of densely haired skin containing relatively few sebaceous and sweat glands. At the anterior lid margin, **eyelashes** (cilia) are embedded deep in the connective tissue of the lid, surrounded by sweat and sebaceous glands. Eyelashes are absent on the lower eyelids of dogs and pigs, and are usually lacking altogether in cats.

Beginning at the posterior eyelid margin, the **posterior surface** of the eyelid is lined by non-glandular mucosa, the **palpebral conjunctiva** (tunica conjunctiva palpebrae). The conjunctiva covers the internal surface of the eyelid and reflects at the fornix conjunctivae onto the sclera as the **bulbar conjunctiva** (tunica conjunctiva bulbi).

The conjunctiva has a stratified epithelial lining incorporating solitary goblet cells. In the horse and carnivore, the epithelium is usually stratified columnar; in cloven-hoofed animals it may be stratified squamous. The lamina propria contains diffuse lymphatic tissue that contributes to the **immune function** of the conjunctiva. At the fornix, a blind pouch (conjunctival sac) containing mucosal folds is formed. The bulbar conjunctiva overlying the sclera gradually transforms into the stratified squamous epithelium of the cornea.

Species variation

Birds: In pigeons, cormorants and other species, the lid margin (limbus palpebralis) may be completely bare. It is sparsely feathered in chickens, while in parrots, raptors and ostriches it is lined with 'hair feathers' (cilia palpebralia), characterised by the absence of vanes. Meibomian glands, located in the eyelid margin of mammals, are absent in birds. In many bird species, the lid margins, and sometimes also the external surface and surroundings of the eyelids, are accentuated with bright colours.

Third eyelid (nictitating membrane, palpebra tertia)

The third eyelid, located at the nasal angle of the eye, consists of a vertically oriented **conjunctival fold** (plica semilunaris conjunctivae) (Figure 16.35). The conjunctiva is supported by cartilage which may be hyaline or elastic. The loose connective tissue of the lamina propria contains clusters of lymphatic nodules and **conjunctival glands** (glandulae palpebrae tertiae). These are subdivided into:

- **superficial glands** (glandula palpebrae tertiae superficialis):
  - serous in the horse and cat,
  - seromucous in the ox, sheep and dog,
  - mucous in the pig, and
- a mixed **deep gland** (**Harderian gland**, glandula palpebrae tertiae profunda) in the pig.

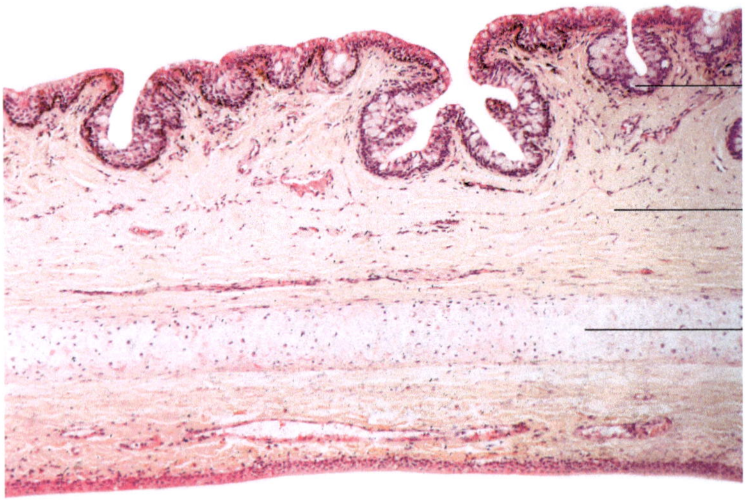

16.35 Third eyelid (horse). Haematoxylin and eosin stain (x70).

> **Species variation**
>
> **Birds**: In contrast to mammals, the third eyelid extends over the cornea from the dorsonasal to the ventrotemporal quadrant of the eye. Its free, often pigmented margin is lined with feather-like epithelial processes that sweep the surface of the cornea clean. The third eyelid is translucent in some birds and white in owls. Most water birds, especially diving species, have a transparent third eyelid that serves as an additional refractive medium, akin to a dive mask, when the animal is underwater.

Lacrimal apparatus (apparatus lacrimalis)

The lacrimal apparatus consists of the lacrimal gland and the structures through which tears drain – the lacrimal canaliculi, the lacrimal sac and the nasolacrimal duct.

The **lacrimal gland** is a compound tubulo-acinar serous or mixed gland (predominantly mucous in pigs). The secretory end pieces have wide lumina and are extensively branched. Glandular secretions pass via ducts into the conjunctival sac at the dorsotemporal aspect of the eye.

The **lacrimal canaliculi** are lined with simple squamous epithelium. Connective tissue containing collagen and elastic fibres is present in the canalicular wall. The **lacrimal sac** has stratified columnar epithelium and contains numerous lymphatic tissue deposits. The **nasolacrimal duct** is also infiltrated with lymphatic cells and contains a well-developed venous plexus. Towards the end of the duct, the lamina propria contains mucous glands.

> **Species variation**
>
> **Birds**: In domestic birds, the **lacrimal gland** is located at the temporal angle of the eye, between the periorbita and the palpebral conjunctiva. It empties by a narrow duct (or ducts) into the **conjunctival sac** near the conjunctival fornix. Owls, which produce only a small volume of tears, do not have a lacrimal gland.

In most bird species the **gland of the third eyelid** is more than double the size of the lacrimal gland. It lies at the nasal angle of the eye, on the caudo-ventromedial aspect of the bulb. As well as producing mucoid tears, the gland of the third eyelid has an important role in cell-mediated immunity (secretion of immunoglobulin A, aggregates of lymphocytes and plasma cells).

The **nasal gland** is a modified lacrimal gland located dorsonasally within the orbit. In certain seabirds, it functions alongside the kidney as an additional means of salt excretion. Thus, the increased lacrimation often observed in seagulls represents a physiological mechanism for ridding the body of salt (e.g. after ingestion of sea water).

Tear drainage occurs at the **nasal angle** via either one (e.g. penguins) or more commonly two openings, the **ostia canaliculi lacrimalis**. These are located on the internal surface of the upper and lower eyelids, clearly separated from the lid margin. Short lacrimal canaliculi (canaliculi lacrimales), only a few millimetres long, convey the tears into the **nasolacrimal duct** (ductus nasolacrimalis) that opens into the nasal cavity beneath the nasal conchae. From there, the tears flow through the choana directly into the oral cavity.

Ear (organum vestibulocochleare)

Within the ear, a close anatomical and functional association exists between the organs of balance and hearing, both of which are housed in the petrous temporal bone. The ear is divided into the following components:

- **external ear** (auris externa):
  - pinna (auricle, auricula),
  - external acoustic meatus (meatus acusticus externus),
  - tympanic membrane (membrana tympanica),

- **middle ear** (auris media):
  - tympanic cavity (cavitas tympanica),
  - auditory ossicles (ossicula auditus):
    - malleus,
    - incus,
    - stapes,
  - auditory tube (tuba auditiva),
- **inner ear** (auris interna):
  - osseous labyrinth (labyrinthus osseus) and
  - membranous labyrinth (labyrinthus membranaceus):
    - vestibular apparatus – sensory cells for balance and
    - cochlear duct – sensory cells for hearing (Figure 16.38).

External ear (auris externa)

The external ear consists of the pinna, the external acoustic meatus and, as the boundary between the external and middle sections of the ear, the tympanic membrane. This portion of the ear collects and conveys sound.

Pinna (auricle, auricula)

A **plate of elastic cartilage** forms the structural core of the pinna. The shape of the pinna varies with species and breed. Both surfaces of the pinna are lined with skin, which is bound to the cartilage by the perichondrium. The hairy skin of the inner surface of the pinna is relatively mobile. It bears long, **protective hairs** (tragi) that become thinner and more sparse in the deeper portion of the pinna. Conversely, the number of sweat and sebaceous glands increases towards the interior of the external ear.

External acoustic meatus (meatus acusticus externus)

The peripheral semicircular portion of the external acoustic meatus consists of elastic cartilage (Figure 16.36). The inner section, which ends at the **tympanic membrane** (membrana tympani) is an osseous ring. The cartilaginous and osseous segments are lined with stratified squamous epithelium. While solitary **hairs** (tragi) are present in the outer regions of the external acoustic meatus, the innermost section is hairless. The lamina propria contains sebaceous glands and pigmented, tubular apocrine sweat glands (**ceruminous glands, glandulae ceruminosae**). The secretion of the ceruminous glands combines with sebum to form **cerumen** (ear wax). These glands are present in the cartilaginous portion of the external acoustic meatus in horses and ruminants, and throughout the length of the meatus in carnivores.

Tympanic membrane (membrana tympani)

The tympanic membrane separates the external ear from the middle ear. It spans the space circumscribed by the annulus tympanicus at the base of the external acoustic meatus. The tympanic membrane is composed of three layers:

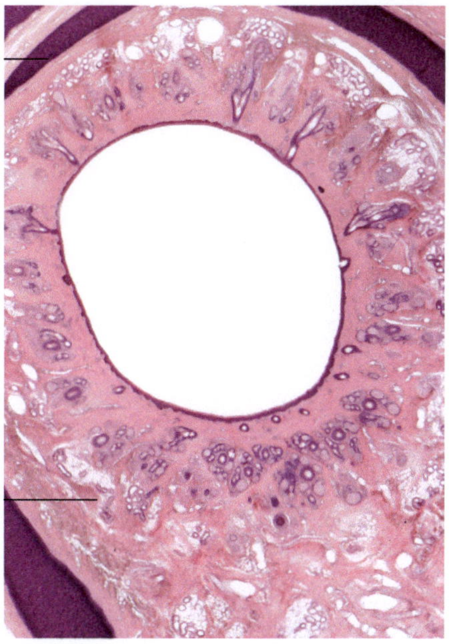

16.36 Cross-section of external acoustic meatus (pig). Haematoxylin and eosin stain (x25).

- outer layer – epithelium of the external acoustic meatus,
- middle layer – connective tissue and
- inner layer – squamous to cuboidal epithelial lining of the tympanic cavity.

The **outer layer** (stratum cutaneum) consists of squamous epithelium. This is underlaid by connective tissue containing collagen and elastic fibres (stratum proprium). The peripheral fibres of the connective tissue layer are arranged radially; the inner fibres have a circular orientation. The connective tissue is highly vascular and receives sensory innervation.

The inner epithelial layer, usually **simple squamous** in type (stratum mucosum), is continuous with the surface of the malleus, which is tightly bound to the connective tissue layer. Vibrations of the tympanic membrane are transmitted by the handle of the malleus to the more proximal ossicles, the incus and the stapes, from whence they pass to the inner ear.

Species variation

Birds: The external ear of birds comprises the external acoustic meatus and the tympanic membrane. There is **no pinna**. In the chicken, the **auditory aperture (apertura auris externae)**, or external ear opening, is 4–5 mm in diameter and is situated above a red or white ear lobe. The ear opening of most birds is covered by **modified contour feathers** (auricular feathers; pennae auriculares) arranged in concentric rows on an annular fold. In the long-eared owl (*Asio otis*), the ears are covered by a rostral **skin fold**. This contains striated muscle that enables the fold to be moved to assist with localisation of sound. Examination of the auditory aperture is an important component of ophthalmic examination in birds.

The **external acoustic meatus** (**meatus acusticus externus**) lies caudal to the quadrate bone. It is approximately 4–7 mm long.

A small mound in the ventral wall contains an opening for the underlying **auricular glands** (**glandulae auriculares**). The opening of the duct draining these glands can be visualised under magnification.

The **tympanic membrane** bulges slightly into the external ear canal. In the chicken it is 0.012 mm thick with a surface area of approximately 25 mm^2. The tympanic membrane is attached to the surrounding bone and its margins are reinforced by elastic fibres. Rostroventrally it incorporates a small, air-filled cavity, the **sinus pneumaticus marginalis**. The tympanic membrane is tensed by the **m. columellae**. This muscle is equivalent to the m. stapedius in mammals and is innervated by the facial nerve. The internal surface of the tympanic membrane is attached to the cartilaginous processes of the **columella**.

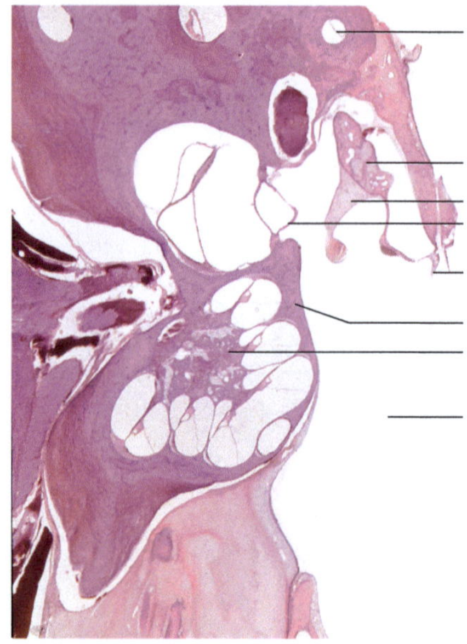

16.37 Middle and inner ear *in situ* within petrous temporal bone (pig). Haematoxylin and eosin stain (x16).

Middle ear (auris media)

The components of the middle ear include the tympanic cavity, the auditory ossicles and the auditory tube. In the horse, each auditory tube has a large expanded portion, the guttural pouch.

The **tympanic cavity** lies within the petrous temporal bone. It is lined by simple squamous epithelium. This epithelial lining covers the ossicles, the tympanic membrane and the vestibular window (Figure 16.37). At the opening of the auditory tube, and throughout this passage, the epithelium is ciliated pseudostratified. In the sheep and carnivore, mixed glands are scattered throughout the lamina propria. The connective tissue contains abundant capillaries and nerves.

The **auditory ossicles** (**malleolus, incus and stapes**) develop through endochondral ossification into lamellar bone in which cartilage remnants may be present. Articulations are present between the bones. The ossicles are covered with simple squamous epithelium. The striated m. tensor tympani and m. stapedius regulate the tension of the tympanic membrane and modify the movement of the ossicles.

The narrow **auditory tube** connects the tympanic cavity with the pharynx. Its ciliated pseudostratified epithelium contains goblet cells. The epithelium rests upon connective tissue containing collagen and elastic fibres, and numerous lymphatic cells. In ungulates, a tubal tonsil is present near the ostium pharyngicum. Initially the auditory tube is surrounded by a short bony collar. This transforms into a **cartilaginous tube**.

The **guttural pouch** of the horse is lined by ciliated pseudostratified epithelium with goblet cells. The lamina propria contains bundles of elastic fibres, smooth muscle cells and glands. A loose, displaceable tunica adventitia lines the external surface.

Species variation

Birds: The middle ear contains the air-filled tympanic cavity (cavitas tympanica), which is connected to the oropharynx by the **auditory tube** (**tuba auditiva**) via the infundibular cleft. The auditory tube is approximately 6 mm long in the chicken. A **single auditory ossicle**, the **columella**, spans the tympanic cavity. Three flexibly interconnected cartilaginous extra-columellar processes project from the columella to the tympanic membrane as the **cartilago extracolumellaris**. Resembling a tripod, the cartilago extracolumellaris is positioned caudally, ventrally and rostrally against the tympanic membrane. The **shaft of the columella** (**scapus columellae**) expands proximally to form the basis columellae, which closes the vestibular window (Figure 16.45). Lateral to the opening of the auditory tube, the tympanic cavity houses a small, curved **vesicular structure**, the **organum paratympanicum**. Lying parallel to the longitudinal axis of the head, the organum paratympanicum contains ciliated sensory cells and is presumed to register changes in air pressure. The left and right tympanic cavities are connected by air-filled spaces. In birds, the **vestibular window** is located immediately adjacent to the **cochlear window**. Pressure from sound waves striking the tympanic membrane is transmitted by the base of the columella to the perilymph within the inner ear. Compression of the perilymph results in bulging of the **secondary tympanic membrane** (**membrana tympanica secundaria**) at the cochlear window.

Internal ear (auris interna)

The internal (inner) ear comprises a system of fluid-filled sacs and ducts. This **membranous labyrinth** lies within osseous excavations termed the **osseous labyrinth**. The two labyrinths are separated by a fluid-filled space, the **spatium perilymphaticum**, which communicates with the subarachnoid space via the ductus perilymphaticus. The perilymphatic space is lined with simple squamous epithelium. It contains **perilymph**, a fluid similar in composition to cerebrospinal fluid. Perilymph is low in K^+ ions and rich in Na^+ ions.

In particular regions of the membranous labyrinth, the epithelium is differentiated to form (secondary) sensory receptor cells. Secondary sensory cells associated with balance are found in the **vestibule**, within the **macula of the sacculus** and the **macula of the utriculus**, and in the **semicircular ducts** (ductus semicirculares) within the **crista ampullaris**. In the cochlea, the **spiral organ** (**organ of Corti**) contains sensory cells for the detection of sound. The space within the membranous labyrinth is filled with **endolymph**. The composition of endolymph is similar to that of intracellular fluid. The vestibular and cochlear components of the membranous labyrinth are connected by the ductus reuniens.

Vestibular apparatus (pars statica labyrinthi, labyrinthus vestibularis)

The organ of balance comprises the **sacculus** and the **utriculus**, located within the osseous vestibule, and **three semicircular ducts**, each with an **ampulla** (**ampullae membranaceae**) that opens into the utriculus (Figure 16.38).

SACCULUS AND UTRICULUS

The lumina of the sacculus and utriculus are lined with simple squamous epithelium underlaid by loose connective tissue. Oval-shaped thickenings of the connective tissue in the wall of these compartments form the foundation for the **macula sacculi** and **macula utriculi**. In these regions, the lamina propria is extensively vascularised and innervated by fibre bundles of the vestibular part of the vestibulocochlear nerve. The maculae contain two cell types:

- supporting cells and
- sensory cells (hair cells) (Figure 16.39).

The **supporting cells** are columnar with a basal nucleus and superficial microvilli. They support the sensory cells that lie between them.

The **sensory cells** are modified epithelial cells (secondary sensory cells) that are not in contact with the basal lamina. The cell surface bears bundles of stereocilia (50–100) and a single non-motile kinocilium (hair cells). Basally, these receptor cells synapse with non-myelinated nerve fibres. Based on cell shape, number of mitochondria and synapse morphology, the sensory cells are subdivided into **types I** and **II**.

The sensory cells are covered with a gelatinous glycoprotein-rich layer, the **otolithic membrane**, into which the stereocilia and kinocilia project. **Calcium carbonate crystals**, termed **otoliths** or **statoconia**, line the surface of the membrane. The hair cells of the maculae are responsive to linear movement (vertical or horizontal). Stimulation results from shifting of the otoliths within the gelatinous membrane. The cells thus act as mechanorecep-

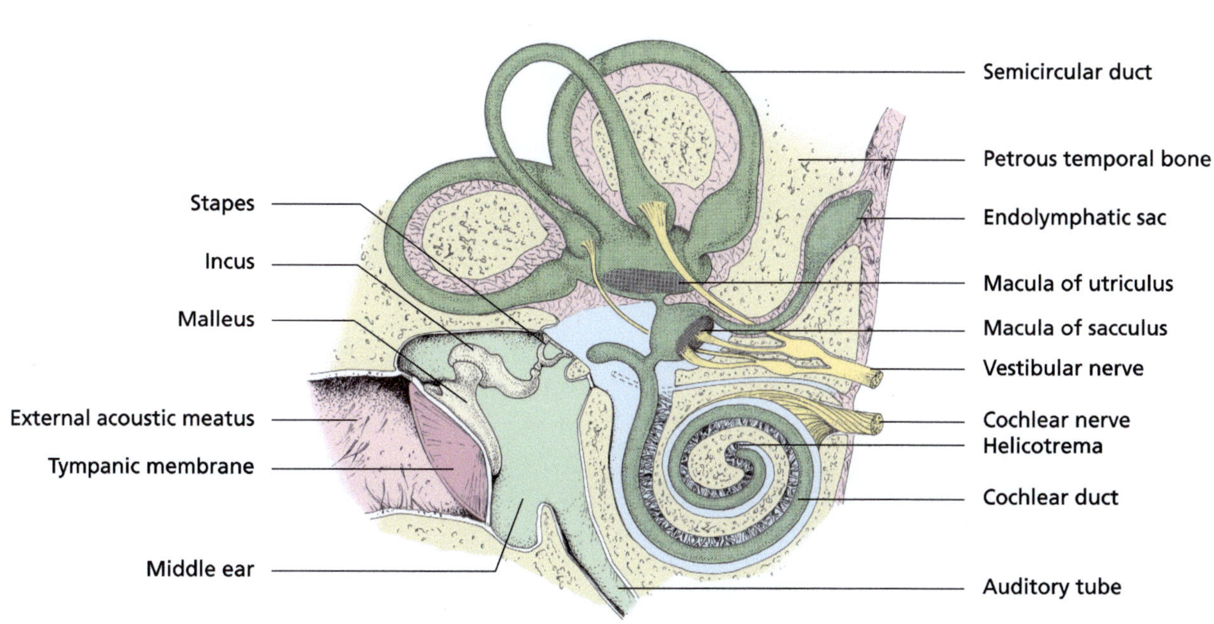

16.38 External acoustic meatus and middle and inner ear (schematic).

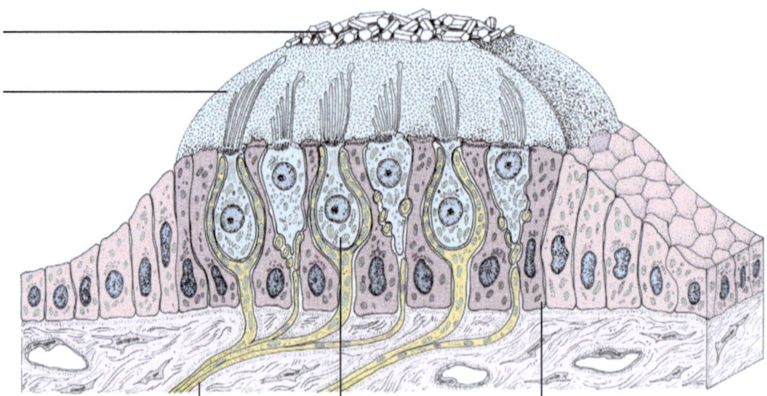

16.39 Macula (schematic).

tors, responding to pressure or tension on the stereocilia. The resulting change in electric potential elicits a neural impulse.

SEMICIRCULAR DUCTS (DUCTUS SEMICIRCULARES)

The epithelial lining of the semicircular ducts resembles that of the sacculus and utriculus. Near their opening into the utriculus, the three semicircular ducts expand into an **ampulla** (ampulla membranacea) (Figure 16.38). There, the loose connective tissue thickens to form a transverse ridge that projects into the lumen as the core of the **crista ampullaris**. The ridge is overlaid by a neuro-epithelial layer of **supporting** and **sensory** cells, similar to those of the maculae sacculi and utriculae.

In contrast to the maculae, the surface of the crista ampullaris is covered by a club-shaped cupula. This layer, composed of glycoproteins, is not coated with crystals. The crista ampullaris responds to **rotational movement**. Neural signals are generated by displacement and deformation of the cupula, brought about by movement of endolymph.

Auditory apparatus (pars auditiva labyrinthi, labyrinthus cochlearis)

In the strictest sense, the organ of hearing consists of the **cochlea** and the **spiral organ** (**organ of Corti**). These internal components of the auditory apparatus are preceded by the outer and middle ear, which convey sound waves to the inner ear through the vestibular window (Figures 16.37 and 16.40 to 16.43). The **cochlea** is a **spiral-shaped osseous canal** (canalis spiralis cochlea). The spirals (2.5 revolutions in the horse, 3.5 in the ox, 4 in the pig, 3 in carnivores) wind around a central axis composed of spongy bone (modiolus). The spiral ganglion of the cochlear nerve lies at the outer edge of the modiolus (Figures 16.37, 16.40 and 16.41).

An **osseous spiral shelf** (lamina spiralis ossea) projects from the modiolus into the spiral canal of the cochlea

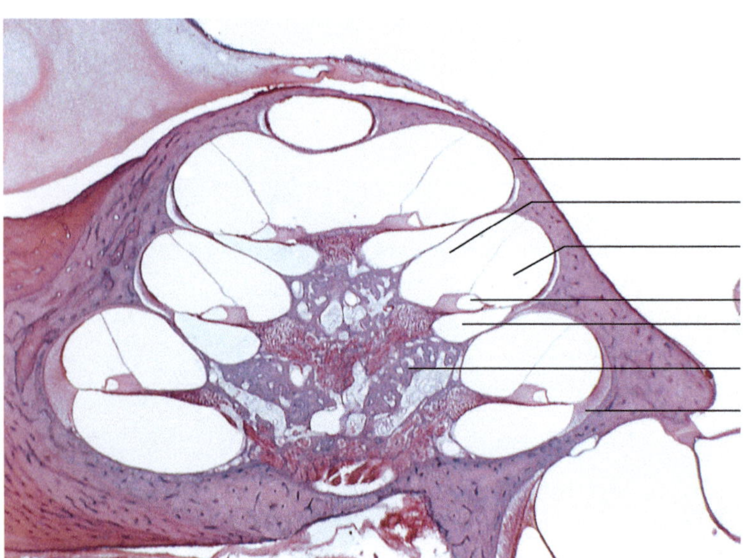

16.40 Cochlea (pig). Haematoxylin and eosin stain (x32).

(Figures 16.40 to 16.42), incompletely dividing its interior. Membranes extending from the osseous spiral lamina to the wall of the cochlea divide the spiral canal into three fluid-filled channels (Figures 16.40 and 16.41) termed the:

- scala vestibuli,
- cochlear duct (ductus cochlearis) and
- scala tympani.

The **scala vestibuli** begins at the base of the stapes at the vestibular window and extends through the spiral canal of the cochlea to its tip, where it is continuous with the scala tympani at the helicotrema. The scala tympani passes through the spiral canal to the cochlear (round) window at the base of the cochlea. Both scalae are lined with epithelium (usually simple squamous) and are filled with perilymph.

The **cochlear duct** lies between the scala vestibuli and scala tympani, accompanying these on their course through the cochlea. It is connected proximally to the saccule by the ductus reunions. At the tip of the cochlea, the cochlear duct ends in a blind sac. In contrast to the scala vestibuli and scala tympani, the cochlear duct contains endolymph.

COCHLEAR DUCT (DUCTUS COCHLEARIS)

The cochlear duct is a triangular spiral passage. At the apex of the triangle, the duct is connected to the free edge of the **lamina spiralis ossea** of the **modiolus** (Figures 16.40 and 16.41). The wall of the cochlear duct is divided into

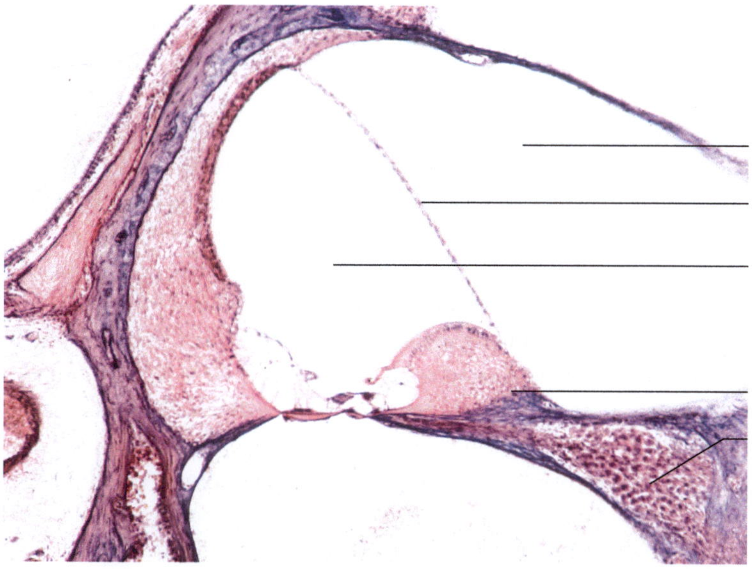

16.41 Cochlear duct in cochlea (pig). Haematoxylin and eosin stain (x320).

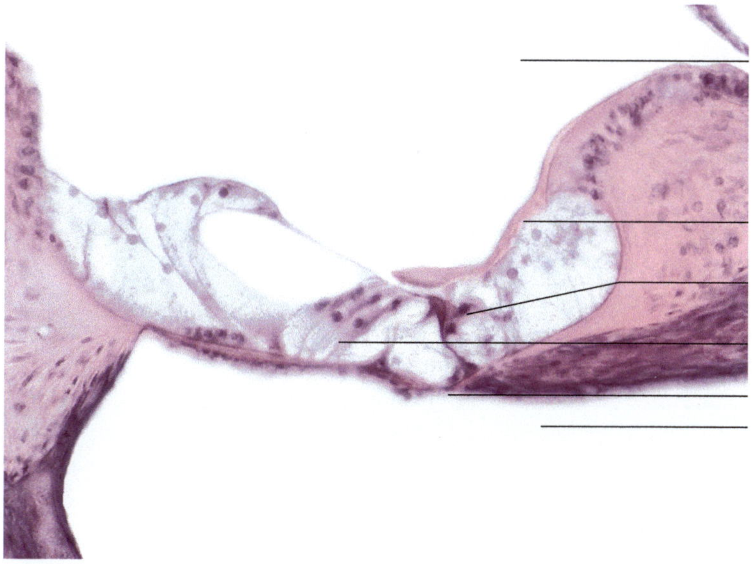

16.42 Spiral organ (pig). Haematoxylin and eosin stain (x1200).

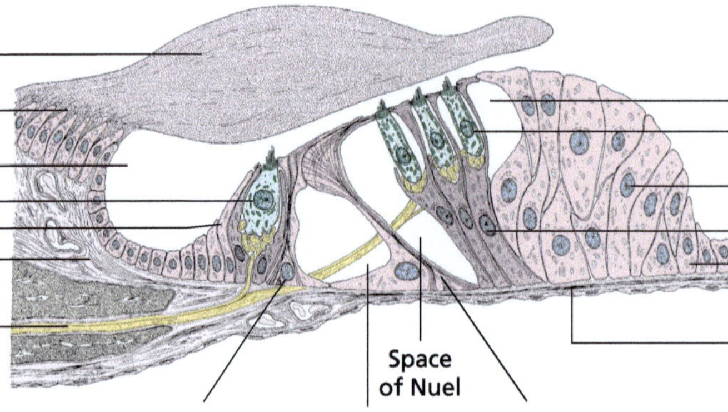

16.43 Spiral organ (organ of Corti; schematic).

three structurally different regions: **vestibular**, **outer** and **tympanic**.

The **vestibular region** (paries vestibularis ductus cochlearis, vestibular [Reissner's] membrane) is very thin. It consists of a narrow fibrous layer lined on both sides with simple squamous epithelium. The membrane is in contact with the perilymph of the scala vestibuli and the endolymph of the cochlear duct. The **outer region** (paries externus) is formed by the **spiral ligament** (**ligamentum spirale**). Constituting an extension of the basilar membrane (see below), the spiral ligament spreads out over the bone of the cochlea and is firmly bound with the periosteum (Figure 16.40). Parts of the spiral ligament are richly vascularised. In the outer region, the cochlear duct is lined by irregular pseudostratified epithelium.

The epithelial cells are characterised by abundant mitochondria and infoldings of the basal plasmalemma (basal striations).

A particular feature of this region is the presence of **intra-epithelial capillaries** (stria vascularis). These contribute to the synthesis and release of endolymph into the cochlear duct. Maintenance of low Na^+/high K^+ ion concentrations is important for perception of auditory signals. Disruption of the ion balance interferes with hearing.

The **tympanic region** (paries tympanicus) is the most extensively differentiated portion of the wall of the cochlear duct. The connective tissue foundation of the tympanic region is the **basilar membrane** (lamina basilaris), which extends from the lamina spiralis ossea to the outer wall of the cochlea, where it merges with the **spiral ligament**. The collagen fibres of the basilar membrane gradually increase in length and breadth from the base to the apex of the cochlea. Resting upon the basilar membrane is a layer of modified epithelium, the **spiral organ** (**organ of Corti**) (Figures 16.42 and 16.43).

SPIRAL ORGAN (ORGANUM SPIRALE, ORGAN OF CORTI)

The spiral organ (Figure 16.43) follows a winding course, extending throughout most of the length of the cochlear duct (**ductus cochlearis**). Its inner section (nearest the modiolus) rests against a raised layer of connective tissue (spiral limbus) on the lamina spiralis ossea. A relatively stiff, gelatinous **glycoprotein-rich membrane** (**tectorial membrane, membrana tectoria**) extends from the epithelial edge of the spiral limbus over the surface of the spiral organ (Figures 16.42 and 16.43). The space thus formed is the internal spiral sulcus. The spiral organ contains the following cell types:

- supporting cells,
  - pillar cells,
  - phalangeal cells and
- sensory cells (hair cells).

Inner and outer **pillar cells** are separated by a space termed the inner tunnel (Corti's tunnel). The pillar cells are flanked by phalangeal cells (inner phalangeal cells lie on the inner aspect of the inner pillar cells; outer phalangeal cells lie on the outer side of the outer pillar cells) (Figure 16.43). Between the outer pillar and phalangeal cells is the space of Nuel.

The pillar cells (modified epithelial cells) have a broad base that rests on the basilar membrane. Their apical cytoplasm is filled with tonofibrils (supporting fibrils). Towards the epithelial surface, the pillar cells become more slender. A characteristic plate is formed at the apices of the cells. The terminal plates of the inner and outer pillar cells are connected.

The **phalangeal cells** are arranged in a single row of inner cells and two to five rows of outer cells. These extend towards the lumen to embrace the **sensory cells** (**hair cells**). Processes extending from the apices of the phalangeal cells form plates that join with the hair cells and plates of the pillar cells to form the mosaic-like reticular lamina (membrana reticularis).

Adjoining the outer phalangeal cells are columnar outer limiting cells (Hensen's cells). Further outward, the cells become cuboidal (external supporting cells, Claudius cells)

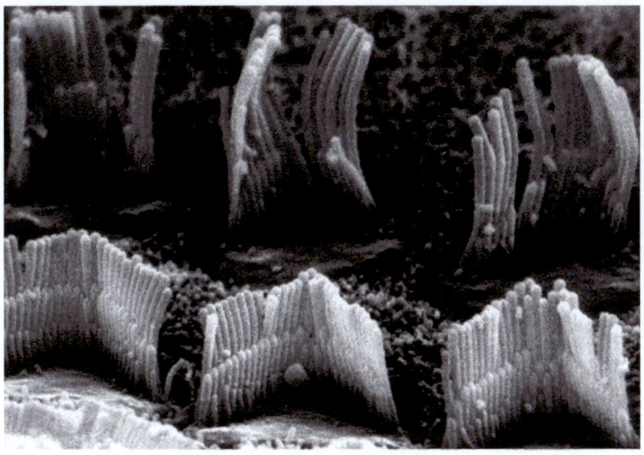

16.44 Scanning electron micrograph of stereocilia on the surface of hair cells in the spiral organ (courtesy of S. Breit).

and eventually merge with the stria vascularis. At the internal spiral sulcus, the inner phalangeal cells are continuous with the spiral limbus.

Sensory cells (hair cells) are arranged in a single inner and several outer rows. The base of these elongated cylindrical receptor cells synapses with an afferent nerve fibre (outer hair cells) or with several afferent and efferent fibres (inner hair cells). Up to 100 stereocilia (sensory hairs) project from the sensory cells between the spaces of the reticular lamina (Figure 16.44). The longest of these contact the tectorial membrane.

Species variation

Birds: As in mammals, the inner ear consists of the **osseous labyrinth** and, within it, **the membranous labyrinth**. The space between the membranous and osseous labyrinth is filled with **perilymph**, while the membranous labyrinth contains the somewhat viscous **endolymph**.

The **osseous labyrinth** (**labyrinthus osseus**) is comprised of the central **vestibule** (**vestibulum**), the ventrally positioned osseous **cochlea** and the caudodorsally projecting **semicircular canals** (**canales semicirculares ossei**). The avian cochlea is shaped like a blunt, slightly medially concave and rostrally convex club. The **semicircular** canals are arranged perpendicular to one another. Based on their plane of orientation, they are termed the rostral vertical (anterior), caudal vertical (posterior) and lateral horizontal (lateral) canals. An **ampulla** is located at one end of each canal.

The **membranous labyrinth** (**labyrinthus membranaceus**) is an extensively partitioned replica of the osseous labyrinth. It is surrounded by **perilymph** and filled with **endolymph**. The central section of the membranous labyrinth contains the larger, dorsally positioned tubular **utriculus**, as well as the smaller, ventrally situated **sacculus**. A small tube, the **ductus utriculosaccularis**, connects the two chambers. The narrow **ductus endolymphaticus** projects from the

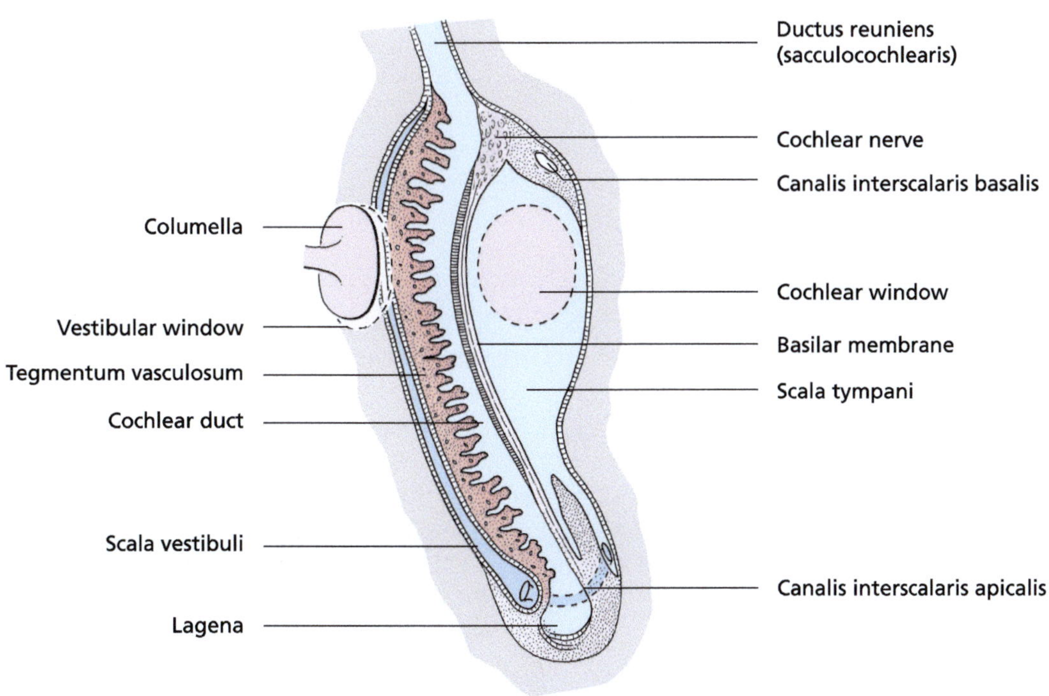

16.45 Inner ear (chicken; schematic; adapted from Evans, 1982).

sacculus, ending blindly between the meninges within the cranial cavity.

The utriculus gives rise to the semicircular ducts, each bearing an expanded ampulla at one end. Considerably smaller in diameter than the semicircular canals in which they lie, the semicircular ducts occupy a slightly eccentric position within the canals. These are attached to the periosteum of the canals by delicate fibres that pass through the perilymph.

The **sensory cells** of the **vestibular apparatus** form the **cristae ampullares** (within the ampullae), the **macula utriculi** and **crista neglecta** (within the utriculus), and the **macula sacculi** in the sacculus. The hair cells of the macula utriculi and the macula sacculi are in contact with **statoconia**. In contrast, the cristae ampullares and the crista neglecta are covered in a **dome-shaped membrane devoid of statoconia**. Movement of endolymph, induced by inertia, stimulates the hair cells, which are connected with fibres of the **vestibular ganglion** and the **vestibular nerve**.

The tubular **cochlear duct** (**ductus cochlearis**) emerges ventrally from the sacculus. In the chicken it measures approximately 6 mm in length. Its blind end, the lagena, reaches the tip of the cochlea (Figure 16.45).

Lying within the centre of the cochlea, the cochlear duct is framed by rostral and caudal cartilaginous ledges. This arrangement gives rise to two channels, the narrow **scala vestibuli** and the **scala tympani**. The two scala communicate at the apex of the cochlea via the apical **interscalar canal** (**canalis interscalaris apicalis**), the equivalent of the helicotrema in mammals.

The cochlear duct is separated from the scala vestibuli by the thick, folded **tegmentum vasculosum**. The **basilar membrane** (**membrana basilaris**) separates the cochlear duct from the scala tympani. Resting upon the basilar membrane, the **papilla basilaris** carries the **sensory cells of the cochlea**. These cells have stereocilia that are anchored in an overlying gelatinous layer, the tectorial membrane (membrana tectoria). Bipolar neurons of the **cochlear ganglion** form a delicate network of nerve fibres at the base of the sensory cells.

A further group of sensory cells is located within the lagena, forming the macula lagenae. Sensory hairs projecting from these cells are in contact with otoconia. The function of the macula lagenae has not been established. Auditory sensitivity in birds is greatest between 1000 and 6000 Hz.

Nervous system (systema nervosum)

17

The processes that take place within the body are controlled by systems that perceive external stimuli and coordinate internal responses. In addition to the regulatory functions performed by the endocrine and immune systems, the nervous system is specialised for detecting, transmitting, processing, storing and – as appropriate – responding to chemical and physical stimuli. The capacity for excitability is particularly highly developed in nerve cells (neurons) (see Chapter 5, 'Nervous tissue'). Chains of neurons are structurally and functionally linked in a network that, together with the glial cells, constitutes the nervous system.

In its simplest form, transmission of information between neurons involves the delivery of a signal by an afferent neuron (neuron 1) to the spinal cord or brain. The electrical signal is passed on via a synapse to an efferent neuron (neuron 2) that initiates a response by an effector organ.

Synaptic connection of an afferent to an efferent neuron constitutes a **simple reflex arc**. Most neuronal pathways are **more complex systems**, involving signal coordination and integration within the spinal cord and/or brain. This is necessary for ensuring normal functional interaction of the organs of the body in the presence of numerous exogenous and endogenous stimuli.

Divisions of the nervous system

In functional terms, the nervous system is divided into neuronal pathways that transmit information between the **organism** and its **environment**, or that serve to regulate the function of **internal organs**. These pathways act in concert and exert an influence on each other. They comprise the:

- somatic nervous system and
- autonomic nervous system.

The **somatic nervous system** detects sensory and physicochemical stimuli in the animal's environment and transmits these to the central nervous system for integration and processing. A nerve impulse then passes through efferent nerve fibres to the muscles of the locomotor system and initiates an appropriate response.

The somatic system encompasses all components of the nervous system, including the brain, spinal cord, afferent and efferent nerve pathways and ganglia. Hence it is also referred to as the **cerebrospinal nervous system** (Figure 17.1).

The **autonomic nervous system** is responsible for control and coordination of the vital functions of the internal organs. This system also enables the organism to adapt to environmental conditions by controlling functions such as respiration, circulation, metabolism and thermoregulation. The autonomic nervous system operates involuntarily, without conscious input from the organism.

Macroscopically, the nervous system is divided into two components:

- central nervous system (CNS; spinal cord and brain),
- peripheral nervous system (PNS; peripheral nerves and ganglia).

Central nervous system (pars centralis, systema nervosum centrale)

The structural elements of the central nervous system are comprised of **neurons** and **glial cells** (described in detail in Chapter 5, 'Nervous tissue'). These are accompanied by blood vessels and connective tissue.

During **ontogenesis** of the nervous system, **neuroblasts** and **glioblasts** differentiate from the neuroectoderm. Within the neural tube, these cells migrate from the inner proliferative layer to the **mantle layer** where they form the **dorsolateral alar plates** (**sensory**) and **ventrolateral basal plates** (**motor**). Thin floor- and roof-plates connect the alar and basal plates on each side. Axons extend outward from neurons in the mantle layer to form the **marginal layer** of the neural tube.

Differentiation of these components of the embryonic neural tube gives rise to the **central nervous system**, including the **nuclei** and **nerve tracts** (see *Veterinary Anatomy of Domestic Mammals: Textbook and Colour Atlas*).

The **mantle layer**, containing large numbers of unmyelinated nerve cell perikarya, forms the **grey matter**. This is composed of a dense meshwork of nerve cell bodies, axons, dendrites and glial cells (astrocytes). Grey matter interspersed between cell bodies consists of cellular processes of neurons and glial cells and is referred to as **neuropil**.

The marginal layer constitutes the fibre-rich **white matter**, consisting predominantly of **myelinated nerve processes**. Neuroglia of the white matter include **oligodendrocytes**, fibrous astrocytes and microglia. The lighter colour of the white matter is attributable to the **myelin sheaths** (formed by oligodendrocytes) surrounding the nerve processes.

Spinal cord (medulla spinalis)

The characteristic 'H-shape' of the **grey matter** (substantia grisea) is appreciable macroscopically in cross-section of the spinal cord. Passing through the centre of the grey matter is the **central canal** (canalis centralis), the remnant of the lumen of the embryonic neural tube. The **white matter** (substantia alba) surrounds the grey matter, giving the spinal cord its external shape (Figures 17.2 and 17.3).

The spinal cord is permeated by a dense capillary network, accompanied by loose connective tissue. This microvasculature results in fine segmentation of the nervous tissue. Highly vascular connective tissue sheaths, the **meninges**, surround the spinal cord.

The segments of the spinal cord (cervical, thoracic, lumbar, sacral) exhibit species-specific variation in the ratio of grey to white matter and in cross-sectional area (and thus in volume).

Despite these regional differences, the **basic structure** of the spinal cord is relatively consistent (Figure 17.2).

The spinal cord is a bilaterally symmetrical organ, divided by a **deep ventral median fissure** (fissura mediana ventralis) and a shallow **dorsal sulcus** (sulcus medianus dorsalis). The latter continues into the tissue of the spinal cord as the **dorsal median septum** (septum medianum dorsale). A bilateral **dorsolateral sulcus** (sulcus lateralis dorsalis) is present at the level of the **dorsal nerve roots** (radices dorsales) of the spinal nerves. A considerably shallower depression is evident at the **ventral nerve roots** (radices ventrales).

Grey matter (substantia grisea)

In transverse section, the grey matter exhibits an 'H-shaped' profile formed by relatively narrow **dorsal horns** (cornu dorsale) and typically larger **ventral horns** (cornu ventrale) (Figures 17.3 and 17.4). The horns are connected by the **lateral intermediate substance** (pars intermedia lateralis). In the thoracolumbar region, the lateral intermediate substance protrudes into the white matter as the **lateral horn** (cornu lateralis). In the cervical spinal cord, an additional cellular network, the **spinal reticular formation** (formatio reticularis), is present between the dorsal and ventral horns.

The two symmetrical halves of the grey matter of the spinal cord are connected by a thin bridge (commissura grisea). The commissure encloses the **central canal** (canalis centralis) (Figure 17.5), which is lined by ependymal cells (see Chapter 5, 'Nervous tissue'). Surrounding the central canal is a ring of tissue, the **central intermediate substance**, composed of neurons and glial cells.

When regarded in three dimensions, the dorsal, ventral and lateral horns form columns of tissue – the **dorsal column** (cornu dorsale), **lateral column** (cornu laterale) and **ventral column** (cornu ventrale).

The grey matter is composed predominantly of **multipolar neurons** and **glial cells** (astrocytes). Neuron size, number and morphology varies with location in the different segments of the spinal cord. Unmyelinated axons and dendrites (**neurofibrae nonmyelinata**) and astrocyte processes form a dense nervous tissue meshwork (**neuropil**). The overarching purpose of the neurons of the grey substance is to establish a synaptic interconnection between afferent and efferent neuronal pathways.

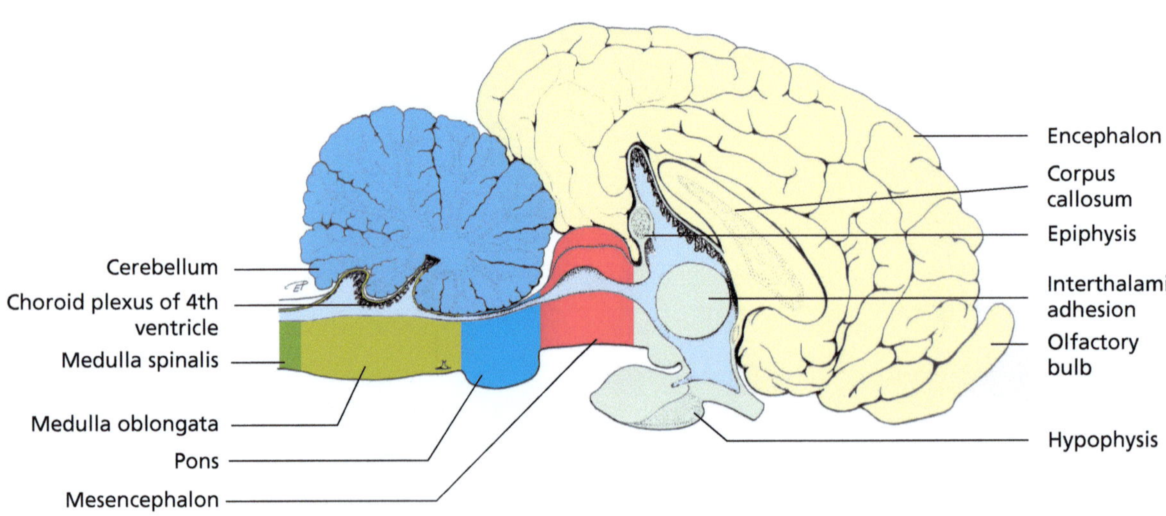

17.1 Brain of a horse (median section; schematic) (König & Liebich, 2009).

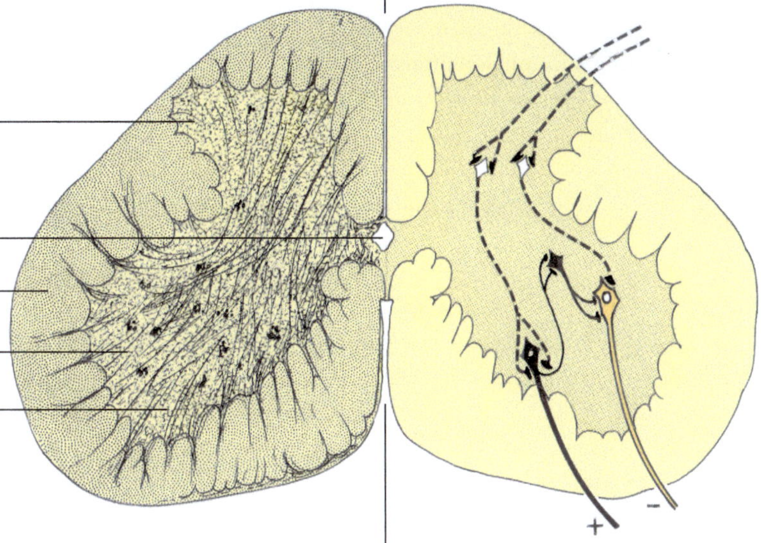

17.2 Lumbar region of the spinal cord in the cat (schematic).

The multipolar cells of the grey matter can be divided into two groups: cells with axons that leave the spinal cord via the ventral horn (fila radicularia) and form the ventral root (**efferent neurons**), and cells that communicate with other neurons within the central nervous system (spinal interneurons and projection neurons).

Efferent neurons may be **somatic** (from the ventral horn) or **autonomic** (sympathetic and parasympathetic).

Interneurons and projection neurons are numerous in the dorsal horn and lateral intermediate substance. These can be subdivided as follows:

- interneurons that transmit impulses within spinal segments,
- interneurons that cross the commissura grisea to the corresponding contralateral segment,
- interneurons that divide into ascending and descending branches, acting ipsilaterally or contralaterally upon efferent cells and
- projection neurons that send axons into the white matter and transmit impulses over long distances (as far as the brain).

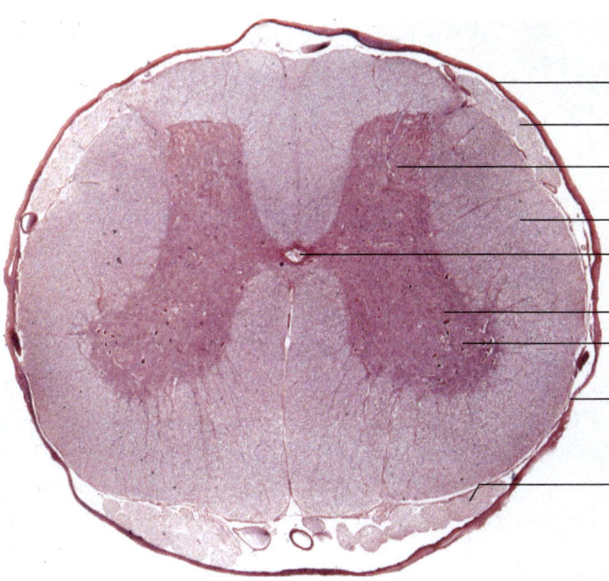

17.3 Transverse section of the spinal cord (sheep). Bodian stain (x8).

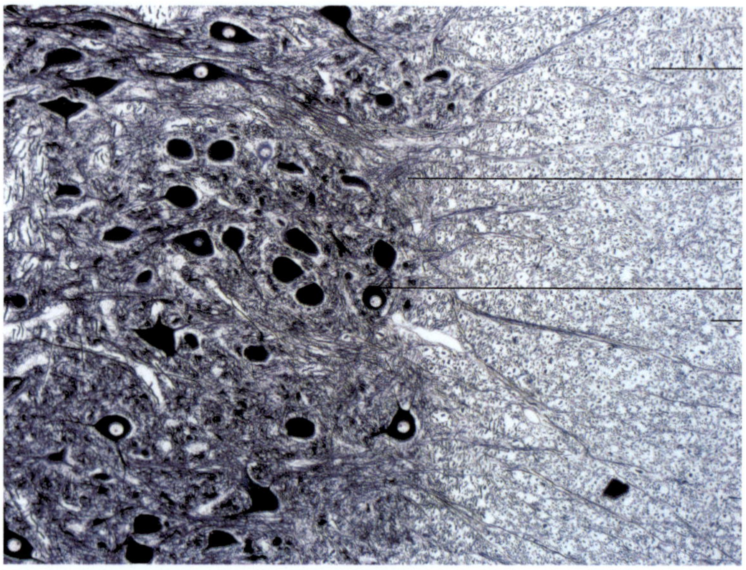

17.4 Partial section of the ventral horn of the spinal cord (dog). Iron haematoxylin stain (x120).

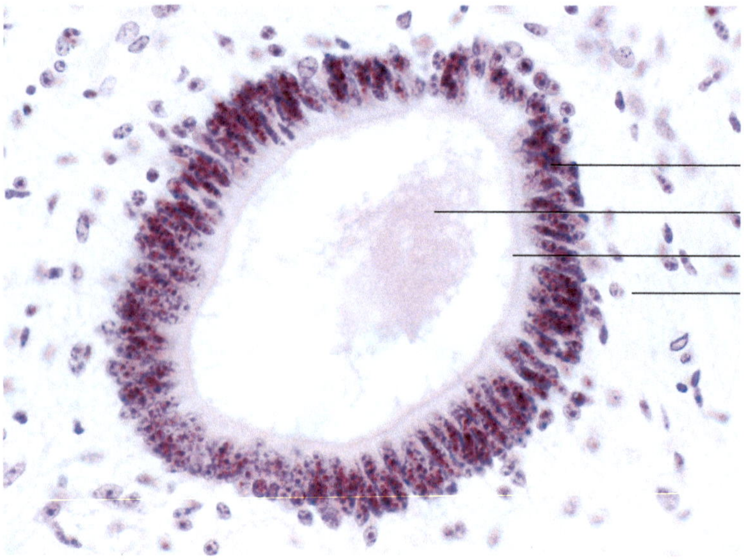

17.5 Transverse section of the central canal of the spinal cord (dog). Haematoxylin and eosin stain (x480).

The grey matter contains variably sized clusters of multipolar neuronal cell bodies referred to as **nuclei**. According to their location within the grey matter, these are designated as dorsal horn nuclei, ventral horn nuclei and nuclei of the pars intermedia lateralis.

Ventral horn nuclei contain motor neurons. Located in the lateral intermediate substance are the neurons of the nucleus sympathicus (intermediolateral nucleus) and nucleus parasympathicus (nucleus intermediomedialis). Axons of these neurons leave the spinal cord mainly through the ventral roots, particularly in the sacral spinal segments where they combine to form the nervi pelvini (pelvic nerves). In some cases, axons pass from the spinal cord via the dorsal roots. The dorsal horn contains large numbers of projection neurons, including those forming nuclei of ascending and descending spinal tracts (e.g. nucleus thoracicus).

White matter (substantia alba)

White matter is composed predominantly of longitudinally oriented **myelinated nerve fibres** (**neurofibrae myelinata**) and glial cells, particularly oligodendrocytes that form the myelin sheath within the central nervous system. A single oligodendrocyte surrounds several axonal processes (see Chapter 5, 'Nervous tissue'). Isolated astrocytes are also found in the white matter.

White matter is divided into regions known as **funiculi**. The cross-sectional diameter of funiculi varies according to function. Based on their position within the white matter, and their relationship to the dorsal and ventral horns, these are termed the dorsal funiculus (funiculus dorsalis), lateral funiculus (funiculus lateralis) and ventral funiculus (funiculus ventralis). The funiculi contain ascending and descending nerve tracts.

Cerebellum

The surface of the cerebellum features numerous convoluted ridges (folia cerebelli) separated by deep fissures. The substantial **medulla** (corpus medullare cerebelli) arborises to form fibre-rich white matter lamellae. These are coated in a thin layer of **cerebellar cortex** (cortex cerebelli) composed of grey matter (Figures 17.6 and 17.7). Due to its characteristic appearance, the radiating white matter is referred to as the **tree of life** (arbor vitae). From exterior to interior, the **cerebellar cortex** is composed of the following layers:

- molecular layer (stratum moleculare),
- Purkinje cell layer (piriform cell layer, stratum neuronorum piriformium, stratum ganglionare) and
- granule cell layer (stratum granulosum) (Figure 17.8).

Molecular layer

The molecular layer is composed of largely unmyelinated nerve fibres, abundant strongly branched dendrites (including those from Purkinje cells, see below) and sparse cell bodies of neurons and neuroglia. Microglia and astrocytes are the most commonly encountered glial cells. The neuron population comprises basket cells (neuronum corbiferum) and stellate cells (neuronum stellatum).

Basket cells are found predominantly in the inner third of the molecular layer. Their dendrites are extensively branched and extend vertically through the cerebellar folia. Basket cells also give off long axons oriented parallel to the surface of the cerebellum. These form a dense network (or 'basket') of fibres around the soma of Purkinje cells (see below). Basket cells have an inhibitory influence on the Purkinje cell layer.

Stellate cells resemble basket cells. These are located mainly in the outer half of the molecular layer. Stellate cells receive nerve impulses from parallel (axonal) fibres and collaterals of small granule cells. The horizontally oriented axons of stellate cells synapse on the dendrites of Purkinje cells, upon which they exert an inhibitory effect.

Purkinje cell layer

The narrow Purkinje cell layer consists of motor **neurons** characterised by **pear-shaped** perikarya (diameter 30–35 µm). Originally named after the neurophysiologist J.E. Purkinje (1787–1869), they are now referred to as piriform cells (*sing.* neuronum piriforme). In deference to tradition, the term **Purkinje cell** is also still used.

Purkinje cells give off an axon into the granule cell layer and send two or, less frequently, three large dendrites into the molecular layer. The dendrites arborise into networks that extend to the surface of the cerebellum. The axons, which become myelinated within the Purkinje cell layer, are the only efferent fibres of the cerebellum and extend into the nuclei in the cerebellar medulla (Figure 17.7).

Purkinje cells receive input from climbing fibres and, via synapses on granule cells, from mossy fibres. Climbing fibres project from the olivary nuclei (nuclei olivares), while mossy fibres originate from various sources including the spinal cord and vestibular nerve.

Granule cell layer

The granule cell layer contains numerous small neurons, a few larger nerve cells, glial cells and nerve fibres, some of which are myelinated (Figure 17.8).

The **small, multipolar granule cells** (perikaryon 5 µm) are characterised by a single axon and three to six dendrites. Their morphology determines the appearance of this layer. The granule cells (neurona granuliformia) can be seen to form clusters, separated by acellular islets (glomeruli cerebellares). In these regions, afferent mossy fibres synapse with dendrites of the granule cells. Granule cell axons extend vertically into the molecular layer, where they undergo a T-shaped bifurcation and pass parallel to the surface (longitudinal or parallel fibres). These axons synapse on basket cells, stellate cells and Purkinje cells.

The **large granule cells** (neuronum stellatum magnum), also referred to as **Golgi cells**, give off short axons that form synapses with dendrites of small granule cells.

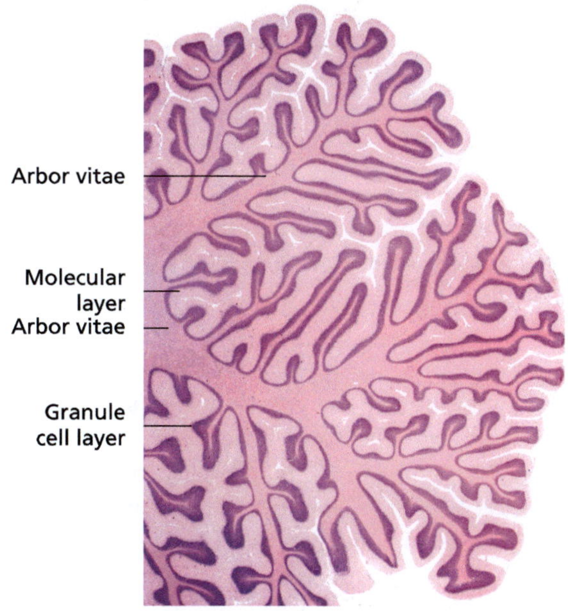

17.6 Cerebellum with arbor vitae (cat). Haematoxylin and eosin stain (x8).

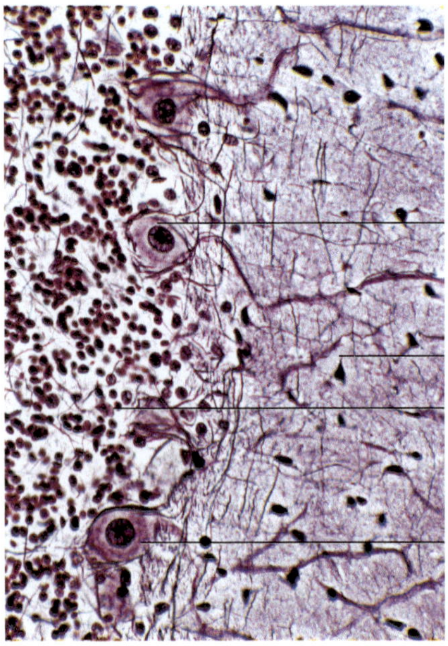

17.7 Grey matter of the cerebellum (cat). Bodian stain (x300).

Golgi cell dendrites extend into the molecular layer where they divide into branches.

Cerebrum

The neural components of the cerebrum vary in size, density, morphology and structure, reflecting the number and complexity of the functions performed by this part of the central nervous system. This accounts for the considerable differences in cyto-architecture observed within individual layers in some parts of the brain. Marked variation also occurs in the organisation of glial tissue, vessels and nerve fibres.

Like the cerebellum, the cerebrum has an **external cortex** composed of **grey matter** (this contrasts with the spinal cord and brain stem, where the nerve fibre-rich white matter is located superficially while the grey matter lies internally, adjacent to the central canal and ventricles). The basal nuclei of the cerebrum are also composed of grey matter. White matter makes up the interior of the cerebrum. The fibres of the white matter establish connections within the main bulk of the brain. Tracts formed by processes extending from efferent cells and interneurons of cranial nerves, and from projection neurons from the spinal cord, connect the components of the brain to form an integrated functional system.

Cerebral cortex (cortex cerebri)

The structure of the cerebral cortex (**neocortex**, **isocortex**) (Figures 17.9 to 17.11) exhibits regional variation in nerve cell, fibre bundle and glial cell architecture, and in the organisation of blood vessels. Nevertheless, all regions conform to a basic structural plan. In mammals, the cerebral cortex is composed of six layers. From superficial to deep, these are the:

- molecular layer (stratum moleculare),
- external granular layer (stratum granulare externum),
- external pyramidal layer (stratum neuronorum pyramidalium externum),
- internal granular layer (stratum granulare internum),
- internal pyramidal layer (stratum neuronorum pyramidalium internum) and
- multiform layer (stratum neuronorum multiformium) (Figure 17.9).

The outermost **molecular layer** is covered by the pia mater. Scattered small neurons (neurona horizontalia) give off myelinated axons that course parallel to the

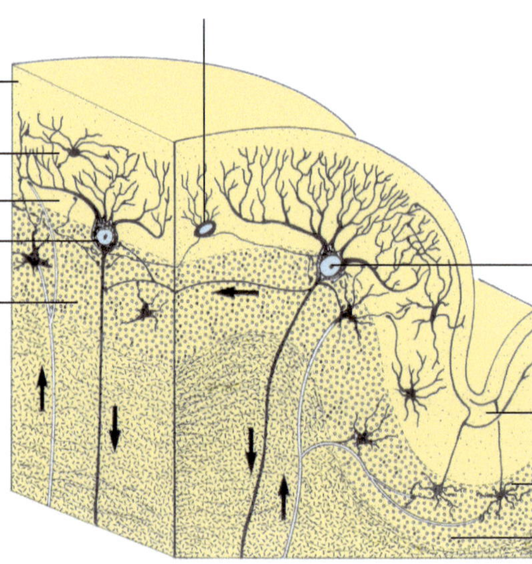

17.8 Layers of the cerebellum (schematic).

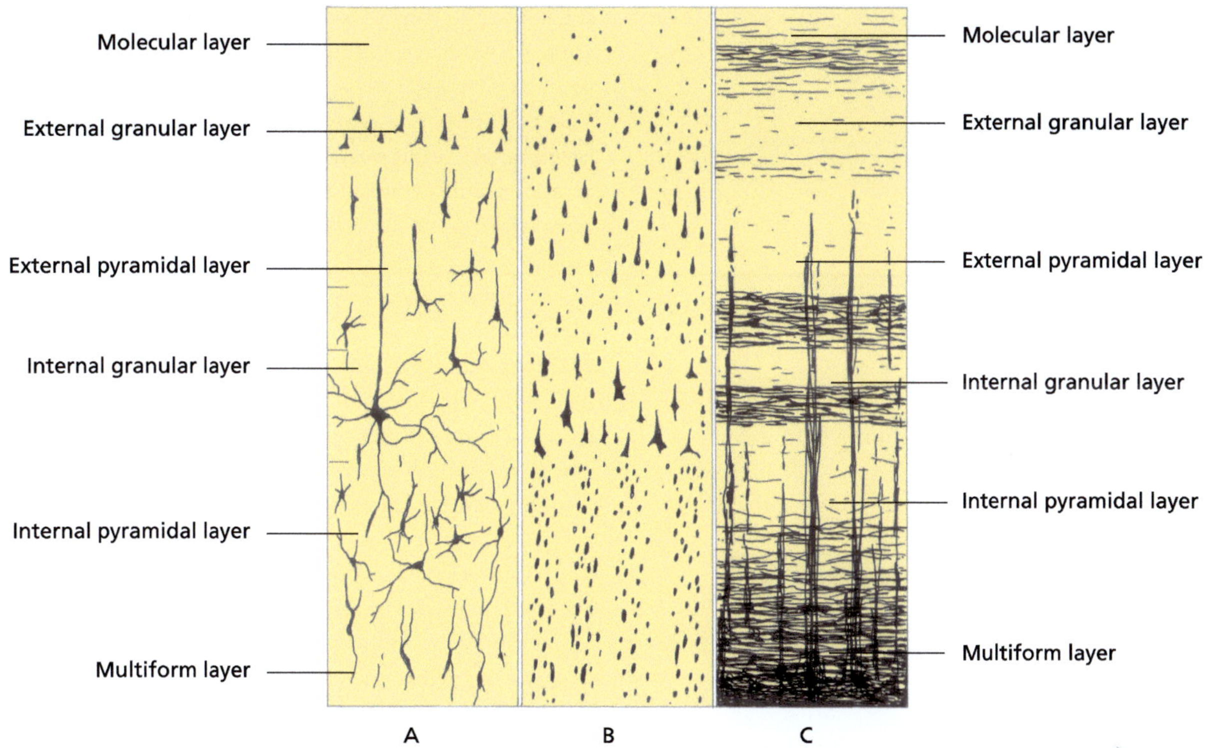

17.9 Layers of the cerebrum (schematic). A: Golgi silver impregnation method showing branching of nerve processes, B: Nissl stain showing neuronal endoplasmic reticulum, C: staining of myelin sheath to illustrate the architecture of myelinated nerve fibres.

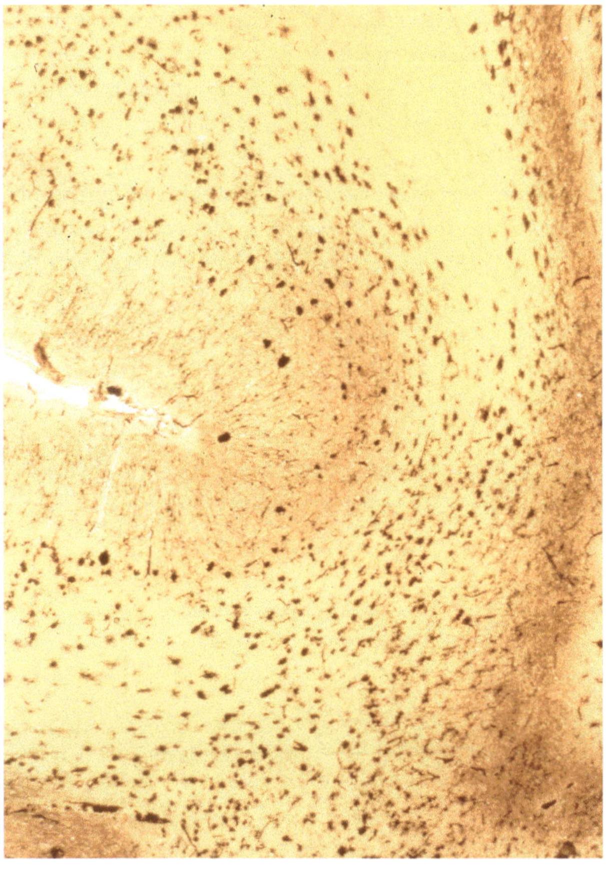

17.10 Cerebrum (dog). Golgi stain (x10).

surface. Together with the terminal branches of association and commissural fibres, these give rise to a tangentially oriented meshwork. The nerve cells act as interneurons. Also present in the molecular layer are dendrites of pyramidal cells located in deeper layers of the cortex. Fibrous astrocytes form the superficial glial limiting membrane (membrana limitans gliae superficialis).

The external granular layer consists of numerous small (10–12 µm) pyramidal nerve cells (neurona pyramidalia parva). The processes of these cells pass into the superficial and deeper cortical layers. In addition to small collateral branches, the cells have a principal dendrite that gives rise to the pyramidal shape of the cell. The external pyramidal layer contains mid-sized and large pyramidal cells (neurona pyramidalia), the size of the cell increasing towards the inner portion of the layer (20–40 µm). The external pyramidal layer is generally the thickest layer of the cerebral cortex. The internal granular layer is composed of small neurons of variable morphology. These cells serve as interneurons, their processes forming macroscopically visible stria that run parallel to the surface.

The internal pyramidal layer is characterised by large pyramidal neurons (neurona pyramidalia magna, 80–120 µm). The axons given off by these cells form a component of the pyramidal tracts. Structurally, the pyramidal neurons of the internal pyramidal layer resemble those of the ventral horn of the spinal cord. Regional accumulations of

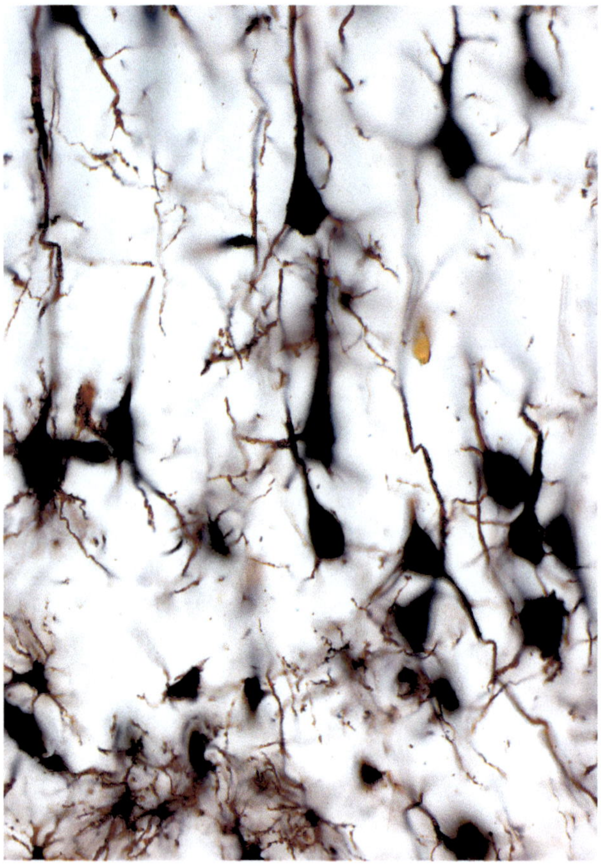

17.11 External granular layer of the cerebrum (cat). Silver impregnation (x250).

mid-sized pyramidal cells (neurona pyramidalia media) are also found in this layer.

The neurons of the **multiform layer** are polymorphic and blend without obvious demarcation with the white matter. This inner region contains many fibres passing to and from the cortex.

In domestic mammals, the layers of the cerebral cortex are not always clearly distinguishable. Particularly the inner layers are frequently merged into one.

Cerebral white matter (corpus medullare cerebri)

The size of the brain is influenced considerably by the **cerebral white matter**. The greater the degree of development of the cerebrum, the more developed the white matter relative to the cerebral cortex. As with the spinal cord, the white matter of the cerebrum is composed of nerve fibres and glial cells. Oligodendrocytes form the myelin sheaths; astrocytes (protoplasmic, fibrous) provide mechanical and metabolic support for the neurons. Association, commissural and projection fibres within the white matter cannot be distinguished with the light microscope (refer to *Veterinary Anatomy of Domestic Animals: Textbook and Colour Atlas*).

Peripheral nervous system (pars peripherica, systema nervosum periphericum)

The **peripheral nervous system** is composed primarily of nerve fibres and their associated ganglia. Anatomically, its two components – the **somatic** (cerebrospinal) and **autonomic** (visceral) nervous systems – are closely associated within nerve fibre bundles. In functional terms, the somatic nerve fibres are designated as sensory or motor. Autonomic nerve fibres are classified as sympathetic or parasympathetic.

With the exception of the cranial nerves, peripheral nerve fibres have a segmental embryonic precursor and are connected with the spinal cord via dorsal and ventral roots. Efferent motor and autonomic fibres leave the spinal cord through the ventral root to act upon target organs in the periphery. Peripheral nerve fibres convey nerve impulses to the central nervous system via afferent (sensory) pathways. These fibres pass into the dorsal horn of the spinal cord (see *Veterinary Anatomy of Domestic Animals: Textbook and Colour Atlas*).

At specific locations within the peripheral nervous system, clusters of nerve cell bodies (perikarya) form localised thickenings. Outside the central nervous system, such accumulations of neuronal cell bodies are referred to as **ganglia**. Ganglia are surrounded by a **connective tissue capsule** that continues as the epi- and perineurium of the associated nerve. Reflecting the functional divisions of the peripheral nervous system, there are two types of ganglia:

- sensory ganglia (spinal ganglia and cranial nerve ganglia) and
- autonomic ganglia (ganglia autonomica, vegetative ganglia).

Sensory ganglia

Paired spinal ganglia (ganglia spinalia) reside in the dorsal roots of the spinal nerves, corresponding with the segments of the spinal cord.

Spinal ganglia are composed mainly of **pseudo-unipolar neurons** (neurona pseudounipolaria) that act as relay points within sensory pathways (Figure 17.12).

The perikaryon of the pseudo-unipolar neuron is surrounded by **satellite cells** (amphicytes, gliocyti ganglii) that serve as neuroglia. Within a short distance of the neuronal soma, the common process extending from the nerve cell divides into a central branch, that passes into the dorsal horn as the **axonal component**, and a peripheral branch that serves as the **dendritic portion** of the neuron.

Embryonically, pseudo-unipolar neurons develop as bipolar cells with a separate axon and dendrite. These cell processes migrate to one side of the cell and fuse, giving rise to a common origin and two branches. While the **peripheral branch** exhibits dendritic terminal branching, it is able – once fully myelinated – to conduct afferent impulses and pass them on to the axon. Both the peripheral and central branches thus act as fully functional axons (see Chapter 5, 'Nervous tissue').

Pseudo-unipolar neurons within spinal ganglia are sometimes accompanied by multipolar nerve cells and other small neurons; these may be interneurons or cells of the autonomic nervous system. Spinal ganglia are subdivided by sheets of loose connective tissue (endoneurium) containing delicate capillary networks.

Most sensory ganglia of the cranial nerves are similar in structure to the spinal ganglia. The spiral (cochlear) ganglion and vestibular ganglion associated with the vestibulocochlear nerve are the only sensory ganglia in which the neurons are bipolar.

Autonomic ganglia

The nerve cells found in ganglia of the autonomic nervous system (ganglia autonomica) are **multipolar** (neurona multipolaria) (Figure 17.13). These variably sized cells are surrounded by **satellite cells** (amphicytes, gliocyti ganglii). Autonomic ganglia are permeated by connective tissue septa that give rise to small compartments.

Autonomic ganglia include segmentally positioned swellings within the sympathetic trunk, prevertebral sympathetic ganglia (e.g. coeliac ganglion) and parasympathetic ganglia (e.g. ciliary ganglion).

Meninges

The central nervous system is encased in connective tissue sheaths referred to as the meninges (Figure 17.15). The meninges are composed of the:

- pachymeninx (dura mater),
- leptomeninges, comprising the
  - arachnoid and
  - pia mater.

Pachymeninx (dura mater)

The outermost meningeal layer, the dura mater, consists of a taut meshwork of connective tissue containing few vessels. In the horse, the **dura mater covering the cerebrum** (dura mater encephali, cranial dura mater) is extensively fused with the cranium. This phenomenon is limited to bony protuberances in other domestic mammals. The dura mater encephali contains venous sinuses lined with epithelium (sinus venosi). Externally, these are bounded by fibrous layers of the dura. The sinuses do not contain valves.

The **dura mater surrounding the spinal cord** (dura mater spinalis, spinal dura mater) forms a large tube that is separated from the periosteum of the vertebral canal (endorhachis) by loose connective tissue interspersed with fat. This epidural space (spatium epidurale) is permeated by venous networks. The veins and connective tissue compartments facilitate the resorption of fluid. This is of clinical significance in epidural anaesthesia.

Leptomeninges

The leptomeninges consist of a thin outer membrane, the **arachnoid**, and an inner layer, the **pia mater**, that lies directly adjacent to the underlying brain and spinal cord (see *Veterinary Anatomy of Domestic Animals: Textbook and Colour Atlas*). The **arachnoid** (arachnoidea encephali and spinalis) is a thin, avascular connective tissue layer that lies against the internal surface of the dura mater. Sheets of flattened cells create a mesothelium-like lining of the cavum subdurale (the potential space between the dura mater and arachnoid). This cell layer, termed the **subdural neurothelium**, plays an important role in fluid resorption. In contrast to the dura mater, the arachnoid surrounding the brain features avascular villous projections, **arachnoid granulation villi** (granulationes arachnoideales). These are presumed to participate in metabolic exchange between venous blood and cerebrospinal fluid.

Arachnoid trabeculae (trabecula arachnoidea), composed of collagen fibres, traverse the **subarachnoid space** (cisterna subarachnoidea) between the arachnoid and the pia mater. This fibrous network has a mesothelial-like lining resembling the subdural neurothelium. The subarachnoid space is filled with **cerebrospinal fluid** (liquor cerebrospinalis). The pia mater of the brain and spinal cord (pia mater encephali and spinalis) is an extensively vascularised layer composed principally of loose connective tissue. It lies loosely against the external surface of the central nervous tissue as a single-celled mesothelium, in direct contact with the superficial glial limiting membrane.

Up to a certain depth, the **pia mater** extends into the fissures on the surface of the central nervous system. Blood vessels accompany the connective tissue, giving rise to a perivascular space between the blood vessels and the pia mater. The blood vessels continue into the nervous tissue where, in conjunction with the glial cells, they form the **blood–brain barrier**. This functional barrier to penetration of blood solutes is composed of modified endothelial cells lining the capillaries and the glial limiting membrane.

Ventricles (ventriculi)

The central nervous system encloses a continuous fluid-filled system comprising a series of chambers and a central canal. The walls of these cavities are lined by ependymal cells. This epithelium-like layer is considered part of the neuroglia and is described in Chapter 5, 'Nervous tissue'.

A special feature of the ventricles of the brain is the **choroid plexus** (plexus choroideus). Located in circumscribed regions of the walls of ventricles, the choroid plexuses consist of pial connective tissue and numerous branched, thin-walled vessels. The surface of these vascular tufts is lined by a cuboidal to low columnar epithelium composed of modified ependymal cells (Figure 17.14).

The choroid plexuses produce the **cerebrospinal fluid** (liquor cerebrospinalis) that fills the entire ventricular system of the brain, the central canal of the spinal cord and the subarachnoid space of the meninges. Cerebrospinal fluid is a clear, watery liquid containing few cells, little protein and relatively large quantities of Na^+, Ka^+ and Cl^- ions. The cerebrospinal fluid provides protection for the central nervous system and allows for metabolic exchange.

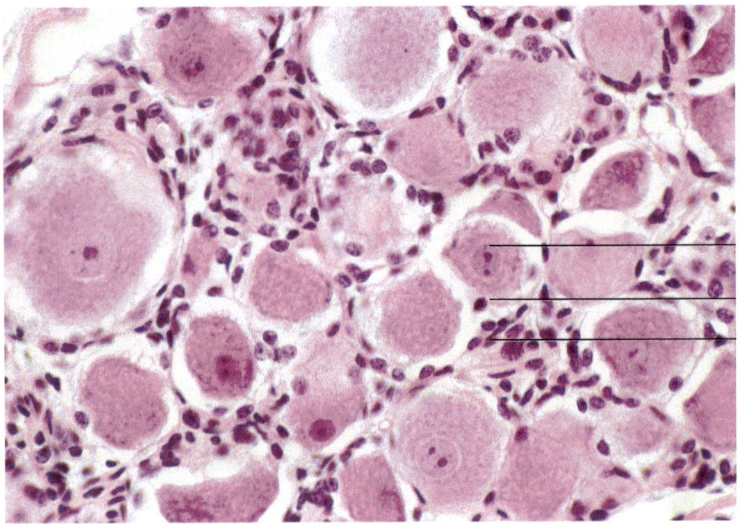

17.12 Spinal ganglion (dog). Haematoxylin and eosin stain (x300).

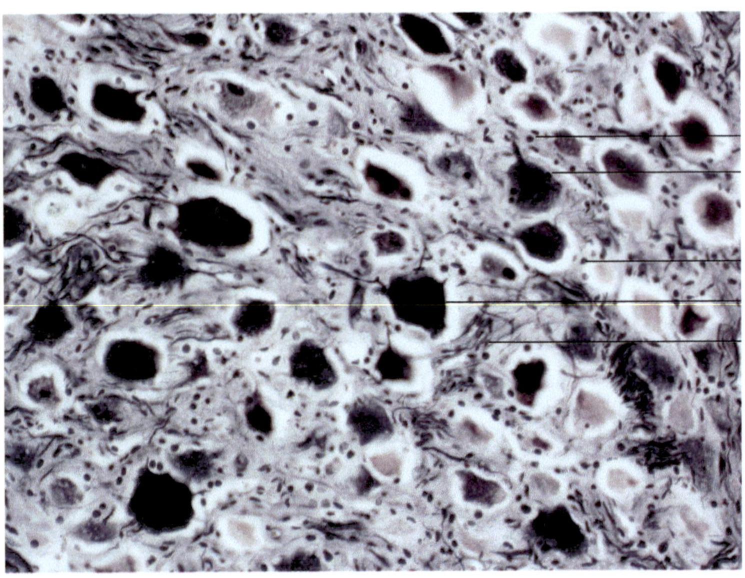

17.13 Autonomic ganglion (dog). Silver impregnation (x250).

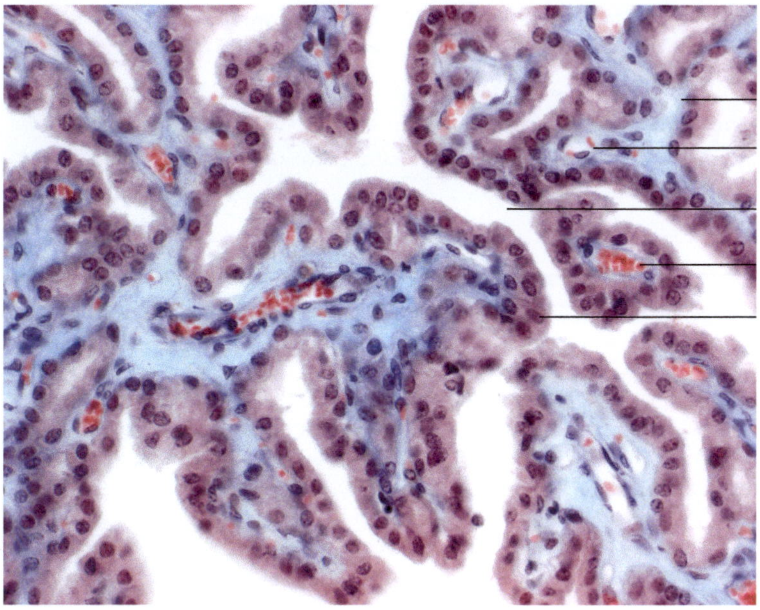

17.14 Choroid plexus (cat). Azan stain (x220).

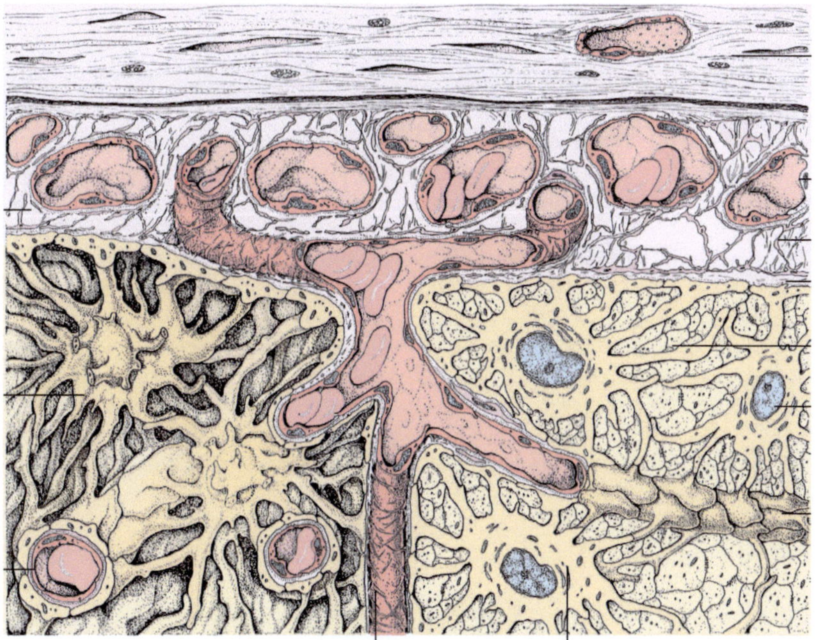

17.15 Meninges (schematic).

Bibliography

Acosta TJ, Miyamoto A. Vascular Control of Ovarian Function: ovulation, corpus luteum formation and regression. Anim Reprod Sci 2004; 82: 127–140.

Adams DR, Hotchkiss KD. The Canine Nasal Mucosa. Zbl Vet Med C Anat Histol Embryol 1983; 12: 109–125.

Altunay H. Fine Structure of the Retinal Pigment Epithelium, Bruch's Membrane and Choriocapillaris in the Horse. Anat Histol Embryol 2000; 29: 135–139.

Amselgruber W. Licht- und Elektronenmikroskopische Untersuchungen zur Ooge- nese der Katze (Felis catus). Zbl Vet Med C Anat Histol Embryol 1983; 12: 193–229.

Amselgruber W, Feder F-H. Licht- und Elektronenmikroskopische Untersuchun- gen der Samenblasendrüse (Glandula vesicularis) des Bullen. Anat Histol Embryol 1986; 15: 361–379.

Amselgruber W, Schäfer M, Sinowatz F. Angiogenesis in the Bovine Corpus Luteum: an immunocytochemical and ultrastructural study. Anat Histol Embryol 1999; 28: 157–166.

Anthauer K, Mülling C, Budras K-D. Membrane-coating Granules and the Intercellular Cementing Substance (Membrane-coating Material) in the Epidermis in Different Regions of the Equine Hoof. Anat Histol Embryol 2005; 34: 298–306.

Arias JL, Cabrera R, Valencia A. Observations on the Histological Development of the Bovine Rumen Papillae – Morphological Changes Due to Age. Zbl Vet Med C Anat Histol Embryol 1978; 7: 140–151.

Arrighi S, Cremonesi F, Bosi G, Domeneghini C. Endocrine-Paracrine Cells of the Male Urogenital Apparatus: a comparative histochemical and immunohistochemical study in some domestic ungulates. Anat Histol Embryol 2004; 33: 225–232.

Augsburger HR. Elastic Fibre System of the Female Canine Urethra. Histochemical Identification of Elastic, Elaunin and Oxytalan Fibres. Anat Histol Embryol 1997; 26: 297–302.

Bacha WJ, Bacha LM. Colour Atlas of Veterinary Histology, 3rd edn. Chichester: John Wiley & Sons Ltd, 2012.

Baer S, Hummel G, Goller H. Feinstruktur des Ammonshornes von Rind, Schaf und Ziege. Zbl Vet Med C Anat Histol Embryol 1985; 14: 242–261.

Belkin AM, Stepp MA. Integrins as Receptors for Laminins. Micros Res Tech 2000; 51: 280–301.

Berens von Rautenveld D, Budras KD. Topography, Ultrastructure and Phagocytic Capacity of Avian Lymph Nodes. Cell Tissue Res 1983; 228: 389–403.

Bergerson W., Amselgruber W, Sinowatz F, Bergerson M. Morphological Evidence of Sperm Maturation in the Ampulla Ductus Deferentis of the Bull. Cell Tissue Res 1994; 275: 537–541.

Bernabé A, Gomez MA, Seva J, Vasquez F, Pallarés FJ, Serrano J. Light and Ultrastructural Immunocytochemical Study of Somatotropic Cells (GH Cells) in Ovine Adenohypophysis: lactation and weaning influences. Anat Histol Embryol 2000; 29: 13–18.

Beyaz F, Asti R. Development of Ileal Peyer's Patches and Follicle Associated Epithelium in Bovine Foetuses. Anat Histol Embryol 2004; 33: 172–179.

Braekevelt CR. Fine Structure of the Choriocapillaris, Bruch's Membrane and Retinal Epithelium of the Cow. Anat Histol Embryol 1986; 15: 205–214.

Braekevelt CR. Retinal Epithelial Fine Structure in the Domestic Cat (Felis catus). Anat Histol Embryol 1990; 19: 58–66.

Braekevelt CR. Fine Structure of the Retinal Photoreceptors of the Domestic Cat (Felis catus). Anat Histol Embryol 1990; 19: 67–76.

Braekevelt CR. Fine Structure of the Feline Tapetum lucidum. Anat Histol Embryol 1990; 19: 97–105.

Bragulla H, Ernsberger S, Budras K-D. On the Development of the Papillary Body in the Feline Claw. Anat Histol Embryol 2001; 30: 211–217.

Buckwalter JA, Cooper RR. Bone Structure and Function. Instr Course Lect 1987; 36: 27–48.

Budras K-D, Berens v. Rautenfeld D. Lymphbildung und Erektion des lymphatischen Kopulationsschwellkörpers beim Hahn (Gallus domesticus). Verh Anat Ges 1978; 72: 565–568.

Budras K-D, Hullinger RL, Berens v. Rautenfeld D. Lymph Heart Musculature in Birds. J Morphol 1987; 191: 77–87.

Casteleyn C, Breugelmans S, Simoens P, Van den Broeck W. The Tonsils Revisited: review of the anatomical localization and histological characteristics of the tonsils of domestic and laboratory animals. Clin Devel Immunol 2011; Article ID 472460 14 pages; https://doi.org/10.1155/2011/472460.

Castranova V, Rabovsky J, Tucker JH, Miles PR. The Alveolar Type II Epithelial Cell: a multifunctional pneumocyte. Toxicol Appl Pharmacol 1988; 93: 472–483.

Cerruti P, Guerrero F. Identification of Positive Cells to Interleukin-4 in Bovine Haemal Nodes. Anat Histol Embryol 2001; 30: 219–223.

Cerruti P, Marcaccini A, Guerrero F. A Scanning and Immunohistochemical Study in Bovine Haemal Node. Anat Histol Embryol 1998; 27: 387–392.

Cesta MF. Normal Structure, Function, and Histology of Mucosa-associated Lymphoid Tissue. Toxicol Pathol 2006; 34: 599–608.

Cooke R. The Sliding Filament Model: 1972–2004. J Gen Physiol 2004; 123: 643–656.

Dabak DO, Aydin G, Ozouner M. Dynamics of Mast Cells in Lymph Node Following Antigenic Stimulation. Anat Histol Embryol 2004; 33: 5–10.

Davis GE, Senger DR. Endothelial Extracellular Matrix. Circ Res 2005; 97: 1093–1107.

De Francischini Carvalho AC, Pacheco MR, Baraldi Artoni SM, Mateus O. Canine Spinal Cord Neuron and Axon Myelin Sheath Morphometry. Anat Histol Embryol 2006; 25: 284–286.

Deeg CA, Amann B, Hauck SM, Kaspers B. Defining Cytochemical Markers for Different Cell Types in the Equine Retina. Anat Histol Embryol 2006; 35: 412–415.

den Haan JM, Mebius RE, Kraal G. Stromal Cells of the Mouse Spleen. Front Immunol 2012; Vol 3 Article 201.

Dyce KM, Sack WO, Wensing CJG. Textbook of Veterinary Anatomy, 3rd edn. Philadelphia: Saunders, 2002.

Egerbacher M, Helmreich M, Probst A, König HE, Böck P. Digital Cushions in Horses Comprise Coarse Connective Tissue, Myxoid Tissue and Cartilage but Only Little Unilocular Fat Tissue. Anat Histol Embryol 2005; 34: 112–116.

Egerbacher M, Mousa EAM, Helmreich M, Böck P, Schuh M. Mammary Gland Secretory Concretions Contain Non-Collagenous Bone Matrix Proteins. Anat Histol Embryol 2006; 35: 343–348.

Eliška O. Purkinje Fibers of the Heart Conduction System. Časopis Lékařů Českých 2006; 145 (4).

Ekstedt E, Söderquist L, Plöen L. Fine Structure of Spermatogenesis and Sertoli Cells (Epitheliocystus sustentans) in the Bull. Anat Histol Embryol 1986; 15: 23–48.

Eurell JA, Frappier BL. Dellmann's Textbook of Veterinary Histology. London: Blackwell Publishing, 2006.

Evans HE. Anatomy of the budgerigar, in Petrak ML (ed.) Diseases of Cage and Aviary Birds. Philadelphia: Lea & Febiger, 1982.

Fazarinc G, Candek-Potokar M, Ursic M, Vrecl M, Poganik A. Giant Muscle Fibres in Pigs with Different Ryr1 Genotype. Anat Histol Embryol 2002; 31: 367–371.

Fink C, Tatar M, Failing K, Hospes R, Kressin M, Klisch K. Serotonin-containing Cells in the Gastrointestinal Tract of Newborn Foals and Adult Horses. Anat Histol Embryol 2006; 35: 23–27.

Flügel-Koch C, Croft MA, Kaufman PL, Lütjen-Drecoll E. Anteriorly Located Zonular Fibres as a Tool for Fine Regulation in Accommodation. Ophthalm Physiol Optics 2016; 36(1): 13–20.

Franca LR, Godinho CL. Testis Morphometry, Seminiferous Epithelium Cycle Length and Daily Sperm Production in Domestic Cats (Felis catus). Biol Reprod 2003; 68: 1554–1561.

Frewein J, Sinowatz F. Sehorgan. In: Nickel R, Schummer A, Seiferle E. Lehrbuch der Anatomie der Haustiere. Bd. V. Vollmerhaus B (Hrsg). Anatomie der Vögel. 3. Aufl. Berlin, Hamburg: Parey, 2004.

Fukumoto S, Yamada Y. Review: Extracellular Matrix Regulates Tooth Morphogenesis. Connect Tissue Res 2005; 46: 220–226.

Gargiulo AM, Pedini V, Ceccarelli P. The Process of Secretion in Swine Apocrine Sweat Glands. Anat Histol Embryol 1990; 19: 264–268.

Garside P, Millington O, Smith KM. The Anatomy of Mucosal Immune Response. Ann N Y Acad Sci 2004; 1029: 9–15.

Gebert A, Pabst R. M Cells at Locations outside the Gut. Semin Immunol 1999; 11: 165–170.

Geiger G, Hild A. Mikromorphologische Untersuchungen an den Odontoblasten des Schafs in verschiedenen Entwicklungs- bzw. Reifestadien. Anat Histol Embryol 1991; 20: 320–333.

Goldring MB, Tsuchimochi K, Ijiri K. The Control of Chondrogenesis. J Cell Biochem 2006; 97: 33–44.

Gomez MA, Navarro JA, Gomez S, Camara P, Gomez JC, Bernabé A. Cytological, Immunocytochemical and Ultrastructural Study of the Adenohypophyseal Pars Distalis of the Kid (Capra hircus): the THS cell. Anat Histol Embryol 1989; 18: 305–315.

Grau H, Walter P. Grundriß der Histologie und vergleichenden mikroskopischen Anatomie der Haussäugetiere. Berlin, Hamburg: Parey, 1967.

Habel ER. Applied Veterinary Anatomy. Philadelphia: Saunders, 1978.

Haenisch-Woehl A, Kölle S, Neumüller C, Sinowatz F, Braun J. Morphology of Canine Cumulus-Oocyte Complexes in Prepubertal Bitches. Anat Histol Embryol 2003; 32: 373–377.

Halata Z, Grim M, Bauman KI. Friedrich Sigmund Merkel and his Merkel Cell, Morphology, Development and Physiology: review and new results. Anat Rec A Discov Mol Cell Evol Biol 2003; 271: 225–239.

Halpern M, Martinez-Marcos A. Structure and Function of the Vomeronasal System: an update. Prog Neurobiol 2003; 70: 245–318.

Hansson E. Ronnback L. Glial Neural Signaling in the Central Nervous System. FASEB J 2003; 17: 341–348.

Hartenstein V. Blood Cells and Blood Cell Development in the Animal Kingdom. Annu Rev Cell Der Biol 2006; 22: 677–712.

Hartmann FD. Zur topographischen Anatomie des Gleichgewichts- und Gehörorgans der Hauskatze. Diss med vet, München, 1992.

Hartwig JH. The Platelets: form and function. Semin Hematol 2006; 43: 94–100.

Hashimoto Y, Reese S, Bragulla H, Budras K-D. Eine lectinhistochemische Untersuchung der Epidermis von Haut und Huf des Pferdes. Anat Histol Embryol 1992; 21: 238–245.

Heinz M, Michel G. Zum Bau der Milchdrüse des Rindes während der Trockenstehperiode unter besonderer Berücksichtigung der Involutionsprozesse. 2. Elektronenmikroskopische Untersuchungen. Anat Histol Embryol 1991; 20: 193–204.

Hinterhofer C, Zoscher M, Gabler C, Stanek C. The Hardness of Horn in Different Segments of the Bovine Claw. Berl Münch Tierärztl Wochenschr 2005; 118: 334–340.

HogenEsch H, Felsburg PJ. Immunohistology of Peyer's Patches in the Dog. Vet Immunol Immunopathol 1992; 30(2–3): 147–160.

Hraste A, Giurcevic-Kantura V, Jakovac M, Brestovec J. Morphological Investigations of the Glandulae Profundae Plicae Semilunares Conjunctivae in the Domestic Swine (Sus scrofa domesticus) and the Wild Hog (Sus scorfa ferus). Anat Histol Embryol 1995; 24: 223–226.

Hummel G, Hild A, Wenisch S. Entwicklung, Zytoarchitektonik und Feinstruktur des mesencephalen Trigeminuskerns bei Hauswiederkäuern. Anat Histol Embryol 1997; 26: 99–106.

Ikemizu T, Kitamura N, Yamada J, Yamashita T. Is Lamina Muscularis Mucosae Present in the Ruminal Mucosa of Cattle? Immunohistochemical and Ultrastructural Approaches. Anat Histol Embryol 1994; 23: 177–186.

Irving-Rodgers HF, Mussard ML, Kinder JE, Rodgers RJ. Composition and Morphology of the Follicular Basal Lamina during Atresia of Bovine Antral Follicles. Reproduction 2002; 123: 97–106.

Irving-Rodgers HF, Rodgers RJ. Ultrastructure of the Basal Lamina of Bovine Ovarian Follicles and its Relationship to the Membrana Granulosa. J Reprod Fertil 2000; 118: 221–228.

Irving-Rodgers HF, Rodgers RJ. Extracellular Matrix of the Developing Ovarian Follicle. Semin Reprod Med 2006; 24: 195–203.

Ishizuya-Oka A. Epithelial-Connective Tissue Cross-Talk is Essential for Regeneration of Intestinal Epithelium. J Nippon Med Sch 2005; 72: 13–18.

Ji RC. Lymphatic Endothelial Cells, Lymphangiogenesis and Extracellular Matrix. Lymphat Res Biol 2006; 4: 83–100.

Junqueira LC, Carneiro J, Gratzl M. Histologie. Heidelberg: Springer, 2005.

Karasek M, Swiltoslawski J, Zieliniska A. Ultrastructure of the Central Nervous System: the basics. Folia Neuropathol 2004; 42: 1–9.

Keating A. Mesenchymal Stromal cells. Curr Opin Hematol 2006; 13: 419–425.

Kielty CM, Sherratt MJ, Shuttleworth CA. Elastic Fibres. J Cell Science 2002; 115: 2817–2828.

King AS, McLelland J. Anatomie der Vögel. Grundzüge und vergleichende Aspekte. Stuttgart: Verlag Eugen Ulmer, 1978.

Kitamura N, Yoshiki A, Sasaki M, Baltazar ET, Hondo E, Yamamoto Y, Agungriyono S. Immunohistochemical Evaluation of the Muscularis Mucosae in the Ruminant Forestomach. Anat Histol Embryol 2003; 32: 175–178.

Klein-Nulend J, Nijweide PJ, Burger EH. Osteocyte and Bone Structure. Curr Osteoporos Rep 2003; 1: 5–10.

Kleiss C, Liebich HG. Puentes Intercellulares entre las Células Sexuales en el Testículo del Toro. Zbl Vet Med C Anat Histol Embryol 1983; 12: 230–244.

Knolle PA. Cognate Interaction between Endothelial Cells and T-cells. Results Probl Cell Differ. 2006; 43: 151–173.

Knospe C, Plendl J. Histochemical Demonstration of Lipase Activity in the Gastric Mucosa of the Cat. Anat Histol Embryol 1997; 26: 303–304.

Knothe Tate ML, Adamson JR, Tami AE, Bauer TW. The Osteocyte. Int J Biochem Cell Biol 2004; 36: 1–8.

König HE and Liebich H-G. Veterinary Anatomy of Domestic Mammals Textbook and Colour Atlas. 4th Edition. Stuttgart: Schattauer, 2009.

König HE, Amselgruber W, Rüsse I. Zur Mikrozirkulation in Follikeln und Corpora Lutea des Rinderovarseine Korrosionsanatomische Studie. Tierärztl Prax 1988; 16: 25–31.

König HE, Macher R, Polsterer-Heindl E, Sora M-C, Hinterhofer Chr, Helmreich M, Böck P. Stoßbrechende Einrichtungen am Zehenendorgan des Pferdes. Wien Tierärztl Mschr 2003; 90: 267–73.

König HE, Popescu A, Polsterer-Heindl E, Hinterhofer Chr. Arteriovenöse Koppelung im Zehenendorgan des Pferdes. Pferdeheilkunde 2003; 19: 459–462.

König HE, Wissdorf H, Probst A, Macher R, Voß S, Polsterer E. Zur Funktion der mimischen Muskulatur und des Organum Vomeronasale beim Flehmen des Pferdes. Pferdeheilkunde 2005; 21: 297–300.

Koy T. Untersuchungen zur Anatomie der Synovialmembran beim Kalb. Diss med vet, München, 1999.

Kraehenbuhl JP, Neutra MR. Epithelial M Cells: differentiation and function. Annu Rev Cell Der Biol 2000; 16: 301–320.

Krause WJ. Brunner's Glands: a structural, histochemical and pathological profile. Prog Histochem Cytochem 2000; 35: 259–367.

Kreidberg JA. Podocyte Differentiation and Glomerulogenesis. J Am Soc Nephrol 2003, 4: 806–814.

Kressin M, Koob B. Actin in Stratified Squamous Keratinized Epithelium. Anat Histol Embryol 1993; 22: 300–308.

Kressin M, Koob B, Schnorr B. Actinfilaments in the Ruminal Epithelium of Cattle. Anat Histol Embryol 1993; 22: 151–159.

Kressin M, Sommer U. Die Differenzierung der Oberflächenzellinie im Labmagen adulter Rinder. Anat Histol Embryol 1996; 25: 177–186.

Krijgsman D, Hokland M and Kuppen PJK. The Role of Natural Killer T Cells in Cancer—A Phenotypical and Functional Approach. Front Immunol 2018; https://doi.org/10.3389/fimmu.2018.00367.

Kumar P, Timoney JF. Histology and Ultrastructure of the Equine Lingual Tonsil. II. Lymphoid Tissue and Associated High Endothelial Tonsils. Anat Histol Embryol 2005; 34: 98–104.

Kumar P, Timoney JF. Histology and Ultrastructure of the Equine Lingual Tonsil. I. Crypt Epithelium and Associated Structures. Anat Histol Embryol 2005; 34: 27–33.

Kumar P, Timoney JF. Histology, Immunhistochemistry and Ultrastructure of the Equine Tubal Tonsil. Anat Histol Embryol 2005; 34: 141–148.

Kumar P, Timoney JF. Histology, Immunohistochemistry and Ultrastructure of the Equine Palatine Tonsil. Anat Histol Embryol 2005; 34: 192–198.

Kumar P, Timoney JF. Histology, Immunohistochemistry and Ultrastructure of the Tonsil of the Soft Palate of the Horse. Anat Histol Embryol 2006; 35: 1–6.

Kumar P, Timoney JF, Southgate HHP, Sheoran AS. Light and Scanning Electron Microscopic Studies of the Nasal Turbinates of the Horse. Anat Histol Embryol 2000; 29: 103–109.

Kuo KH, Seow CY. Contractile Filament Architecture and Force Transmission in Swine Airway Smooth Muscle. J Cell Sci 2004; 11: 1503–1511.

Lauwers H, Nicaise M, Simoens P, De Vos NR. Morphology of the Vesicular and Bulbourethral Glands in Barrows and the Changes Induced by Diethylstilboestrol. Zbl Vet Med C Anat Histol Embryol 1984; 13: 50–63.

Lemasters JJ. Dying a Thousand Deaths: redundant pathways from different organelles to apoptosis and necrosis. Gastroenterology 2005; 129: 351–360.

Liebhold M, Wendt M, Kaup F-J, Drommer W. Lichtund Elektronenmikroskopische Studien zur Struktur des Normalen Blasenepithels beim Weiblichen Schwein. Anat Histol Embryol 1995; 24: 42–52.

Liebich HG, Scharrer E. Entwicklungsbedingte Veränderungen von Struktur und Funktion des Pansenepithels. 2. Morphologische Differenzierung der Epithelschranke bei Lämmern Innerhalb der ersten Lebenswochen. Anat Histol Embryol 1984; 13: 25–41.

Lloyd RV. Endocrine Pathology: differential diagnosis and molecular advances, 2nd edn. New York: Springer, 2010.

López-Rivero JL, Diz AM, Monterde JG, Agüera E. Intramuscular Distribution of the Fibre Types in the Gluteus Medius of the Horse: a histochemical analysis. Anat Histol Embryol 1993; 22: 233–240.

Ludewig T. Licht- und Elektronenmikroskopische Untersuchungen an der Blut- Milchschranke der Laktierenden Milchdrüse des Rindes. Anat Histol Embryol 1996; 25: 121–126.

Lynch CD, O'Sullivan VR, Dockery P, McGillycuddy CT, Sloan AJ. Hunter-Schreger Band Patterns in Human Tooth Enamel. J Anat 2010; 217(2): 106–115.

Lynch C, O'Sullivan VR, Dockery P, McGillycuddy CT, Rees JS, Sloan AJ. Hunter-Schreger Band Patterns and Their Implications for Clinical Dentistry. J Oral Rehab 2011; 38(5): 359–365.

Mabbott NA, Donaldson DS, Ohno H, Williams IR, Mahajan A. Microfold (M) cells: important immunosurveillance posts in the intestinal epithelium. Mucos Immunol 2013; 6(4); 666–677.

Maierl J. Die Aufhängung des Klauenbeins – Funktionelle Anatomie und Bio-mechanik der Rinderklaue. Tierärztl Prax 2004; 32 (G): 239–244.

Marks SC Jr, Seifert MF. The Lifespan of Osteoclasts: experimental studies using the giant granule cytoplasmic marker characteristic of beige mice. Bone 1985; 6(6): 451–455.

McDougal DH, Gamlin PD. Autonomic Control of the Eye. Comp Physiol 2015; 5(1): 439–473.

Metha D, Malik AB. Signaling Mechanisms Regulating Endothelial Permeability. Physiol Rev 2006; 86: 279–367.

Mimoda T, Kitamura N, Hondo E, Yamada J. Immunohistochemical Colocalization of Serotonin, Substance P and Met-enkephalin-Arg6-Gly7-Leu8 in the Endocrine Cells of the Ruminant Duodenum. Anat Histol Embryol 1998; 27: 65–69.

Moller M, Baeres FM. The Anatomy and Innervation of the Mammalian Pineal Gland. Cell Tissue Res 2002; 309: 139–150.

Mukherjee S, Ghosh RN, Maxfield FR. Endocytosis. Physiol Rev 1997; 77: 759–803.

Mülling C, Bragulla H, Budras K-D, Reese S. Strukturelle Faktoren mit Einfluss auf die Hornqualität und Prädilektionsstellen für Erkrankungen an der Fus- sungsfläche der Rinderklaue. Schweiz Arch Tierheilk 1994; 136: 49–57.

Mülling C, Bragulla H, Reese S, Budras K-D, Steinberg W. How Structures in Bovine Hoof Epidermis Are Influenced by Nutritional Factors. Anat Histol Embryol 1999; 28: 103–108.

Myojin T, Kitamura N, Hondo E, Baltazar ET, Pearson GT, Yamada J. Immunohistochemical Localization of Neuropeptides in Bovine Pancreas. Anat Histol Embryol 2000; 29: 167–172.

Nagai T, Yasuoka Y, Izumi Y, Horikawa K, Kimura M, Nakayama Y, Uematsu T, Fukuyama T, Yamazaki T, Kohda Y, Hasuike Y, Nanami M, Kuragano T, Kobayashi N, Obinata M, Tomita K, Tanoue A, Nakanishi T, Kawahara K, Nonoguchi H. Reevaluation of Erythropoietin Production by the Nephron. Biochem Biophys Res Commun 2014; 449 (2).

Nickel R, Schummer A, Seiferle E (Hrsg). Lehrbuch der Anatomie der Haustiere. Bd. I. Frewein J, Wille K-H, Wilkens H (Hrsg). Bewegungsapparat. 8. Aufl. Stuttgart: Parey bei MVS, 2004.

Nickel R, Schummer A, Seiferle E (Hrsg). Lehrbuch der Anatomie der Haustiere. Bd. II. Frewein J, Gasse H, Leiser R, Roos H, Thomé H, Vollmerhaus B, Waibl H. (Hrsg). Eingeweide. 9. Aufl. Stuttgart: Parey bei MVS, 2004.

Nickel R, Schummer A, Seiferle E (Hrsg). Lehrbuch der Anatomie der Haustiere. Bd. III. Habermehl K-H, Vollmerhaus B, Wilkens H, Waibl H (Hrsg). Kreislaufsystem, Haut und Hautorgane. 4. Aufl. Stuttgart: Parey bei MVS, 2005.

Nickel R, Schummer A, Seiferle E (Hrsg). Lehrbuch der Anatomie der Haustiere. Bd. IV. Böhme G. Nervensystem, Sinnesorgane, endokrine Drüsen. 4. Aufl. Stuttgart: Parey bei MVS, 2004.

Nickel R, Schummer A, Seiferle E (Hrsg). Lehrbuch der Anatomie der Haustiere. Bd. V. Vollmerhaus B (Hrsg). Anatomie der Vögel. 3. Aufl. Stuttgart: Parey bei MVS, 2004.

Nicolson GL. The Fluid—Mosaic Model of Membrane Structure: still relevant to understanding the structure, function and dynamics of biological membranes after more than 40 years. Biochim Biophys Acta 2014; 1838(6): 1451–1466.

Nilsson O, Matino R, De Luca F, Phillip M, Baron J. Endocrine Regulation of Growth Plate. Horm Res 2005; 64: 157–165.

Nurse CA, Piskuric NA. Signal Processing at Mammalian Carotid Body Chemoreceptors. Semin Cell Devel Biol 2013; 24 (1): 22–30.

Nutt SL, Hodgkin PD, Tarlinton DM, Corcoran LM. The Generation of Antibody-secreting Plasma Cells. Nat Rev Immunol 2015; 15(3): 160–171.

Okada H, Shigeta Y, Un-No Y. C-cell Distribution in Ovine Thyroid Gland. Anat Histol Embryol 1994; 24: 281–284.

Oswald IP. Role of Intestinal Epithelial Cells in the Innate Immune Defence of the Pig Intestine. Vet Res 2006; 37: 359–368.

Paape MJ, Bannerman DD, Zhao X, Lee JW. The Bovine Neutrophil: structure and function in blood and milk. Vet Res 2003; 34: 597–627.

Paik DY, Janzen DM, Schafenacker AM, Velasco VS, Shung MS, Cheng D, Huang J, Witte ON, Memarzadeh S. Stem-like Epithelial Cells Are Concentrated in the Distal End of the Fallopian Tube: a site for injury and serous cancer initiation. Stem Cell 2012; 30 (11): 2487–2497.

Palma GA, Tortonese DJ, Sinowatz F. Development Capacity In Vitro of Prepubertal Oocytes. Anat Histol Embryol 2001; 30: 295–300.

Pavelka M, Roth J. Descemet's Membrane. In: Functional Ultrastructure. Vienna: Springer, 2010; 184–185.

Pavenstadt H. Roles of the Podocyte in Glomerular Function. Am J Renal Physiol 2000; 278: 173–179.

Pearse G. Normal Structure, Function and Histology of the Thymus. Toxicol Pathol 2006; 34: 504–514.

Perera RM, Zoncu R. The Lysosome as a Regulatory Hub. Ann Rev Cell Devel Biol 2016; 32: 223–253.

Pfeiffer CJ, Levin M, Lopes MAF. Ultrastructure of the Horse Tongue: further observations on the lingual integumentary architecture. Anat Histol Embryol 2000; 29: 37–43.

Pickett JA, Edwardson JM. Compound Exocytosis: mechanisms and functional significance. Traffic 2006; 7: 109–116.

Plendl J. Angiogenesis and Vascular Regression in the Ovary. Anat Histol Embryol 2000; 29: 257–266.

Plendl J, Stierstorfer B, Sinowatz F. Growth Factors and Their Receptors in the Olfactory System. Anat Histol Embryol 1999; 28: 73–79.

Prelle K, Zink N, Wolf E. Pluripotent Stem Cells – Model of Embryonic Development, Tool for Gene Targeting, and Basis of Cell Therapy. Anat Histol Embryol 2002; 31: 169–186.

Pries AR, Kuebler WM. Normal Endothelium. Handb Exp Pharmacol 2006; 176 Pt 1: 1–40.

Probst A, Sora M-C, Böck P, Budras K-D, Liebich H-G, König HE. Plastinierte Schnitte von Hufpräparaten: eine didaktisch wertvolle Ergänzung zur Darstellung anatomischer Feinstrukturen. Wien Tierärztl Mschr 2006; 93: 98–102.

Randall TD. Bronchus-associated Lymphoid Tissue (BALT) Structure and Function. Adv Immunol 2010; 107: 187.

Reese S, Dalamani G, Kaspers B. The Avian Lung-associated Immune System. Rev Vet Res 2006; 37: 311–324.

Ribeiro AC, Elias CF, Liberti EA, De Lima Guidi W, Souza RR. Structure and Ultrastructure of the Celiac-Mesenteric Ganglion Complex in the Domestic Dog (Canis familiaris). Anat Histol Embryol 2002; 31: 344–349.

Rolink AG, Massa S, Balciunaite G, Ceredig R. Early Lymphocyte Development in Bone Marrow and Thymus. Swiss Med Wkly 2006; 136: 679–683.

Roodman GD. Regulation of Osteoblast Differentiation. Ann N Y Academic Sci 2006; 1068: 100–109.

Rooney SA, Young ST, Mendelson CR. Molecular and Cellular Processing of Lung Surfactant. FASEB J 1994; 8: 957–967.

Ross MH, Pawlina W. Histology – a Text and Atlas. London: Lippincott Williams & Wilkins, 2006.

Ross MH, Pawlina W. Histology: A Text and Atlas with Correlated Cell and Molecular Biology, 7th edn. Philadelphia: Wolters Kluwer Health, 2016.

Roughley PJ. The Structure and Function of Cartilage Proteogylcans. Eur Cell Mater 2006, 12: 92–101.

Rüsse I. Oogenesis in Cattle and Sheep. Bibliotheca Anatomica 1983; 24: 77–92.

Salazar I, Quintero PS, Cifuentes JM. The Soft-tissue Components of the Vomeronasal Organ in Pigs, Cows and Horses. Anat Histol Embryol 1997; 26: 179–186.

Samuelson DA. Textbook of Veterinary Histology. New York: Saunders Elsevier, 2007.

Sanchez B, Flores JM, Pizarro M, Garcia P. Histological and Immunohistochemical Study of the Cat Epididymis. Anat Histol Embryol 1998; 27: 135–140.

Saunders CJ, Reynolds SD, Finger TE. Chemosensory Brush Cells of the Trachea. A stable population in a dynamic epithelium. Am J Respir Cell Mol Biol 2013; 49(2): 190–196.

Schaller O. Illustrated Veterinary Anatomical Nomenclature, 2nd edn. Stuttgart: Enke, 1992.

Schams D, Berisha B. Regulation of Corpus Luteum Function in Cattle – an Overview. Reprod Domest Anim 2004; 39: 241–251.

Schneider C, Kressin M, Schnorr B. Zur Morphologie der Zungenrandpapillen Neugeborener Ferkel. Anat Histol Embryol 1996; 25: 95–100.

Schonhoff SE, Giel-Moloney M, Leiter AB. Minireview: Development and Differentiation of Gut Endocrine Cells. Endocrinology 2004; 145: 2639–2644.

Schubert ML. Gastric Secretion. Curr Opin Gastroenterol 2005; 21: 636–643.

Schweiger M, Erhard MH, Amselgruber WM. Cell-specific Localization of the Cholecystokinin A Receptor in the Porcine Pancreas. Anat Histol Embryol 2000; 29: 357–361.

Senoo H. Structure and Function of Hepatic Stellate Cells. Med Electron Microsc 2004; 37: 3–15.

Sinowatz F, Hees H. Histologie – Kurzlehrbuch der Zytologie und mikroskopischen Anatomie, 4. Aufl. Eigenverlag 2006.

Sinowatz F, Kölle S, Töpfer-Petersen E. Biosynthesis and Expression of Zona Pellucida Glycoproteins in Mammals. Cell Tissue Organs 2001; 168: 24–35.

Sinowatz F, Schams D, Habermann F, Berisha B, Vermehren M. Localization of Fibroblast Growth Factor I (Acid Fibroblast Growth Factor) and its mRNA in the Bovine Mammary Gland during Mammogenesis, Lactation and Involution. Anat Histol Embryol 2006; 35: 202–207.

Sinowatz F, Töpfer-Petersen E, Kölle S, Palma G. Functional Morphology of the Zona Pellucida. Anat Histol Embryol 2001; 30: 257–263.

Sinowatz F, Wessa E, Neumüller C, Palma G. On the Species Specificity of Sperm Binding and Sperm Penetration of Zona Pellucida. Reprod Domest Anim 2003; 38: 141–146.

Sobotta J (Hrsg). Anatomie des Menschen. Der Komplette Atlas in einem Band. Putz R, Pabst R (Hrsg). Allgemeine Anatomie, Bewegungsapparat, Innere Organe, Neuroanatomie. 22. Aufl. München: Urban & Fischer bei Elsevier, 2007.

Sommer U, Schlechta C, Kressin M, Schnorr B. Intraepitheliale Nervenendigun- gen in den Zungenrandpapillen neugeborener Ferkel. Anat Histol Embryol 1997; 26: 121–126.

Spencer TE, Bazer FW. Uterine and Placental Factors Regulating Conceptus Growth in Domestic Animals. J Anim Sci 2004; E-Suppl: E4–13.

Sykaras AG, Demenis C, Case RM, McLaughlin JT, Smith CP. Duodenal Enteroendocrine I-Cells Contain mRNA Transcripts Encoding Key Endocannabinoid and Fatty Acid Receptors. PLoS ONE 2012; August; 10.1371/journal.pone.0042373.

Takehana K, Abe M, Yamada O, Ida-Abe M, Abe-Ishioka N, Hiraga T, Iwasa K, Hiratsuka T. Morphological Study of Bovine Pregnant Corpus Luteum Cells. Anat Histol Embryol 1997; 26: 231–235.

Takehana K, Masty J, Yamaguchi M, Kobayashi A, Yamada O, Kuroda M, Park YS, Iawasa K, Abe M. Fine Structural and Histochemical Study of Equine Paneth Cells. Anat Histol Embryol 1998; 27: 125–129.

Tizard IR. Veterinary Immunology. An Introduction. New York: Saunders, 2004.

Turner JR. Molecular Basis of Epithelial Barrier Regulation: from basic mechanism to clinical application. Am J Pathol 2006; 169: 1901–1909.

Ushiki T. Collagen Fibres, Reticular Fibres and Elastic Fibres. A comprehensive understanding from a morphological viewpoint. Arch Histol Cytol 2002; 65: 109–126.

Väänänen HK, Zhao H, Mulari M, Halleen JM. The Cell Biology of Osteoclast Function. J Cell Sci 2000; 113: 377–381.

Van Cruchten S, Van den Broeck W. Morphological and Biochemical Aspects of Apoptosis, Oncosis and Necrosis. Anat Histol Embryol 2002; 31: 214–223.

Van Geet C. Thrombopoiesis: new concepts. Verh K Acad Geneeskd Belg 2004; 66: 5–24.

Vodenicharov A. Peculiarities of the Connection between Mesangial and Glomerular Endothelial Cells in the Domestic Swine Kidney. Anat Histol Embryol 1995; 24: 227–231.

Vodenicharov A, Chouchkov C. Morphological Study of Mast Cell Localization in the Wall of the Proximal Tubule in the Domestic Swine Kidney. Anat Histol Embryol 1999; 28: 85–88.

Vodenicharov A, Simoens P. Morphologic Peculiarities of the Renal Cortical Vasculature Connected with Blood Redistribution in the Kidney of the Domestic Pig. Anat Histol Embryol 1998; 27: 257–262.

Von Engelhardt W, Breves G. Physiologie der Haustiere. Stuttgart: Enke Verlag, 2005.

Walde I, Nell B, Schäffer EH, Köstlin RG (Hrsg). Augenheilkunde. Lehrbuch und Atlas. Hund, Katze, Kaninchen und Meerschweinchen. 3. Aufl. Schattauer 2008.

Wang J, Laurie GW. Organogenesis of Exocrine Gland. Dev Bio 2004; 273: 1–22.

Watnabe T, Hiramatsu K, Ohmori Y, Paik Y-K. Histo- and Cytochemical Studies on the Distribution of Acetylcholinesterase-positive Nerve Fibres in the Goat Adrenal Gland. Anat Histol Embryol 1990; 19: 245–254.

Welsch U. Lehrbuch Histologie. Amsterdam: Urban & Fischer, 2006.

Willard-Mack CL. Normal Structure, Function and Histology of Lymph Nodes. Toxicol Pathol 2006; 34: 409–424.

Wille K-H. Über die Adenosintriphospahtasen des Fetalen Dickdarmepithels. Licht- und elektronenmikroskopische Untersuchungen am Caecum des Rindes (Bos primigenius taurus). Anat Histol Embryol 1987; 16: 21–36.

Wille K-H. Zytoplasmastrukturen der Schleimbildung in der Fetalen Becherzelle des bovinen Darmes. Anat Histol Embryol 1987; 16: 351–356.

Wille K-H. Zur funktionellen Morphologie der Dickdarm-Mukosa von Rind (Bos primigenius f. taurus), Schaf (Ovis ammon f. aries) und Ziege (Capra aegagrus f. hircus). Anat Histol Embryol 2001; 30: 65–76.

Wille K-H, Nakov C. Über die Funktionelle Morphologie der Dickdarm-Mukosa vom Pferd (Equus przewalskii f. caballus) unter Besonderer Berücksichtigung ihres Epithels. Anat Histol Embryol 1999; 28: 355–365.

Wille K-H, Winkler F. Ein weiterer Beitrag über die Feinstruktur der Fetalen Becherzelle. Untersuchungen am Dünndarm des Rindes. Anat Histol Embryol 1999; 28: 49–53.

Wisse E, Braet F, Luo D, De Zanger R, Jans D, Crabbe E, Vermoesen A. Structure and Function of Sinusoidal Lining Cells in the Liver. Toxicol Pathol 1996; 24: 100–111.

Witter K. Frühe Odontogenese beim Hausschaf (Ovis aries). Diss med vet, München, 1999.

Wray S, Burdyga T. Sarcoplasmic Reticulum Function in Smooth Muscle. Physiol Rev 2010; 90: 113–178.

Yamamoto Y, Kitamura N, Yamada J, Andrén A, Yamashita T. Morphological Study of the Surface of the Omasal Laminae in Cattle, Sheep and Goats. Anat Histol Embryol 1994; 23: 166–176.

Yildiz D, Gultiken ME, Karahan S. The Scanning Electron and Light Microscopic Structure of Bovine Tactile Hair. Anat Histol Embryol 2004; 33: 304–308.

Yu M, Yue Z, Wu P, Wu DY, Mayer JA, Medina M, Widelitz RB, Jiang TX, Chuong CM. The Biology of Feather Follicles. Int J Dev Biol 2004; 48: 181–191.

Zengerling G. Struktur und Entwicklung des Immunsystems der Hühnerlunge. Diss med vet, München, 2006.

Index

The suffixes f and t indicate a figure or table on that page, respectively

complication of aortic valve stenosis and indicates left ventricular failure. Most patients with passive pulmonary hypertension will benefit from relief of the left heart obstruction.

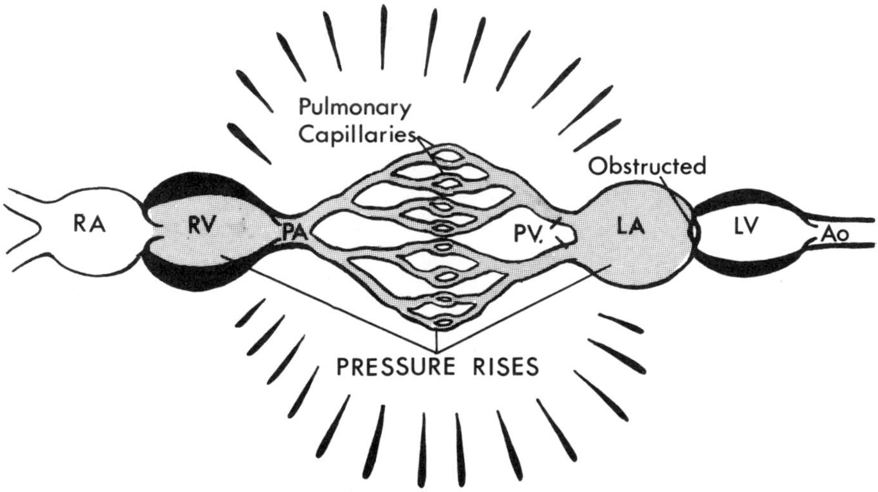

Fig. 2.10. With the two sides of the heart and the lungs represented as a single tube, it is seen that the pressure rises in that part of the circulation intervening between the obstructed valve and the active right ventricle. PV, Pulmonary vein; LA, Left atrium; LV, Left ventricle; Ao, Aorta; RA, Right atrium; RV, Right ventricle.

Active Pulmonary Hypertension. This is somewhat more complicated than passive pulmonary hypertension. A less commonly used term, it helps to identify a group of conditions where raised pulmonary artery pressure results from underlying heart disease, with increased flow or pressure in the pulmonary vascular bed. Both factors may be operative. Pulmonary hypertension arising from increased flow is known also as hyperdynamic pulmonary hypertension.

A common cause of an increased flow of blood through the lungs is a left-to-right shunt, such as occurs with an atrial or ventricular septal defect or persistent ductus arteriosus. Reduction of the flow to physiological levels by closure of the defect should restore the pulmonary artery pressure to normal if no changes have occurred in the lung vessels themselves. It should be noted that these cases therefore have a normal pulmonary vascular resistance, the rise in pressure being simply a flow phenomenon.

More often, however, patients with a left-to-right shunt, from a ventricular septal defect for example, have not only an increased flow but also increased pulmonary vascular resistance due to underlying changes in the lung vessels. It is important to try to assess how much of the increased pressure is attributable to increased flow and how much relates to the increased resistance, because correction of the shunt removes the flow factor but will not necessarily restore the pulmonary artery pressure to normal. Measurements made at cardiac catheterisation are used to calculate pulmonary blood flow and resistance, and, in a general way, resistance estimated from haemodynamic measurements correlates with the histological changes in the lung vessels or the degree of pulmonary vascular disease.